RHINITIS

SECOND EDITION

RHINITIS
SECOND EDITION

Edited by:

Guy A. Settipane, M.D.

Clinical Professor of Medicine, Brown University and Director, Division of Allergy, Department of Medicine, Rhode Island Hospital

SECOND EDITION
with 121 illustrations and 12 color plates.

OceanSide Publications, Inc.

Providence, Rhode Island 1991

OceanSide Publications, Inc.

Second Edition

Library of Congress Catalog Card Number 90-64470

Published by OceanSide Publications, Inc., 95 Pitman Street, Providence, Rhode Island 02906

Printed in the United States of America
ISBN 0-936587-04-0

Contributors

Irving Bailit, M.D.
Associate in Allergy
Children's Hospital
Clinical Instructor in Pediatrics
Harvard Medical School
Boston, Massachusetts

James N. Baraniuk, M.D.
Allergic Diseases Section
Laboratory of Clinical Investigations
National Institute of Allergy & Infectious Diseases
National Institutes of Health
Bethesda, Maryland

John J. Ballenger, M.D.
Associate Professor
Northwestern University Medical School
Chief, Emeritus
Division of Otolaryngology-Head & Neck Surgery
Evanston Hospital
Evanston, Illinois

Peter Borum, M.D.
Otopathological Laboratory
Department of Otorhinolaryngology
Rigshospitalet, Copenhagen, Denmark

Sidney S. Braman, M.D.
Professor of Medicine
Bio-Med Medicine
Brown University
Director, Division of Pulmonary Diseases
Rhode Island Hospital
Providence, Rhode Island

Philip Cole, M.D.
Department of Otolaryngology Airflow Laboratory
St. Michael's Hospital
Toronto, Ontario

John T. Connell, M.D.
Director, Nasal Diseases Study Center
Holy Name Hospital
Englewood, New Jersey

James W. Cooper, Jr., Ph.D.
Associate Professor
Head, Department of Pharmacy Practice
   University of Georgia School of Pharmacy
Athens, Georgia

T. Dietmer, M.D.
Universitat Munster
Klinik und Poliklinik fur Hals-Nasenund
   Ohrenheilkunde
Munster, Federal Republic of Germany

William K. Dolen, M.D.
Clinical Assistant Professor of Medicine
University of Colorado Health Sciences Center
Denver, Colorado

Howard M. Druce, M.D.
Assistant Professor of Internal Medicine
Director, Nasal & Paranasal Sinus Physiology
   Laboratory
St. Louis University School of Medicine
St. Louis, Missouri

Jack E. Farnham, M.D.
Clinical Associate Professor of Medicine
Allergy & Clinical Immunology Unit
Massachusetts General Hospital
Boston, Massachusetts

William Franklin, M.D.
Associate Physician
Massachusetts General Hospital
Assistant Clinical Professor of Medicine
Harvard Medical School
Boston, Massachusetts

Nathan Geurkink, M.D.
Associate Professor of Surgery
Section of Otolaryngology, Head & Neck Surgery
Dartmouth Medical School
Hanover, New Hampshire

James S. Haight, M.D.
Department of Otolaryngology Airflow Laboratory
St. Michael's Hospital
Toronto, Ontario, Canada

John H. Haines, Ph.D.
Biological Survey
The New York State Museum
Albany, New York

Mindy Hauptschein-Raphael, M.S., R.D.
Allergic Diseases Section
Laboratory of Clinical Investigation and
    Clinical Nutrition Service
National Institutes of Health
Bethesda, Maryland

Othon Iliopoulos, M.D.
Division of Clinical Immunology
Department of Medicine
The Johns Hopkins University School of Medicine
Baltimore, Maryland

Alfredo A. Jalowayski, Ph.D.
Director, Pediatric Respiratory Unit
    & Rapid Diagnostic Laboratory
Department of Pediatrics
University of California
San Diego, California

Anne Kagey-Sobotka, Ph.D.
Assistant Professor of Medicine
Division of Clinical Immunology
Department of Medicine
The Johns Hopkins University School of Medicine
Baltimore, Maryland

Michael A. Kaliner, M.D.
Head, Allergic Diseases Section
Laboratory of Clinical Investigations
National Institute of Allergy and Infectious Diseases
National Institutes of Health
Bethesda, Maryland

David W. Kennedy, M.D.
Department of Otolaryngology
Head and Neck Surgery
University of Pennsylvania Medical Center
Philadelphia, Pennsylvania

T. P. King, Ph.D.
Professor
Rockefeller University
New York, New York

Donald E. Klein, M.D.
Clinical Associate Professor of Pediatrics
Brown University Program in Medicine
Director, Division of Allergy
Department of Medicine
Rhode Island Hospital
Providence, Rhode Island

Walter Kucharczy, M.D.
Department of Radiology
The Toronto Hospital
Toronto, Ontario, Canada

Lawrence Lichtenstein, M.D.
Professor of Medicine
The Johns Hopkins University School of Medicine
Baltimore, Maryland

Frank E. Lucente, M.D.
Professor and Chairman
Department of Otolaryngology
Long Island College Hospital
Long Island, New York

Donald N. MacKay, M.D.
Clinical Associate Professor of Medicine
Stanford University Medical Center
Stanford, California

Jan Malat, M.D.
Clinical Assistant Professor
Yale University School of Medicine
MRI and Neuroradiology Consultant
Southern Massachusetts Hospitals Consortium
Fall River, Massachusetts

Kenneth P. Mathews, M.D.
Adjunct Member, Scripps Clinic and
    Research Foundation
La Jolla, California
Professor Emeritus of Internal Medicine
University of Michigan
Ann Arbor, Michigan

James A. McLean, M.D.
Professor Emeritus of Internal Medicine
Division of Allergy
The University of Michigan Medical Center
Ann Arbor, Michigan

Lawrence Z. Meiteles, M.D.
Department of Otolaryngology
New York Medical College
New York Eye & Ear Infirmary
New York, New York

Eli O. Meltzer, M.D.
Clinical Professor of Pediatrics
Division of Allergy & Immunology
University of California
Allergy & Asthma Medical Group and Research Center
San Diego, California

George M. Meredith, M.D.
Assistant Clinical Professor of Otolaryngology
Eastern Virginia Medical School
Norfolk, Virginia

Scott D. Meredith, M.D.
Allergic Diseases Section
Laboratory of Clinical Investigations
National Institutes of Health
Bethesda, Maryland

S. David Miller, M.D.
Assistant Instructor in Medicine
Brown University
Providence, Rhode Island

Richard P. Millman, M.D.
Associate Professor of Medicine
Brown University Program in Medicine
Director, Pulmonary Function Laboratory and
  Sleep Disorder Laboratory
Rhode Island Hospital
Providence, Rhode Island

David L. Mulcahy, Ph.D.
Botany Department
University of Massachusetts
Amherst, Massachusetts

Michael F. Mullarkey, M.D.
Head, Allergy & Clinical Immunology
Virginia Mason Clinic
Seattle, Washington

Niels Mygind, M.D.
Otophatological Laboratory
Department of Otolaryngology & Internal
  Medicine TTA
Copenhagen, Denmark

Robert M. Naclerio, M.D.
Associate Professor of Medicine & Otolaryngology
Division of Clinical Immunology
Department of Medicine
The Johns Hopkins University School of Medicine
Bethesda, Maryland

Kensei Naito, M.D.
Department of Otolaryngology Airflow Laboratory
St. Michael's Hospital
Toronto, Ontario

Minoru Okuda, M.D.
Department of Otolaryngology
Nippon Medical School
Tokyo, Japan

S. Phadhana-anek, M.D.
Universitat Munster
Klinik und Poliklinik fur Hals-Nasenund
  Ohrenheilkunde
Munster, Federal Republic of Germany

Ulf Pipkorn, M.D.
Ent Department
University Hospital
Lund, Sweden

Donald F. Proctor, M.D.
Emeritus Professor of Environmental Health Sciences
Otolaryngology, Anesthesiology
The Johns Hopkins Medical Institutions
The Johns Hopkins School of Hygiene & Public Health
Baltimore, Maryland

David Proud, M.D.
Associate Professor of Medicine
Division of Clinical Immunology
Department of Medicine
The Johns Hopkins University School of Medicine
Baltimore, Maryland

Gordon D. Raphael, M.D.
Allergic Disease Section
Laboratory of Clinical Investigation
National Institute of Allergy & Infectious Diseases
National Institutes of Health
Bethesda, Maryland

Ira F. Salkin, Ph.D.
Division of Laboratories & Research
New York State Department of Health
Albany, New York

Philip S. Schoenfeld, B.S.
Department of Otolaryngology
New York Medical College
New York Eye & Ear Infirmary
New York, New York

John C. Selner, M.D.
Clinical Professor of Pediatrics
University of Colorado Health Sciences Center
Head, Section of Allergy
Children's Hospital
Denver, Colorado

Guy A. Settipane, M.D.
Clinical Professor of Medicine
Brown University Program in Medicine
Director, Division of Allergy
Department of Medicine
Providence, Rhode Island

Sheldon C. Siegel, M.D.
Clinical Professor of Pediatrics
UCLA School of Medicine
Los Angeles, California

F. Estelle R. Simons, M.D.
Professor & Head,
Section of Department of Pediatrics & Child Health
University of Manitoba
Winnipeg, Manitoba, Canada

J. Montgomery Smith, M.D.
Department of Internal Medicine
University of Iowa Hospitals & Clinic
Iowa City, Iowa

Sheldon L. Spector, M.D.
Clinical Professor of Medicine
UCLA School of Medicine
Co-director, Allergy Research
Los Angeles, California

Alkis G. Togias, M.D.
Instructor in Medicine
Division of Clinical Immunology
Department of Medicine
The Johns Hopkins University School of Medicine
Baltimore, Maryland

Robert G. Townley, M.D.
Professor of Medicine
Associate Professor of Microbiology
Creighton University
Omaha, Nebraska

Joel K. Weltman, M.D., Ph.D.
Clinical Associate Professor of Medicine
Division of BioMedical Sciences
Brown University
Providence, Rhode Island

S. James Zinreich, M.D.
Assistant Professor
Neuroradiology Division of the
    Russell H. Morgan Department of
    Radiology and Radiological Sciences
The Johns Hopkins University School of Medicine
Baltimore, Maryland

FOREWORD

Rhinitis—who among us has not had it or been treated for it? The practice of allergy/immunology and otolaryngology depends to a great extent on the frequent occurrence of upper airway disease. Most physicians, regardless of their specialty, periodically are asked by their patients, "By the way, my sinuses are bothering me. Could you prescribe something for me?" Therefore, it behooves all physicians to know how to diagnose and treat the variety of diseases covered in *Rhinitis*.

When lecturing on upper airway disease, I sometimes state that more is known about the pathophysiology of heart, liver, or kidney disease than is known about such diseases as sinusitis, allergic rhinitis, or vasomotor rhinitis. To this day, that remains true. However, great strides are being made to better understand the pathophysiology and to improve the treatment of the varied diseases that affect the upper airway.

Guy Settipane, M.D., editor, and the other authors of *Rhinitis* are to be congratulated. This book should be in every physicians' personal library inasmuch as chronic rhinitis affects one of five individuals. For the most part rhinitis is not life threatening, therefore, not enough research and attention has been given to its pathophysiology, diagnosis, and treatment. This is changing, as reflected by the chapters included in this book: immunopharmacology and mediators of rhinitis, mucosal physiology, pollen and molds, and the clinical diseases that affect the upper airways. Methods to measure upper airway physiology are included as well as discussions on the relationship between upper and lower airway disease. In 1844, Adam, Herck, and Freiberg recognized the importance of sinus disease as a contributing factor to asthma. In 1871, Voltolini first demonstrated the beneficial effects of sinus surgery on asthma. Today, no physician who regularly treats asthma would deny the importance of treating upper airway disease to control asthma, a recurrent theme throughout *Rhinitis*. Even HIV infection can present as rhinitis, as explored in a separate chapter.

A variety of new procedures have revolutionized our approach to the diagnosis and treatment of upper airway disease. The computed tomography scan and magnetic resonance imaging have greatly improved our evaluation of sinusitis and the anatomical abnormalities that sometimes accompany this disease. Flexible fiberoptic endoscopy also is effective, enabling the physician to diagnose and assess problems with much greater accuracy than was possible by traditional diagnostic modalities. Endoscopic surgery, an outpatient procedure, has enabled the otolaryngologist to routinely visualize and surgically treat various parts of the upper airway with improved results as well as reduced trauma and morbidity. Medical treatment also has improved with the development of new antihistamines (including nonsedating ones), decongestants, and innovative treatments, such as topical anticholinergics, sodium cromolyn, and glucocorticosteroids. These diagnostic and treatment modalities are thoroughly covered in this book. Modified allergens for immunotherapy and immunotherapy also are reviewed.

Much has changed since Blackley in 1873 started his systematic study of "hay fever" by personal observations and experimentation. Today, the explosion of scientific knowledge has allowed upper airway disease to be better defined and understood. These advances enable physicians to more appropriately diagnose, treat, and even eliminate illnesses that cause so much discomfort. This book, one-of-a-kind, goes a long way in summarizing this important new and revolutionary information.

Richard F. Lockey, M.D.
Professor of Medicine, Pediatrics and
  Public Health
Director, Division of Allergy and Immunology
University of South Florida College of Medicine
Tampa, Florida

BIBLIOGRAPHY

Blackley CH. Experimental Researches on the Causes and Nature of Catarrhus Aestivus (Hay-Fever or Hay-Asthma). Abington, GB. Oxford Historical Books, 1988 (reissued).
Cooke RA. Allergy in Theory and Practice. Philadelphia: W.B. Saunders, Company, 1947.

PREFACE

The second edition of *Rhinitis* has been greatly expanded from 28 to 42 chapters. The list of contributors has increased from 34 to 60 authors. The new chapters include Immunopharmacology of Nasal Reactions, Airway and Dentofacial Development, Olfaction, Physiology and Pathology, Nasal Reflexes, Sleep Apnea and Patency, Chronic Sinusitis and Nonallergic Rhinitis, Gustatory Rhinitis, Nasal Manifestations of Acquired Immunodeficiency Syndrome, New Nonsedating Antihistamine, Cromolyn and Anticholinergic Drug Chapters, Functional Endoscopic Approach to Inflammatory Sinus Disease, Allergy Testing, Nasal Cytology, CT Scan, MRI, Rhinometry: Patency and Assessment, Rhinoscopy, Nasal Provocation Testing, and Ciliary Beat Frequency: Physiology and Counting Methods.

Contributing authors include international experts from America, Europe, and Japan. The topics are also cosmopolitan with chapters on epidemiology and pollen-and-mold surveys reviewed on a worldwide basis.

Guy A. Settipane, M.D.

Acknowledgment: I wish to thank our publishing staff: Cynthia Burke, Carole Fico, Virginia Loiselle, Sally Martone, and Joseph Settipane for their help in publishing this book.

RHINITIS—2nd Edition

Editor, Guy A. Settipane, M.D.

TABLE OF CONTENTS

PROCEDURES

CHAPTER I
INTRODUCTION

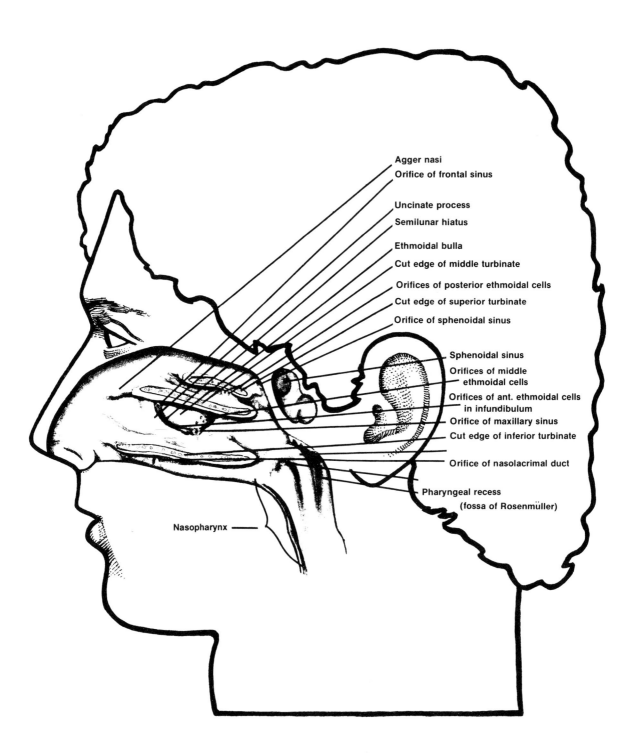

Agger nasi
Orifice of frontal sinus
Uncinate process
Semilunar hiatus
Ethmoidal bulla
Cut edge of middle turbinate
Orifices of posterior ethmoidal cells
Cut edge of superior turbinate
Orifice of sphenoidal sinus
Sphenoidal sinus
Orifices of middle
  ethmoidal cells
Orifices of ant. ethmoidal cells
  in infundibulum
Orifice of maxillary sinus
Cut edge of inferior turbinate
Orifice of nasolacrimal duct
Pharyngeal recess
  (fossa of Rosenmüller)
Nasopharynx

Nasal Anatomy

Chapter I

Rhinitis: Introduction

Guy A. Settipane, M.D.

A llergic rhinitis is one of the most frequent diseases of allergy seen in the general population. About 20% of the population has hay fever and another 5% has nonseasonal allergic rhinitis.[1-3] Therefore, over 25% of the population suffers from some form of nasal allergy. If the nonallergic components of rhinitis, such as vasomotor rhinitis, nasal polyps and NARES (non-allergic rhinitis eosinophilic syndrome), are added to these figures, the overall frequency approaches 30% of the general population. Indeed a significant portion of the population is afflicted with a nonsurgical form of chronic or recurrent rhinitis.

Symptoms of rhinitis are nonspecific for a particular diagnosis. They include nasal congestion, rhinorrhea, postnasal drip, frequent sneezing, itchy nose, watery itchy eyes, and headaches over the paranasal sinus areas. If symptoms are severe or continuous, loss of smell (anosmia) and taste (ageusia) will result.

The association of allergic rhinitis with asthma and atopic eczema is well known. Rackemann[4] and Buffum[5] have noted this association and have found that atopic eczema beginning within the first year of life is followed by asthma and then allergic rhinitis. In our study[1-3] of Brown University students, the mean ages of onset of asthma, nonseasonal allergic rhinitis, and hay fever were 6.9, 9.1, and 10.6 years respectively. However, rhinitis at times may begin before the onset of asthma. Cumulative frequency of nonseasonal allergic rhinitis and hay fever by age of onset (years) are shown in Figures 1 and 2. In a prospective study of 1,352 college students, the frequency of developing hay fever in the three-year interval between the freshmen and senior years was found to be 3.1%. Of the 614 asymptomatic freshmen, 4.4% developed hay fever as seniors.[2,3]

Allergy skin tests positive to pollens precede the development of clinical hay fever and may be used as a prognostic sign for developing hay fever. In a three-year follow-up study, the risk of developing hay fever in asymptomatic college freshmen with positive skin tests to pollens is over 10 times higher than in asymptomatic students with negative tests to pollens (18.2% vs 1.7%), Table I.[2] This relationship was also present in a seven-year follow-up study, Table II.[3] In addition, the risk of developing hay fever increases with the degree of positive reactivity to pollen skin testing, Table III.

In college students, asthma occurs in about 17–19% of patients with allergic rhinitis; however, 56–74% of patients with asthma have allergic rhinitis, Table IV.[1-3,6,7] As discussed in later chapters by both Braman and Townley, a large number of patients with allergic rhinitis but no overt symptoms of lung disease and no history of asthma have abnormal methacholine tests. In a seven-year follow-up study done on Brown University students, Hagy and Settipane[3] found that about 6% of the college students with allergic rhinitis developed asthma, compared to 1.3% of students with no allergic rhinitis, Table V.

This risk factor of 6% for developing asthma compares favorably with Townley and Braman's prediction that 5–7.5% of patients with allergic rhinitis will develop asthma at a later date. Townley's prediction is based on methacholine challenge studies. He states that although 50% of patients with allergic rhinitis show a greater than 20% decrease in FEV$_1$, many of these patients reached a "plateau" and further increases in methacholine dosage do not result in a further decrease in FEV$_1$. Only 5% show a positive response without a plateau phenomenon, and these 5% of allergic rhinitis patients are at risk for developing asthma at a later time. Townley believes that a partial beta adrenergic

Clinical Professor of Medicine, Brown University School of Medicine, and Director, Division of Allergy, Department of Medicine, Rhode Island Hospital

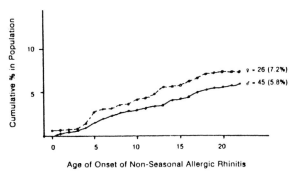

Figure 1. *Cumulative frequency of nonseasonal allergic rhinitis by age of onset in college students.*

blockage exists in patients with allergic rhinitis but not to the degree found in asthmatic patients. Braman et al.[8] followed prospectively 40 ragweed hay fever patients with no history of asthma and normal spirometry and found that three (7.5%) developed asthma within five years. These three patients were in a group of 16 patients who initially had hyperresponsiveness to methacholine.

There are five functional biochemical receptors in the nose: the alpha adrenoceptor, beta$_2$ adrenoceptor, cholinoceptor, histamine (H$_1$) receptor, and irritant receptor, Table VI. The H$_2$ histamine receptor is essentially nonfunctional.[9,10] Stimulation of receptors found in the nose, pharyngeal, and sinus areas may produce bronchospasm through neural reflexes. The receptors involved are the histamine (H$_1$) and irritant receptors which send afferent neural impulses through the trigeminal, facial, and glossopharyngeal nerves to the medulla

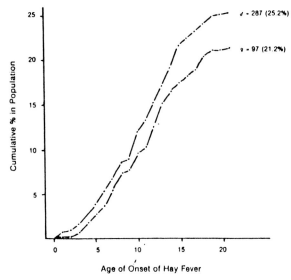

Figure 2. *Cumulative frequency of seasonal hay fever by age of onset in college students. Hagy GW & Settipane Ga. J Allergy Clin Immunol 48:200, 1971.*

oblongata where the vagal nucleus is stimulated. The efferent arm of this reflex is the vagal nerve with its ramifications sending neural impulses to the bronchial tree causing bronchospasm in much the same way as a methacholine inhalation challenge.

Kaufman and Wright[11] demonstrated that increased airway resistance in the lung produced by exposing the nasal and nasopharyngeal area to silica particles, which stimulated the irritant receptors, was prevented by pretreatment with atropine. Ogura et al.[12] reported that functional compliance in the lung is increased by the use of nasal sprays (vasoconstrictors) or following nasal surgery where an airway obstruction is removed. They also noted that functional lung compliance, measured through the mouth, decreased with increasing grades of nasal obstruction.

Clinically, the treatment of acute or chronic sinusitis with antibiotics, decongestants, or surgical procedures (both removal of polyps or sinus operations) has been found to improve asthmatic episodes to a degree that corticosteroids are able to be discontinued or greatly reduced in certain cases.[13-16] As far back as 1947, Robert A. Cooke[17] suggested that sinusitis may aggravate an existing asthma and improvement of the sinus condition may improve the asthma. His observations were based on clinical observation.

The mechanism by which acute or chronic sinusitis or rhinitis aggravates asthma is probably through the rhinosino-bronchial reflex. However, the questions about rhinobronchial reflex still are unresolved.[18] What is apparent is that it is important to treat the nose and sinus areas in patients with asthma, especially since chronic sinusitis and rhinitis frequently co-exist with asthma.

About 64% of patients with allergic rhinitis and asthma have a positive family history of these conditions in first-degree relatives compared to 35% found in controls with no allergies.[1,2] In a direct interview and questionnaire study of 599 families done at Brown University where the study group (probands) were obtained either from a private pediatric practice or from college freshmen, Hagy and Settipane[19] demonstrated that individuals with hay fever have a significantly higher family history of hay fever in first-degree relatives than do asthmatics or normal individuals, Table VII. Although both allergic rhinitis and asthma are diseases of the respiratory tract, they are separate entities and appear to have different genetic transmission mechanisms. However, the definite relationship existing between these two conditions is more than just a chance occurrence.

Evidence suggests that in addition to an inherited predisposition for developing specific IgE to certain antigens, the atopic individual also may have a mucous membrane defect. Apparently, both this genetic predisposition and a membrane defect are needed to express

2

TABLE I

Asymptomatic College Freshmen Who Later Developed Hay Fever: A 3-Year Follow-up Study

Status of Freshmen	Total No.	No. with New Hay Fever	%	P Value
Positive pollen scratch tests	99	18	18.2	
				<0.01
Negative pollen scratch tests	515	9	1.7	
Total	614	27	4.4	

Hagy GW, Settipane GA. J Allergy Clin Immunol 48:200, 1971.

clinically the allergy in the form of hay fever, asthma, or food allergy.

In a series of experiments beginning in 1964, Salvaggio et al.[20–22] showed that intranasal instillation of purified protein and polysaccharide antigens more readily induce wheal-and-flare skin reactivity in atopic individuals than in normals. However, in studies on individuals with vasomotor rhinitis or on those with rhinitis due to "intrinsic allergy," attempts to sensitize such individuals in a similar fashion by intranasal instillation of purified protein antigens failed.[23]

Disturbance of mucus membranes by low or absent IGA[24–29] or by previous challenge with another antigen in a sensitized individual[30] increases the risk of sensitivity of allergy. Jackson et al.[31] have shown that individuals with atopic eczema absorb larger size molecules from the gastrointestinal tract than do nonatopic individuals. Bloch et al.[32] reported that during acute local anaphylaxis of the GI tract, the mucous membranes are disturbed and larger size molecules are absorbed than under normal conditions.

When the mucous membranes are circumvented by applying the antigen parenterally (such as in insect stings or penicillin), the frequency of anaphylaxis to these parenterally applied antigens is similar in atopic

and nonatopic individuals.[33,34] These data suggest that parenterally applied antigens may produce anaphylaxis by a different mechanism than that found in atopy. Antigens applied through the mucous membranes may stimulate production of specific IgE if two conditions are present: (1) a membrane defect allowing the antigen to be absorbed and (2) the presence of a genetic factor leading to production of IgE in response to this antigen. The location of the membrane defect may be related to the manifestation of allergy: food allergy-gastrointestinal membranes, asthma-bronchial membranes, and hay fever-nasal membranes.

In the basic science part of this book, Dr. Mathews, in Chapter II on mediators of anaphylaxis, describes the ever-growing list of substances that are released for formed to produce anaphylaxis. There are at least four separate sources from which mediators of anaphylaxis are derived:

1. Mast cell granules are discharged intact and on interacting with tissue fluids release certain water-soluble preformed mediators.

2. These preformed mediators generate secondary mediators on interacting with target tissue.

3. Neurohormones are discharged in response to mediators.

TABLE II

Asymptomatic College Freshmen Who Later Developed Hay Fever: A 7-Year Follow-up Study

Status of Freshmen	Total No.	No. with New Hay Fever	%	P Value
Positive pollen scratch tests	91	29	31.9	
				<0.001
Negative pollen scratch tests	467	36	7.7	
Total	558	65	11.6	

Hagy GW, Settipane GA. J Allergy Clin Immunol 58:330, 1976.

TABLE III

New Cases of Hay Fever and Degree of Pollen Reaction in Students Who Initially Had No Clinical Manifestations of Allergy

Maximum degree of scratch test reactions to any of 7 pollens	A 3-Year Follow Up Of Asymptomatic Freshmen			
		New cases of hay fever		
	No. followed up	No.	%	P Value
Negative (all pollens)	515	9	1.7	
1+	31	2	6.5	
2+	38	6	15.8	<0.01*
3+	23	7	30.4	<0.01**
4+	7	3	42.9	
Total	614	27		

*Compared to negative pollen test group. ** Compared to the 1+ positive test group.*
Hagy GW, Settipane GA. J Allergy Clin Immunol 48:200, 1971.

4. The matrix from mast cell granules in a belated response solubilizes, releasing preformed constituents.[35] These mast cell-derived mediators are listed by Mathews's in Chapter II of this book.

When mast cells degranulate, they directly produce several prostaglandins (PGD_2 12-HETE) which cause target tissues to produce other prostaglandins, HETE, and leukotrienes. Mediator release is regulated by cAMP, cGMP, CA++, neurohormones, and negative and positive feedback loops. Various drugs or substances interact at different stages in this regulatory system to affect the clinical expression of anaphylaxis.

Mathews also points out that an important late-phase reaction occurs as a consequence of the immediate reactivity. These late-phase reactions involve complex cellular interactions that include mast cells, basophils, neutrophils, eosinophils, lymphocytes, macrophages, and platelets. A new discovery about anaphylactic mediators is that anaphylactic deaths now can be documented by measuring mast cell tryptase levels in postmortem sera up to 12 hours after death.[36]

In Chapter III, Johns Hopkins investigators led by Naclerio and Lichtenstein report on the pharmacology and pathophysiology of the upper airway allergic reaction after studying lavage fluid following nasal provocation. They found that administration of systemic steroids inhibited mediator release, improved symptoms, inhibited accumulation of eosinophils and mononuclear cells but not neutrophils during the late-phase reaction. Steroids had no effect on mediators or symptoms of the early reaction except for kinins.

The advantages and disadvantages of allergy skin tests compared to *in vitro* tests, RAST, or ELISA are described by Weltman. For routine allergy practice,

TABLE IV

Asthma in College Students

Investigators and Population Source	Year of Study	Total No. Students	% Asthma with Allergic Rhinitis	% Allergic Rhinitis with Asthma
Van Arsdel and Motulsky Univ. Washington	1959	5,818	57	19
Maternowski and Mathews Univ. Michigan	1962	434	56	19
Hagy and Settipane Brown Univ.	1969	1,836	74	17

TABLE V

Risk of Developing Asthma: A 7-Year Follow-up Study

Diagnosis of Freshmen	No. of Students in Group	No. with New Asthma	%	P Value
Allergic Rhinitis (both seasonal and nonseasonal)	215	13	6.0	
				<0.001
No allergic rhinitis	628	8	1.3	
Total	843	21	2.5	

scratch or intracutaneous skin tests are simple, sensitive, rapid, less expensive and clinically valid. There are special situations in which *in vitro* solid-phase immunoassay for IgE may be preferred. These special situations include skin rashes, life-threatening allergic symptoms, and those with nonreactive skin to histamine.

The pollen and mold section of this book represent an important etiology of allergic reactions. Farnham describes in great detail atmospheric pollen and molds on a worldwide basis, including microspores and biochemical characteristics of these airborne allergens as well as methods of pollen and mold collection and counting techniques. Indoor aeroallergens also are dis-

cussed. A recently discovered indoor allergen is the house dust mite, found on a global basis. Usually the mites *Dermatophagoides pteronyssinus* (Dp) and *Dermatophagoides fairnae* (Df) are the important allergens, but storage mites and predator mites also have been implicated. Their feces contain the allergen. Factors such a high humidity, wall-to-wall carpeting overlying a concrete slab, pets, old overstuffed furniture and beddings, skin scales, and mold spores promote the growth of mites. Currently, commercial extracts are not available for testing skin reaction to mite species other than Dp and Df. Cross-reactivity exists between antigens of these species. Extracts of Dp and Df are available

TABLE VI

Nasal Receptors

	Type of Receptor	Drug	Action	Nasal Airway Resistance	Remarks
1	Alpha Adrenoceptor	Neosynephrine Norepinephrine	Stimulation	Decreased	Reserpine depletes norepinephrine causing increased nasal airway resistance
2	Beta$_2$ Adrenoceptor	Isoproterenol	Stimulation	Increased	Blocked by propranolol
3	Cholinoceptor	Methacholine	Stimulation	Increased	Causes profuse rhinorrhea blocked by atropine
4	Histamine (H$_1$) Receptor	Histamine	Stimulation	Increased	60% of action is through neuro-reflexes, H$_1$ receptor blocked by H$_1$-antihistamines
5	Histamine (H$_2$) Receptor	Histamine	Stimulation	Slightly increased	H$_2$ receptor blocked by cimetidine, which has slight to no effect
6	Irritant Receptor	Nonspecific (dust, histamine, NH$_3$, etc.)	Stimulation	Increased	Reflex abolished by atropine. Antihistimines have no effect

Antihistamines do not improve nasal airway resistance, but do suppress sneezing, itching, and hypersecretion.

TABLE VII

Frequency of Hay Fever Observed in Living Relatives of Allergic and Nonallergic Individuals

| Probands Diagnosis | No. | Parents & Sibs | | | | P Value Control Group vs. Allergic |
		Total	#HF	%HF	SE	
No Allergy	267	1096	101	9.22	.008	
Intrinsic Asthma*	35	135	20	14.81	.030	N.S.
Extrinsic Asthma†	75	288	40	13.89	.020	<0.05
Extr. Asthma & HF	70	283	69	24.38	.025	<0.01
Hay Fever	152	522	125	23.95	.018	<0.001
Total	599	2324				

SE = Standard error.
* Extrinsic Asthma = one or more positive skin tests to pollens, dander and mold.
† Intrinsic Asthma = negative skin tests to pollens, dander and mold.

for immunotherapy. Tests for detecting and chemicals for eradicating mite antigens have been developed. Mite antigens are known causes of allergic rhinitis and asthma.

In the next chapter, Mulcahy discusses the genetic determinants of pollen phenotype. Competition among a vast number of pollen grains for a limited number of ovules creates the opportunity for very intense natural selection. This chapter is followed by Drs. Haines and Salkin who discuss the biology and identification of fungi, which may be unicellular (yeastlike), filamentous (moldlike), or both (dimorphic). Fungi are classified as a separate kingdom primarily on the basis of their ability to absorb nutrients and their multinucleate character.

Chapter VIII by Geurkink initiates the anatomy and physiology section. He discusses the variety of functions of the nose related to its unique anatomy and the vascular tone of the mucous membrane. The basic functions of the nose reviewed are airflow resistance (about 30% of the total resistance to inspiration), conditioning of the air by temperature and humidity, filtration of the inspired air, olfaction, contribution of vocal resonance, and the initiation of nasal reflex activity (some of which results in bronchospasm).

One of the most important functions of the nose is the filtration and removal of foreign particles larger than 15 μ in size. Only 5% of 1 μ particles are removed by the mucous membrane. The mucous blanket aids in this removal, and the two constituents of the mucous blanket are the enzyme muramidase (lysozyme) and secretory immunoglobulins (IgA, IgE). The movement of foreign particles by ciliary activity is 1–2 mm per hour in front of the nose and 10 mm each minute in the posterior aspect of the nose.

In Chapter IX, airway and dentofacial development are reviewed. Chronic rhinitis in children can produce long-standing mouth-breathing that in turn places abnormal stimulation on facial muscles, affecting the facial skeletal system and leading to the "long-face" syndrome.

Dr. John J. Ballenger discusses anatomy, physiology, pathology, and treatment of olfaction. Abnormalities of olfaction including congenital, endocrine, mechanical, infectious, trauma, neoplasms, drugs, and toxins etiologies and different types of olfaction testing procedures are reviewed.

The olfactory neuroepithelium cells are unique in that receptor cells are regularly replaced when injured through trauma, viral infections, and neurotoxic chemicals. These receptor cells regenerate from basal cells, which reestablish contact with the olfactory bulb. Olfactory neuroepithelium is gradually replaced with respiratory epithelium as part of the aging process and probably correlates with the diminution in olfactory sensitivity that occurs with aging. The olfactory neuroepithelium is located in the area of the cribriform plate and the superior portions of the lateral walls and nasal septum. The differences between the olfactory and the respiratory epithelium are: the olfactory epithelium is thicker, contains Bowman's glands, and lacks the dynein arms in the cilia. The olfactory receptors number 6 million and contain a functional protein, olfactory marker protein. These receptor sites are found on the cilia. The mechanisms for olfaction are: odorant chemicals are absorbed in the mucus, diffuse on the dentritic processes of the cilia to the olfactory receptor cell, and reversibly bind the olfactory marker protein causing a neurologic stimulation. Loss of smell (anosmia) frequently results in mental depression especially in those individuals with dysosmia or dysgeusia.

In Chapter XI, McLean discusses rhinomanometry and experimental nasal challenges including the effect of physiologic buffered saline (PBS), ragweed, histamine, methacholine, NH_3, polymyxin B, and isoproterenol on nasal airway resistance (NAR). He also describes the inhibiting effects of atropine, chlorpheniramine, aspirin, indomethacin, and sodium salicylate on the ragweed and NH_3-induced increase in nasal airway resistance.

Next, Proctor points out that nasal infections are associated with desquamation of respiratory epithelium, and on patient recovery, mucociliary function is restored in two to six weeks. In allergic rhinitis, nasal congestion and rhinorrhea may interfere with nasal airflow either directly or through mediators of anaphylaxis such as leukotrienes, slow-reactive substance of anaphylaxis (SRS-A), and histamine. Chemical pollutants such as dioxide and formaldehyde can impair mucociliary clearance.

A thorough review and discussion of nasal reflexes occurs in Chapter XV by the National Institute of Allergy and Infectious Diseases investigators headed by Kaliner. This review discusses nasal innervation, neuropeptides, and summarizes different types of nasal reflexes including the rhino-bronchial reflexes. Littel et al.[18] recently demonstrated that local application of histamine and methacholine do not produce this reflex, a finding opposite to that of Yan and Salome.[37] Less controversial is the fact that treatment of sinusitis or nasal obstruction such as polyps improves asthma on a long-term basis.[13–17,38]

In Chapter XVI, on sleep apnea and nasal patency, Millman states that partial or complete nasal obstruction even in normal subjects can cause sleep disruption, hyponoia, and apnea. Daytime drowsiness in patients with chronic rhinitis may be explained by nasal obstruction occurring during sleep.[39]

Chapter XVII initiates the clinical section wherein Smith reviews various epidemiologic studies in allergic rhinitis throughout the world. She explains that some of the differences in these studies are due to methods of investigation and type of population studied as well as to environmental factors. She states that allergic rhinitis is a hereditary disorder that affects about 10–20% of Americans and 10 to 15% of northern Europeans.

Next, Dr. Connell categorizes the various diseases of the nose. He reviews his experience with over 1,500 nasal mucosa biopsies in various types of nasal disorders. In 1968 he was the first to describe the "priming effect" where nasal mucosa becomes hyperresponsive to antigen when the challenges are done on consecutive days. This is a local phenomenon and is not antigen specific. Priming is reproducible and transient, becoming progressively less by days 8 through 15. The irritant NH_3 does not cause a similar effect. Under abnormalities not associated with the immune system, Connell lists neurogenic disease (vasomotor rhinitis), epithelial abnormalities (replacement of ciliated columnar epithelium by cuboid cells or squamous cells), rhinitis medicamentosa, rhinitis of endocrine origin (hypothyroidism), nasal mastocytosis, and eosinophilic nonallergic rhinitis. He also reviews nasal diseases caused by immunological mechanisms, the major one being allergic rhinitis.

In Chapter XIX Dr. Mullarkey describes in detail the relatively new syndrome, nonallergic rhinitis eosinophilic syndrome (NARES) comparing its characteristics with allergic rhinitis and vasomotor rhinitis. NARES is associated with negative allergy skin tests, normal IgE, nasal eosinophilia, and an excellent response to corticosteroids. He also restricts this definition to exclude those patients with nasal polyps or aspirin sensitivity.

We recently studied 68 consecutive patients with nonallergic rhinitis (negative allergy skin tests).[40] Those with nasal polyps, aspirin intolerance, anatomical nasal obstruction, rhinitis medicamentosa, asthma/bronchitis, and elevated serum IgE were excluded from this study. We found that 61% had vasomotor rhinitis, 33% had NARES, and one patient (2%) had hypothyroidism. Three (4%) other patients with characteristics of NARES also had elevated blood eosinophilia averaging 951 mm^3. This may be a new syndrome and we called it BENARS (blood eosinophilic nonallergic rhinitis syndrome).

Chapter XX is a comprehensive review on nasal polyps. Nasal polyps are found most frequently in patients with aspirin intolerance and intrinsic asthma, especially in those over 40 years of age. Children 16 years or younger with nasal polyps should be evaluated for cystic fibrosis. Nasal polyps are frequently bilateral, multiple, freely movable, pale-gray, and usually arise from the middle meatus of the nose. Histologically, they have pseudo-stratified, ciliated columnar epithelium, thickening of the epithelial basement membrane, high stromal eosinophil count, mucin with neutral pH, few glands, and essentially no nerve endings. Cells consist of a mixture of lymphocytes, plasma cells, and eosinophils. Chemical mediators found in nasal polyps are histamine, serotonin, SRS-A, ECF-A, and norepinephrine.

There is more histamine in nasal polyps than in normal nasal mucosa. The concentration of IgA and IgE, and in some cases IgG and IgM, are greater in polyp fluid than in serum. IgE-mediated disease is not the cause of nasal polyps, but when present, may contribute to episodes of exacerbation. Despite medical or surgical management, a significant number of nasal polyps are recurrent. Polypectomy does not increase the risk of developing asthma or making asthma worse. For treatment systemic corticosteroids should be tried before polypectomy.

Our recent investigations suggest that the time between recurrence of polyps is greater after surgical polypectomy than after oral corticosteroid treatment.

It also was noted that patients with aspirin intolerance have frequent exacerbations and recurrence of nasal polyps. At the present time, the pathogenesis of polyp formation is unknown.

In the next chapter, Druce discusses chronic sinusitis and nonallergic rhinitis. He states that clinical diagnoses must be differentiated from those made solely on radiographic criteria. However, with the advent of the CAT scan, radiographic criteria have become much more important. Contributing factors to symptom pathogenesis are vascular reactivity, cellular infiltration, modifications of nasal secretions, anatomic abnormalities, deficiency of mucociliary clearance, immunodeficiency, and nasal reflexes. Symptoms attributed to sinusitis are postnasal drainage, facial fullness or swelling, head pressure, and nasal congestion. There is question whether nonallergic rhinitis is a disease or an exaggerated physiologic response.

In Chapter XXII, Raphael, Hauptschein-Raphael, and Kaliner from the National Institutes of Health explain the newly recognized syndrome of gustatory rhinitis, which is described as a profuse, watery rhinorrhea produced by consumption of certain spicy hot foods. There was additional evidence of increased secretion of albumin and total protein in nasal lavage fluid. They state that nasal pretreatment with atropine clinically blocked the positive food-induced rhinorrhea and significantly reduced albumin and total protein secretion. It appears that gustatory rhinitis is stimulated through atropine-sensitive muscarinic receptors.

Chapter XXIII is on systemic diseases associated with nasal symptoms. Rhinitis associated with asthma is probably the most common with leprosy and fungal infections being the rarest. A careful history and nasal examination in a patient with rhinitis may lead to the discovery of more significant systemic diseases. Proper treatment of systemic disease often will cure or improve the associated rhinitis and may reduce systemic complaints such as asthma. At times, identification of the cause of rhinitis (as in cerebral spinal fluid rhinorrhea, Wegener's syndrome, etc.) alerts one to a life-threatening entity.

It is apparent that the nose is an excellent mirror of some systemic diseases and that identifying and understanding the differential diagnosis of nasal symptoms may help in diagnosing the disease and treating the whole patient.

Rhinologic manifestations of acquired immunodeficiency syndrome have assumed immense importance, and this disease also has nasal manifestations including infections and tumors of the sinuses and nasal pharyngeal areas. *Haemophilus influenzae* and *S. pneumoniae* are the most common bacterial organisms encountered in AIDS patients with sinusitis, and *Pseudoallescheria boydii* is the most common fungal pathogen. Other disease entities encountered in the nasal pharyngeal areas are Kaposi's sarcoma, large cell lymphoma, candidiasis, herpes zoster, and herpes simplex. Precautions and specific guidelines for safeguarding health care procedures are reviewed.

Chapters XXV to XXXIV constitute the treatment section, starting with an in-depth discussion of the pharmacology of antihistamines and decongestants by Dr. James Cooper, Director of the Department of Pharmacy Practice, the University of Georgia's School of Pharmacy. He lists various types of nasal spray, classes of antihistamines, and a combination of antihistamines/decongestants and stresses side effects and adverse reactions. Decongestant drugs either should be avoided or used with caution in patients with high blood pressure, cardiovascular disease, diabetes, and thyroid disease. The interaction of antihistamine/decongestant, with neurological and psychologic drugs is stressed. For example, severe blood pressure increases may be seen in patients taking monoamine oxidase inhibitors (MAOI) and phenylpropanolamine or pseudoephedrine.

New non-sedating antihistamines are reviewed by Simons in Chapter XXVI. These include terfenadine, astemizole, cetirizine, loratadine, levocabastine, ketotifen, and azelastine all of which have diverse pharmacokinetics, pharmacodynamics, and potency. Astemizole is the most long-acting antihistamine. Cetirizine (the carboxylic acid metabolite of hydroxyzine) is minimally metabolized in the body and is primarily excreted unchanged in the urine. Levocabastine is the most potent of the new antihistamines and is efficacious topically on the conjunctivae or on the nasal mucosa. Cetirizine, terfenadine, loratadine, ketotifen, and azelastine have other antiallergic effects. For example, cetirizine is a potent anti-inflammatory drug. It is important to emphasize that the new H_1 receptor antagonists appear to be no more effective in relieving nasal congestion than the first-generation H_1 receptor antagonists. Most of the new H_1 receptor antagonists do not have anticholinergic effects. Also, they are relatively nonsedating.

Topical corticosteroids are reviewed by Sheldon Siegel in Chapter XXVII. They include beclomethasone, flunisolide, fluocortin, triamcinolone, betamethasone, and fluticasone. The most potent topical steroid is fluticasone followed by budesonide, and beclomethasone. Some of these newer topical steroids are classified as investigational drugs in the United States. Indications for intranasal topical corticosteroids are allergic rhinitis, nasal polyps, eosinophilic nonallergic rhinitis syndrome (NARES), rhinitis medicamentosa, and vasomotor rhinitis. Needless to say, their use should be limited to properly selected patients using the lowest possible dose for the shortest period of time for the control of symptoms.

Next, Spector discusses the effectiveness of cromolyn

sodium in various clinical situations. He states that ocular cromolyn has been utilized in allergic eye conditions as well as vernal conjuctivitis, atopic keratoconjunctivitis, and giant papillary conjuctivitis. Nasal cromolyn has been used successfully in the treatment of allergic rhinitis of the seasonal and perennial types, and oral cromolyn has been employed in people with multiple food allergies and under unusual conditions such as systemic mastocytosis. An effective blocker of both early and late phase allergic reactions, it essentially lacks side effects.

Chapter XXIX is on anticholinergic drugs for rhinitis. Mygind and Borum state these drugs reach the glandular cholinoceptors in the nose and block the secretory response to methacholine. This type of treatment significantly reduces watery rhinorrhea in patients with perennial rhinitis not responsive to other types of treatment. Anticholinergic drugs have no effect on sneezing or on nasal congestion. The major side effect is nasal dryness, which improves with a lower dose.

In the next chapter, Dr. MacKay discusses the antibiotic treatment of rhinitis and sinusitis. He states that the most common organisms causing bacterial sinusitis are pneumococci and *Hemophilus influenza*. In patients not allergic to penicillin, ampicillin or amoxicillin are the antibiotics of choice. Organisms obtained by culture of nasal secretions do not correlate with organisms obtained from sinuses by direct puncture aspiration; therefore, culture of nasal secretions is not recommended in sinusitis.

In Chapter XXXI, Kennedy and Zinreich of Johns Hopkins review the current status of the diagnosis of chronic inflammatory sinus disease and of functional endoscopic surgical techniques. They present technical modifications made since this type of surgery was introduced and the lessons learned from close postsurgical endoscopic examination. The importance of the ostealmeatal abnormality for sinusitis is emphasized.

The role of hyposensitization is reviewed by Dr. Franklin in Chapter XXXII. He states that evidence from many controlled studies of good experimental design, using the principle of random assignment of patients, placebo control, and blind evaluation supports the conclusion that immunotherapy can be effective in allergic rhinitis and that this effect is specific and dose related. Ragweed, grass, and tree pollen as well as mites (house dust ingredient) have been studied, and the effect is probably more general, involving other allergenic extracts such as danders and molds. Dr. Franklin stresses that immunotherapy is indicated only in those patients who cannot be controlled by other measures such as allergen avoidance procedures and antihistamine/decongestant drugs.

In the next chapter, T. P. King discusses modified antigen and the immune response. He describes various types of modification especially the chemical ones that have been studied as possible reagents for immunotherapy in allergic diseases. Modified antigens retain the property of native antigens to induce suppression of specific IgE levels in sensitized mice, and this suppression is dependent on the dose and on the immune state of the mice.

Patients usually can be treated with larger doses of the modified antigens than of the native antigens because of their reduced allergenicity, and these patients demonstrate similar changes in specific IgE and IgG levels as do native antigens. Modified antigens for immunotherapy still are in the investigational stage of development.

Pediatric aspects of allergic rhinitis are discussed by Bailit. He stresses that rhinitis in childhood is likely to be of allergic origin and therefore more responsive to both medical management and immunotherapy. Rhinitis may predispose the child to an increased incidence of otitis media, serous otitis, chronic sinusitis, and asthma. He also discusses pediatric aspects of various modalities of treatment such as antihistamines/decongestants, cromolyn sodium, and topical corticosteroids.

The last section of this second edition of *Rhinitis* deals with procedures used for the diagnosis and treatment of rhinologic-related disorders. Miller and Klein start this section with a detailed review of methodology of allergy diagnostic tests for detection of specific IgE antibodies. They describe hands-on methods for testing and interpretation of results. They compare *in vivo* and *in vitro* testing procedures outlining the advantages and pitfalls of each method. They emphasize that correlating test results with a comprehensive history and physical examination is essential for the proper diagnosis and treatment of allergic disease.

In the next chapter, Meltzer and Jalowayski correlate nasal cytology to pathophysiology and response to therapy. They review the technique for obtaining and interpreting cytology nasal specimens. Specific types of epithelial and inflammatory cells are seen in various disease patterns. They present an excellent guide for grading various cells seen on a quantitative basis. Specifically, they list epithelial cells, eosinophils, neutrophils, basophils, goblet cells, and bacteria.

In Chapter XXXVII, the computer tomography (CT) scan is described as the most accurate procedure for evaluating the paranasal sinuses and especially the osteomeatal complex. A direct coronal CT image of the sinus should be obtained for best results. Paradoxical rotation of the middle turbinates, lateral deviation of the uncinate process, and excessive ethmoidal bulla formation may be responsible for abnormal drainage of the osteomeatal complex resulting in chronic sinusitis. We prefer not to use the opaque contrast media with CT scan especially in atopic individuals.

In Chapter XXXVIII, Cole and his colleagues review the magnetic resonance imaging (MRI) of the nasal airways. The advantages of the MRI are that multiple orthogonal views may be obtained without changing the patient's position, and lesions of the brain or orbits are better demonstrated by MRI than by CT scan. Fungal infections and tumors are better visualized with MRI, which is not optimal for bony structures.

In Chapter XXXIX, Cole outlines the practical aspects of rhinomanometry in clinical situations. He states that there is a gradual trend toward lower nasal airways resistance (NAR) throughout adult life. Normally, nasal airway resistance is reduced approximately half by topical decongestants. In children with abnormal nasal airway resistance, 15% demonstrated fixed adenoidal obstruction and 40% revealed obstructive mucosal swelling, which responded to decongestants. Of interest is that 20% of the adult patients complaining of subjective nasal obstruction have normal nasal airway resistance. As a rule, patients self-assessment of the severity of any obstruction correlated poorly with objective findings of nasal airway resistance. Rhinomanometry before and after topical decongestants may be useful to determine if a nasal septal repair is necessary for physiological reasons.

During exercise, it usually is necessary to supplement the nasal airway with oral nasal breathing. This occurs when the nasal ventilation volume exceeds 30 to 40 L/min. A marked decrease in nasal resistance takes place immediately or within 30 minutes of exercise averaging about 4 minutes after exercise. In 22–30% of the cases, this decrease in NAR is followed by unilateral exercise-induced nasal obstruction.[41,42] This phenomenon has been reported only in allergic individuals and is thought to be due to an enhancement of the nasal cycle where the alternating changes in patency peak at 1.5–6 hours.

The development of a flexible rhinolaryngoscope has made use of this instrument safe. A physician can easily integrate fiberoptic rhinolaryngoscopy into an office practice. Patients with continuous irreversible nasal obstruction or unsatisfactory response to treatment may be candidates for rhinoscopy.

In Chapter XL, Dolan and Selner review specific indications for rhinoscopy and pathology that could be discovered by rhinoscopy. Complications are minimal and consist of syncopy, coughing spasms, and rare, transient, easily controlled epistaxis. In our office, rhinometry and rhinoscopy frequently are used together. The former procedure allows us to determine if there is reversibility of abnormal increased airway resistance after nasal decongestants. Those patients who do not have a significant reversal of NAR need further diagnostic procedures such as rhinoscopy, nasal cytology, and nasal circulation time.

In Chapter XLI, Okuda from the Nippon Medical School, Tokyo, Japan reviews nasal provocation testing. This procedure is mostly employed as a research tool but is progressively being used in certain clinical situations. Okuda has developed a paper disk that can be impregnated with various concentrations of allergens or drugs. It gives semiquantitative results in the form of local visible reactions, rhinomanometry measurements, frequency of sneezing, and an analysis of nasal secretions. Side effects include systemic reactions if the dose of allergen or drug is too high and local nonspecific irritation on the site of the control disk. Dr. Okuda states that this paper disk method of nasal provocation has been widely and safely used in Japan for 25 years. Clinically, this procedure may be useful when allergy skin tests or RAST are equivocal and when there is a need to establish the clinical relevance of an allergen or the efficacy of a topical medication in a particular problem patient.

In Chapter XLII, Deitmer and Phadhana-Anek from Germany describe *in vitro* tests for counting ciliary beats. Their samples are obtained by cytologic brush biopsy of the respiratory epithelium and by using a microphotometric apparatus for counting purposes. This *in vitro* procedure is mostly used for research purposes. Practically, cilia beats are measured through nasal circulation time using saccharine. In this procedure, a few grains of saccharine are placed on the middle one-third of the inferior turbinate by means of a small round wooden applicator that has been moistened in water and dipped into powdered saccharine. The patient is told to sit upright without head movement and to breath through the mouth. It normally takes the nasal cilia about 20 minutes (average about 5–7 minutes) to push the saccharine particles posteriorly until it reaches the base of the tongue. The end point is a sudden sweet taste. The distance transversed is about 60 mm in adults, shorter in children. Each ciliated cell has about 12 to 20 cilia that beat several hundred times per minute. The beat is a quick and forceful forward stroke followed by a slower recovery stroke. These cilia propel a film of mucus made up of two layers: an outer viscous layer and an inner thin layer. Foreign inhaled particles that escape through nasal hairs (vibrissae) adhere to the mucous film by impaction or by electrostatic surface change. In the front part of the nose there are few cilia and mucous movement is slow.

Cilia physiology is easily impaired leading to mucus retention and impaction. Hypotonic saline solutions inhibit ciliary motion and hypertonic solutions as well as a pH of 6.4 or less will stop ciliary motion altogether. Adrenaline and cocaine will ultimately cause irreversible inhibition, but ephedrine has little effect on ciliary motion. Pollutants, such as sulfur dioxide and formaldehyde, and viral infections also inhibit ciliary clearance. Mucociliary clearance is inhibited or absent in patients with dyskinetic cilia syndrome such as Kartagener's syndrome.

In summary, it is apparent that the nose not only represents an extension of the lower respiratory tract but also may be a reflection of pathogenic processes occurring in other parts of the body. Although a great deal of aberrant findings are limited to the nasal pharyngeal area, the nose is analogous to the tip of an iceberg alerting a careful and astute physician to possibilities of systemic diseases that lie in incipient stages presenting with insidious symptoms.

REFERENCES

1. Hagy GW, Settipane GA. Bronchial asthma, allergic rhinitis and allergy skin tests among college students. J Allergy 44:323–332, 1969.
2. Hagy GW, Settipane GA. Prognosis of positive allergy skin tests in an asymptomatic population. J Allergy Clin Immunol 48:200–211, 1971.
3. Hagy GW, Settipane GA. Risk factors for developing asthma and allergic rhinitis: a 7-year follow-up of college students. J Allergy Clin Immunol 58:330–336, 1976.
4. Rackemann FM. The natural history of hay fever and asthma. N Engl J Med 268:415–419, 1963.
5. Buffum WP, Settipane GA. Prognosis of asthma in childhood. Am J Dis Child 112:214–217, 1966.
6. Van Arsdel PP Jr, Motulsky AG. Frequency and hereditability of asthma and allergic rhinitis in college students. Acta Genet 9:101–114, 1959.
7. Maternowski CJ, Mathews KP. The prevalence of ragweed pollinosis in foreign and native students at a midwestern university and its implications concerning methods for determining the inheritance of atopy. J Allergy 33:130–140, 1962.
8. Braman SS, Barrows AA, DeCotiis BA, Settipane GA, Corrao WM. Airway hyperresponsiveness in allergic rhinitis: a risk factor for asthma. Chest 91:671–674, 1987.
9. Mygind N. Mediators of nasal allergy. J Allergy Clin Immunol 70:149–159, 1982.
10. Brooks CD, Butler D, Metzler C. Effect of H_2 blockade in the challenged allergic nose. J Allergy Clin Immunol 70:373–376, 1982.
11. Kaufman J, Wright GW. The effect of nasal and nasopharyngeal irritation on airway resistance in man. Am Rev Resp Dis 100:626–630, 1969.
12. Ogura JH, Nelson JR, Dammkoehler R, Kawasaki M, Togawa K. Experimental observations of the relationships between upper airway obstruction and pulmonary function. Ann Oto Rhinol Laryngol 73:381–403, 1964.
13. Slavin RG. Relationship of nasal disease and sinusitis to bronchial asthma. Ann Allergy 49:76–80, 1982.
14. Slavin RG, Linford PA, Friedman WH. Sphenoethmoidectomy (SE) in the treatment of nasal polyps, sinusitis and bronchial asthma. J Allergy Clin Immunol 71:(Part 2) 156, 1983 (abst).
15. Friedman R, Ackerman M, Wald E, Friday G, Reilly J, Casselbrant M, Fireman P. Bacterial sinusitis exacerbating asthma. J Allergy Clin Immunol 71:(part 2) 155, 1983 (abst).
16. Rachelefsky G, Siegel S, Katz R. Chronic sinus disease with associated induced reactive airways disease in children. J Allergy Clin Immunol 71:(Part 2) 156, 1983 (abst).
17. Cooke RA (ed). Allergy in theory and practice. Philadelphia and London: W. B. Saunders Co, 1947.
18. Littell NT, Carlisle CC, Millman RP, Braman SS. Changes in airway resistance following nasal provocation. Am Rev Resp Dis 141:580–583, 1990.
19. Hagy GW, Settipane GA. Unpublished data, United States Public Health Service Grant A102632.
20. Salvaggio JE, Cavanaugh HHA, Lowell FC, Leskowtiz S. A comparison of the immunologic responses of normal and atopic individuals to intranasally administered antigen. J Allergy 35:62–69, 1964.
21. Salvaggio JE, Kayman H, Leskowtiz S. Immunologic responses of atopic and normal individuals to aerosolized dextran. J Allergy 38:31–40, 1966.
22. Kontou-Karakitsos K, Salvaggio JE, Mathews KP. Comparative nasal absorption of allergens in atopic and nonatopic subjects. J Allergy Clin Immunol 55:241–248, 1975.
23. Schwartz HJ, Leskowitz S, Lowell FC. Studies on "intrinsic" allergic respiratory disease with an hypothesis concerning its pathogenesis. J Allergy Clin Immunol 42:169–175, 1968.
24. Taylor B, Norman AP, Orgel HA et al. Transient IgA deficiency and pathogenesis of infantile atopy. Lancet 2:111–113, 1973.
25. Orgel HA, Hamburger RN, Bazaral M et al. Development of IgE and allergy in infancy. J Allergy Clin Immunol 56:296–307, 1975.
26. Settipane RJ, Hagy GW. Effect of atmospheric pollen on the newborn. R I Med J 62:477–482, 1979.
27. Bjorksten F, Suoniemi I. Dependence of immediate hypersensitivity on month of birth. Clin Allergy 6:165–171, 1976.
28. Pearson DJ, Freed DL, Taylor G. Respiratory allergy and month of birth. Clin Allergy 7:29–33, 1977.
29. Smith JK, Springett VH. Atopic disease and month of birth. Clin Allergy 9:153–157, 1979.
30. Connell JT. Quantitiative intranasal pollen challenges III. The priming effect in allergic rhinitis. J Allergy 43:33–44, 1969.
31. Jackson PG et al. Intestinal permeability in patients with eczema and food allergy. Lancet 1:1285–1286, 1981.
32. Block KJ, Kleinman R, Walker WA. Effects of local intestinal anaphylaxis on antigen uptake. Abstracts of papers presented at the 37th Annual Meeting of the American Academy of Allergy, March 7–11, 1981.
33. Settipane GA, Newstead GK, Boyd GK. Frequency of Hymenoptera allergy in an atopic and normal population. J Allergy Clin Immunol 50:146–150, 1972.
34. Stember RJ, Levine BB. Prevalence of allergic diseases, penicillin hypersensitivity and aeroallergen hypersensitivity in various populations. J Allergy Clin Immunol 51:100, 1973 (abst).
35. Kaliner M. Mast cell mediators and prostaglandin formation in human lung tissues. N Engl Soc Allergy Proc 3:239–240, 1982.
36. Jones RT, Nelson DR, Schwartz LB, Holley KE, Squillace DL, Sturner WQ, Sweeney KG, Yunginger JW. Elevated mast cell-derived tryptase levels in post-mortem sera from victims of fatal anaphylaxis. J Allergy Clin Immunol 85:154, 1990 (abstr).
37. Yan K, Salome C. The response of the airways to nasal stimulation in asthmatics with rhinitis. Eur J Respir Dis 64:105–108, 1983.
38. Settipane GA. Nasal polyps: Epidemiology, pathology, immunology and treatment. Am J Rhinol 1:119–126, 1987.
39. Connell JT, Settipane GA. Drowsiness associated with antihistamine therapy. J Allergy Clin Immunol 73:137, 1984 (abst).
40. Settipane GA, Klein DE. Nonallergic rhinitis: Demography of eosinophils in nasal smear, blood total eosinophil counts and IgE levels. New Engl Reg Allergy Proc 6:363–366, 1985.
41. Ohki M, Hasegawa M, Sakuma A. Exercise-induced nasal obstruction in patients with allergic rhinitis. Am J Rhinol 3:1–4, 1989.
42. Hasegawa M, Kabasawa Y, Ohkl M, Watanabe I. Exercise-induced change of nasal resistance in asthmatic children. Otolaryngol-Head and Neck Surg 93:772–776, 1985.

BASIC SCIENCE

Chapter II

Mediators of Anaphylaxis, Anaphylactoid Reactions, and Rhinitis

Kenneth P. Mathews, M.D.

ABSTRACT

Besides histamine, a large and increasing number of mediators of allergic reactions are being found to be released by mast cells or basophils during anaphylactic reactions. Many of these same substances are released by stimuli other than allergen-IgE interactions, and this type of phenomenon (anaphylactoid or pseudo-allergic reaction) may account for some nasal symptoms that simulate allergy. In addition to rapidly developing reactions of these types, numerous recent investigations have emphasized the importance of late-phase reactions that occur as a consequence of the immediate reactivity. Besides mast cells and/or basophils, these late effects seem to involve a complex network of cellular interactions, which may include neutrophils, eosinophils, lymphocytes, macrophages, and platelets.

Studies of nasal washings following allergen challenges in humans have provided cogent in vivo support of earlier hypotheses about mediator release based on in vitro experimentation.

Anaphylaxis usually results from the interaction of antigens with antibodies, generally IgE, residing on mast cells or basophils and the subsequent release of various biologically active materials. The term most often is applied clinically to instances of systemic symp-

toms, often of severe degree, but the same processes frequently result in only local manifestations. It is in this broader context that this brief discussion will consider IgE-dependent reactivity of both systemic and local types with emphasis on recent information and human rhinitis. More comprehensive reviews of the mediators of immediate hypersensitivity and factors affecting their release have been provided elsewhere.[1, 2]

Seasonal allergic rhinitis (hay fever) might be regarded as an example *par excellence* of IgE-mediated disease. Nevertheless, until recently there was a paucity of information directly relating to the mediators released by sensitized human nasal tissue upon exposure to allergens. In addition, there is the possibility that secretion of these mediators might be induced by initiating events other than allergen-IgE interactions. When this occurs in other tissues or results in systemic symptoms, such phenomena often are referred to as "anaphylactoid" or "pseudo-allergic" reactions. Recent evidence indicates such phenomena also may occur in the nose.

The list of potential mediators of allergic reactions has expanded very rapidly in the last few years, and it is likely that more will be added. There has not as yet been time to assess the relative importance of all these various mediators in causing allergic inflammation in different tissues, such as the nose versus the lung or skin. Since allergens are known to react with IgE antibodies on the surface of the mast cells or basophils, the focus of attention has been on mediators liberated from these cells. However, it is clear that some of these

Adjunct Member, Scripps Clinic and Research Foundation, La Jolla, CA, and Professor Emeritus of Internal Medicine, University of Michigan, Ann Arbor, MI

mediators are liberated by other types of cells. The situation is further complicated by the fact that some mast cell products can secondarily induce the generation of additional biologically active materials. Another important development is the realization that in many tissues IgE-allergen initiated reactions can lead to late inflammatory responses as well as to immediate reactions. Amid these complexities a definitive assessment of the role of various mediators in producing nasal disease must await further studies, but briefly reviewing the substantial progress in this field does provide a good measure of insight into the mechanisms likely to be operative.

As reviewed more extensively elsewhere,[3] there is cogent evidence that the induction of liberation of mediators by mast cells or basophils in a variety of tissues and species requires the cross-linking or bridging of two or more IgE molecules at the cell membrane with one molecule of antigen or other ligand. More recent studies have indicated that the critical event is the aggregation of IgE receptor molecules, which occurs secondarily to the cross-linking of IgE. Consequently there is activation of several membrane-associated enzymes including (1) serine protease(s), which are inhibited by agents such as diisopropylfluorophosphate or trypsin and chymotrypsin substrates; (2) two methyl transferases, which convert phosphatidylethanolamine to phosphatidylcholine; (3) phospholipases, which can cleave arachidonic acid (see below) and inositol triphosphate from membrane phospholipids; and (4) adenylate cyclase, which generates cAMP from ATP. Products of these enzymatic cleavages play important roles in the subsequent steps leading to mediator release; e.g., inositol triphosphate mobilizes intracellular calcium, which is required for several of these processes, and di- and monoacylglycerol activate protein kinase C and enhance fusion of granule and cytoplasmic membranes. Another important participant in these processes is calmodulin, a calcium-binding protein that plays an essential role in the activation of adenylate cyclase, phospholipase A_2 and cAMP phosphodiesterase as well as regulating microtubule assembly.[2] Conversely, lipocortin (lipomodulin or macrocortin) plays an important role as a phospholipase A_2 inhibitor, and part of the effect of glucocorticosteroids can be attributed to its capacity to stimulate lipocortin production.

The activation of mast cells and basophils is modulated by intracellular cyclic nucleotides via protein kinase activation. In contrast to some endocrine organs, elevated cAMP leads to decreased secretion of histamine and other mediators whereas in some tissues elevated cGMP leads to increased mediator secretion. Accordingly, the many agents that affect cyclic nucleotide levels have a predictable effect on mediator release; i.e., cAMP levels increase and mediator release decreases after *in vitro* or *in vivo* exposure to theophylline or agents that stimulate adenylate cyclase to enhance cAMP production from ATP, such as β-adrenergic compounds and prostaglandins of the E series. α-Adrenergic stimuli, however, tend to produce decreased cAMP levels. Conversely, in some tissues stimulation of mediator release occurs through the enhanced production of cGMP from GTP by guanylate cyclase activation by acetylcholine or by prostaglandin $F_{2\alpha}$.

It is evident from these observations that the autonomic nervous system can directly or indirectly influence mediator release in addition to its effects on peripheral tissues involved in allergic reactions. Studies of mono- and dizygotic twins indicate there also is a genetic factor controlling the releasability of histamine from basophils that is independent of the surface density of IgE.[4] In addition, enhanced histamine-releasing activity secreted by mononuclear cells has been reported to occur in asthmatic patients.[5] Interferon also can enhance histamine release.[6]

The secretory phase of mediator release from mast cells or basophils requires energy, which is derived largely from glycolytic sources, as well as Ca ions. It is increased by deuterium oxide and is inhibited by colchicine, which prevents microtubule aggregation. As shown in Figure 1, the final step is the fusion of granule membranes with the cell membranes, thus exteriorizing the granule contents. Readily soluble contents of the latter diffuse rapidly, while the granule matrix remains associated with the cell for a time.

THE MEDIATORS

Table I lists some of the potential mediators of allergic reactions of anaphylactic, atopic, or anaphylactoid types. Although thought of by allergists as mast cell- or basophil-derived products, some of these agents also are released by other cells. There also are some differences between mast cells and basophil mediator-releasing activities; e.g., prostaglandin D_2 is released by mast cells but not basophils, corticosteroids suppress histamine release only from basophils (after prolonged incubation), mast cells lack the H_2-histamine receptor present on basophils, and adenosine has opposite effects on mediator release from these two types of cells.

HISTAMINE

Secreted histamine may exert its physiologic effects either locally or occasionally at distant sites. These actions include stimulation of smooth muscle contraction and increased permeability of venules with subsequent edema formation. Such effects can account for many symptoms of atopic disease, including allergic rhinitis. Additionally, histamine can produce reflex bronchoconstriction through afferent and efferent vagal impulses and initiate cutaneous flare reactions via axon

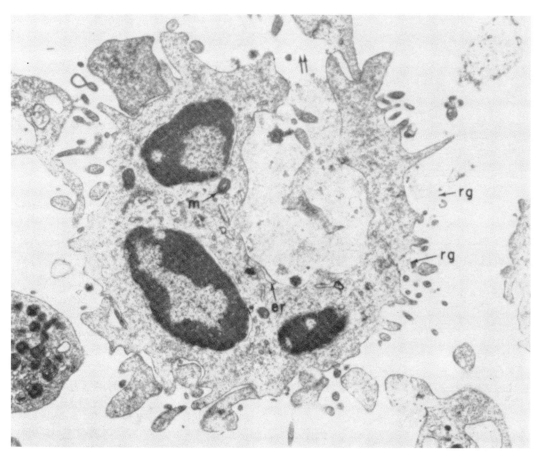

Figure 1. *Degranulated human basophil after incubation with rye grass group I antigen. Note the irregular cell surface to which projections platelets or other leukocytes are adherent. No basophilic granules can be seen, but a large membrane-bound cavity is evident, which contains residual granular material and communicates widely with the exterior (double arrows). Two smaller masses of residual granular material can be seen at the cell surface (rg). Several cisternae of smooth endoplasmic reticulum (er) are seen near the exocytotic cavity. (Reprinted with permission from Hastie R, Levy DA, Weill L. The antigen-induced degranulation of basophil leucocytes from atopic subjects studied by electron microscopy. Lab Invest 36:173, 1977.)*

reflexes. The delineation of H_1- and H_2-receptors in various tissues[7] has led to a renaissance of interest in histamine that is too extensive for review here. The most relevant aspects of this information are the observations that in addition to H_1-receptors on smooth muscle cells, vascular endothelium, and respiratory mucosae, through H_2-receptors histamine can stimulate mucus secretion (as well as gastric acid secretion) and cAMP formation. It also inhibits basophil histamine release, lymphokine release, neutrophil enzyme release, eosinophil migration, and T-lymphocyte mediated cytotoxicity. The presence of H_2- as well as H_1-receptors in vascular tissues implies that the former may play a role in the vasodilation, hypotension, flushing, headache, and cardiac effects produced by histamine in some patients during anaphylaxis. Based on the effects of histamine on nasal airway resistance, there is evidence for the presence of H_2-receptors in the nasal vasculature;

clinically, however, the addition of an oral H_2 antagonist to H_1 antihistamines has only a small effect on the nasal congestion associated with hay fever.[8] In addition to its direct action, histamine also produces indirect reflex effects on the nasal mucosa.[9]

EOSINOPHIL CHEMOTACTIC FACTORS OF ANAPHYLAXIS

Many substances are chemotactic for eosinophils including agents derived from the complement system, arachidonic acid, lymphocytes, neutrophils, tumors, infectious agents, and histamine. Stimulated mast cells secrete two low molecular weight peptides that are chemotactic for eosinophils:[10] Val-Gly-Ser-Glu or Ala-Gly-Ser-Glu. Possibly these tetrapeptides may account, at least in part, for the presence of eosinophils seen in the nasal secretions of hay fever patients.

TABLE I

Mast Cell- or Basophil-Derived Mediators of Anaphylactic, Atopic, and Anaphylactoid Reactions

Preformed, rapidly released mediators
  Histamine
  High molecular weight neutrophil chemotactic factor
  Eosinophil chemotactic factors of anaphylaxis
  Kininogenase(s)
  Prekallikrein activator
  Hageman factor "activator"
  Arylsulfatase A
  Serotonin*
  Exoglycosidases (β-hexoseaminidase, β-glucuronidase,* β-galactosidase)
  Lymphocyte chemotactic factors*
  Eosinophil chemotactic factor oligopeptides
Granule matrix-associated materials
  Heparin or other proteoglycans
  Tryptase and chymotryptic proteases
  Arylsulfatase B
  Inflammatory factors of anaphylaxis*
  Peroxidase*
  Superoxide dismutase*
Newly generated or secondary agents
  Arachidonic acid derivatives
    Leukotrienes C_4, D_4, and E_4 (slow reacting substance of anaphylaxis)
    Hydroperoxyeicosatetraenoic acids
    Hydroxyeicosatetraenoic acids
    Prostaglandins
    Thromboxanes
  Platelet-activating factor
    Superoxide, H_2O_2, free hydroxyl radicals, singlet oxygen, and activated halides
  Adenosine
  Bradykinin
  Prostaglandin-generating factor of anaphylaxis

Documented in species other than humans.

KININOGENASE, PREKALLIKREIN ACTIVATOR, AND HAGEMAN FACTOR ACTIVATOR

In addition to the kallikreins found in glandular secretions and plasma, it has been shown that stimulated mast cells and basophils secrete an enzyme with kininogenase activity that acts on low molecular weight kininogen. Other enzymes in sensitized lung tissue can activate prekallikrein[11] or cleave Hageman factor. These are important observations in that they provide mechanisms whereby the kinin system can secondarily become activated in anaphylactic reaction. The gener-

ation of kinins in nasal secretions is discussed in Chapter III.

LEUKOTRIENES C_4, D_4, AND E_4 (SLOW-REACTING SUBSTANCE OF ANAPHYLAXIS), HYDROPEROXYEICOSATETRAENOIC ACIDS, AND HYDROXYEICOSATETRAENOIC ACIDS

More than 40 years ago it was recognized that certain snake venoms generated material that produced a slow, sustained contraction of smooth muscle in a variety of species. Later it was found that supernatants of tissues from sensitized animals exposed to antigen *in vitro* or *in vivo* contained a similar activity referred to as slow-reacting substance of anaphylaxis (SRS-A). Clinical interest in this material was heightened by the observations that it was very potent in causing contraction of human bronchiolar smooth muscle and that it was released in relatively large quantity when appropriate allergens were added to chopped lung tissue from asthmatic patients specifically sensitive to those allergens. For many years it was apparent that it was a low molecular weight lipid-like substance, and it finally was characterized as arachidonic acid metabolites. After arachidonic acid is cleaved by phospholipase A_2 or diacyl glycerol lipase from membrane phospholipids, it is metabolized by cyclooxygenase to prostaglandins and thromboxanes (see below) or by the lipoxygenase pathway to hydroperoxyeicosatetraenoic acids (HPETEs) and monohydroxyeicosatetraenoic acids (HETEs) (Figure 2). The 5-HPETE and 5-HETE compounds can augment histamine release from basophils while 15-HPETE inhibits the synthesis of prostaglandin (PG) I_2, which is a potent vasodilator. The 5-HPETE alternatively can be converted into leukotriene (LT) A_4, and the addition of glutathione to the latter generates LTC_4. Cleavage of the glutamyl group then yields LTD_4, and removal of glycine gives LTE_4. LTC_4, LTD_4, and LTE_4 produce the SRS-A activities, which include alteration of vascular permeability and stimulation of mucus secretion in addition to its very potent capacity to constrict smooth muscle (particularly in small airways). The LTs can be derived from basophils and mast cells, but they also are produced by many other cells, particularly macrophages. In some cells 5-lipoxygenase predominantly generates LTB_4, which provides a very potent inflammatory stimulus, and subsequent to 15-lipoxygenase activity there may be generation of lipoxins, which can produce contraction of bronchial smooth muscle as well as protein kinase C activation and inhibition of human IVK cell activity.[12] Leukotriene release by allergen challenge of sensitized nasal tissue is discussed in Chapter III. The very large literature on the biology of the leukotrienes recently has been reviewed including their central nervous system,

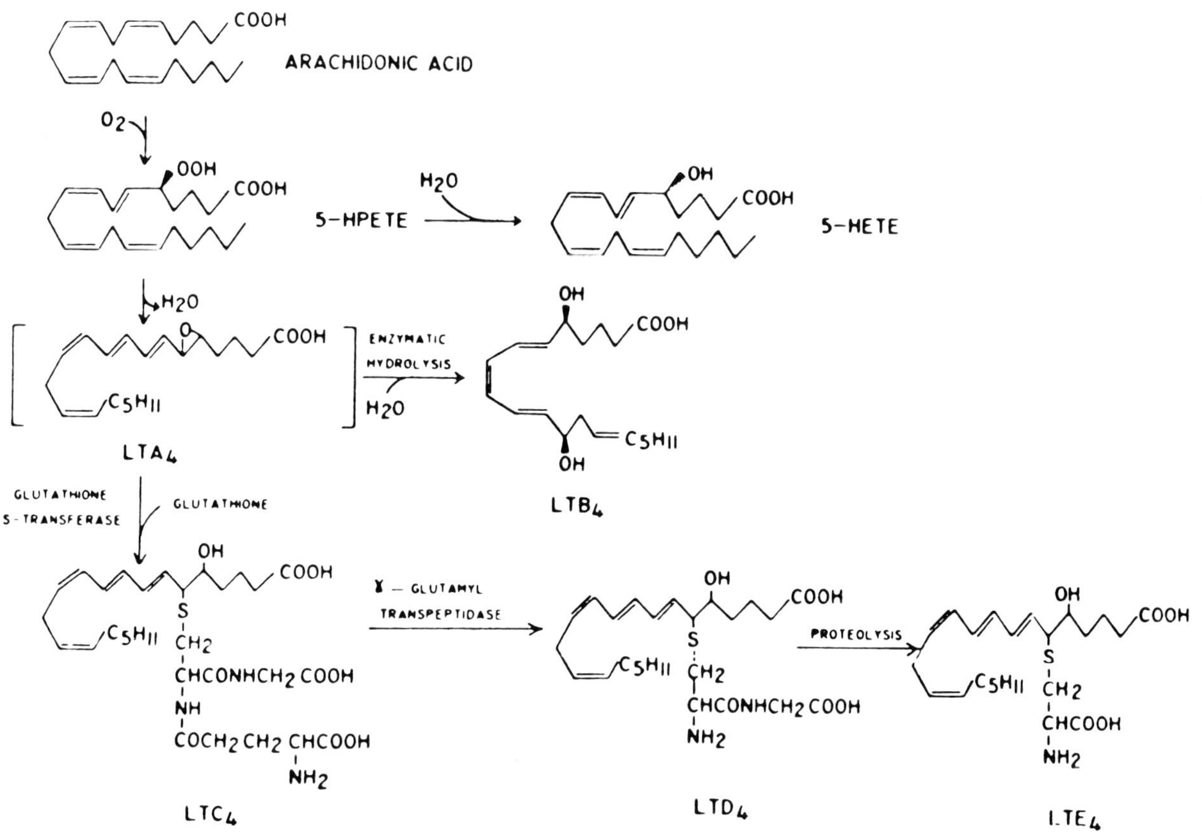

Figure 2. Metabolism of arachidonic acid via the lipoxygenase pathway. (Reprinted with permission from Burka JF. The products of the lipoxygenase pathway of arachidonic acid metabolism. NER Allergy Proc 2:62, 1981.)

cardiovascular and immunologic effects, their receptors, and the development of antagonists.[13]

PROSTAGLANDINS, THROMBOXANES, AND PROSTAGLANDIN-GENERATING FACTOR OF ANAPHYLAXIS

By way of the cyclooxygenase pathway a variety of other arachidonic acid metabolites may be found in supernatant fluids derived from sensitized tissues challenged by allergens. Prostaglandins may be derived from mononuclear cells, eosinophils, platelets, endothelial cells, or epithelial cells, but PGD_2 is especially likely to be derived from mast cells, its metabolites being prominent in the urine of patients with mastocytosis.[14] It is a potent vasodilator and constrictor of bronchial smooth muscle as well as causing mucus secretion. Among the other cyclooxygenase metabolites, $PGF_{2\alpha}$, PGG_2, and thromboxane A_2 are bronchoconstrictors, primarily in the periphery, while PGE_2 and PGI_2 are bronchial dilators; $PGF_{2\alpha}$, PGI_2, PGE, and PGA_2 stimulate mucus secretion, and PGE can cause mucosal edema. Besides these direct effects on peripheral tissues, as noted above PGE and $PGF_{2\alpha}$ potentially can moderate mediator release via their effects on cytoplasmic cyclic nucleotide levels. In ad-

dition, there is evidence that mast cells secrete a 1,450-dalton prostaglandin-generating factor that can induce surrounding tissues to generate prostaglandins secondarily.[15] Histamine itself can stimulate prostaglandin synthesis in some tissues, whereas aspirin and other nonsteroidal anti-inflammatory drugs impair prostaglandin synthesis through cyclooxygenase inhibition. Prostaglandin release from nasal tissue following allergen challenge is described in Chapter III.

PLATELET-ACTIVATING FACTOR

In rabbits, histamine is present in platelets rather than in basophils, and immunologists studying anaphylactic reactions in this species accordingly have been very interested in the platelet activating factor secreted by rabbit basophils, thereby stimulating platelets to secrete histamine and other biologically active materials. As in the case of SRS-A, interest in platelet-activating factor (PAF) in humans has been greatly stimulated by its chemical characterization as 1-o-alkyl-2-acetyl-sn-glycero-3-phosphorylcholine (PAF-acether). It may be derived from neutrophils, eosinophils, monocytes, macrophages, mast cells, basophils, platelets, fibroblasts, bacteria, and stimulated endothelial cells and can be carried piggyback on serum lipoproteins.[16]

Some effects of PAF may result secondarily from the stimulation of platelets to secrete their α-granule contents including serotonin, platelet factor 4, and perhaps β-thromboglobulin, PF4 being a mediator releaser. PAF also has many other potent, direct biologic effects. These include smooth muscle contraction, mucosal edema, histamine release, stimulation of neutrophil aggregation, chemotaxis, lysosomal enzyme release and superoxide formation, eosinophil chemotaxis and activation, decreased CD2 and CD3 antigen expression on human T cells, and modulation of c-fos and c-myc gene in human monocytes.[16] *In vivo* effects include hypotension, a negative cardiac inotropic effect, decreased coronary flow, and arrhythmias. Some of its *in vivo* effects arise secondarily from activation of eosinophils, platelets, or neutrophils. Of particular relevance to allergic rhinitis is the observation that PAF and more prominently lyso-PAF are released into nasal secretion following allergen challenge.[17] PAF itself is reported to produce dual response in human skin[18] but not in the bronchi,[19] and a PAF antagonist can inhibit late allergen-induced bronchial responses in experimental animals.[20] For obvious reasons much effort is being expended on the development of PAF inhibitors.[21]

NEUTROPHIL CHEMOTACTIC FACTOR

This material has been identified in plasma of patients with cold, solar, or cholinergic urticaria or in asthmatics following allergen or exercise challenge.[22] It is of higher molecular weight than most of the other substances that are chemotactic for neutrophils and may provide one explanation for the presence of neutrophils late in the course of allergic inflammatory reaction initiated by IgE-mediated mechanisms (see below).

EOSINOPHIL CHEMOTACTIC FACTOR OLIGOPEPTIDES

In addition to the very low molecular weight eosinophil chemotactic factor substances mentioned above, anaphylactic-type reactions can be accompanied by the liberation of chemotactic factors with a molecular weight in the range of 1,500–3,000 daltons.[1]

SUPEROXIDE AND OTHER REACTIVE OXYGEN SPECIES

The generation of superoxide, free hydroxyl radicals, H_2O_2, activated halides, and singlet oxygen has been widely studied in activated neutrophils,[23] and there is evidence that these toxic substances also are generated by stimulated mast cells. These could contribute to allergic inflammation and damage epithelial surfaces.

HEPARIN AND OTHER PROTEOGLYCANS

The staining properties of mast cells and basophil granules are substantially due to their significant content of these materials. Heparin is the predominant proteoglycan in connective tissue mast cells; chondroitin 4- and 6-sulfates are predominant in basophils. These substances tend to remain with the granule matrix following cell degranulation. Heparin has been thought to produce some manifestations of anaphylaxis in dogs, but its role in human immediate hypersensitivity is uncertain. It potentially can activate the contact system and can interact with the complement system in several ways. It binds tryptase, histamine, and platelet factor 4.

TRYPTASE, CHYMOTRYPTIC PROTEASE, AND ARYLSULFATASES A AND B

These enzymes would be expected to be additional factors contributing to allergic inflammation. Some of these enzymes, like heparin, remain associated with the granule matrix and stay in the vicinity of the cell for a period.[24] Tryptase comprises up to 40% of the total granular protein of mast cells. Of particular relevance is its capacity to generate anaphylatoxins and to cleave high molecular weight kininogen into inactive fragments. Of practical interest is the fact that following human anaphylaxis plasma tryptase levels may remain elevated for several hours[25] in contrast to the fleeting elevations of plasma histamine.

INFLAMMATORY FACTORS OF ANAPHYLAXIS AND LYMPHOCYTE CHEMOTACTIC FACTORS

As discussed below, the great importance of late-phase allergic reactions has been recognized only relatively recently. In some species these may be attributed in part to a 1,400-dalton peptide referred to as inflammatory factor of anaphylaxis.[26] Activated rat mast cells also release three types of chemotactic factors for various populations of lymphocytes,[27] but further study is needed regarding such factors in humans. Kallikrein and plasminogen activator also have been reported to be chemotactic for mononuclear cells.[28]

ADENOSINE

As reviewed elsewhere,[29] the role of adenosine is complex, being both an inhibitor or activator of mediator release or a product thereof under various conditions.

KININS

Besides the previously mentioned kinogenase activity derived from mast cells or basophils, the kinin system potentially could become activated when histamine or other vascular permeability enhancing factors permit the egress of kininogen into the airways or extravascular compartment where cleavage of kinins by kallikrein may occur (see Chapter III regarding kinin generation in the nasal airways after allergen challenge).

20

Among its several *in vivo* biologic effects in humans, bradykinin produces bronchoconstriction,[30] nasal obstruction,[31] rhinorrhea, and cutaneous edema. It also is reported to release histamine and arachidonate from murine mast cells.[32] Kallikrein has the further potential of activating plasminogen and affecting the coagulation system through cleavage of Hageman factor (XII) with subsequent activation of factor XI.

INHIBITORS OF MEDIATORS OR THEIR RELEASE

Maintenance of homeostasis requires that there must be counterbalancing checks on mediators or their release to terminate allergic reactions that otherwise might become very destructive to the host. Some of these protective mechanisms are as follows.

1. Eosinophils, which are attracted into areas of allergic inflammation by mechanisms mentioned above, may be protective in that they contain histaminase (diamine oxidase), they can inhibit histamine release through the action of PGE_2, and their Charcot-Lyden crystal protein is a lysophospholipase that potentially could inactivate lysophospholipids generated by phospholipase A_2. On the other hand, earlier suggestions of inactivation of leukotrienes and PAF have not been confirmed, and indeed there is cogent evidence that, in general, eosinophils contribute to allergic inflammation as discussed below.

2. Agents that activate adenylate cyclase inhibit mediator release (see above).

3. Serum albumin and adenosine can inhibit histamine release under some conditions.

4. A potent PAF inactivator (acetyl hydrolase) is present in normal human plasma.

5. The major proteolytic enzyme inhibitors will tend to protect against this type of secreted enzyme: α_1-protease inhibitor, α_1-antichymotrypsin, α_2-macroglobulin, inter-α inhibitor and antithrombin III.

6. C1 inhibitor would tend to protect against activated kallikrein (as well as against activated C1, plasmin and XIa, the latter two to a lesser extent).

7. Serum carboxypeptidase N would protect against secondarily generated anaphylatoxins and perhaps kinins.

8. α_2-Antiplasmin would inhibit plasmin.

9. Superoxide dismutase protects against superoxide effect.

OTHER POTENTIAL INITIATORS OF MAST CELL AND BASOPHIL SECRETION

In addition to stimulation of mast cells or basophils by IgE-dependent mechanisms (e.g., by allergen or anti-IgE), there are several other clinical and experimental circumstances under which the same mediators are liberated. As mentioned previously, these reactions may simulate anaphylaxis and therefore are referred to as "anaphylactoid" or "pseudo-allergic" reactions. It is tempting to speculate that in a number of clinical conditions where no allergen can be found as the cause for apparently allergic reactions, this mechanism could be operative. This includes rhinitis as well as bronchial and cutaneous conditions. Experimentally, it is clear that the following can stimulate mast cell or basophil secretion under suitable conditions.

1. *Anaphylatoxins (C5a, C3a, and C4a).* The capacity of these active materials to produce anaphylactoid reactions has been documented *in vitro* and *in vivo* in both man and experimental animals. This observation provides an important link between the complement and mast cell-dependent systems.

2. *Calcium ionophores.*

3. *Concanavalin A and other lectins.*

4. *Anti-IgG and anti-light chain sera.*

5. *Protein A.*

6. *Formylmethionyl peptides.*

7. *Compound 40/80, morphine, codeine, meperidine, polymyxin antibiotics, thiamine, d-tubocuraine, stilbamidine, muscle depolizers, dextran, and other histamine-releasing drugs.* Pharmacologists have known for decades that a large number of drugs, including those just mentioned, release histamine from perfused animal tissues.[33] This occurs with the first exposure to the compound, and in general there is no good reason to believe that immune mechanisms are involved. However, this matter has not been studied sufficiently to determine why some patients experience reactions to these drugs at dosage levels well tolerated by others. Tissue mast cell content may be one relevant factor, since patients with mastocytosis are prone to anaphytoid reactions from these types of drugs.

8. *Neuropeptides.* Substance P is involved in the flare phenomenon in wheal-and-flare skin reactions. It is liberated from cutaneous neural tissue in the course of the axon reflex initiated by the reaction to the allergen and produces a further histamine release in the surrounding area. Substance P also is liberated from guinea pig tracheobronchial nerve endings and appears to mediate the bronchospasm induced by vagal stimulation either by a direct effect on bronchial smooth muscle, by releasing mediators from lung mast cells or macrophages, or by enhancing the response to other mediators.[32] In addition to substance P, neurotensin, dymorphin, and β-endorphin also produce human cutaneous mast cell degranulation, and somatostatin and vasoactive intestinal peptide can produce wheal-and-flare reactions by stimulating substance P release from nerve endings.[34] The propensity of various narcotic drugs, noted above, to produce histamine release may well be related to the capacity of endorphins to produce this same effect.

9. *Radiographic contrast media.* Ionic media in sufficiently high concentrations may cause histamine re-

lease *in vitro* and *in vivo*; the *in vitro* effect is enhanced in the presence of complement. However, histamine release occurs in nonreactors to radiographic contrast media as well as reactors.

10. *Eosinophil-derived substances.* The four principal proteins derived from eosinophil granules are the major basic protein (MBP), eosinophil peroxidase (EPO), the eosinophil cationic protein (ECP), and the eosinophil-derived neurotoxin (EDN). MBP also is found, in much smaller amounts, in basophils. MBP can produce non-cytolytic histamine release from human basophils and rat mast cells at concentrations comparable to those present in body fluids of patients with eosinophilia. EPO binds to mast cells and in combination with H_2O_2, and halide can induce mast cell degranulation and histamine release. ECP can enhance the activation of factor XII, kallikrein, and plasminogen. A major function of eosinophils has been to damage helminth parasites, a process involving ECP, MBP, and EPO. Unfortunately, however, eosinophils in allergic inflammatory reactions may cause tissue injury, e.g., MBP in concentrations occurring pathophysiologically *in vivo* can impair ciliary function and cause exfoliation of respiratory epithelial cells. Eosinophils' prominent LT production also could result in bronchospasm, edema, and mucus secretion. Eosinophil degranulation is enhanced by IL-5 and partly downregulated by IF-γ-effects that are similar to the actions of these cytokines on eosinophil differentiation and proliferation.[35] There also is a monokine that specifically enhances human eosinophil cytotoxicity.[36] The presence of low affinity receptors for IgE on eosinophils further implicates a role in allergic inflammation. The extensive literature on eosinophils has been reviewed elsewhere.[37]

11. *Histamine-releasing activity (HRA) derived from lymphocytes, neutrophils, eosinophils, macrophages, and platelets.* Several laboratories have confirmed the important observation of Thueson et al.[38] that there is a lymphokine that can produce histamine release. This provides a possible link between anaphylactic phenomena and cell-mediated immunity. One could speculate that it might be relevant to chronic idiopathic urticaria where there is a lymphocytic infiltrate in skin rich in mast cells. As discussed below, HRA is of great interest in connection with late-phase allergic reactions characterized by substantial numbers of polymorphonuclear cells in the afflicted tissues. Secretion of HRA by these cells could produce a positive feedback phenomenon that could provide one explanation for a prolonged course of late-phase reactions. HRA clearly is heterogenous; some types require the presence of a certain type of IgE to release histamine from basophils.[39]

12. *Interleukins and granulocyte-macrophage colony-stimulating factor (GMCSF).* Interleukin 1 has been reported to release histamine from human basophils and mast cells,[40] and GMCSF and IL-3 produce histamine release from human basophils.[41] The IL-3 effect seems to require some level of pre-existing basophil activation such as with D_2O_2 or a specific type of IgE.[42]

13. *Other serum factors.* British investigators recently have reported the presence of a 10–15 kd protein in chronic urticaria patients' serum that produces a wheal-and-flare reaction and a neutrophilic infiltrate at the site of injection into the patient's own skin.[43]

14. *Several other factors including hyperosmolarity, exercise, hypoosmolarity, hypoxia, and perhaps vasoactive peptides arising from the gastrointestinal tract.* The latter possibility is suggested by the capacity of gastrin and pentagastrin to produce cutaneous wheals in some humans.[44] It is intriguing to speculate whether this type of observation could relate to the development of anaphylactoid reactions in some individuals after eating any type of food.

LATE-PHASE ALLERGIC REACTIONS

The immediate hypersensitivity reactions described above usually begin with a few minutes after antigen exposure, peak at 10–20 minutes, and grossly resolve within about one hour. However, there frequently ensues a late-phase reaction having similar features often beginning about two hours after antigen exposure and peaking at about four to eight hours; occasionally it persists for a prolonged period. In contrast to Arthus reactions and delayed hypersensitivity of the tuberculin test type, this phenomenon is a consequence of an initial IgE-dependent reaction or similar reactions leading to the release of mediators from mast cells/basophils.[45] Following the initial mast cell degranulation, late-phase reactions (LPRs) are characterized by a polymorphonuclear leukocyte infiltration after which mononuclear cells become more dominant as the reaction wanes.

For investigative purposes, LPRs can be induced by injecting anti-IgE, mast cell activators (e.g., compound 48/80) or large doses of allergen into human skin, and clinically they are seen as recurrent asthma or rhinitis after spontaneously occurring or induced symptoms. Prior administration of corticosteroid drugs can inhibit LPRs but not immediate reactivity. β-adrenergic agents have the opposite effect, and cromolyn sodium and ketotifen may inhibit both immediate and late-phase reactions.

Besides their importance in producing clinical difficulty per se, the prolonged allergic inflammation associated with LPRs may predispose patients to heightened reactivity upon subsequent exposure to allergens or various irritants. Thus, asthmatic patients may show enhanced bronchial reactivity to histamine or methacholine for a substantial time following allergic reactions, but this is limited to patients who exhibit a late-phase component.[46] Likewise, LPRs may explain in part the "priming" phenomenon in rhinitis patients[47] (i.e., nonspecific increased nasal reactivity to pollen challenges in sensitive patients for several days following an allergic reaction). As noted above, LPRs may result, at least in part, from liberation of histamine-releasing factors and other inflammatory substances from the cells (neutrophils, eosinophil, basophils, and mononuclear cells) accumulating in the inflamed tissue as a consequence of the immediate allergic reaction. The stimulated mast cells or basophils might again liberate a new wave of mediators. There is the possibility that this could be a self-perpetuating phenomenon for a substantial period. The complexity of these cellular networks is emphasized even further by the report that histamine can stimulate endothelial cells to produce a lipid substance that has neutrophil chemoattractant activity.[48] Also, human respiratory tract epithelial cells and eosinophils produce 15-HETE, which enhances murine and canine mast cell leukotriene production and canine tracheal mucus secretion.[32] The large body of information relative to LPCR has been reviewed elsewhere.[49]

MEDIATOR RELEASE IN HUMAN RHINITIS

In spite of the vast amount of *in vitro* and experimental animal data concerning mediators of anaphylaxis that has accrued over more than 20 years and has been very briefly summarized above, its direct relevance to human rhinitis remained an assumption rather than an established fact until relatively recently. Suggestive *in vitro* evidence was provided by the observations that inflammatory mediators are released when specific allergens are added to minced nasal polyps[50] or nasal scrapings.[51] The *in vivo* observation that mast cell degranulation can be observed in nasal biopsies taken before and after nasal challenge with specific allergens supports the assumed role of these cells.[52] Of special importance are the series of reports, largely from investigators at Johns Hopkins University, indicating the release of several mediators of anaphylaxis into nasal washings, after intranasal challenge with various allergens. It may seem surprising that this was not accomplished sooner, but specific methods for detecting minute quantities of some of the mediators have been perfected only relatively recently, and special procedures were developed to obtain satisfactory nasal washings. As described in Chapter III, these methods have provided much information about both the immediate and the late-phase release of mediators from the nasal mucosa following allergen challenge of sensitive humans. Also of major importance is the observation that nasal challenge with cold dry air leads to the presence of histamine, kinins, TAME-esterase, PGD_2, LTC_4, LTD_4, and LTE_4 in the nasal washings only in patients who develop symptoms after such exposures.[53] Thus, this syndrome is appropriately classified as a pseudo-allergic reaction (assuming no cold-related IgE is in-

volved), and this finding raises the intriguing possibility that other types of idiopathic rhinitis also may involve a similar mechanism.

SKIN TESTING

In the everyday clinical evaluations of patients with rhinitis, skin testing provides the most feasible method of gleaning information about whether IgE-initiated mediator release is likely to be playing a role in the patient's disease. The evidence provided is indirect, but, acknowledging its limitations, skin testing has withstood the test of time and promptly provides potentially useful information with minimal equipment. The presumed sequence of events is that the test allergens react with specific IgE antibodies on the surface of cutaneous mast cells thereby stimulating them to secrete various mediators. Among the latter, histamine is likely to be important in producing these immediate skin reactions.

A major problem is that some patients give positive skin test reactions to allergens that are not responsible for their current symptoms. Sometimes these reflect past clinical allergies (e.g., to egg) or potential future difficulties. Lack of exposure to reactive test allergens or the use of irritant concentrations of testing materials also could be important. Another possible explanation for "false positive" reactions is that antibodies of low avidity may stimulate mediator release when the skin is exposed to high concentrations of allergens, as in skin testing, whereas since natural exposures usually involve only minute amounts of allergens, perhaps only highly avid antibodies produce nasal symptoms. The comparative numbers of mast cells in the nasal mucosa and skin and their relative saturation with specific IgE antibodies also may be significant factors. In any case, it is mandatory that the results of either skin testing or *in vitro* tests be correlated with a very carefully obtained history to avoid serious clinical errors. In cases of uncertainty about such correlations, some type of challenge test should be considered. This is particularly important (indeed usually mandatory) in assessing the significance of positive skin tests to foods, since many of these are not of clinical significance. On the other hand, negative skin test reactions to potent food extracts are quite reliable indicators of the lack of atopic allergy thereto.

There also may be "false negative" skin tests. Most commonly these arise from the administration of antihistamines prior to testing (but theophylline, corticosteroids, and terbutaline do not affect skin test reactions). Even without medications some older persons have rather unreactive skins. Errors from this source can be averted by routinely using positive control skin tests with codeine and histamine. Inactive test materials also may cause errors.

REFERENCES

1. Wasserman SI. Mediators of immediate hypersensitivity. J Allergy Clin Immunol 72:101–119, 1983.
2. Marone G. The role of basophils and mast cells in the pathogenesis of pulmonary diseases. Int Arch Allergy Appl Immunol 76(suppl 1):70–82, 1985.
3. Ishizaka T. Analysis of triggering events in mast cells for immunoglobulin E-mediated histamine release. J Allergy Clin Immunol 67:90–96, 1981.
4. Marone G, Poto S, Celestino D, Bonini S. Human basophil releasability. III. Genetic control of human basophil releasability. J Immunol 137:3588–3592, 1986.
5. Grant JA, Lett-Brown A, Warner JA, Lichtenstein LM, Haak-Frendscho M, Kaplan AP. Activation of basophils. Fed Proc 45:2653–2658, 1986.
6. Ida S, Hooks JJ, Siraganian RP, Natkins AL. Enhancement of IgE-mediated histamine release from human basophils by viruses; role of interferon. J Exp Med 145:892–906, 1977.
7. Black JW, Duncan WA, Durrant CJ, Ganellin CR, Parsons EM. Definition and antagonism of histamine H2-receptors. Nature 236:385–390, 1972.
8. Carpenter GB, Bunker-Soler AI, Nelson HS. Evaluation of combined H1- and H2-receptor blocking agents in the treatment of seasonal allergic rhinitis. J Allergy Clin Immunol 71:412–417, 1983.
9. Mygind N, Anggard A. Anatomy and physiology of the nose—pathophysiologic alterations in allergic rhinitis. Clin Rev Allergy 2:173–188, 1984.
10. Austen KF. Biologic implications of the structural and functional characteristics of the chemical mediators of immediate-type hypersensitivity. Harvey Lect 73:93–161, 1978.
11. Meier HL, Kaplan AP, Lichtenstein LM, Revak SD, Cochrane CG, Newball H. Anaphylactic release of a prekallikrein activator from human lung in vitro. J Clin Invest 72:574–581, 1983.
12. Samuelsson B, Dahlen SE, Lindgren JA, Ronzer CA, Serhan CN. Leukotrienes and lipoxins: Structures, biosynthesis, and biological effects. Science 237:1171–1176, 1987.
13. Levi R, Krell RD (eds) Biology of the leukotrienes. Ann NY Acad Sci 524:1–464, 1988.
14. Roberts LJ, Sweetman BJ, Lewis RA, Austen KF, Oates JA. Increased production of prostaglandin D2 in patients with systemic mastocytosis. N Engl J Med 303:1400–1404, 1980.
15. Steel L, Kaliner M. Prostaglandin-generating factor of anaphylaxis. Identification and isolation. J Biol Chem 256:12692–12698, 1981.
16. Benveniste J. PAF-acether (platelet-activating factor). Adv Prostaglandin Thromboxane Leukotriene Res 19:355–357, 1989.
17. Miadonna A, Tedeschi A, Arnoux B, Sala A, Zanussi C, Benveniste J. Evidence of PAF-acether metabolic pathway activation in antigen challenge of upper respiratory airways. Am Rev Respir Dis 140:141–147, 1989.
18. Archer CB, Page CP, Morley J, MacDonald DM. Actions of disodium cromoglycate (DSCG) on human skin responses to histamine, codeine and Paf-acether. Agents Actions 16:6–8, 1985.
19. Rubin AE, Smith LJ, Patterson R. The bronchoconstrictor properties of platelet activating factor in humans. Am Rev Respir Dis 136:1145, 1987.
20. Abraham WM, Stevenson JS, Garrido R. A possible role for PAF in allergen-induced late responses: Modification by a selective antagonist. J Appl Physiol 66:2351–2357, 1989.
21. Braquet P, Touquil L, Shen TY, Vargaflig BB. Perspectives in platelet-activating factor research. Pharmacol Rev 39:97–145, 1987.
22. Lee TH, Brown MJ, Nagy L, Causon R, Walport MJ, Kay AB. Exercise-induced release of histamine and neutrophil chemotactic factor in atopic asthmatics. J Allergy Clin Immunol 70:73–81, 1982.
23. Hurst NP. Molecular basis of activation and regulation of the phagocyte respiratory burst. Ann Rheum Dis 46:265–272, 1987.
24. Schwartz LB, Riedel C, Caufield JP, Wasserman SI, Austen KF. Cell association of complexes of chymase, heparin proteoglycan, and protein after degranulation by rat mast cells. J Immunol 126:2071–2078, 1981.
25. Schwartz LB, Yunginger JW, Miller J, Bokhari R, Dull D. Time course of appearance and disappearance of human mast cell tryptase in the circulation after anaphylaxis. J Clin Invest 83:1551–1555, 1989.
26. Oertel HL, Kaliner M. The biologic activity of mast cell granules. III. Purification of inflammatory factors of anaphylaxis (IF-A) responsible for causing late phase reactions. J Immunol 127:1398–1402, 1981.
27. Center DM. Identification of rat mast cell-derived chemoattractant factors for lymphocytes. J Allergy Clin Immunol 71:29–35, 1983.
28. Gallin JI, Kaplan AP. Mononuclear cell chemotactic activity of kallikrein and plasminogen activator and its inhibition by C1 inhibitor and alpha2-macroglobulin. J Immunol 113:1928–1934, 1974.
29. Holgate ST, Mann JS, Cushley MJ. Adenosine as a bronchoconstrictor mediator in asthma and its antagonism by methylxanthines. J Allergy Clin Immunol 74:302–306, 1984.
30. Fuller RW, Dixon CMS, Cuss FMC, Barnes PJ. Bradykinin-induced bronchoconstriction in humans. Am Rev Respir Dis 135:176–180, 1987.
31. Proud D, Reynolds CJ, LaCapra S, Kagey-Sobotka A, Lichtenstein LM, Naclerio RM. Nasal provocation with bradykinin induces symptoms of rhinitis and a sore throat. Am Rev Respir Dis 137:613–616, 1988.
32. Goetzl EJ. Asthma; new mediators and old problems. N Engl J Med 311:252–253, 1984.
33. Paton WDM. Histamine release by compounds of simple chemical structure. Pharmacol Rev 9:269–328, 1957.
34. Goetzl EJ, Chernov T, Renold F, Payan DG. Neuropeptide regulation of the expression of immediate hypersensitivity. J Immunol 135:802s–805s, 1985.
35. Fujisawa T, Abu-Ghazaleh R, Kita H, Sanderson CJ, Gleich GJ. Regulatory effect of cytokines on eosinophil degranulation. J Immunol 144:642–646, 1990.
36. Silberstein DS, Ali MH, Baker SL, David JR. Human eosinophil cytotoxicity-enhancing factor. J Immunol 143:979–983, 1989.
37. Gleich GJ, Adolphson CR. The eosinophilic leukocyte: Structure and function. Adv Immunol 39:177–253, 1986.
38. Thueson DD, Speck LS, Lett-Brown MA, Grant JA. Histamine-releasing activity (HRA): I. Production by mitogen- or antigen-stimulated human mononuclear cells. J Immunol 123:626–632, 1979.
39. MacDonald SM, Lichtenstein LM, Proud D, Plaut M, Naclerio RM, MacGlashan DW, Kagey-Sobotka A. Studies of IgE-dependent histamine-releasing factors: Heterogeneity of IgE. J Immunol 139:506–512, 1987.
40. Subramanian N, Bray MA. Interleukin 1 releases histamine from human basophils and mast cells in vitro. J Immunol 138:271–275, 1987.
41. Haak-Frendscho M, Arai N, Arai K-I, Baeza ML, Finn A, Kaplan AP. Human recombinant granulocyte-macrophage colony-stimulating factor and interleukin 3 cause basophil histamine release. J Clin Invest 82:17–20, 1988.
42. MacDonald SM, Schleimer RP, Kagey-Sobotka A, Gillis S, Lichtenstein LM. Recombinant IL-3 induces histamine re-

lease from human basophils. J Immunol 142:3527–3532, 1989.

43. Grattan CEH, Hamon CGB, Cowan AM, Leeming RJ. Preliminary identification of a low molecular weight serological mediator in chronic idiopathic urticaria. Br J Dermatol 119:179–184, 1988.

44. Tharp MD, Thrilby R, Sullivan TJ. Gastrin induces histamine release from cutaneous mast cells. J Allergy Clin Immunol 74:159–165, 1984.

45. Solley GD, Gleich GJ, Jordan RE, Schroeter AL. Late phase of the immediate wheal and flare skin reactions: Its dependence on IgE antibodies. J Clin Invest 58:408–420, 1976.

46. Cockcroft DW, Ruffin RE, Dolovich J, Hargreave FE. Allergen-induced increase in non-allergic bronchial reactivity. Clin Allergy 7:503–513, 1977.

47. Connell JT. Quantitative intranasal pollen challenges. III. The priming effect in allergic rhinitis. J Allergy 43:33–44, 1969.

48. Farber HW, Weller PF, Rounds S, Beer DJ, Center DM. Generation of lipid neutrophil chemoattractant activity by histamine-stimulated cultured endothelial cells. J Immunol 137:2918–2924, 1986.

49. Zweiman B. Mediators of allergic inflammation in the skin. Clin Allergy 18:419–433, 1988.

50. Kaliner M, Wasserman SI, Austen KF. Immunologic release of chemical mediators from human nasal polyps. N Engl J Med 289:277–281, 1973.

51. Ohtsuka H, Okuda M. Important factors in the nasal manifestations of allergy. Arch Otorhinolaryngol 233:227–235, 1981.

52. Gomez E, Corrado OJ, Baldwin DL, Swanson AR, Davies RJ. Direct in vivo evidence for mast cell degranulation during allergen-induced reactions in man. J Allergy Clin Immunol 78:637–645, 1986.

53. Peters SP, Naclerio RM, Togais A, et al. In vitro and in vivo model systems for the study of allergic and inflammatory disorders in man. Chest 87:1625–1645, 1985.

Chapter III

Immunopharmacology of Nasal Allergic Reactions

Othon Iliopoulos, M.D., David Proud, Ph.D., Alkis G. Togias, M.D., Ulf Pipkorn, M.D.,
Anne Kagey-Sobotka, Ph.D., Lawrence M. Lichtenstein, M.D., and Robert M. Naclerio, M.D.

ABSTRACT

The technique of nasal provocation followed by lavage was used to study the pharmacology and pathophysiology of upper airway allergic reactions. The levels of histamine, TAME-esterase activity, kinins, and arachidonic acid metabolites were measured in the recovered nasal lavage fluid obtained during the early and, in certain cases, the late phase and rechallenge reactions to antigen. Leukocytes contained in the lavage were counted and differentiated. Topical application of azatadine and systemic administration of theophylline reduced both mediators and symptoms during the early reaction, probably by inhibiting antigen-induced mast cell activation. Pretreatment with aspirin decreased the concentration of cyclooxygenase products during the early reaction without ameliorating symptoms. Administration of systemic steroids ablated the increase of mediators and symptoms and the mucosal accumulation of eosinophils and mononuclear cells, but not of neutrophils during the late phase reaction, without affecting the mediators or symptoms of the early reaction, with the exception of kinins. Topical steroids reduced both the amount of mediators and the severity of symptoms during the early, late, and rechallenge reactions. The accumulation of eosinophils, basophils, neutrophils, and mononuclear cells during the late phase reaction was also significantly reduced. Thus, this nasal challenge model has helped us to gain insights into the pathophysiology of allergic reactions and the pharmacology of their treatment and can be used to examine the efficacy of pharmacologic agents designed for the treatment of such reactions.

Since the identification of IgE as the major reaginic antibody in humans, studies have shown that the severity of mucosal allergic reactions is dependent on an impressive variety of factors. It is believed that these reactions are initiated by the interaction of allergen with specific IgE antibodies on the surface of mast cells that leads to the cross-linking of high affinity IgE receptors.[1] The subsequent mast cell activation results in degranulation and the release of a panel of preformed, as well as newly generated, inflammatory mediators with the concomitant generation of allergic symptomatology.[2]

One approach to treatment of this IgE-mediated disease concentrated on the pharmacologic manipulation of mast cell activation, with the goal of identifying chemical compounds that would prevent the release of mediators. Therefore, *in vitro* models were developed using conveniently obtainable mast cells: rat pleural and peritoneal mast cells, guinea pig lung fragments and human lung fragments, as well as mechanically or enzymatically dispersed human lung mast cells.[3-4] The latter can be purified and used to study various aspects of allergenic activation. These models have been useful in identifying the mediators released in the supernatant of the challenged cells. In spite of similarities between animal and human tissues, there are considerable differences in biologic behavior. Consequently, pharmacologic findings cannot always be extrapolated directly from one species to another, e.g., sodium cromoglycate significantly reduces rat peritoneal mast cell histamine release after antigen challenge under optimum conditions, but fails to do so in purified human lung mast cells. Recently heterogeneity, even between human mast cells obtained from different tissues, became apparent, underscoring the fact that pharmacologic ma-

Publication 036 from the Johns Hopkins Asthma and Allergy Center, 301 Bayview Boulevard, Baltimore, MD 21224

Department of Medicine, Division of Clinical Immunology, and Department of Otolaryngology, Johns Hopkins University School of Medicine, Baltimore, MD 21205

nipulation of mast cell activation may bear tissue specificity.[5-7]

Although mast cells sensitized with specific IgE antibodies play a central role in the initiation of allergic reactions, a series of data has accumulated from *in vitro* experimentation suggesting that the *in vivo* microenvironment in which the encounter between the allergen and the IgE molecule on the surface of the mast cell takes place influences the severity of the host's reaction. In the case of allergic rhinitis, a variety of parameters may be operative. The pH of nasal secretions affects the type of allergenic molecules extracted from the inhaled pollen grain.[8] The osmolality of the mucous blanket is thought to affect the response of mast cells to antigen,[9] particularly at the range of low antigen concentrations thought to occur naturally. Nerve excitation due to released inflammatory mediators contributes to the induction of hay fever symptomatology directly,[10] and probably indirectly by the action of neuropeptides,[11] which in turn could potentially induce or regulate the release of inflammatory mediators from mast cells. Structural cells of the nasal mucosa (epithelial, endothelial, fibroblasts) both produce, and respond to, inflammatory mediators *in vitro*, and could possibly affect the allergenic response *in vivo*.[12] This cellular milieu can be enriched by cells that leave the intravascular compartment and infiltrate the nasal mucosa, as has been shown to occur under different inflammatory conditions. Basophils, as well as eosinophils and mononuclear cells, bearing high and low affinity IgE receptors, respectively, may actively participate in the generation of the allergic symptomatology after exposure to antigen.[13] Other interfering factors include differences in mast cell "releasability,"[14] as well as the rate of inflammatory mediator catabolism. One can thus conceive of the existence of a fine network of humoral and cellular elements dictating the outcome of an allergic reaction.

Given the complexity of the IgE-mediated response, the need to develop a model for studying the allergic reaction *in vivo* is clear. It would be desirable for such a model to bear both species and organ specificity in order to: 1) confirm the *in vivo* participation and relative importance of the various mediators of allergic inflammation; and 2) study the mechanisms of pharmacologic and immunologic intervention (immunotherapy) in the allergic reaction.

We feel that in order to confirm the importance and direct participation of a mediator in the generation of allergic symptomatology, the following criteria should be fulfilled: 1) the mediator of interest should be specifically generated during the response of an atopic subject's target organ to the relevant allergen; 2) exposure of a nonallergic person to the same allergen under identical experimental conditions should not induce generation of the mediator; 3) significant reduction of mediator release following antigen challenge or the presence of a specific antagonist at the time of exposure and under optimal concentration should result in amelioration of symptoms; and finally, 4) appropriate application of the mediator on the nasal mucosa should generate the symptomatology for which the mediator is suspected to be responsible. Within this context of experimentation it is important to consider the possibility that a mediator, independent of its direct effect on the generation of symptoms, may exert a synergistic effect with other mediators or may have a chemoattractive or immunoregulatory role, and through this, indirectly influence the severity of the allergic reaction.

We have developed a model, based on nasal antigen provocation with subsequent collection of nasal secretions, that allows us to evaluate the role of mediators in the allergic response.[15] By studying the humoral and cellular content of these secretions and relating them to the clinical response of the subjects, we have attempted to dissect the mode of action of drugs currently used in the treatment of allergic rhinitis and to attribute their beneficial effect to one or more of the following: 1) reduction of the amount of mediators generated after contact with the antigen; 2) reduction of tissue response to the same level of mediators; and 3) reduction of the inflammatory process that follows the early reaction (ER) to the antigen. We believe that this model will help us to establish the differences between local and systemic administration of a drug, to study its *in vivo* effective concentration and duration of action, and to test new chemical compounds purported to interfere with allergic reactions. This model could also address questions regarding systemic or local immunotherapy with a variety of naturally extracted or modified antigens.[16] Moreover, the use of such agents will help to elucidate the various steps in the pathophysiology of allergic rhinitis as a humoral and cellular inflammatory response. The description that follows will present experimental work on the mode of action of drugs that have been widely used for allergy treatment, as well as insights into the pathophysiology of the allergic inflammation based on this work.

METHODS

Nasal provocation involves gently delivering antigen extracts into one nostril using a tuberculin syringe. The protocols of nasal challenge vary according to each study's purpose and the duration of action of the particular drug used. Subjects are premedicated with either the active drug or placebo in a double-blind fashion, and a nasal challenge with antigen follows. Challenges are separated by at least 1 week to prevent any effect of one challenge on the other and to allow for drug "washout." Alternatively, when immediate effects of a topically applied drug are to be investigated, the active compound or placebo is administered following an initial antigen challenge and is followed shortly thereafter by a second, identical, challenge. The total amount of mediators generated after the second challenge is compared to the amount generated after the initial challenge.

The nasal challenge technique has been described elsewhere in detail.[15] Generally, initial lavages to establish a baseline precede the topical application of oxymetazoline hydrochloride, an α-adrenostimulator, that prevents excessive congestion of the nasal mucosa after antigen challenge and allows for the continuation of nasal lavages. We have shown that oxymetazoline has no influence on mediator release. Challenges with the vehicle used for the antigen (diluent) are performed to rule out nonspecific reactivity to the delivery system and are followed by a series of challenges with increasing doses of antigen [usually 1, 10, 100, and 1000 protein nitrogen units (PNU)] at standard time intervals (usually 12 minutes). Nasal lavages are performed 10 minutes after each challenge.

Nasal secretions are obtained according to the following method: the volunteer extends his neck backwards while holding his breath, and 2.5 or 5 ml of saline, prewarmed to 37°C, are instilled into each nostril. Approximately 10 seconds later the fluid, a mixture of mucus and saline, is expelled into a tray and centrifuged at $3,000 \times g$ for 15 minutes, at a temperature of 4°C, to separate cells and mucus (gel phase) from the supernatant (sol phase). The supernatant is then aliquoted and treated appropriately for subsequent mediator assays. Histamine is measured by an automated fluorometric assay sensitive to 1 ng/ml. Prostaglandin and leukotriene measurements are performed by using radioimmunoassays sensitive to approximately 30 and 200 pg/ml, respectively. High-pressure liquid chromatography analysis combined with radioimmunoassay is used to establish the identity of specific leukotrienes.

When the cellular content of the pellet was to be studied, lactated Ringer's solution was used for nasal lavages instead of saline. The pellet obtained by centrifugation was resuspended in RPMI 1640 medium containing 0.1 mM EDTA and 8 mg/ml of N-acetylcysteine as a mucolytic agent. It was then incubated at 37°C for 45 minutes, washed twice in phenylacetylglutamine medium, and resuspended in RPMI 1640. The cells were counted in a hemocytometer, and a slide differentiation among eosinophils, neutrophils, and mononuclear cells was made by using Diff-Quick, a modified Wright's stain. The percentage of histamine-containing cells (mast cells and basophils) was estimated using alcian blue staining.

RESULTS AND DISCUSSION

Nasal challenge of atopic volunteers with the appropriate antigen confirmed the *in vivo* generation of a panel of inflammatory mediators. Challenge of either nonallergic volunteers with antigens or of allergic subjects with saline or diluent did not lead to generation of inflammatory mediators or symptoms.[15] This crossover observation controls the specificity of mediator generation.

The levels of histamine in the recovered lavage fluid increased during nasal challenge.[15] We believe that this increase represents mast cell activation, since morphologic studies of the nonstimulated mucosa have identified mast cells to be the majority of histamine-containing cells residing in the epithelium and stroma; basophils are essentially absent from the nasal mucosa or secretions when antigen stimulation has not taken place within a week.

Both cyclooxygenase and lipoxygenase pathway metabolites of arachidonic acid were identified in lavage samples following antigen challenge.[17] (Prostaglandin (PG) D_2 is formed by mast cells, but not basophils, upon antigenic stimulation,[18] and its significant increase offers support to the concept that the early outcome of the contact of a previously nonstimulated mucosa with antigen is a mast cell-mediated phenomenon. Additionally, PGE_2, $PGF_{2\alpha}$ and 6-keto-$PGF_{1\alpha}$ clearly increase in the postchallenge nasal secretions, but the potential sources of these prostanoids are broader than the ones for PGD_2: epithelial, endothelial, and mononuclear cells, as well as eosinophils and platelets, have been shown both to produce them *in vitro* and to be implicated in their metabolism.[19]

Of the sulfidopeptide leukotrienes (LT), only LTC_4 is shown to be produced by purified human lung mast cells upon antigen challenge. Lung fragments, however, have been shown to generate $LTC_4/D_4/E_4$, pointing to the participation of a broader cell population in the production and/or metabolism of these inflammatory mediators.[20] Likewise, nasal antigenic provocation confirmed the *in vivo* formation of $LTC_4/D_4/E_4$.[21] LTB_4 is detected in relatively lower concentrations following antigen challenge of both lung mast cells and the nasal mucosa.[22, 23]

Postchallenge nasal secretions also contain high concentrations of the potent vasoactive peptides bradykinin and lysylbradykinin[24] that may play a role in the pathogenesis of the allergic reaction. In the process of delineating the biochemical events responsible for the formation of these peptides during the allergic response *in vivo*, we noted increased concentrations of peptide kininogens in nasal secretions collected after challenge.[25] These kininogens, which enter nasal secretions by transudation from plasma, provide the substrates from which the powerful kinin-generating enzymes, plasma and glandular kallikreins, liberate kinins. The concentrations of these enzymes also increase postchallenge and contribute to the TAME-esterase activity detected in lavages.[26,27] The synthetic substrate, N-α-p-tosyl-L-arginine methyl ester, is used to detect the presence of enzymes with arginine esterase activity in nasal lavages. The principal contributor to this activity during the immediate allergic response is the complex formed between plasma kallikrein and α_2-macroglobulin.[26] The other enzyme which represents a significant component of the TAME-esterase activity in postchallenge lavages is the mast cell granule protease, tryptase. The increased concentration of this protease following antigen challenge is one more indication of mast cell activation. Since the principal component of the measured TAME-esterase activity is a kinin-forming enzyme, it is not surprising that a close correlation exists between this activity and kinin concentrations.

Recently we investigated whether the potent pro-inflammatory molecule, platelet-activating factor (PAF), was present in postchallenge nasal secretions. Although the concentration of PAF was not increased following challenge, its metabolite, lyso-PAF, was found in significant quantities.[28] This finding emphasizes the dynamic nature of the postchallenge events which include the generation of a complex network of inflammatory mediators, their interaction with the target organ, and the rate of their catabolism.

In a subpopulation of atopics, the response to the antigen does not consist of an early reaction only. Eosinophils, neutrophils, basophils, and mononuclear cells infiltrate the nasal mucosa following the ER and can be identified in increased numbers in the nasal lavages for the next 24 hours. The cellular infiltrate is accompanied by a second wave of all the inflammatory mediators described above, with the exception of PGD_2. Mediator elevation correlates with the reappearance of symptoms of congestion, rhinorrhea, and sneezing.[29] This phenomenon, known as the late phase reaction (LPR), is of significant interest because it is considered to more closely represent the nature of the ongoing allergic reaction than does the early response to antigen. This is due to its longer duration compared to the early phase, the presence of a mixed cellular infiltrate in the inflamed mucosa, and its sensitivity to systemic steroids.[30] Moreover, in certain subjects, if the nasal mucosa is rechallenged with antigen as the LPR subsides, the ensuing levels of mediators are significantly greater than those induced by the same antigen dose during the early response, although these two phenomena are not obligatorily linked (Fig. 1). Our interest thus evolved towards the study of the pharmacology of the ER, LPR, and rechallenge reaction (RCR) by monitoring the levels of mediators and the cellular content of nasal lavages and relating these to symptom scores reported by our challenged volunteers. The relationship between these different phases and the mechanism(s) of their generation are currently under investigation.

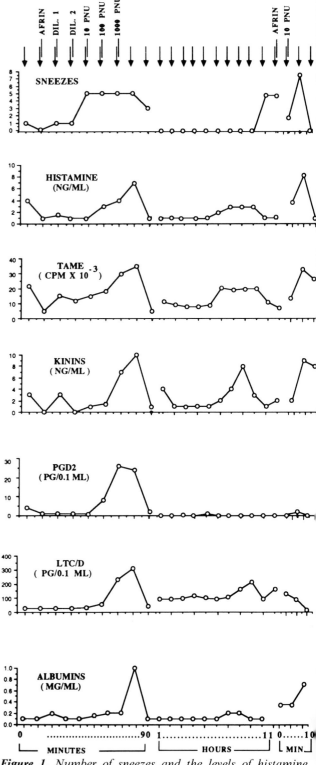

Figure 1. *Number of sneezes and the levels of histamine, TAME-esterase activity, kinins, prostaglandin D_2, leukotrienes C/D, and albumin in the recovered nasal lavages of a volunteer obtained during early, late, and rechallenge reactions to antigen. Arrows represent nasal lavages. The induction of sneezes by diluent, shown in this particular subject, occurs rarely in some individuals and should not be considered representative.*

H1 Receptor Antagonists

Antihistamines have been the cornerstone of the available treatment for mild allergic disease for a long time. Well-performed, double-blind clinical trials have proved their efficacy in reducing the pruritus, sneezing, and runny nose that accompanies the natural exposure to allergen, without significantly affecting nasal congestion.[31] H1-type antihistamines also have anticholinergic, antiserotonin, sedative, and local anesthetic properties that may contribute significantly to their clinical efficacy.[32]

More recently, our attention has shifted to the consideration of another mode of action of selected antihistamines. It has been found that preincubation of peripheral blood basophils, as well as dispersed human lung mast cells, *in vitro* with tricyclic H1 antihistamines, reduces the antigen-induced release of histamine.[33, 34] Therefore, we selected the H1 antagonist azatadine to investigate whether such an "antirelease" property was operative on human nasal mast cells *in vivo*. To achieve a concentration thought necessary to inhibit release *in vivo*, we administered this agent topically.

The challenge consisted of administration of an individual antigen dose (100 or 200 PNU, based on the subject's sensitivity) given three times at 30-minute intervals. Mediators were measured, as described above, every 10 minutes after each dose of antigen. A volume of 0.125 ml of either a 0.4% solution of azatadine base or placebo was administered, in a double-blind crossover fashion, into each nostril 10 minutes before the second antigen challenge. Eight volunteers participated in the study. Figure 2 presents the mediator levels and symptoms of a patient on two different occasions of treatment, one with placebo and one with the drug. On the drug administration day, TAME-esterase activity generated after the second and third challenge was significantly lower than the activity generated during the first challenge ($p < 0.01$). The same was true for the corresponding levels of histamine and kinins, as well as for the number of sneezes ($p < 0.05$, $p < 0.01$, and $p < 0.01$, respectively). On the placebo day, there was no change in the levels of histamine, TAME-esterase activity, and kinins generated after each of the three challenges. Sneezes decreased in number ($p < 0.02$) only after the third challenge, probably due to receptor tachyphylaxis.

Using the nasal provocation model, we confirmed the *in vivo* antirelease properties of H1 antihistamines when applied topically in high concentrations.[34] This agreement between *in vitro* and *in vivo* results supports the concept that mast cell activation is a central event in the early reaction to antigen. It is unlikely, though, that systemically administered antihistamines achieve such high concentrations in the nasal mucosa with conventional doses. However, if there were preferable

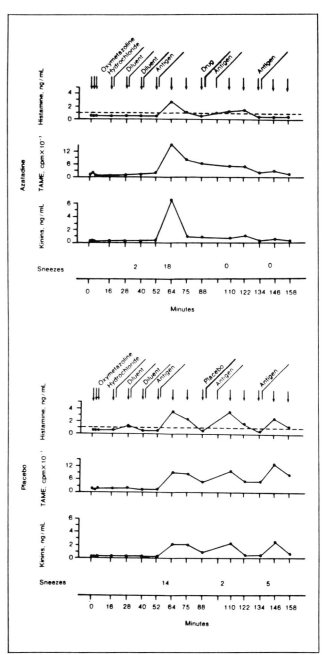

Figure 2. *Levels of histamine, TAME-esterase activity, and kinins and number of sneezes of a volunteer challenged according to the protocol illustrated at the top of the figure. In the first case (top), azatadine was given between the first and second antigen doses. In the second case (bottom), placebo was sprayed instead of drug. Reproduced with permission.*[34]

accumulation of the drug locally, it is possible that the beneficial action of H1 antihistamines would derive primarily from inhibition of the release of a whole panel of mast cell-derived mediators, not just from histamine antagonism. This interesting aspect of systemic H1 blocker effects is currently under investigation. Additional questions concerning the mode of action and the suggested use (dose, frequency of administration, route of application) of antihistamines to achieve an optimum inhibition of mediator release, while minimizing the side effects, can be addressed using this model. Furthermore, the antirelease properties of new compounds and their potential effect on the LPR will be easily determined following protocols similar to the one described above.

Theophylline

Since the early 1890s when Salter suggested that "two large cups of coffee is the best remedy for asthma," a variety of nonmutually exclusive mechanisms responsible for the beneficial effect of theophylline on the asthmatic reaction have been proposed:[35] Direct relaxation of smooth muscle, inhibition of mediator release from human mast cells and basophils, inhibition of adenosine production, adenosine receptor antagonism, antiprostaglandin activity, prevention of increases in the permeability of postcapillary venules after exposure to inflammatory mediators, and, finally, increase in diaphragmatic contractility. The initial observation that theophylline possesses bronchodilating and antirelease properties, mediated through an elevation of the intracellular levels of cyclic adenosine monophosphate, was confounded by the fact that these actions required *in vitro* concentrations much higher than those clinically achieved. In addition, wheal and flare reactions after intradermal injection of antigen were not reduced by pretreatment of subjects with theophylline, casting doubt on the hypothesis that theophylline acts by inhibiting mast cell activation. Since our model allows us to study the antirelease potential of a drug, we decided to investigate whether theophylline, a widely used antiasthmatic drug, inhibited mediator release at therapeutic concentrations.[36]

Sixteen volunteers entered a double-blind, randomized crossover study to compare the effect of 400 mg of theophylline, administered orally twice a day, with placebo treatment. A nasal challenge was performed on every volunteer on three separate occasions: as a screen for entry into the study and following a week of treatment with the active drug or placebo. As shown in Figure 3, the total levels of histamine, TAME-esterase activity, and kinins and the total number of sneezes were significantly reduced after treatment with theophylline ($p < 0.03$); there was no significant difference between the screening and placebo challenges. The mean serum concentration of the drug at the time of challenge for the treated group was within therapeutic range (13.8 μg/ml), and this concentration was effective in reducing mediator release.

Although we cannot exclude the possibility that theophylline (or one of its metabolites) inhibited mediator release after antigen challenge indirectly (e.g., by acting on cells other than mast cells or by affecting nerve reflexes or blocking the adenosine receptors), it is tempting to speculate that it directly affected resident mast cells of the nasal mucosa. Whatever the mechanism of action, these experiments clearly demonstrate that administration of theophylline in clinically relevant pharmacologic concentrations reduces the generation of inflammatory mediators after antigen challenge. These findings do not exclude other mechanisms through which theophylline might be clinically operative, such as some anti-inflammatory action and/or the possibility of affecting the LPR that may follow an ER.

In both the studies with antihistamines and with theophylline, a reduction in the amount of mediators generated during the early reaction to antigen was accompanied by a reduction in the symptoms. According to the criteria set at the introduction of this review,

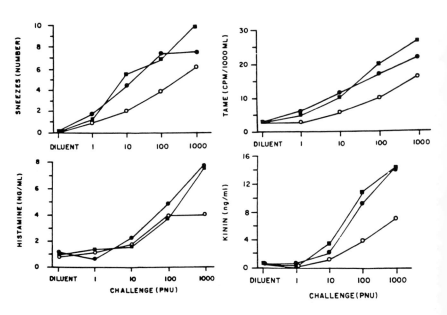

Figure 3. Number of sneezes and mediator concentration per antigen administered dose after treatment with theophylline (open circles) or placebo (solid circles) and after antigen challenge without any premedication (boxes). (Reproduced with permission from Am J Med 79(6A):43–47, 1985).

such an observation strengthens the concept that a cause and effect relationship exists between the generation of inflammatory mediators and the symptomatology of the ER. This picture was not obtained when a histamine synthesis inhibitor and aspirin were studied.

α-Fluoromethylhistidine

The use of α-fluoromethylhistidine, an irreversible histamine decarboxylase inhibitor, offered us the possibility of investigating the role of a single mediator, histamine, in the ER. Three weeks of pretreatment with the inhibitor reduced the synthesis of histamine, as evidenced by the reduced level of the major histamine metabolite excreted in the urine. The pre- and post-challenge histamine concentrations in nasal secretions were also reduced by 60% without significant effect on the concentration of TAME-esterase activity and kinins or on the severity of symptoms.[38]

Although the drug is unlikely to be used therapeutically due to its side effects, it served as an effective experimental tool to reduce the levels of one mediator and observe the consequences of this manipulation. In reference to the criteria set at the introduction regarding the participation of a mediator in the allergic reaction, these findings question the importance of histamine in the induction of the symptomatology of the ER. This provides more evidence that antihistamines may not solely or even primarily work through histamine antagonism but rather through their anticholinergic and/or antirelease properties. Alternatively, it is possible that low levels of a mediator are operative and that the 60% reduction in histamine achieved in these experiments was not sufficient to produce significant symptomatic relief.

Aspirin

The levels of cyclooxygenase metabolites of arachidonic acid in nasal lavages were found to be increased in a group of volunteers subjected to nasal challenge with antigen. A week later all subjects underwent an identical challenge preceded by a 2-day course of oral aspirin, 650 mg 3 times a day. Aspirin significantly inhibited the increase in PGD_2, PGE, $PGF_{2\alpha}$, and thromboxane, but did not affect the amount of sneezing or the levels of histamine, TAME-esterase activity, and leukotrienes.

The above pattern indicates that prostaglandins generated during the early nasal allergic reactions do not significantly contribute to the induction of early symptomatology.[17] However, we cannot disregard the possibility that prostaglandins are more important in other elements of the nasal allergic reaction, such as induction of a LPR,[38] nonspecific hyperreactivity following an antigen challenge, or specific priming of the nasal mucosa to the antigen. These hypotheses are the object of current research, the results of which may have significant consequences in the treatment of allergic inflammation.

Sulfidopeptide leukotrienes were also measured in the course of this study and, as with *in vitro* human lung mast cells, pretreatment with a cyclooxygenase inhibitor did not increase their production. This observation strengthens the concept that the ER to antigen is mediated by mast cells of the nasal mucosa, since pretreatment of peripheral blood basophils with a cyclooxygenase inhibitor does, on the contrary, increase the production of sulfidopeptide leukotrienes after antigenic stimulation.

Steroids

Clinical observations on the effective use of corticosteroids in the treatment of severe asthma were followed by intense research aimed at understanding the mode of action of these compounds both at the clinical and molecular levels.[39] In allergic rhinitis, extensive use of systemic steroids is limited by the serious side effects associated with their administration. Renewed interest in their use was stimulated by reports on the effectiveness of local application.[40] We designed a series of double-blind, crossover, randomized studies to investigate the effects of systemic and local corticosteroids on nasal challenge with antigen.

After 48 hours of treatment with 60 mg/day of oral prednisone or placebo, a nasal provocation was performed in volunteers selected on the basis of a previously demonstrated LPR. Our interest was primarily stimulated by observations, made after bronchoprovocation and skin challenge with antigen, that systemic steroid administration preferentially reduced the LPR but did not decrease the ER. We therefore extended our observation of the events that follow the ER to antigen by studying both the mediators and the cellular content of nasal lavages performed hourly up to the 11th hour after the ER.[41]

In agreement with observations made in other models, the systemically administered steroids did not decrease the intensity of the ER to antigen. The increase in the levels of histamine, TAME-esterase activity, and LTC_4/D_4, as well as the number of sneezes and other symptoms, did not differ between drug and placebo treatment. Only the amount of kinins generated during the ER was diminished after steroid treatment, indicating a possible effect of steroids on the propagation of inflammation by the vascular contact activation system.

After placebo treatment, the ER was followed by an accumulation of eosinophils, neutrophils, and mononuclear cells in the nasal lavage fluid. This cellular infiltrate was accompanied by a second wave of symptoms and of all mediators, except PGD_2 (Fig. 1). Systemic steroids dramatically ablated this accumulation of eosinophils and mononuclear cells as well as the late increase in mediators.[42] The number of neutrophils did not decrease significantly after treatment. Although we cannot exclude the possibility that steroids prevented their activation, this observation questions the importance of neutrophils in the pathogenesis of the LPR. We did not look for the presence of basophils among the leukocytes that infiltrated the nasal mucosa in this particular study, but we have recently found that basophils do accumulate during the LPR in the nasal mucosa and that their number significantly increases over prechallenge baseline in the collected lavage fluid.[43]

In vitro experimentation failed to demonstrate inhibition of mediator release from mast cells after long-term incubation with pharmacologic concentrations of steroids,[44] whereas basophil histamine release was reduced after similar treatment.[45] Such a difference places the basophil in a central position regarding the pathogenesis of the LPR and may explain the preferential reduction of the LPR, thought to be mediated by the basophil, after systemic administration of steroids over the ER, which seems to be mediated by the mast cell.

Natural exposure to antigen during pollinosis increases the intensity of a subsequent response to the same antigen, and this increased responsiveness may be responsible, in part, for the allergic symptoms during the pollen season.[46] In an attempt to study this phenomenon, we rechallenged our volunteers, after the LPR had subsided, with the lowest antigen dose used during the ER. Placebo-treated subjects responded to rechallenge with an increase in mediators and symptoms much higher than that seen during the ER. This enhanced response was also ablated by systemic steroids. It is possible that this effect was mediated through the reduction of the LPR and/or that it was due to a direct

inhibitory effect of steroids on the rechallenge reaction. In either case, the reduction of both the LPR and rechallenge reaction by steroids stresses the importance of these responses in allergic inflammation.

Topical steroids were assessed in a similarly designed study, in which 1-week intranasal administration of 200 μg/day of flunisolide was compared to placebo. Interestingly enough, the effects of the topically administered steroids differed from those of systemic steroids:[47] not only were the mediators and symptoms of the LPR (Fig. 4) and rechallenge reactions reduced but a significant inhibition of the ER was also observed. The numbers of eosinophils, basophils, neutrophils, and mononuclear cells collected during LPR after pretreatment with local steroids were also significantly reduced as compared to placebo.[43]

That 1-week pretreatment with topical steroids effectively reduces ER, LPR, and RCR opens an interesting area of investigation. Longer exposure to a high concentration of steroids, achieved with local application, appears to influence components of the nasal mucosa that determine the intensity of the ER: a reduction in mucosal permeability to the antigen, a direct effect on the number and/or mediator release from mast cells, or functional alterations in the behavior of other cell types that affect mast cell mediator release are among the possibilities that warrant investigation.

Our nasal provocation model approach provided us, in the case of steroids, with the ability to detect differences in the mode of action of the same class of drugs when given topically and systemically and to extend our observations on the inflammatory events that follow the early encounter with antigen.

Moreover, major progress in understanding the pathophysiology of the LPR was made: the lack of PGD_2 from the group of mediators generated during

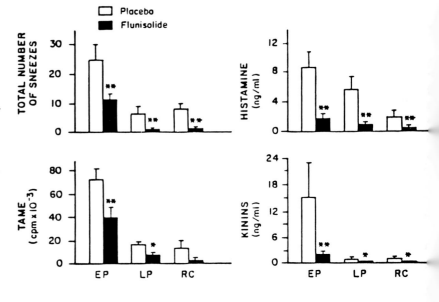

Figure 4. *Levels of histamine, TAME-esterase activity, and kinins and number of sneezes during ER, LPR, and RCR to antigen after pretreatment with flunisolide (solid bar) or placebo (open bar).* **p < 0.05, *p < 0.01. (Reproduced with permission from N Engl J Med 316:1506-1510, 1987.)

34

LPR, combined with the presence of histamine, pointed to basophils as the probable source of late mediator generation. Indeed, morphologic studies of the cellular content of nasal lavages confirmed the influx of basophils into the nasal mucosa during LPR. Support for their direct activation in the area of inflammation was provided by the ability of steroids, which, *in vitro*, inhibit basophil mediator release, to reduce the phenomenon of LPR. All the above observations suggest a role for the basophil in the pathogenesis of the LPR and, probably, in chronic allergic disease as well.

Evaluation of the Nasal Mucosal Response to Challenge with Various Mediators

The rather unexpected results of the study of a histamine synthesis inhibitor on nasal challenge with antigen, where the lower levels of histamine did not correlate with a clinical improvement, underscore the necessity of a multipathway approach in the evaluation of the role of a mediator in inflammation. Direct *in vivo* application of the mediator to the organ or tissue of interest should be included in the strategy of this evaluation.

Along this line of investigation, several groups have performed nasal challenges with histamine in concentrations high enough to induce sneezing, pruritus, and rhinorrhea. To confirm and ascribe the induced symptoms to the presence of histamine, H1 blockers alone or in combination with H2 antagonists were administered before histamine challenge.[48] These treatments significantly reduced the severity of symptoms, supporting the notion that histamine was, indeed, the inducing mediator.

Recently LTD$_4$, LTC$_4$, or bradykinin, mediators shown to be generated after nasal antigen challenge, were reintroduced in the nasal cavity in an effort to study the nasal response to an individual mediator. LTD$_4$ increased nasal airway resistance and nasal blood flow of nonatopic subjects in a dose-response manner, as recorded by rhinomanometry and laser-Doppler flowmetry, but no pruritus, sneezing or profuse rhinorrhea was apparent.[49] LTC$_4$ produced similar results: nasal obstruction, which began later and lasted longer than the obstruction produced by histamine challenge.[50] Proud et al.[51] challenged a population of atopic and nonatopic volunteers with intranasal bradykinin. The challenge was followed mainly by nasal obstruction, which remained lateralized on the challenged side, rhinorrhea, and sore throat. The ipsilateral presence of the obstruction suggests that no neural reflexes were involved in the generation of this symptom, while rhinorrhea was due, in part, to vascular leakage, as indicated by an increase of the albumin concentration in nasal secretions.

Since different symptoms are induced by various mediators, more methods need to be developed for further dissection of the action of each mediator and the evaluation of its contribution to allergic disease. Objective ways to quantify specific tissue responses will be of great help. There have been efforts to measure nasal blood flow by laser flowmetry[52] and radiolabeled xenon uptake[53] has been used to evaluate vessel and/or mucosal permeability, based on the albumin concentration of nasal secretions or the tissue uptake of radiolabeled macromolecular compounds,[54,55] and to quantify mucus production. Refinement of the above and the establishment of other, more accurate, techniques will help us obtain detailed knowledge of the role of each mediator and of the complex network of inflammation in general.

EPILOGUE

The study of inflammatory mediators after antigen challenge reveals that the complex events following an acute allergenic insult, as presented by the late and the rechallenge reactions, are undoubtedly implicated in the disease process. At the same time, it allows a more in-depth understanding of the inflammatory cascade and its pharmacologic modulation. Our next challenge is to creatively reconstitute all these defined steps in a picture of the pathophysiology of naturally occurring allergic rhinitis and to use this knowledge in developing effective methods of prevention and treatment of the disease.

ACKNOWLEDGMENT

This work was supported by Grants NS 22488, AI 07290, and AI 08270 from the National Institutes of Health, Bethesda, MD.

REFERENCES

1. Plaut M, Lichtenstein LM. Cellular and chemical basis of the allergic inflammatory response. Component parts and control mechanism. In: Middleton E, Ellis E, Reed CE, eds. Allergy: Principles and Practice. St. Louis: CV Mosby Co, 1978, pp 115–138.
2. Lichtenstein LM, Schleimer RP, McGlashan DW, Peters SP, Schulman ES, Proud D, Creticos PS, Naclerio RM, Kagey-Sobotka A. *In vitro* and *in vivo* studies of mediator release from human mast cells. In: Kay AB, Austen KF, Lichtenstein LM, eds. Asthma III: Physiology, Immunopharmacology and Treatment. London: Academic Press, 1984, pp 1–18.
3. Church MK. Mast cell models. In: Delvin JP, ed. Pulmonary and Antiallergic Drugs. New York: John Wiley and Sons, 1985, pp 73–82.
4. Schulman ES, MacGlashan DW, Peters SP, Schleimer RP, Newball HH, Lichtenstein LM. Human lung mast cells: purification and characterization. J Immunol 129:2662–2667, 1982.
5. Schulman ES, Kagey-Sobotka A, MacGlashan DW, Adkinson NF, Peters SP, Schleimer RP, Lichtenstein LM. Heterogeneity of human mast cells. J Immunol 131:1936–1941, 1983.
6. Tharp MD, Kagey-Sobotka A, Fox CC, Marone G, Lichtenstein LM, Sullivan TJ. Functional heterogeneity of human mast cells from different anatomical sites: *in vitro* response to morphine sulfate. J Allergy Clin Immunol 79:599–604, 1987.
7. Lawrence ID, Warner JA, Cohan VL, Hubbard WC, Kagey-

Sobotka A, Lichtenstein LM. Purification and characterization of human skin mast cells: evidence for human mast cell heterogeneity. J Immunol 139:3062–3069, 1987.

8. Marsh DG, Belin L, Bruce CA, Lichtenstein LM, Hussain R. Rapidly released allergens from short ragweed pollen. I. Kinetics of release of known allergens in relation to biologic activity. J Allergy Clin Immunol 67:206–216, 1981.

9. Eggleston PA, Kagey-Sobotka A, Schleimer RP, Lichtenstein LM. Interaction between hyperosmolar and IgE-mediated histamine release from basophils and mast cells. Am Rev Respir Dis 130:86–91, 1984.

10. Eccles R. Neurological and pharmacological considerations. In: Proctor DF, Andersen IB, eds. The Nose: Upper Airway Physiology and the Atmospheric Environment. New York: Elsevier Biomedical Press, 1982, pp 191–214.

11. Barnes PJ. Neural control of human airways in health and disease. Am Rev Respir Dis 134:1289–1314, 1986.

12. Atkins FM, Friedman MM, Subba Rao PV, Metcalfe DD. Interactions between mast cells, fibroblasts and connective tissue components. Int Arch Allergy Appl Immunol 77:96–102, 1985.

13. Gleich GJ, Loegering DA. Immunobiology of eosinophils. Annu Rev Immunol 2:249–259, 1984.

14. Marone G. Modulation of mast cell/basophil function *in vivo*: the releasability concept. In: Proceedings of the XII International Congress of Allergology and Clinical Immunology. St. Louis: CV Mosby Co, 1985, pp 175–181.

15. Naclerio RM, Meier HL, Kagey-Sobotka A, Adkinson NF, Meyers DA, Norman PS, Lichtenstein LM. Mediator release after nasal airway challenge with allergen. Am Rev Respir Dis 128:597–602, 1983.

16. Norman PS. Challenge techniques in the evaluation of immunotherapy. In: Proceedings of the XII International Congress of Allergology and Clinical Immunology. St. Louis: CV Mosby Co, 1985, pp 319–322.

17. Brown MS, Peters SP, Adkinson NF Jr, Proud D, Kagey-Sobotka A, Norman PS, Lichtenstein LM, Naclerio RM. Arachidonic acid metabolites during nasal challenge. Arch Otolaryngol Head Neck Surg 113:179–183, 1987.

18. Peters SP, MacGlashan DW Jr, Schulman ES, Schleimer RP, Hayes EC, Rokach J, Adkinson NF Jr, Lichtenstein LM. Arachidonic acid metabolism in purified human lung mast cells. J Immunol 132:1972–1979, 1984.

19. Goetzl EJ. Oxygenation products of arachidonic acid as mediators of hypersensitivity and inflammation. Med Clin North Am 65:809–828, 1981.

20. Peters SP, Schulman ES, Schleimer RP, MacGlashan DW Jr, Newball HH, Lichtenstein LM. Dispersed human lung mast cells: pharmacologic aspects and comparison with human lung tissue fragments. Am Rev Respir Dis 126:1034–1039, 1982.

21. Creticos PS, Peters SP, Adkinson NF Jr, Naclerio RM, Hayes EC, Norman PS, Lichtenstein LM. Peptide leukotriene release after antigen challenge in patients sensitive to ragweed. N Engl J Med 310:1626–1630, 1984.

22. Freeland HS, Schleimer RP, Schulman ES, Lichtenstein LM, Peters SP. Generation of LTB$_4$ by human lung fragments and purified human lung mast cells. Am Rev Respir Dis, in press.

23. Freeland HS, Pipkorn U, Naclerio RM, Adkinson NF, Lichtenstein LM, Peters SP. The role of leukotriene B$_4$ (LTB$_4$) in human allergic late phase reactions: lack of LTB$_4$ inhibition by systemic glucocorticoids (Abstract). J Allergy Clin Immunol 77(suppl):244, 1986.

24. Proud D, Togias A, Naclerio RM, Crush SA, Norman PS, Lichtenstein LM. Kinins are generated *in vivo* following nasal airway challenge of allergic individuals with allergen. J Clin Invest 72:1678–1685, 1983.

25. Baumgarten CR, Togias AG, Naclerio RM, Lichtenstein LM, Norman PS, Proud D. Influx of kininogens into nasal secretions after antigen challenge of allergic individuals. J Clin Invest 76:191–197, 1985.

26. Baumgarten CR, Nichols RC, Naclerio RM, Lichtenstein LM, Norman PS, Proud D. Plasma kallikrein during experimentally induced allergic rhinitis: role in kinin formation and contribution to TAME-esterase activity in nasal secretions. J Immunol 137:977–982, 1986.

27. Baumgarten CR, Nichols RC, Naclerio RM, Proud D. Concentrations of glandular kallikrein in human nasal secretions increase during experimentally induced allergic rhinitis. J Immunol 137:1323–1326, 1986.

28. Ramesha C, Peters S, Naclerio R, Lichtenstein L, Pickett W. Decreased PAF concentration in nasal secretions following antigen challenge (Abstract). Fed Proc 45:1530, 1986.

29. Naclerio RM, Proud D, Togias AG, Adkinson NF Jr, Meyers DA, Kagey-Sobotka A, Plaut M, Norman PS, Lichtenstein LM. Inflammatory mediators in late antigen-induced rhinitis. N Engl J Med 313:65–70, 1985.

30. Gleich GJ. The late phase of the immunoglobulin E-mediated reaction: a link between anaphylaxis and common allergic disease? J Allergy Clin Immunol 70:160–169, 1982.

31. Valentine MD, Norman PS, Lichtenstein LM. Evaluation of an antihistamine in ragweed hay fever. In: McMahon FG, ed. Principles and Techniques of Human Research Therapeutics, vol 9. New York: Futura Publishing Company, 1974, pp 227–237.

32. Douglas WW. Histamine and antihistamines. In: Goodman LS, Gilman A, eds. The Pharmacological Basis of Therapeutics, ed 5. New York: Macmillan Publishing Co, 1975, pp 590–613.

33. Lichtenstein LM, Gillespie E. The effects of the H1 and H2 antihistamines on "allergic" histamine release and its inhibition by histamine. J Pharmacol Exp Ther 192:441–450, 1975.

34. Togias AG, Naclerio RM, Warner J, Proud D, Kagey-Sobotka A, Nimmagadda I, Norman PS, Lichtenstein LM. Demonstration of inhibition of mediator release from human mast cells by azatadine base. *In vivo* and *in vitro* evaluation. JAMA 255:225–229, 1986.

35. Perrson CGA. Overview of effects of theophylline. J Allergy Clin Immunol 78:780–786, 1986.

36. Naclerio RM, Bartenfelder D, Proud D, Togias AG, Meyers DA, Kagey-Sobotka A, Norman PS, Lichtenstein LM. Theophylline reduces histamine release during pollen-induced rhinitis. J Allergy Clin Immunol 78:874–876, 1986.

37. Pipkorn U, Granerus G, Proud D, Kagey-Sobotka A, Norman PS, Lichtenstein LM, Naclerio RM. The effect of a histamine synthesis inhibitor on the immediate nasal allergic reaction. Allergy 42:496–501, 1987.

38. Grönneberg R, Zetterström O. Inhibition of the late phase response to anti-IgE in humans by indomethacin. Allergy 40:36–41, 1985.

39. Schleimer RP. The mechanisms of antiinflammatory steroid action in allergic diseases. Annu Rev Pharmacol Toxicol 25:381–412, 1985.

40. Mygind N. Topical steroid treatment for allergic rhinitis and allied conditions. Clin Otolaryngol 7:343–348, 1982.

41. Pipkorn U, Proud D, Lichtenstein LM, Schleimer RP, Peters SP, Adkinson NF Jr, Kagey-Sobotka A, Norman PS, Naclerio RM. Effect of short term systemic glucocorticosteroid treatment on human nasal mediator release after antigen challenge. J Clin Invest 80:957–961, 1987.

42. Bascom R, Pipkorn U, Lichtenstein L, Naclerio RM. The influx of inflammatory cells into nasal washings during the late response to nasal antigen challenge: effect of systemic steroid pretreatment. Am Rev Respir Dis 138:406–412, 1988.

43. Bascom R, Wachs M, Naclerio RM, Pipkorn U, Galli SJ, Lichtenstein LM. Basophil influx occurs after nasal antigen

challenge: effects of topical corticosteroid pretreatment. J Allergy Clin Immunol 81:580–589, 1988.

44. Schleimer RP, Schulman ES, MacGlashan DW Jr, Peters SP, Hayes EC, Adams GK III, Lichtenstein LM, Adkinson NF Jr. Effects of dexamethasone on mediator release from human lung fragments and purified human lung mast cells. J Clin Invest 71:1830–1835, 1983.

45. Schleimer RP, Lichtenstein LM, Gillespie E. Inhibition of basophil histamine release by anti-inflammatory steroids. Nature 292:454–455, 1981.

46. Connell JT. Quantitative intranasal pollen challenges. III. The priming effect in allergic rhinitis. J Allergy 43:33–38, 1969.

47. Pipkorn U, Proud D, Lichtenstein LM, Kagey-Sobotka A, Norman PS, Naclerio RM. Inhibition of mediator release in allergic rhinitis by pretreatment with topical glucocorticosteroids. N Engl J Med 316:1506–1510, 1987.

48. Secher C, Kirkegaard J, Borum P, Maansson A, Osterhammel P, Mygind N. Significance of H_1 and H_2 receptors in the human nose: rationale for topical use of combined antihistamine preparations. J Allergy Clin Immunol 70:211–218, 1982.

49. Bisgaard H, Olsson P, Bende M. Effect of leukotriene D_4 on nasal mucosal blood flow, nasal airway resistance and nasal secretion in humans. Clin Allergy 16:289–297, 1986.

50. Miadonna A, Tedeschi A, Leggieri E, Lorini M, Folco G, Sala A, Qualizza R, Froldi M, Zanussi C. Behavior and clinical relevance of histamine and leukotrienes C_4 and B_4 in grass pollen-induced rhinitis. Am Rev Respir Dis 136:357–362, 1987.

51. Proud D, Reynolds CJ, LaCapra S, Kagey-Sobotka A, Lichtenstein LM, Naclerio RM. Nasal provocation with bradykinin induces symptoms of rhinitis and a sore throat. Am Rev Respir Dis 137:613–616, 1988.

52. Druce HM, Bonner RF, Patow C, Choo P, Summers RJ, Kaliner MA. Response of nasal blood flow to neurohormones as measured by laser-Doppler velocimetry. J Appl Physiol 57:1276–1283, 1984.

53. Bende M, Flisberg K, Larsson I, Ohlin P, Olsson P. A method for determination of blood flow with ^{133}Xe in human nasal mucosa. Acta Otolaryngol 96:277–285, 1983.

54. Boucher RC, Pare PD, Gilmore NJ, Moroz LA, Hogg JC. Airway mucosal permeability in the *Ascaris suum*-sensitive rhesus monkey. J Allergy Clin Immunol 60:134–140, 1977.

55. Bisgaard H, Krogsgaard OW, Mygind N. Measurement secretions in nasal lavage. Clin Sci 73:217–222, 1987. □

Chapter IV

In vitro Detection and Quantitation of IgE Antibodies

Joel K. Weltman, M.D., Ph.D.

ABSTRACT

Measurement of total and allergen-specific IgE antibodies helps to identify atopic individuals and to pinpoint allergens which may be provoking symptoms. Solid-phase radio-immunoassays possess the requisite sensitivity for detection of IgE antibodies at the subnanogram level. Enzyme-immunoassays can be as sensitive as their corresponding radio-immunoassay, but avoid the use of unstable and dangerous radio-isotopes. Results of immunoassays for allergen-specific IgE antibodies in serum correlate with clinical history, skin tests, bronchial provocation and nasal provocation.

Antibodies of IgE isotype are the major immunological mediators of allergic inflammation.[1] Mast cells and basophils possess plasma membrane receptors for the Fc regions of IgE molecules. Cross-linking or polymerization of membrane-bound IgE causes exocytosis of granules and release of the pharmacologically active chemical mediators of allergic inflammation.[2] Cross-linking of membrane IgE may be induced by allergen with two or more antigenic sites per allergen molecule. The equilibrium concentration of cross-linked membrane IgE and the probability of degranulation are a function of concentrations of serum total IgE and of specific IgE antibody. The IgE in plasma and other extracellular

Clinical Associate Professor of Medicine.
Division of BioMedical Sciences.
Brown University,
Providence, RI 02912

fluids is in equilibrium with IgE non-covalently bound to receptors on the plasma membranes of basophils and mast cells. Expression of allergic inflammation is regulated by the quantitative relationships between total and allergen-specific IgE, and membrane IgE-Fc receptors.[3] It has been reported that the binding constant of the membrane receptor for IgE-Fc is higher in allergic than in non-allergic individuals,[4] providing yet another mechanism for regulation of allergy. Synthesis of IgE and of IgE-Fc receptor (CD23) is regulated by IL-4.[5,6]

Measurement of total and allergen-specific IgE concentration in the blood yields clinically useful data. A significantly elevated total IgE concentration is associated with atopy.[7,8] Furthermore, elevated allergen-specific IgE can help to identify allergens which are provoking allergic symptoms in a particular case. The clinical expression of asthma may be directly correlated with antibodies of IgE isotype.[9b] The serum of patients with food-related hypersensitivity has been reported to contain a special form of IgE, called IgE+, which sensitizes basophils to a histamine-releasing factor produced by mononuclear leukocytes.[10,11] Immunoglobulins of IgE isotype comprise less than 0.01% of the total immunoglobulin concentration of the blood. For this reason, sensitive methods are needed to detect and quantitate IgE. Radio-immunoassay and enzyme-immunoassay techniques possess the requisite sensitivity. Solid phase immunosorbents facilitate separation of bound from unbound reagents. Practicable solid phase radio-immunoassays[12] and enzyme-immunoassays[8] have been reported for detecting total and specific IgE, and versions of these are now available commercially.

Solid-phase immunoassay of IgE is outlined in Figure 1. For detection of serum total IgE, the solid phase immunosorbent is insolubilized anti-IgE. For detection

Figure 1.

SOLID-PHASE IMMUNOASSAY OF IgE

Solid Phase Immunosorbent	+	IgE	<=======>	Adsorbed IgE	(Step 1)
Wash Immunosorbent to remove Unadsorbed IgE					(Step 2)
Adsorbed IgE	+	Labelled anti-IgE	<=======>	Adsorbed Labelled anti-IgE	(Step 3)
Wash Immunosorbent to remove Unadsorbed Labelled anti-IgE					(Step 4)
Assay Immunosorbent for Adsorbed Label					(Step 5)

of allergen-specific IgE antibodies, the solid phase immunosorbent is insolubilized allergen. The label used to tag the anti-IgE is either radioactive iodine, as in the RAST,[7] or galactosidase, as in the GIST.[13]

Enzyme immunoassays, such as the GIST, are as sensitive as their counterpart radio-immunoassays, but avoid the use of unstable and dangerous radioisotopes. Enzyme-immunoassays are simple to perform and yield colored products which are even visually detectable. Enzyme-immunoassays for IgE, therefore, can be office procedures.

The solid-phase immunoassays for total and allergen-specific IgE possess the requisite sensitivity for detection of IgE antibodies at the subnanogram level. The use of monoclonal anti-IgE antibodies may extend the sensitivity even further.

Solid phase enzyme and radio-immunoassays for total and allergen-specific IgE yield useful data which aid in diagnosis and which help guide clinical decision-making.[14] Application of Bayes' Theorem may strengthen this decision-making.[15] Results of immunoassays for allergen-specific IgE antibodies in serum correlate with clinical history,[16,17] with skin tests,[16-18] with bronchial provocation tests[19] and with nasal provocation tests.[20] However, for routine allergy practice, *in vivo* scratch and intradermal skin tests are simple, sensitive, rapid, less expensive, and clinically valid tools. Nevertheless, there are special situations in which *in vitro* solid phase immunoassays for IgE may be preferable to skin tests. These special situations include: skin rashes, life threatening allergic symptoms and unreactive skin.

REFERENCES

1. Ishizaka K, Ishizaka T. Identification of IgE antibodies as a carrier of reaginic activity. J Immunol 99:1187–1198, 1967.
2. Siraganian RP, Hook WA, Levine BB. Specific *in vitro* histamine release from basophils by bivalent haptens: Evidence for activation by simple bridging of membrane bound antibody. Immunochem 12:149–157, 1975.
3. Weltman JK, Senft AW. An analysis of allergy. Immunoglobulin E and diagnostic skin tests in schistosomiasis. Parasit Immunol 3:157–163, 1981.
4. Malveaux FJ, Bui-Tran MT, Herry VE. Correlation of serum IgE, association constant, and IgE receptors on human basophils in allergic and non-allergic donors. J Allergy Clin Immunol Suppl Abstr 69:33, 1982.
5. Mizel SB. The interleukins. FASEB J 3:2379–2388, 1989.
6. Paul WE, Ohara J. B-cell stimulating factor-1/interleukin 4. Annu Rev Immunol 5:429–460, 1987.
7. Johansson SGO. Serum IgND levels in healthy children and adults. Int Arch Allergy Appl Immunol 34:1–8, 1968.
8. Gleich GJ, Averback AK, Swedlund HA. Measurement of IgE in normal and allergic serum by radio-immunoassay. J Lab Clin Med 77:690–698, 1971.
9. Burrows B, Martinez FD, Halonen M, Barbee RA, Cline MG. Association of asthma with serum IgE levels and skin-test reactivity to allergens. N Engl J Med 320:271–277, 1989.
10. Sampson HA, Broadbent KR, Bernhisel-Broadbent J. Spontaneous release of histamine from basophils and histamine-releasing factor in patients with atopic dermatitis and food hypersensitivity. N Engl J Med 321:228–323, 1989.
11. Metcalfe DD. Diseases of food hypersensitivity. N Engl J Med 321:255–257, 1989.
12. Wide L, Bennich H, Johansson SGO. Diagnosis of allergy by an *in vitro* test for allergen antibodies. Lancet ii:1105–1107, 1967.
13. Weltman JK, Frackelton AR, Jr., Szaro RP, Rotman B. A Galactosidase Immunosorbent Test (GIST) for human Immunoglobulin E. J Allergy Clin Immunol 58:426–431, 1976.
14. Hamburger RN. A cautious view of the use of RAST in clinical allergy. Immunology and Allergy Practice 3:10–16, 1981.
15. Weltman JK. Laboratory tests for total and allergen-specific immunoglobulin E. N Engl Reg Allergy Proc 9:129–133, 1988.
16. Stenius B, Wide L, Seymour WM, Holford-Stevens V, Pepys J. Clinical significance of specific IgE to common allergens. Clin Allergy 1:37–55, 1971.
17. Aas K, Johansson SGO. The Radioallergosorbent Test

(RAST) in the *in vitro* diagnosis of reaginic allergy. A comparison of diagnostic approaches. J Allergy Clin Immunol 48:134–141, 1971.

18. Norman PS, Lichtenstein LM, Ishizaka K. Diagnostic tests in ragweed hayfever: a comparison of direct skin tests. IgE antibody measurements, and basophil histamine release. J Allergy Clin Immunol 52:210–224, 1973.

19. Berg T, Bennich H, Johansson SGO. *In vitro* diagnosis of atopic allergy. 1. A comparison between provocation tests and the Radioallergosorbent Test (RAST). Int Arch Allergy Appl Immunol 40:770–778, 1971.

20. Hunt KJ, Valentine MD, Sobotka AK, Lichtenstein LM. Diagnosis of allergy to stinging insects by skin testing with Hymenoptera venoms. Ann Int Med 85:56–59, 1976.

Chapter V

Atmospheric Pollen and Fungi

Jack E. Farnham, M.D.

ABSTRACT

This chapter deals with the atmosphere, aeroallergens within it, and factors influencing these. An overview of current sampling techniques is presented, and current aeroallergen networks are described briefly. Discussion of pollen grains, their interrelationships, and dynamics is presented along with an outline of geographic differences in several areas of the world. The most common fungal spores, diseases associated with them, and methods of collection are discussed. The difference between indoor and outdoor spores and a comparison of allergenicity to spore prevalence is reviewed. A brief discussion of indoor air contamination by microbiological agents is presented.

Any discussion of the study of airborne particles such as pollen and fungal spores must take into account the atmosphere surrounding the earth. Into this envelope of water vapor and gases that is essential for the stability of the earth's ecosystem, the pollen and fungal spores are released, transported, and become interactive with human life.

For our purpose, the most important atmospheric layers are (1) the trophosphere, from the earth's surface to a height of 11 Km, (36,000 feet) and (2) the stratosphere from 11 Km height up to 80 Km (260,000 feet).[1] The trophosphere, particularly the micro climate (3 meters above the surface), is where most human and aerobiologic activity occurs and where weather factors such as moisture, wind, temperature, and electrostatic charges have the greatest effect on terrestrial plants and animals, including man.[2] The stratosphere, with its jet streams, has a dampening effect on the oftimes violent activity of the trophosphere. Some aerobiologic particles have been recovered from the lower stratosphere;

Allergy Immunology Associates, Chelmsford, MA. Clinical Associate, Allergy & Clinical Immunology Unit, Massachusetts General Hospital

the upper reaches of the stratosphere contain the ozone layer.

Since time immemorial the atmosphere of the earth has never been clear of particles, water vapor, or gaseous matter. Even before manmade pollutants and the ozone paradox (too much in the trophosphere and too little in the stratosphere), the natural ecological cycle allowed continuous discharge of viable and nonviable materials into the atmosphere, some highly reactive and some relatively inert. Aerobiology is the study of the formation, transmission, and fate of atmospheric biological materials.

Inhalation of these materials by air-breathing creatures may cause either no reaction or a whole gamut of changes ranging from minor irritation of the respiratory tract to overwhelming inflammation and mortality; in humans, hypersensitivity, infection, or toxicity may result. It is primarily with the hypersensitivity reactions that the study of allergy concerns itself, even though infections and toxicity may coincidentally occur in allergic individuals.

ATMOSPHERIC CONTAMINANTS

Many contaminants, almost all invisible to the naked eye, are present in the air even on a pristine day. Fluctuations occur, depending on weather factors, seasonal variations, botanical cycles, and, at times, human activity. Some of the more important contaminants are listed in Table I. These components are innocuous to most people, but may be irritating to many, antigenic to some, and allergenic to a significant percentage. Reactions may occur when a susceptible individual is exposed to a critical concentration for a sufficient period of time. These aeroallergens, which may be viable or nonviable, can be identified by means of microscopy, culture, and immunoassay.

The remainder of this chapter deals with atmospheric pollen and fungi that comprise the major antigens responsible for allergic rhinitis (along with dust mite and animal dander).

TABLE I

Atmospheric Contaminants

1. Particulate, fixed structure
   a. pollens
   b. fungus spores and algae
   c. animal products
   d. insect products
   e. vegetable products
   f. bacteria and viruses
2. Particulate, changeable structures
   a. dust
   b. solid crystals
3. Amorphous
   a. gases
   b. liquids

ATMOSPHERIC FACTORS

The circulation of atmospheric contaminants is purely passive; that is, it is influenced by factors completely unrelated to the materials in question such as physical factors, insects, and human activity. Of the several known influencing factors, six are of upmost importance: moisture, wind, temperature, sunlight, particle size, and electrostatic force (see Table II).

Of all the influencing factors, moisture in the form of relative humidity, dew, fog, or rain is the most critical. The anthers of oak trees remain closed if the relative humidity is over 45% at the time of pollination,[3] likewise, ragweed anthers remain closed if relative humidity is above 80%.[4] Generally, increasing moisture will lower airborne pollen and fungal contamination (except for some fungi such as *Ascomycetes*, which only ejaculate spores in the presence of free water). The finer the moisture, the greater the dampening effect (e.g. fog versus thunderstorms). Splash effect and convection currents associated with downpours may at times increase the concentration of aeroallergens.

Because most pollen and fungal spores are windborne (anemophilous), wind speeds of over 4 meters per second will lift the particles free of deposited surfaces; at 10–20 meters per second wind speed, there is no lag at

TABLE II

Factors Influencing Aeroallergens

1. Moisture
2. Wind
3. Temperature
4. Sunlight
5. Particle size
6. Electrostatic forces

all from anther release to the airborne state.[5] Studies have shown that not all pollen from a source becomes airborne: even under ideal conditions only 6% of the pollen in a ragweed stand became entrained in the air in the Sheldon and Hewson study.[4]

Nighttime low temperature is an extremely important factor affecting the following day's pollen release. All other factors being equal, oak anthers remained closed the following morning if night low is below 10° C (50° F),[3] and ragweed anthers remain closed if the previous night's low is less than 4° C (39° F). Generally, the subsequent day's high must rise above 24° C (75° F) for ragweed anthers to open.[4]

Sunlight, more importantly the angle of the sun and the length of daylight (actually the length of the night) is extremely important in influencing the time of pollination. Experiments with light have shown that altering the length of light exposure will determine whether ragweed anthers will release pollen before or after the plant's usual pollination date.[5]

Particle size, especially the square of the diameter, determines the falling velocity, even in turbulent air. This influences the collection frequency of both pollen and fungal spores. Entrained particles tend to drop out of an air stream in a direct relationship to their size: the large drop earliest and smallest much later.[6]

Inasmuch as all pollen and fungal spores are electrically charged, ambient electrostatic forces will attract or repel these particles to or from objects and humans. Benninghoff's[7] and Corbet's[8] studies and our Alpine Slide hypothesis[9] suggest the electrostatic forces have strong influences.

SAMPLING TECHNIQUES, AN OVERVIEW

As soon as it was realized that particulate matter was present in the atmosphere, attempts were made to capture, identify, and count the material. As early as 1776 Spallanzani was able to capture and identify airborne particles; subsequently Pasteur, Tyndell, Miguel, and others carried out original observations with volumetric samplers in the mid 1800s. No practical method was described until Blackley carried out his work in 1865,[10] and this afforded the means of qualitatively analyzing the fallout.

By 1946 Durham systematically collected and identified pollen, using a device that prevented vertical fallout and allowed linear deposition of particles on glass microslides but that still was not capable of measuring the volume of air sampled.[11] In the 1970s, a practical rotating arm impactor was developed, allowing volumetric assessment (particles per cubic meter).[12] Subsequently, a whole new technology of sampling devices was developed.

Basically, all sampling devices rely on the fallout velocity of the airborne particle that, in turn, is related to its size, weight, and shape. In addition, all devices must enable the investigator to recognize the particle based on microscopic morphology, culture characteristics, or immunologic properties. Table III shows a brief listing of important sampling techniques.

Historically (and probably the most widely used standard gravimetric fallout collector from 1950 to 1980) was the Durham sampler that consisted of a collecting surface mounted one inch above a nine-inch circular disk floor with a similar disk as a roof three inches above. Horizontal air flow through the collector allowed particulate matter to fall out on a greased micro slide or culture plate. The advantages were its economy in cost and maintenance, ease of operation, and lack of dependence on an external power source. The disadvantages were the inability to determine the volume of air sampled, low catch (particularly small particles), and dependence on wind speed, orientation, and turbulence. Its usefulness was limited to determining aeroallergen qualitative trends.

Since 1980, the use of volumetric impaction samplers has become widespread, and it is considered one of the accepted methods of aeroallergen sampling by the Aerobiology Committee of the American Academy of Allergy and Clinical Immunology.

The intermittent rotating arm impaction sampler is based on the principle of moving an adhesive-coated surface rapidly through an arc of known diameter at a known speed. Examples of this are the rotorod, rotobar, rotoslide, and rotodisc. The Intermittent Retracting Head Rotorod, now available commercially, is in widespread use. Advantages are that it is independent of wind, the volume of air sampled can be calculated, it enables a high catch for large particles (may miss small

---

TABLE III

Aerobiological Sampling Techniques

1. Gravitational fallout
   a. particulate
   b. viable
2. Volumetric impactors
   a. rotating arm
   b. suction type
      1. particulate
      2. viable
      3. filtration
3. Volumetric impinger
   a. suction into liquid
   b. suction unto surface
4. Immunoassay by impactor or impinger
   a. Histamine release
   b. RAST inhibition
   c. radioimmunoassay (RIA)
   d. enzyme linked immunoassay (ELISA)

---

ones), and the collecting surface (lucite rod) may be intermittently shielded. Disadvantages are greater cost and maintenance than the gravitational samplers, external power source needed (although new portable models are battery operated) and special apparatus needed for microscopy. In addition, once stained, the rotorods are not easily preserved for future reference. Information and equipment may be obtained from Sampling Technologies, Inc., 26338 Esparanza Drive, Los Altos Hills, CA 94022.

There are several suction type volumetric impactors in use, all based on the principle that a known volume of air is drawn across the collecting membrane (coated adhesive tape, micro slide, or a culture media) to allow deposition of particles on the collecting surface.

Particulate matter may be collected by the Burkard modification of the Hirst spore trap in which a steady flow of air is drawn across an adhesive coated tape slowly rotating on a horizontal drum behind the slit orifice. Outdoor, indoor, and personal modifications of this device are available. A recent modification also makes viable material collection possible with a Burkard sampler. Advantages are that a known volume of air is sampled, continuous hourly record is available, and easy storage of micro slide or tape is possible. Disadvantages are its cost, external power source and suction required, no accessible North American service available, and necessity to orient the device to the wind source in the outdoor type. Information and equipment may be obtained from the Burkard Manufacturing Co, Ltd, Woodcock Hill Industrial Estate, Richmansworth, Hertfordshire, England WD3 IPJ.

Viable material may be collected by Bourdillon slit sampler or the Anderson Cascade sieve sampler. In the former, air is pulled through a slit onto the culture medium in a plate slowly rotating under the orifice; in the Anderson Cascade sampler, the air stream is drawn through successive stages (usually 2 to 6) that contain sieves of smaller and smaller orifices as the lower stage is reached. Large particles fall out of the top, the smaller particles are entrained in the airflow and are deposited in the lower stages, each passing through the sieve to the culture medium in plates below. The Bourdillon collector allows one to determine time differentials in maximum deposition of viable particles; the Anderson sampler allows size differentiation, separating respirable (under 5 micron) from nonrespirable (over 5 micron) particles. Disadvantages of both are the cost, specialized growth media plates required, and the necessity for external power and a source of suction. Information and equipment may be obtained from Anderson Samplers, Inc., 45 Wendall Ave, Atlanta, GA 30336.

Filtration suction impactors work on the principle of pulling air at a steady rate through filters of various materials and porosity. Either particulate or viable materials entrapped in the filter can be analyzed directly or washed off, concentrated by centrifugation, and examined microscopically or by culture. Advantages are ease of handling the filter cassettes and the machine's ability to handle large numbers of particulate material without overload. Disadvantages are the special disposable filters, equipment, and wash material needed. Information and equipment may be obtained from E.I. DuPont deNemours & Company, Wilmington, DE., 19898 and Nuclcopore Corp, 7035 Commerce Circle, Pleasanton, CA 94506-3294.

Volumetric impinges of the all-glass type draw air through a cascade of tubes of diminishing sized orifices, directing particles into a collecting fluid, depending upon size. The collecting fluid is then removed and evaluated by microscope, culture, or immunoassay. This type collector is used primarily for indoor air studies, especially immunoassays. Information and equipment may be obtained from Ace Glass, Vineland, NJ.

Because some aeroallergens (dust mite, animal dander, and urine) are in a nonviable form or are submicronic, nondescript fragments, other means of collecting are needed for identification. Within the past ten years, the development of practical immunoassay techniques has made identification of this type of aeroallergen possible. In principle, atmospheric material is collected by cascade impactors onto a solid medium or by liquid impingers into a solute, then analyzed by immunochemical means. Several assays have been developed to measure total antigen load by histamine release or RAST inhibition. Single antigens can be detected by radioimmunoassay (RIA) or enzyme-linked immunoassay (ELISA) using monoclonal antibodies.

It is beyond the scope of this chapter to address the various sampling techniques in detail. The interested reader is referred to articles by Muhlenberg[13] and Platts-Mills[14] for a definitive discussion of this topic.

POLLEN AEROALLERGENS AND INTERRELATIONS

Pollen grains are the male gamete of plants containing the haploid number of chromosomes. The pollen grains are able to form seeds only by fertilizing the ovum. The size of pollen grains may vary from 2 to 250 μm, but most antigenic pollen is in the 6 to 40 μm range. Pollen grains may be disseminated by wind (anemophilous), insects (entomophilous), or both (amphiphilous). Most allergenic pollen is wind transmitted, usually being carried a few hundred meters but occasionally 30 to 60 Km or more. All pollen has three coats: exine, intine, and protoplast (see Figure I). The exine, the outermost layer, can resist heat to 500° F., is a hard polymer (sporopollenin) with many furrows, pores, or sculptured features. Most of the pollen allergens are located in this layer. The intine layer, immediately in contact with the inner surface of the exine, is mostly composed of cellulose; however, it may contribute somewhat to the antigenicity of the pollen. The innermost layer (protoplast) contains starch and genetic material and is believed not to contribute much to the allergenicity of the pollen grain.

Usually pollen is only viable (able to extend a ger-

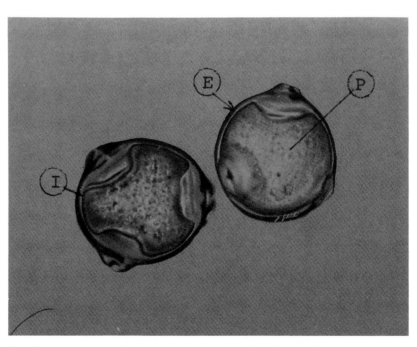

Figure 1. Birch pollen (27 micron) showing exine (E), intine (I) and protoplast (P). Courtesy Hollister-Stier.

minal tube) for a few hours or days after being released from the pollen anther. Optimum ragweed germination occurs two hours after release,[15] pine within three hours, and maple within eight hours.[16] It is believed the antigenicity residing in the exine long outlasts the viability of the pollen grain, but the exact duration of the antigenicity has not been determined.

Pollen antigens are small proteins (10,000–40,000 daltons) that are rapidly eluted from the exine onto human mucous membranes. Within minutes the mast cells in the mucosa of IgE sensitized people will release histamine and other vasoactive and smooth muscle active components in response to this antigen-antibody reaction. The antigenic material in the intine is slowly released through the pores of the exine.

The intensity of the allergenicity varies with the species of the pollen. In New England, birch, oak, and maple are the most potent tree pollens, and ragweed is the most potent weed pollen, based on skin reactivity. Concentrations of the pollen at the time of exposure may have great influence on the severity of the patient's symptoms.

Threshold levels above which symptoms of pollenosis occur undoubtedly exist for all allergenic pollens, but very few have been determined. Davies and Smith found that grass pollen levels of 50 gr/M³ elicited symptoms in virtually all of their grass-sensitive patients.[17] Studies with ragweed pollen have shown thresholds ranging from 50–800 gr/M³.[18] Comtois and Gag-

non have determined that 8–23 gr/M³ of tree pollen and 4–12 gr/M³ of grass pollen can cause symptoms in allergic patients.[19] "Priming," the condition of continued or exacerbated pollinosis symptoms upon exposure to lower and lower concentrations of airborne pollen, has been demonstrated for ragweed exposure[20] and probably exists with other pollens as well. Because of this, absolute threshold levels may vary considerably from time to time.

CROSS-REACTIVITY

The fact that plants and the pollen produced by them have antigens is not surprising. The amazing thing is that so many of these morphologically different plants are phylogenetically related (Figure II) and may have identical or very similar antigenic structure. Some of these antigens can be allergenic to susceptible individuals. Because of cross-reactivity, pollen from a related species may cause allergic reactions in people known to be sensitized to a completely different pollen (e.g. birch pollen producing symptoms in a known oak-sensitive patient).

Pollen total cross-antigenicity can be measured by using animal antisera in gel diffusion and hemagglutination techniques and crossed immunoelectrophoresis (CIE). Cross-allergenicity (which demonstrates IgE) can be measured by comparative skin testing, RAST inhibition, and a crossed radioimmunoelectrophoresis (CRIE) and P-K neutralization.[21]

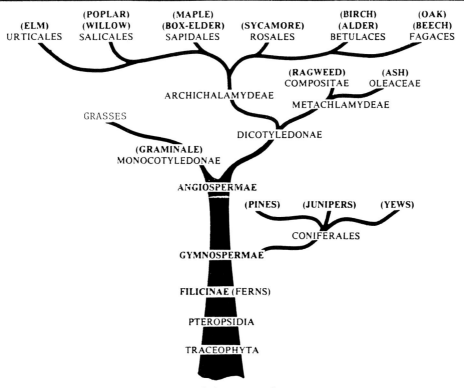

Figure 2. Phylogenetic schema.

Generally, the more primitive the botanical class, the less allergenic the pollen will be to humans. For instance, fern spores from the ancient class *Filicinae* have shown no skin test reactivity in our series, although Geller-Bernstein[22] has proposed such reactivity. Eastern white pine (class *Gymnospermae*) shows less skin test reactivity than trees such as birch in the more advanced *Angiosperm* class.

Generally, there is no cross-reactivity between the three major classes of allergenic plants; that is, class *Filicinae* (ferns), class *Gymnospermae* (conifers) and class *Angiospermae* (flowering plants), although cross-reactivity does occur between species within each genus.

Within the class Conifer, plants within the Cupressaceae (cyprus, juniper, and cedar) all demonstrate allergenicity. Cross-reactivity between species in these genuses has been reported. Dirksen and Osterballe[23] found no skin test association between juniper and pine or spruce. Our own skin test results showed no correlation between juniper and Eastern white pine.[24]

Several angiosperm tree pollens, particularly in the orders Fegales (oak and beech) and Betulales (birch and alder) demonstrate strong allergenicity and strong cross-reactivity. For correlations, RAST testing and PK-neutralization studies from many investigators have shown there is strong cross-reactivity within and between these orders. PK-neutralization studies by Rackemann and Wagner show complete cross desensitization by birch antigen to oak, maple, and willow.[25] This appeared to show that birch contains all the major allergens of oak, maple, and willow and one unique allergen of its own, inasmuch as the other three antigens were not able to completely desensitize birch. Maple appeared to have the fewest shared allergens of the four trees.

In the order Salicales (containing poplar, aspen, and willow), strong cross-reactivity among these three trees and moderate cross-reactivity to oak and beech (order Fegales) has been shown.[26] In 1981, our evaluation of 2,000 patients by prick skin testing demonstrated a strong cross-reactivity between oak, beech, and birch and also a separate strong cross-reactivity between willow and poplar.[27]

Within the grass (Poaceae) family are five subfamilies of differing allergenic potency that show some, but not intense, cross-reactivity. The subfamily Festucoidae constitutes the common grasses of Canada, Northern United States, and Europe (timothy, blue grass, fescue, rye, orchard, brome, sweet vernal, and red top). Members of this group show intense cross-reactivity with each other but only variable cross-reactivity with other subfamilies. Subfamily Eragrostoideae contains Bermuda grass, a strong allergen in the southern United States and other warm-weather areas. This does not cross-react generally with the Festucoids. Subfamily Panicoideae contains Bahia and Johnson grasses, which grow in the extremely limited areas of southern United States, are allergenic and show cross-reactivity with each other and some cross-reactivity with members of the Festucoid and Eragrostoid families. At present purified grass allergens have been studied for rye grass, timothy grass, blue grass (subfamily Festucoideae), and Bermuda grass (subfamily Eragrostoidae).

The allergenic weeds consist of a vast group of loosely related families. The family Chenopodiaceae contains lamb's quarters, Russian thistle, and the artiplex genus (wind scale, lens scale, and annual salt bush). The family Amaranthaceae contains the amaranths and pigweed. Both of these families are the source of much allergenic pollen production, particularly in the West. The family Polygonaceae contains sorrel and dock (both in the genus Rumex).

The Chenopods and Amaranth families are closely related; strong cross-reactivity exists especially between the Amaranth family and the atriplex genus (Chenopod family). Russian thistle seems to be the most important allergenic plant in these groups. Two allergens, 30,000 and 42,000 daltons, have been identified and appear to be identical by RAST inhibition.

The Compositae family of weeds consists of three tribes, Heliantheae (the sunflower group), the Anthemideae tribe which consists of mugwort (sage), and the Ambrosia tribe containing the ragweeds. Nine purified allergens have been isolated from the ragweeds, (short, tall, Western, and false). Antigen E (38,000 daltons) is the most important of the ragweed allergens. There is strong cross-reactivity and almost identical allergenicity between short, tall, Western, and false ragweed. Ragweed cross-reacts with many other members of the Compositae family.

In view of cross-reactivity and shared antigens many observers have reported the association of oral and pharyngeal burning and irritation associated with ingestion of tree fruits (pears, peaches, and apples) in patients who are allergic to birch pollen. Similar symptoms have been reported in patients who are allergic to ragweed pollen upon ingestion of watermellon.

Because of cross-antigenicity present in many species of pollen, the possibility exists of administering a select number of antigens for immunotherapy (rather than a large number of individual antigens) that would afford adequate immunologic protection. Thus Timothy extract could protect against all the Festicoides, and birch could protect against oak, maple, willow. This requires further study.

For a more complete discussion of pollen allergens and cross reactivity, the reader is referred to the review article by Weber and Nelson.[21]

POLLEN DYNAMICS

Once pollen is released, its main purpose is to land on the stigma of a female plant of the appropriate species. On impact with the stigma, a chemical reaction occurs that stimulates protrusion of the germinal tube. The haploid number of cells travels down the germinal tube to reach the ovum in the female flower, thus assuring fertilization. If the pollen grain strikes a mucous membrane of a sensitized patient, the germinal tube is not extended, but antigen is extruded from the exine and intine.

From year to year, there is a predictable orderly succession of tree, grass, and weed pollen in the temperate climate (see Figure III), the only alterations being caused by unusual weather factors or plant pathology. In tropical areas, a more continuous pollen succession occurs, resulting in less variation in total pollen load seasonally. These variations will be discussed in the section on geography of pollen.

In addition to the annual seasonal cycles, there appears to be a diurnal cycle for each pollinating species. The dramatic effect of sunlight on anther release of pollen was demonstrated in our 1981 study of oak, birch, and ragweed pollen[27] and in our 1989 study of oak and birch pollen in northeastern Massachusetts. In both instances, there was an increased hourly pollen concentration of all species within 60 to 90 minutes following sunrise. In the case of tree pollen, the airborne concentration then declined for several hours, but in the case of ragweed, the concentration continued to rise to a peak within a few hours. Our studies have shown that ragweed pollen in the northeast peaks between 7 a.m. and 9 a.m., grass pollen peaking between early and late morning (although fescue may pollinate in the afternoon), and tree pollen peaking late morning and early afternoon.

By observing the influencing factors during the pollination seasons, in addition to data on the previous year's pollen cycles, we and others have proposed a working model for the prediction of severity and duration of ragweed[28] and oak pollen[29] concentrations. This theoretically can be transferred to other pollinating plants as well.

GEOGRAPHIC AEROALLERGEN NETWORKS

Since the late 1970s, individual isolated aerobiologic collection stations gradually have been augmented by network stations that cooperate by making concurrent collections and assessments over regional and national areas. Generally, all networks have established their own guidelines of standardized collecting methods, quality control, reporting protocol, and dissemination of information. The end result is uniform, scientifically accurate data.

Initially in the late 1950s through the 1960s, Agriculture Canada carried out a nationwide airborne pollen study in all Canadian provinces by means of gravity fallout collections.[30–34]

For over 20 years, the Aerobiology Committee of the American Academy of Allergy and Immunology has recorded data received from many American, Canadian, Latin American, European, and Asian collectors who use a variety of collecting devices. Since the late 1980s, a quality control certified aeroallergen network has been established. Sixty-nine stations are in this network, 24 of these stations have been certified, and all are using volumetric collecting devices—predominantly roto-rod samplers, although one station is using a Burkhard suction sampler. Quality control and data tabulation are done through the University of Michigan Allergy Research Laboratory.

Starting in 1981, the New England Society of Allergy operated a five-station rotorod collecting network with all samples sent by mail to one paleonologist for uniform counting. Subsequently, the number of collecting sites was increased to ten, scattered throughout the six New England states, with quality control and data tabulation done by the University of New Hampshire, Department of Plant Pathology.

Aerobiological data has been analyzed for allergenic taxa present and total allergenic load from station to station and year to year. In both United States networks, data is analyzed as received, but because of lack of computer and facsimile linkages, rapid sharing of the information between stations and to mass media has not been considered feasible or desirable.

In Europe, 21 countries joined in a working group to form the European Aeroallergen Network (EAN) in late 1986. At present, this group is compiling regional and national pollen calendars. Among 21 countries in the network, there is a vast range in the number of stations from one in some countries to as many as 63 in the Italian Allergenic Pollen Monitoring Network. This network is perhaps the most ambitious of all of the European countries and consists of a large number of collecting stations, using Hirst type samplers and transmitting data by phone to regional and central recording stations for entry into the pollen data bank. Information is released weekly to mass media and to the European Aeroallergen Server Network for the central data bank in Vienna, Austria. At present, the EAN is working to determine the most important allergenic pollen-producing plants and the most prevalent skin test reactions at various centers. This will enable some assessment of true allergenicity to be made.

GEOGRAPHIC POLLEN DIFFERENCES

Airborne pollen varies in taxa and concentration throughout the world, depending on regional weather, topography and botanical species present. Because of this there can be no uniform, worldwide pattern, but instead one must rely on regional assessments to determine the significant pollens. Not only is it important for the allergist to recognize the botanical allergenic plants in his/her area but also he/she should be familiar with some of the most common pollen grains. The following brief overview of the major regional pollens includes some comments about allergenicity.

The United States can be subdivided arbitrarily into seven geographical regions for purposes of this discussion: 1. The Northeast (Connecticut, Delaware, Maine, Maryland, Massachusetts, New Hampshire, New Jersey, New York, Pennsylvania, Rhode Island, Vermont). 2. Southeast (Alabama, Florida, Georgia, Louisiana, Mississippi, North Carolina, South Carolina, Tennessee, Virginia, and West Virginia). 3. The Midwest (Illinois, Indiana, Kentucky, Michigan, Ohio, and Wisconsin). 4. The North Central (Iowa, Minnesota, Nebraska, North Dakota, and South Dakota). 5. The South Central (Arkansas, Kansas, Missouri, Oklahoma, and Texas). 6. The Mountain States (Arizona, Colorado, Idaho, Montana, Nevada, New Mexico, Utah and Wyoming). 7. West Coast (California, Oregon, and Washington).

The Northeast and Midwest

Generally, in the Northeast and Midwest, an orderly progression of trees, grass, and weed pollens starts in late March or early April and lasts until early to mid-October, usually becoming minimal before frost appears. The earliest tree pollen to appear, even before snow is completely gone in the northern areas, is that of the Cupressaceae family (probably juniper species) by mid-March. This is followed (in New England at least) by rapid overlap of willow, elm, cottonwood, then maple peaking by mid-April, followed by birch species

early in May, ash, and then massive oak species pollination by late May. By far and away the heaviest pollinator, eastern white pine (Pinus Strobus) releases its pollen in late May and early June.

Many of these highly antigenic trees pollinate in overlapping cycles resulting in the presence of several different types of airborne pollen simultaneously. This demonstrates the concept of total pollen load in which the additive effects of several individual antigens can lead to clinical symptoms not caused by any of the individual pollens. This is especially important in view of the fact that multiple sensitivities are common in tree allergic patients.

In New England, the heaviest tree pollinators are oak (Quercus), ash (Fraxinus), pine (Pinus), birch (Betula), juniper (Juniperus), cottonwood (Populus), maple (Acer), alder (Alnus), willow (Salix), and beech (Fagus) (Figure 3). The five most allergenic, based on skin prick testing of over 2,000 patients, are birch, oak, beech, maple, and ash (Table IV).[35] Although among the heaviest pollinators, the conifers, (juniper and pine) do not cause a significant clinical allergenic response. Our interest in Eastern white pine (Pinus Strobus) allergy arose when many patients complained they were allergic to pine pollen and demonstrated rhinitis symptoms coincident with pine pollination. Until then all formal teaching stressed that pine was nonallergic because of its waxy coat and huge size (100 micron). We skin tested 2,067 patients by prick (and, if negative, by intradermal) methods to Pinus Strobus; 201 (9.7%) reacted positively by prick test and 256 (12.4%) by

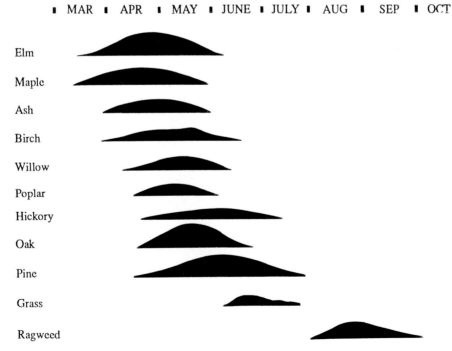

Figure 3. New England major pollen seasons. Length of line corresponds to length of pollen season. Height of hump corresponds to approximate concentration of pollen in atmosphere.

TABLE IV

Prevalence of New England Tree Pollen and Skin Tests

Top Ten Trees (1982–87)	Prick Test (2,067 pts)	
Pine (Pinus)	Birch	31.1%
Oak (Quercus)	Oak	28.5%
Birch (Betula)	Beech	25.2%
Ash (Fraxinus)	Maple	22.3%
Juniper (Juniperus)	Ash	21.6%
Cottonwood (Populus)	Willow	21.1%
Maple (Acer)	Hickory	18.8%
Alder (Alnus)	Elm	13.6%
Willow (Salix)	Cottonwood	11.6%
Beech (Fagus)	Pine	9.7%

intradermal for a total of 22.1% positive reactions. To eliminate the possibility of false-positive reactions based on irritation, we discarded all intradermal tests, leaving only the prick test reactors as truly positive. This still revealed a significantly higher reaction rate (9.7%) than demonstrated in other studies. Coincident with this, Kalliel and Settipane found that nasal challenge with Eastern white pine was able to induce pollinosis symptoms.[36] Our present explanation for that is that a large population is exposed to the massive pollination of Eastern white pine in the New England area each June, thus increasing the potential for sensitization of a significant segment of atopics.

In the northern Northeast, the grasses (mainly in the subfamily Festucoidae) consist mostly of timothy (Phleum), blue grass (Poa), orchard grass (Dactylis), fescue (Festuca), rye grass (Lolium), red top (Agrostis), sweet vernal (Anthoxanthum), and brome grass (Bromus). The grasses form a background of relatively low airborne pollen but do show peaks in July. It is difficult to differentiate the grass pollen grains morphologically, but it is assumed that the peaks represent different grass species. In the Midwest, grass pollen reaches much higher concentrations than in the Northeast and can be a significant allergenic problem.

The significant allergenic weed pollens are English plantain (Plantago) May through August, ragweed (Ambrosia) and mugwort (Artemesia) mid-August to late September. At times, mugwort pollen counts are higher than ragweed in New England. Secondary pollinators are sorrel-dock (Rumex) in June and July, lamb's quarters (Chenopodium), cocklebur (Xanthium), pigweed (Amaranthus) in mid-August through late September. As with grass pollen, the northern Northeast has much lower ragweed counts than the southern portions of this area or the Midwest. Russian thistle (Salsola) may be a problem in western portions of the Midwest in the fall, as is Kochia.

The Southeast

In the Southeast region, tree pollen appears as early as mid-January (Cupressaceae) lasting into June. Major pollinators are elm (Ulm), oak (Quercus), pecan (Carya), walnut, (Juglans), hickory (Carya), maple (Acer), cottonwood (Populus), and pine (Pinus).

According to Jelks, the pines, cypresses, and junipers may pollinate as early as mid-December in Florida.[37] About 25 percent of the allergic population in Florida will react to skin tests of cypress (Taxodum) and juniper species. Elm may also pollinate in September.

The grass season in the Southeast is long (April through November in some areas) and is accompanied by relatively high pollen counts. In southern Florida, grass may pollinate year round. Grasses of the Festucoid family grow well in addition to Bermuda grass (Cynodon) and Johnson grass (Sorghum) in many areas and are strongly allergenic. Weeds of the Southeast usually pollinate intensely from July through October in the southern areas especially. Ragweed (Ambrosia) may be extremely troublesome, but secondary allergens are Kochia, Plantain (Plantago), dock-sorrell (Rumex), lamb's quarters (Chenopodium) and pigweed (Amaranthus). In Louisiana, Russian thistle (Salsola) and marsh elder (Xanthifolia) may be troublesome.

North Central

In the North Central region, tree pollen is significant from March through May. The major trees in this area are elm (Ulmus), oak (Quercus), box elder (Acer), cottonwood (Populus), sycamore (Platanus), ash, birch, and the Cypressaceae. Grasses pollinate from May through September in the southern regions of Iowa and during June and July in the northern areas of this region. The main grasses are those of the Festucoid subfamily, although wheat (Agropyron), is a problem in Nebraska and North and South Dakota. The major weed pollination season stretches from July through September and consists of ragweed, Russian thistle, sage (Artemisia), Kochia, and hemp (Cannabis), and in Minnesota, the amaranth group.

South Central Region

The tree pollination season in the South Central area ranges from December through April in Texas to February through May and June in Arkansas and Kansas. In Texas, mountain cedar (Juniperus Asheii) is a heavy pollinator in December and January. Mesquite (Prosopis) is also a major source of allergenic pollen in regions of Texas from March through July. Generally, elm, live oak, cottonwood, sycamore, and pecan are the most significant pollinating trees in this area. Local areas of walnut pollinosis occur in Oklahoma in April; birch pollen may be a problem in Arkansas. Oak, birch, the Cupressaceae, and pecan are significant pollinators in Missouri. Grass season lasts all year in south Texas and usually lasts from May through June in Kansas with varying seasons of May through September in areas in between. Grasses of the Festucoid families grow well in irrigated areas and Bermuda grass is also a heavy pollinator. The weed season lasts from July through September in the northern areas of this region and may actually be manifest by ragweed pollen in the air from May through November in southern Texas. The major pollinators in addition to ragweed are plantain, Chenopod, and amaranth families. Russian thistle, kochia, and lamb's quarters of the Chenopod family and pigweed of the Amaranth family are major pollinators.

Mountain States

Tree season in the mountain states ranges from February to April in the south (Arizona and New Mexico) to March through May in the north (Idaho). Significant trees range from cottonwood, juniper, and mosquite in the south to elm, oak, and maple in Colorado and aspen and birch in Idaho and Montana. In addition willow, sycamore, elm, and box elder are secondary pollinators throughout this area. Grass pollination ranges from April through October in the southern sections to June and July in Wyoming. In the states of Wyoming, Utah, and Montana, most of the grass is of the Festucoid subfamily. In New Mexico, Arizona, and Nevada, Bermuda grass grows as well as Johnson grass (especially in New Mexico and Arizona). Colorado and Idaho have the Festucoid grass subfamily.

The weed pollination is very complex in the Mountain State area, and several species cause a great deal of allergies. Ragweed pollinates from April through October in the southern part of this area but may only pollinate from August through early September in Wyoming. Russian thistle is a major allergen in the south and central areas from June through September and may be a problem in Wyoming, Idaho, Montana, and Utah in July and August. Kochia is also a major allergen in June through September, especially in Arizona and Colorado. Salt bush (Atriplex) is a major allergen in June through September, and sage can be a significant problem in August through October. Marsh elder is often high in Idaho and Montana.

West Coast

Tree pollination season varies from January and February in southern California to February through May in Oregon. East of the Cascades in Oregon, and in eastern Washington, tree pollination usually is from mid-March through mid-April, although elm pollinates in September and October in the south. Major pollinators in southern California according to Ellis and Gallup are olive,[38] chinese elm, mulberry, ash, oak, cottonwood, and the Cupressaceae. In northern California, similar trees are significant such as olive, elm,

and oak, in addition to birch and cottonwood. In Oregon and Washington, trees are birch, cottonwood, box elder, willow, and the Cupressaceae. Alder predominates in Oregon and aspen in Washington. The grass season ranges from June to September in the northern areas of this region and from March through November in the southern areas. The Festucoids plus Bermuda grass are the predominating pollinating grasses in the northern area. In the southern areas, not only are the above grasses present, but also Johnson grass and oats (Avena) are significant grass family pollinators. The weed pollinating seasons in the West Coast area may range from April through November in the south to July through September in the north. Russian thistle is a heavy pollinator in the southern areas of this region from July through October and does extend along the eastern portions of the northern regions from July through September. Kochia and sage are also major pollinators at this time. Much of the region remains ragweed free, but it can be a problem in local clusters from July through November in the south and August and September in the north. Amaranth in the south (April through November) and salt bush in the north (July through September) seem to be moderately heavy pollinators in their geographic locale. Plantain and sorrel are at times heavy pollinators in the northern areas of this region, as is the Urtica (Nettle) family.

Of the noncontiguous states, Alaska and Hawaii, very little material is available from the former, but Roth has collected much data from Hawaii. Inasmuch as most plants are insect pollinated in the Hawaiian islands, very few are of allergenic significance. The mesquite tree pollinates from March through September Australian pine (Casuarina) and olive (Olea) have windborne pollens that are allergenic to some. Grasses pollinate year round and include red top, Bermuda, Johnson, sugar cane. Ragweed and false ragweed grow sparsely in a few areas.

Mexico

Trees of the northern section of Mexico are Mesquite and acacia, which pollinate in July and August. In the southern less arid areas are ash, poplar, juniper, and oak trees. Grasses pollinate from October through December and are the highest of the allergenic pollens, the primary grass being Bermuda grass. The weeds are prevalent in July and August and consist of the Chenopods, Amaranth, and Artemisia (sage).

Canada

Trees of the Maritime Provinces (Newfoundland Nova Scotia, Prince Edward Island, and New Brunswick) are similar to those of the American northeast and pollinate just a bit later, usually in late April May, and into early June. The most important trees are birch, maple (the national symbol of Canada), oak cottonwood, and the conifers, spruce and pine. Grasses are those of the Festucoid family and usually pollinate in June and July. Although ragweed is growing in the Maritime Provinces, it is minimal and does not reach significant proportions of airborne pollen.

The central provinces (Quebec, Ontario, and Manitoba), have similar trees to those of the Maritime Provinces and the pollination season is approximately the same. The grass pollens are mainly of the Festucoid family and appear airborne in June and July. Ragweed is the most prevalent weed pollen in this area and exists from mid-August to mid-September. Ragweed counts in the central provinces are the highest in Canada, although there has been a general decline since 1953.

The prairie provinces of Alberta and Saskatchewan have tree pollen in the springtime months of April and May from poplars, box elders, ash, willows, oaks, elms, and birches. Grass is the most significant pollen in this area and is usually airborne in June and July. The weeds consist mainly of Russian thistle, marsh alder, and sage, pollinating in July and August. Ragweed is a minor pollinator in August.

British Columbia has had predominantly conifer pollen, with lesser amounts of alder, box elder, cottonwood, willow, and birch trees. Ragweed is minimal in this area, but the Chenopods and Amaranth weeds are heavy pollinators in August.

Europe

The following current information has been supplied by Frits Th. M. Spieksma, PhD, co-chair of the subcommittee on Aerobiology of the European Academy of Allergy and Clinical Immunology.[39–40] Generally throughout Europe the pollen of grasses (Poaceae) and nettle (Urticaceae) is very common. In western Europe, about half the airborne pollen is from these two families, followed by birch (Betula), pine (Pinacea), oak (Quercus), and alder (Alnus). In central Europe and Scandinavia, tree pollen predominates over grass and weed pollens. In southern Europe in the Mediterranean areas, juniper and cedar (Cupressaceae), wall pellitory (Parietaria), and olive pollen are more important.

On the basis of data generated from collecting sites in several European countries, "the top ten" airborne pollens are:

1. Poaceae (grass)
2. Urticaceae (nettle, wall pellitory)
3. Betulaceae (birch, alder and hazelnut)
4. Pinaceae (pine, spruce)
5. Fagaceae (oak, beech, and chestnut)
6. Cupressaceae (cedar, juniper)
7. Oleaceae (ash, olive)
8. Plantago (plantain)
9. Salcaceae (willow, poplar)
10. Platanus (planetree)

Birch season peaks in April in southern Europe and May in the north. Grass pollen peaks in May in southern Europe, June in west and central countries, and July in the north. Artemisia (mugwort) peaks in July in northern Europe, August in western and central countries, and September in the south.

Skin test observations of allergic patients at Leiden, Montpelier, and Perugia, show grass pollen to be the most allergenic (80–90% of positive reactions) followed by alder and birch in the north with wall pellitory and olive in the south.

With the European Aeroallergen Negwork now operating, complete aeroallergen mapping and skin test correlations will be possible within the next decade.

Great Britain

In the United Kingdom of England, Scotland, and Wales, tree pollens are present from February through May. The most prevalent pollens are those of planetree, birch, oak, and elm. Hazel and alder are early pollinators in February and March: elm, birch, and ash pollinate in March and April; and oak, beech, and planetree pollinate in May.

As in continental europe, grass pollen is the major antigenic pollen in the United Kingdom. Grass pollinates from mid-May to mid-July and consists of grasses in the Festucoid family.

The second most important pollen group, that of the Urticaceae family (nettle and wall pellitory) pollinate from June into early September.

Australia

Tree pollens in Australia are usually not clinically important. Australian pine (Casuarina) pollinates from August to November in many areas. In New South Wales (the most populous industrialized area) the most common tree is the eucalyptus. In Victoria state (the second most populous) the most common trees are birch, sycamore, and oak. The most important pollen is that of the grasses to which over 90% of pollen-sensitive patients are allergic. Pollination peaks from October through December. Much of central and western Australia is extremely arid and very little pollen is present in that area.

China

In south central China, tree pollen from the conifers is present in March, and planetree pollen occurs in April in Shang-hai. In northern China, elm, poplar, and willow pollinate in April. Grass is a perennial pollinator in southern and southeastern China, and it pollinates in July through August in northern China. Sage (Artemisia) is a very significant pollinator in August in the north and September through November in the south. In north China, weeds such as the Chenopods, sage, and hemp (Cannabis) are the most significant fall pollinators.

Japan

Tree pollens occur from March through April and consist of Japanese cedar, oak, ash, birch, beech, juniper, elm, pine, and alder. Grass pollen is extremely antigenic and reaches a peak in June, the common grasses being timothy, orchard grass, rye grass, Fescue, foxtail, and rice grass (Oryzopsis). Weed aeroallergens are rare.

This relatively incomplete summary of worldwide pollen can be augmented by referring to data available in the annual reports of the Aerobiology Committee of the American Academy of Allergy and Immunology, the *Allergy Advocate* newsletter published by the Academy, and in the text, *Allergy in the World*, by Roth.[41] Serious students of airborne pollen are referred to Lewis' definitive work.[42]

FUNGAL SPORES

Airborne fungal spores and mycelial fragments are the most ubiquitous and numerous of all aeroallergens worldwide. Fungal spore counts from collecting surfaces of impaction and suction samplers usually outnumber pollen grains by several hundredfold. Local environmental factors influence the exact type of fungal growth, but generally the most common groups are similar worldwide. Relative humidity, temperature, and the amount of substrate disturbance, seem to be the important factors in controlling airborne concentrations of fungal spores.[43]

Much difficulty is encountered in collection and identification of fungal spores for several reasons: (1) The minute size of some species (basidio spores) require oil immersion microscopy for classification), (2) the similarity in appearance of many genera (*Aspergillus* and *Penicillium* for instance), (3) the difference in morphological stages of the same fungus, and (4) the fact that culture growth on specialized media (such as malt agar, tryptocase, and others) is required.

To add to confusion, not only has the nomenclature changed recently, but also a more fundamental change has occurred in the realization that fungi previously classed as *Deuteromycetes* (which consist of the majority of allergenic species) are really the asexual stage of *Ascomycetes*. This limits to three the classes of medically important fungi; *Zygomycetes* (Mucor, Rhizopus), *Ascomycetes* (Cladosporium, Penicillium, Aspergillus, Epicoccum, Alternaria, and others), and *Basidiomycetes* (rusts, smut, Ganoderma).

A complete description of the biology and identification of fungal aeroallergens can be found in the chapter by Salkin and Haines elsewhere in this text.

DISEASES CAUSED BY FUNGI

Fungi may cause three types of reactions in humans: infection, toxicity, and hypersensitivity depending on fungal concentration and host immune factors.

Infection from tissue invasion by fungi usually occurs in immunocompromised hosts, although massive exposure to *Histoplasma* and *Cryptococcus* may cause respiratory infection in otherwise healthy people.

Toxicity may result from ingestion or even inhalation of fungal metabolites such as aflatoxins from *Aspergillus* and trichothecenes from *Fusarium.*

Hypersensitivity involving IGG as well as IGE antibodies may result in diseases ranging from mild allergic rhinitis to life-threatening bronchopulmonary aspergillosis and hypersensitivity pneumonitis with gradually deteriorating pulmonary function. Spore size and concentration of exposure seem important in determining the exact type of hypersensitivity response. For example, intense exposure to small spores is often related to hypersensitivity pneumonitis while low concentrations of large spores often causes IGE-mediated allergic rhinitis and asthma.

COLLECTION

Collection of airborne fungal spores can be done similarly to that of pollens with some exceptions. With the intermittent rotorod, one tends to underestimate the small particles while rods become overloaded with larger spores. This is somewhat lessened with the Burkhard spore trap but many nondescript spores such as *Aspergillus* and *Penicillium* cannot be identified with certainty by either of these collectors. The Anderson sieve cascade impactor permits the volumetric collection of viable airborne spores on culture media so that individual characteristics can be analyzed and spores identified. This may require several days incubation and subculturing before microscopic analysis is possible. Fungal spore fallout plates do not collect as representative a sample of airborne flora as do volumetric suction devices; this can lead to erroneous assessments.

COMMON AIRBORNE SPORES

Bearing in mind the limitations of fungal spore collection and identification, there seems to be a universal prevalence of common spores reported, with some variation due to local weather and geography. Outdoor collections in New England and eastern Canada show high concentrations of *Cladosporium* followed by *Alternaria*, *Epicoccum*, and *Dreschlera* in April and September with massive intrusion of the *Basidomycetes Ganoderma* and *Ustilago* (smut) in June and July. Other common spores identified from impaction samples are *Pithomyces*, *Stemphyllium*, *Ascospores*, and *Nigrospora.* Table V lists these common outdoor fungal spores that have been recorded from 1985 through 1988.

In subtropical areas such as south Florida and southern California, ascospores are of great importance. Although penicillium and aspergillus spores are very difficult to identify unless culture methods are used, these genera have been reported in Panama, Brazil, and Havana as well as in the tropical arid regions of Kuwait, Iran, and Iraq.[44]

Under normal conditions, the fungal spore concentration indoors is less than half that outdoors, unless an indoor source of contamination is present. Indoor collections usually are done using samplers capable of providing culture growth, although sometimes particulate impaction samples are used as well. Bearing in mind the differences in technique, there appears to be a somewhat different flora indoors than out, but this may be more apparent than real. Indoor culture collections show spores of *Cladosporium, Aspergillus, Penicillium,* yeast, *Aureobasidum, Alternaria, Rhizopus,* and *Mucor.*

ALLERGENICITY

As with pollen, fungal spores demonstrate varying degrees of allergenicity and cross-reactivity. Skin testing, RAST inhibition, and crossed immunoelectrophoresis (CIEP) have been used to identify these factors. Several allergens from *Alternaria, Cladosporium, Aspergillus,* and *Candida* have been isolated; the most important being found in *Alternaria.*[45] Fungal antigens are formed in rodlet structures located in spore wall[45] and in the mycelium.[46] Not much is known about antigenic release.

It is difficult to determine with certainty which fungi are capable of causing allergy:[46] most assumptions are based either on symptoms associated with exposure to areas in which spores have been identified or on skin-test results. Unfortunately, in the former case, the causative spore may not have been recognized, while inci-

dental spores are implicated; in the latter case, purified antigens for testing are either unavailable (for many basidiospores) or are produced in such a fashion that cross-reacting proteins are present. However limited our present capacity is to determine the specific allergenic fungi, assumptions based on skin testing have proved helpful. When testing atopic individuals by the prick technique using fungal antigens, a positive reaction (5 mm wheal, 20 mm flare) is assumed to denote allergy to that allergen. In the face of negative prick-testing results, intracutaneous test using 0.2 ml of a 1-200 aqueous concentration of that antigen can be done, although the possibility of nonspecific irritative (not immunological) reaction is increased. In view of this, our results, plus literature review showed the following fungi to be the most common causes of prick skin test positivity (see Table VI).

Although these results[47,48] show geographic variations in fungal reactions, it should be noted that *Cladosporium,* which is by far the most abundant spore identified in air sampling, is not as antigenic as *Alternaria* or other spores. When one compares the prevalence of positive skin tests to fungal antigens with testing to pollens and environmentals, it is apparent that there is less sensitivity to fungi than to environmentals and pollens.

INDOOR AIR

The topic of atmospheric pollen and fungal spores would not be complete without a brief discussion of indoor air, where American adults spend almost 90% of their time at work or leisure. The late 1970s and early 1980s saw the advent of tighter buildings and more efficient handling of air because of energy restric-

TABLE V

Most Frequent Outdoor Fungi 1986–1988
New England and Southeastern Canada

1. Cladosporium
2. Ganoderma
3. Alternaria
4. Ustilaginales (smut)
5. Epicoccum
6. Ascospore
7. Uredinales (rust)
8. Dreschlera
9. Pithomycetes
10. Nigrospora

TABLE VI

Most Common Fungal Skin Tests

Investigator:	Farnham, MA	Lopez, LA*	Rodriquez, VA**
Patients:	1,700	659	809
Fungus: (% of total)			
Alternaria	14%	29%	28%
Phoma	8	27	23
Aspergillus	7	22	15
Dreschlera	7	23	17
Cladosporium	6.7	29	21
Fusarium	6.7	2	20
Aureobasidium	6	8	20
Curvularia	5	—	25
Mucor	4.9	5	15
Penicillium	4.8	28	13

Lopez M, de Shazo RD, Lehrer SB. Mold induced pulmonary syndromes. In: Current Views on Allergy & Immunology XIV. Augusta: Medical College of Georgia, 1986.

**Rodriquez GE, Dyson MC, Mohagheghi H. The art and science of allergy skin testing. Ann Allergy 61;6:428–432, 1988.*

tions. This led to recycled indoor air into which various contaminants were continuously inadvertently added or remained without being exhausted. As the concentration of these contaminants increased, initially a few sensitive individuals would experience irritation of the respiratory tract and skin. Further increases in concentration led to exacerbations of respiratory allergies (rhinitis and asthma) in atopics, and general nonspecific symptoms of irritation of the eyes, malaise, headache, and fatigue in others. After enough cases became manifest, it was realized that there was a direct relationship between indoor airborne contaminants and morbidity: building-related illness.

A National Institute of Occupational Safety and Health study by Gorman and Wallingford[49] revealed that there were five causes of indoor air contamination: (1) inadequate ventilation, (2) contamination from internal materials (such as fabrics, building materials, and equipment), (3) microbiological contamination, (4) contamination from external sources (outside pollutants being introduced into the building) and (5) undetermined factors. In the majority of cases, improvement of ventilation to 30 cubic feet per person per hour can alleviate the problem.

Microbiological contamination (the third most common source of building-related illness) on the other hand, once established, often requires more definitive action than merely increasing air exchange. Table VII outlines the major types of biological contaminants, their relative concentrations indoors and out (on a scale of 1–4), and the type of diseases possible from each.

As stated before, fungi have the unique ability of causing hypersensitivity, infection, and toxicity. Bacteria of the thermophilic actinomycetes group also may cause hypersensitivity (humidifier fever or hypersensitivity pneumonitis). Often the specific illness is determined by the concentration and type of the organism

TABLE VIII

Health Effects of Microbiologicals

I Allergy or hypersensitivity
  A. IGE mediated
    1. Acute rhinitis, asthma, dermatitis
    2. Allergic bronchopulmonary Aspergillosis
  B. IGG mediated
    1. Humidifier fever
    2. Hypersensitivity pneumonitis
II Infections
  A. Bacterial
    1. Common gram positive and gram negative organisms
    2. Pontiac fever, Legionnaire's Disease
    3. TBC
    4. Brucella
    5. Miscellaneous
  B. Viral
    1. Respiratory viruses
  C. Fungal
    1. Immunologically normal
    2. Immune deficient
III Toxicity
  A. Mycotoxins
  B. Bacterial exotoxins

and the immune status of the host. Demonstrative of this is the fact that spores of the fungus *Aspergillus* may cause acute asthma and/or bronchopulmonary aspergillosis in the atopic person (through IGE antibody), or humidifier fever/hypersensitivity pneumonitis in the nonatopic person (through IGG antibody) (see Table VIII).

Because the normal interface is through the respiratory tract and skin, common symptoms of building-related illness are eye irritation, nasal congestion, sinus pressure, dryness and soreness of the throat, shortness of breath, cough, and skin irritation. More general and vague complaints are headache, dizziness, nausea, and fatigue. Many complaints are so nonspecific that great difficulty is encountered relating them to the specific inhaled microbiologicals. If enough people in a particular building are affected with these complaints, the event is referred to as sick-building syndrome. Usually the situation is corrected by increasing ventilation, reducing relative humidity, and eradicating the cause of microbiological contamination (changing or eliminating the substrate).

Indoor air also contains house dust mites, a potent aeroallergen present on a global basis. Specific details on dust mites are described in the Introduction chapter of this book.

TABLE VII

Microbiologicals

Agent	Out	In	Disease
Pollens	+3	+1	A
Fungal spores, algae	+4	+3	A, I, T
Bacteria, viruses	+2	+3	A, I
Organic dust	+1	+3	A
Insects (mite, vermin)	+1	+3	A
Protozoa	+1	+1	I
Pets and pests	+2	+4	A, I

A—Allergy and hypersensitivity.
I—Infection.
T—Toxicity.

SUMMARY

In summary, this chapter dealt with pertinent facts about the earth's atmosphere, its contaminants, and methods of collecting these. The pollens and fungal spores of particular importance, their dynamics, associated diseases, and geographic differences have been discussed. A brief look at indoor air contamination has been offered.

ACKNOWLEDGMENTS

The author gratefully thanks Jean Champman, M.D. and Paul Comtois, PhD, for their review of the contents of the manuscript. Frits Th. M. Spieksma, PhD, graciously provided information about the European aeroallergens and networks; Clifford Crompton, PhD, Christine Rogers, and Lee Coates supplied detailed aeroallergen data from Canada. Acknowledgment is also given to the American Academy of Allergy and Immunology, especially to Sarah E. Kaluzhy, Communications Manager, for use of various pertinent monographs and newsletters.

REFERENCES

1. Schafer VJ, Day JA. Field Guide to the Atmosphere Boston: Houghton Mifflin Company, 1981, pp 1–44.
2. Geiger R. The Climate Near the Ground. Boston: Harvard University Press, 1980, pp. 480–488.
3. Sharp WM, Chisman HH. Flowering and fruiting in white oaks. Ecology 42:365–372, 1961.
4. Sheldon JM, Hewson EW. Atmospheric Pollution by Aeroallergens, Univ Mich Res Inst Prog Rep 3. Ann Arbor: Univ Michigan, 1959.
5. Soloman AM. Pollen P51. In Edmonds RL (ed). Aerobiology The Ecological Sytems Approach. US/IBP Synthesis Series 10. Stroudsburg, PA: Dowden, Hutchinson & Ross, Inc., 1979.
6. Lippmann MW, Albert RE. The effect of particle size on regional deposition of inhaled steroids in the human respiratory tract. J Am Ind Hyg Assoc 30:257–275, 1969.
7. Benninghoff WS, Benninghoff AS. Considerations of Electro-statics in Aerobiology (Abstr). Second Int Conf on Aerobiology. Seattle, 1982.
8. Corbet SA, Beament J, Eisckowitch D. Are electrostatic forces involved in pollen transfer? Plant Cell Environ 5:125–129, 1982.
9. Spitalny KC, Farnham JE, Witherel LE, et al. Alpine slide anaphylaxis. N Engl J Med 310:103–1037, 1984.
10. Blackley C. Experimental Researches on the Cause and Nature of Catarrhus Aestivas (Hayfever and Hay Asthma). London: Balliere, Tindall & Cox, 1873.
11. Durham OC. The volumetric incidence of airborne allergens. IV. A proposed standard method of gravity sampling, counting and volumetric interpolation of results. J Allergy 17:79–86, 1946.
12. Perkins WA. The rotorod sampler, 2nd Semiannu Rep CML 186 Aerosol Lab, Stanford Univ Stanford CA, 1957.
13. Muilenberg ML. Allergen assessment by microscopy and culture. Immunol Allergy Clin North Am 9:245–268, Aug 1989.
14. Platts-Mills TAE, Chapman NB, Heymann PW, Luczynska CM. Measurements of airborne allergen using immunoassays. Immunol Allergy Clin North Am 9:2, 269–283, Aug 1989.
15. Sheldon JM, Hewson EW. Atmospheric pollution by aeroallergens. Univ Mich Res Inst Prog Rep 4. Ann Arbor: Univ Michigan, 1960.
16. Werfft R. Uber die Lebensdauer der Pollenkroner in der freien Atmosphare. Biol Zentralbl 70:354–367, 1951.
17. Davies RR, Smith SLP. Forecasting the start and severity of the hayfever season. Clin Allergy 3:263, 1973.
18. Solomon WR. Experimental ragweed pollenosis induced during normal respirations in a test chamber: initial observations. J Allergy 43:181, 1969.
19. Comtois P, Gagnon L. Concentration pollenique et frequence des symptomes de pollinose: unc methode pour determiner les seuils cliniques. Rev fr Allergol 28:4 279–286, 1988.
20. Connell JT. Quantitative intranasal pollen challenge III the priming effect in allergic rhinitis. J Allergy 43:33–44, 1969.
21. Weber RW, Nelson HS. Pollen allergens and their interrelationships. Clin Rev Allergy 3:291–318, 1985.
22. Geller-Bernstein C, Keyman N, Bejerano A, et al. Positive skin tests to fern spore extracts in atopic patients. Ann Allergy 58:125–127, 1987.
23. Dirksen A, Osterballe O. Common components in pollen extracts. Allergy 35:611–616, 1980.
24. Farnham JE. A new look at conifer allergy (Editorial) New Engl Reg Allergy Proc 9:3, 237–238, 1988.
25. Rackemann FM, Wagner HC. The desensitization of skin sites passively with serum of patients with hay fever. J Allergy 7:319–322, 1936.
26. Weber RW. Cross reactivity among tree pollens: Skin test correlations (Abstr). Ann Allergy 50:363, 1983.
27. Farnham JE, Vaida GA. A new look at New England tree pollen, New Engl Soc Allergy Proc 3:320–326, 1982.
28. Farnham JE, Mason D, Batchelder GL, Colby FD. Ragweed pollen forecasting aerobiology, health and environment (Symposium Proc). Universite de Montreal, 1989, pp. 15–24.
29. Fairley D, Batchelder GL. A study of oak pollen production and phenology in northern California: prediction of annual variation in pollen counts based on geographic and meterologic factors. J Allergy Clin Immunol 78:300–307, 1986.
30. Bassett IJ. Atmospheric Pollen Studies at Ottawa, Canada. Ottawa, Ont: Can Dep Agr 1956.
31. Bassett IJ. Surveys of air-borne ragweed pollen in Canada with particular reference to sites in Ontario. Can J Plant Sci 39:491–497, 1959.
32. Bassett IJ. Air-borne pollen surveys in Manitoba & Saskatchewan. Can J Plant Sci 44:7–14, 1964.
33. Bassett IJ, Crompton CW. Air-borne pollen surveys in British Columbia. Can J Plant Sci 47:251–261, 1967.
34. Bassett IJ, Crompton CW. Air-borne pollen surveys in eastern Canada. Can J Plant Sci 49:247–253, 1969.
35. Farnham JE. N.E. tree pollen and skin test reactivity - a 3-year study, (abst). Joint Canadian & Panamerican Symp Aerobiol Health Proc Health & Welfare Canada, 1989, p. 11.
36. Kalliel JN, Settipane GA. Eastern pine sensitivity in New England. New Engl Reg Allergy Proc 9:3, 233–237, 1988.
37. Jelks ML. Aeroallergens of Florida. Immunol Allergy Clin North Am 9: Aug 1989. 381–397.
38. Ellis, MH, Gallup J. Aeroallergens of Southern California. Immunol Allergy Clin North Am 9: 365–380, Aug 1989.
39. Spieksma FThM. Allergenic Pollens in Europe. Proc 2nd Natl Congress Italian Assoc Aerobiol Capri: 60–69, 1986.
40. Spieksma FThM. Personal communication.
41. Roth A (ed). Allergy in the World, A Guide for Physicians and Travelers. Univ Press Hawaii, 1978.
42. Lewis WH, Vinay P, Zenger VE. Airborne and Allergenic Pollen of North America. Baltimore: Johns Hopkins Univ Press, 1984.
43. Sneller MR. Mould allergy & climate conditions. In Al-Doory Y, Domson JF. Mould Allergy, Philadelphia, PA: Lea & Febiger, 1984, pp. 244–266.
44. Hoffman DR. Mould allergens. In Al-Doory Y, Domson JF.

Mould Allergy. Philadelphia, PA: Lea & Febiger, 1984, pp. 104–116.

45. Cole GT, Samson RA. The conidia. In Al-Doory Y, Domson JR. Mould Allergy. Philadelphia, PA: Lea & Febiger, 1984, pp. 66–103.

46. Burge MA. Airborne allergenic fungi. Immunol Allergy Clin North Am 9:307–319, Aug 1989.

47. Lopez M, de Shazo RD, Lehrer SB. Mold induced pulmonary syndromes. In: Current Views in Allergy & Immunology XIV. Augusta: Medical College of Georgia, 1986.

48. Rodriquez GE, Dyson MC, Mohagheghi H. The art and science of allergy skin testing. Ann Allergy 61 6:428–432, 1988.

49. Gorman RW, Wallingford KM. The NIOSH approach to conducting indoor air quality investigations in office building. In press.

Chapter VI

Genetic Determinates of Pollen Phenotype

David L. Mulcahy, Ph.D.

ABSTRACT

Competition among a vast number of pollen grains for a limited number of ovules creates the opportunity for very intense natural selection. Such selection, intensified by microbial-like characteristics in the pollen, gains significance from the fact that much of the plant (diplophase) structural genome is expressed in the pollen. As a result of this intense selection, pollen exhibits extremely rapid reactions upon a compatible stigma, releasing large fractions of its total protein content within minutes. These proteins are derived from both haplo- and diplophase cells. The first compounds released are relatively invariant and may serve to initiate species recognition reactions.

In all sexually reproducing organisms, the life cycle includes two major milestones, meiosis and fertilization. These two, respectively, mark the beginning and the end of haploid cells, that is, those which contain only one set of chromosomes. The prominence of this haploid phase varies enormously from one taxonomic group to another. With vertebrates, for example, sperms and eggs are the only haploid cells while in some groups of plants, e.g. the mosses, the haploid phase represents the major portion of the life cycle. The flowering plants (the angiosperms) are found between these two extremes of haplophase development but, as in the vertebrates, here too the diplophase is the conspicuous part of the life cycle. In their angiosperms, the male haplophase (pollen) consists

David L. Mulcahy, Ph.D., Botany Department, University of Massachusetts, Amherst, MA 01003

of only three cells, and two of these, the sperm cells, are contained within the third, the vegetative (or tube) cell. Pollen produces the male gametes, and it also delivers them.

Delivery requires that pollen provides protection during transport from the anther of one flower to the stigma of another, and it requires also a tube through which sperm cells can travel from stigma to ovules. This pollen tube may be hundreds of times longer than the diameter of the pollen grain, and yet it is sometimes produced within less than one hour.[1] This tremendous growth can be accomplished only by a structure that is particularly rich in preformed compounds,[2] and this may help to explain the allergenic potency of pollens.

Because the number of pollen grains produced greatly exceeds the number of eggs,[3] it may be assumed that there is intense competition among pollen grains. This assumption has been tested in recent studies of natural populations, and while pollen is limiting in some cases,[4] it is indeed overly abundant in others.[5]

Haldane[6] pointed out that whenever pollen competition is intense, any gene which causes rapid pollen tube growth will be greatly favored by natural selection, even if it causes moderately disadvantageous changes in the adult (diploid) plant. Thus, he suggested, "A higher plant is at the mercy of its pollen grains." This consideration is perhaps what led Haldane to describe pollen as a suppressed generation with "a physiology of its own, influenced by special genes." Presumably these "special" genes were not expressed in the diploid phase of the life cycle, thus insulating the diplophase from harmful effects of haplophase selection. The distinction between haplophase genes and diplophase genes is seemingly reinforced by the tenets of mendelian genetics. In a segregating individual (Aa), for example, two types of pollen grains are produced in equal frequencies, and almost invariably, we detect no differences in the number of fertilizations accomplished by the gametes of each type. Thus, the success or failure of a pollen tube seems to be independent of its genetic contents. Further apparent confirmation of Haldane's supposition was the fact that in corn *(Zea mays L.)* the expression of a highly studied gene, waxy (Wx/wx), is limited to the haploid portion of the life cycle.[7]

The first evidence that haplo-and diplophase were not independently functioning entities was produced by Ter-Avanesian.[8,9] He reported that the variance in height of offspring was reduced when excessive quantities of pollen were used in pollinations. This implied that the fastest growing pollen tubes were a genetic subpopulation among all pollen tubes, and this haplophase genetic difference was expressed also in the resultant diplophase. A similar study and conclusion was reported by Matthews.[10] These studies were followed by a series of investigations which reported that the quality of a diplophase individual is significantly and positively correlated with the quality of the pollen tubes which gave rise to the individual. Pollen tubes which grow rapidly give rise to diplophase plants which germinate, grow, and flower more rapidly than do other diplophase plants.[11,12] The simplest explanation for these observations is that some of the genes which are expressed (and selected) in the pollen are expressed also in the diplophase.

The first precise evidence that at least some genes were expressed in both parts of the life cycle also came from *Zea mays.* Schwartz[13] showed quite conclusively that the genes for alcohol dehydrogenase were expressed in both haploid and diploid portions of the life cycle. Eventually, Tanksley, Zamir, and Rick,[14] in a survey of 9 different enzyme systems in *Lycopersicon esculentum,* the cultivated tomato, found that 60% of the structural genes which are expressed in the diplophase plant are expressed also in the pollen. Furthermore, 95% of the genes which are expressed in the pollen are expressed also in the diplophase. Thus, in the flowering plants, there is extensive overlap between the haplo- and diplophase genetic systems. Because the correlation between haplo- and diplophase qualities is positive, i.e., good pollen tubes make good plants; Haldane's[6] concern about the possible deleterious effects of such overlap was apparently unnecessary.

The apparent conflict with mendelian tenets is as easily resolved. Consider what qualities we can observe in the phenotype of a pollen tube. There, almost no features can be used as the single gene markers (e.g., round versus wrinkled seeds), so useful in diplophase mendelian genetic studies. In fact, almost the only variable characteristic of a pollen tube is its growth rate, and, in both haplophase and diplophase organisms, growth rate is a highly complex, multigenically determined, quality. Each single locus, therefore, will have a relatively small effect on pollen tube growth rates. There are exceptions, of course. The literature is replete with examples of alleles which are lethal or semi-lethal in pollen, not necessarily because such alleles are very frequent, but rather because they are the ones most easily detected. Can we detect alleles which have small effects? In theory we can, but it is surprisingly difficult. To be 90% certain of detecting a 1% deviation from mendelian expectations of a 1:1 ratio, it is necessary to determine the genotype in at least 26,546 offspring. Smaller samples would probably fail to detect any deviation from expectations.[15] Because small deviations from expectations are rarely detected, it is thus assumed that the segregating alleles have no effect, that is, they are not expressed, in pollen tube growth. However, micromethods of electrophoresis have recently allowed the genetic analysis of single pollen grains, and these methods demonstrate directly that a substantial number of genes are active in pollen.[16]

Consider now the mature pollen grain. It consists of a semi-rigid wall, but one which can expand or contract as the grain is hydrated or dehydrated. The microspores are contained within the floral anther, and, immediately surrounding the mass of microspores, is a layer of diplophase cells, the tapetum. These tapetal cells serve a nutritive function for the microspores. The microspore wall generally consists of two subunits, an inner pectocellulosic layer, the *intine,* and an outer layer, the *exine,* composed of sporopollenin, a complex polymer of carotenoids and carotenoid esters.[17] These two microspore wall layers differ, not only in their chemistry, but also in their structure, their origin and their genetic determinants. The intine is relatively homogeneous in structure although it contains inclusions of proteins[18,19] and, furthermore, cellulosic microfibrils within this layer cause birefringence in polarized light.[20] In contrast to the relative homogeneity of the intine, the outer portions of the exine, while generally isotropic,[21] are often highly sculptured and may contain a complex network of pits and cavities. The intine and its inclusions are produced by the microspore cytoplasm and thus represent haplophase products. The exine is composed of sporopollenin derived from the diplophase tapetum.[20,21] Additionally, the cavities of the exine sculpturing are filled with the products resulting from the last stage of diplophase tapetum breakdown. Because the quality and the reactions of pollen grains are determined by both diplophase material upon the exine, and haplophase proteins within the intine, pollen is a complex structure, influenced by both diplophase and haplophase genotypes.[12,20]

Consider now what happens when a pollen grain touches a wet surface. Within seconds, it begins to hydrate[22] and protein is leached from the pollen. In

Oenothera organensis, this amounts to the loss of 10-12% of total pollen protein within 2.5 minutes and 30-42% within 30 minutes (based on loss to tris-borate buffer, pH 7.6.[23]) Immunofluorescence studies have shown that, in pollen leachates from intact *Gladiolus* and *Ambrosia,* antigens were derived from both the intine (haplophase) and to a lesser extent the surface (diplophase) materials deposited on the *Ambrosia* exine.[18] Considering only antigen E in *Ambrosia* spp. and *Cosmos bipinnatus,* Howlett, Knox, and Heslop-Harrison[24] found that this antigen was released mainly from the exine in *Cosmos* but, in *Ambrosia* species, it originates from the intine.

The possible function of these rapidly released proteins has been suggested by Porter.[25] She studied diffusates from intact pollen of *Zea mays,* and found that three major low molecular proteins (that is, 28-30% of total diffusate protein) represented only 5–6% of all soluble proteins, i.e., those released when pollen grains were crushed. More importantly, Porter found that pollen *diffusates* seemed to be highly conserved throughout a sample of 40 very different races of *Zea mays.* Electrophoretic analysis of *total* soluble proteins from the same 40 races, however, exhibited considerable variation. She thus suggests that rapidly released proteins in *Zea* pollen may play some fundamental part in establishing pollen-stigma recognition reactions. Any changes in them would thus be rigorously eliminated by natural selection.

Once hydrated, and if no incompatibility exists between pollen and stigma or style, then the pollen produces a tube through which two sperm cells are carried toward the ovary and ovules. Brief though it is, this passage through the stylar tissue exposes the haploid genotype to selection and a large fraction of unbalanced genomes are eliminated.[26] Furthermore, selection is not limited to this negative function. Of the many haploid genotypes which are capable of directing a pollen tube through this rigorous course, only the fastest will succeed in entering an unfertilized ovule. The consequences of this intense selection are difficult to assess but we have some basis for judging. Consider how quickly a population of bacteria can respond to selection pressures. Their adaptability exists because their populations are extremely large (thus increasing the probability that at least one individual will be adapted) and also because their haploidy exposes even rare alleles which might not be expressed in a diploid organism. Like bacteria, pollen is found in very large populations, and it too is haploid. Now that it seems that many (60%) of the diplophase structural genes may be exposed to haplophase selection, can we anticipate bacterial-like responsiveness in the flowering plants? The flowering plants apparently arose quite suddenly, about 125×10^6 years ago, displacing the gymnosperms and the ferns from their preeminence in the world flora. In only the angiosperms is pollen subjected to an intense selection. Thus, in no other higher plant is

there good opportunity for haplophase selection. Could this selection have contributed to the angiosperm rise to dominance? This may never be known but, in any case, the expression of diplophase genes in the pollen promises to provide a powerful method for modifying the flowering plant genome. It may already have done so in natural populations.

REFERENCES

1. Heslop-Harrison J. Recognition and response in the pollen-stigma interaction in cell-cell recognition. Symp of Soc for Experimental Biology 32: 121-138, 1978.

2. Brown SW, Cave MS. The detection and nature of dominant lethals in *Librium* I. Effects of x-rays on the heritable component and functional ability of the pollen grain. Am Jour Bot 41: 455-469, 1954.

3. Cruden RW. Pollen-ovule ratios: a conservative indicator of breeding systems in flowering plants. Evolution 31: 32-46, 1977.

4. Bierzychudek P. Pollinator limitation of plant reproductive effort. Am Nat 117: 838-840, 1981.

5. Mulcahy DL, Curtis P, Snow A. Pollen competition in a natural population. In Handbook of Experimental Pollination Biology, ed. by CE Jones and R John Little, Van Nostrand Reinhold Co., NY. In press.

6. Haldane JBS. The Causes of Evolution. Longmans, Green and Co., London. 1932.

7. Akatsuka T, Nelson OE. Studies on starch synthesis in maize mutants. J Japan Soc Starch Sci 17: 99-115, 1969.

8. Ter-Avanesian DV. The influence of the number of pollen grains used in pollination. Bull Appl Genet Plant Breeding Leningrad 28: 119-133, 1949.

9. Ter-Avanesian DV, The effect of varying the number of pollen grains used in fertilization. Theor Appl Genetics 52: 77-79, 1978.

10. Lewis D. Annual Report of the Department of Genetics. Ann Rep John Innes Inst 45: 12-17, 1954.

11. Mulcahy DL. Correlation between speed of pollen tube growth and seedling height in *Zea mays* L. Nature 249: 491-493, 1974.

12. Mulcahy DL. The rise of the angiosperms: a genecological factor. Science 206: 20-23, 1979.

13. Schwartz D. Genetic control of alcohol dehydrogenase — a competition model for regulation of gene action. Genetics 67: 411-425, 1971.

14. Tanksley SD, Zamir D, Rick CM. Evidence for extensive overlap of sporophytic and gametophytic gene expression in *Lycopersicon esculentum.* Science 213: 453-455, 1981.

15. Mulcahy DL, Kaplan SM. Mendelian ratios despite non-random fertilization. Am Nat 113: 419-425, 1979.

16. Mulcahy DL, Robinson RW, Ihara M, Kesseli R. Gametophic transcription for acid phosphatases in pollen of *Cucurbita* species hybrids. Jour Hered 72: 353-354, 1981.

17. Brooks J, Shaw G. Recent developments in the chemistry, biochemistry, geochemistry and post-tetrad ontogeny of sporopollenins derived from pollen and spore exines. In Pollen: Development and Physiology, ed. by J. Heslop-Harrison. 1971. Appleton-Century-Crafts, NY. pp. 99-120.

18. Knox RB, Heslop-Harrison J, Reed C. Localization of antigens associated with the pollen grain wall by immunofluorescence. Nature 225: 1066-1068, 1970.

19. Knox RB, Heslop-Harrison J. Pollen-wall proteins: localization and enzymic activity. J Cell Sci 6: 1-27, 1970.

20. Heslop-Harrison J. The pollen wall: structure and development.

In Pollen Development and Physiology. 1971. Appleton-Century-Crafts, NY. pp. 77-98.

21. Stanley RG, Linskens HG, Pollen: Biology, Biochemistry, and Management 1975. Springer Verlag, NY.

22. Heslop-Harrison J. An interpretation of the hydrodynamics of pollen. Am Jour Bot 66: 737-743, 1979.

23. Lewis D, Burrage S, Walls D. Immunological reactions of single pollen grains, electrophoresis and enzymology of pollen protein exudates. Jour Exp Bot 18: 371-378, 1967.

24. Howlett BJ, Knox RB, Heslop-Harrison J. Pollen-wall proteins: release of the allergen antigen E from intine and exine sites in pollen grains of ragweed and *Cosmos*. J Cell Sci 13: 603-619, 1973.

25. Porter EK Origins and genetic nonvariability of the proteins which diffuse from maize pollen. Environ Health Perspectives 37: 53-59, 1981.

26. Khush GS Cytogenetics of Aneuploids. Academic Press, NY. 1973. pp. 301. □

Chapter VII

The Biology and Identification of Fungal Aeroallergens[†]

John H. Haines, Ph.D* and Ira F. Salkin, Ph.D.**

ABSTRACT

Fungi are a unique group of organisms classified as a separate kingdom primarily on the basis of their ability to absorb nutrients and their multinucleate character. They may be unicellular (yeastlike), filamentous (moldlike), or both (dimorphic). Fungi may form reproductive propagules through an asexual process by mitotic nuclear division (e.g., buds, sporangiospores, or condidia) and/or through a sexual process by meiotic division (e.g., zygospores, ascospores, or basidiospores). The morphologic features of the reproductive mechanism and the propagules are the critical characteristics used to identify fungi. The key features of the spores of several common fungi of interest to allergists, as well as the methods used to qualitatively evaluate airborne spores are described.

BIOLOGY

To appreciate fungi as allergens and to comprehend the methods used for their isolation and identification requires a basic understanding of the biology of this group of microorganisms. A logical point to begin such a general discussion is the relationship of fungi with other living organisms. Mycologists of the late 18th and 19th centuries were primarily concerned with higher land fungi, specifically mushrooms. The "nonmotile" character of mushrooms and their "rooted" manner of growth suggested their classification in the plant kingdom. We still see vestiges of this botanic heritage in mycologic terminology, i.e., the description of the major growing phase of a fungus as the vegetative stage, or the use of the suffix *phyte* (i.e., plant) in the term *saprophyte* to describe a fungus developing on nonliving organic matter.

At the start of the 20th century, however, the classification of fungi and all other living organisms began to change with the work of Haeckel and others. These changes culminated in Whittaker's five-kingdom scheme.[1,2] In that scheme, which is now accepted by most mycologists, fungi are neither plants, nor animals, nor directly related to any other living form. They are simply fungi, a unique kingdom which did not evolve into any other living forms.

What characteristics distinguish fungi and necessitate the establishment of a separate kingdom? All fungi are eukaryotic (possessing a true nucleus), heterotrophic (incapable of forming all of their nutritional requirements), and achlorophyllous (lacking chlorophyll). However, it we use just these three characteristics, many living forms, even man, could be included in the fungi. It is a fourth feature, the ability to release extracellular enzymes which break down nutrient sources and to absorb the nutrients, which distinguishes fungi from most other living organisms.[3] If animals are recognized as a separate kingdom, due in part to their ingestion of nutrients, and if plants are considered a separate kingdom, in part because they photosynthesize or form their own nutrients, it can be logically argued that fungi are a separate kingdom on account of their ability to absorb nutrients.

Finally, a fifth characteristic of fungi differentiates them as a unique group. All fungi are multinucleate, in

*Biological Survey, New York State Museum, The State Department of Education, Albany.
**Wadsworth Center for Laboratories and Research, New York State Department of Health, Albany.
†Contribution #512 of the NYS Science Service.

that "factually or functionally" the entire developing body of the organism lacks crosswalls (septa).[3] In lower or primitive fungi the growing body is wholly interconnected and "factually" devoid of septa, except at the point of formation of the reproductive structures. The growing mat of such a fungus may be thought of as one giant cell, containing thousands of nuclei. Although septa may be formed by higher or advanced fungi, the crosswalls are usually incomplete, containing openings through which cytoplasm and subcellular structures freely migrate. Thus, in a functional sense, the developing body of even such higher forms may be considered to be one multi-nucleate cell.

By combining these five characteristics, i.e., by describing fungi as eukaryotic, heterotrophic, achlorophyllous forms which absorb nutrients into a growing body which lacks crosswalls, one can distinguish fungi and incorporate them as a separate kingdom.

What is the general developmental pattern found in this unique group of living organisms? The first portion of the life cycle of virtually all fungi is a major growing state or vegetative phase. During this stage the fungus establishes its body form, invades the environment, and absorbs and stores nutrients. Mycologists have used the morphology of this vegetative phase to divide fungi into three broad groups. In the vast majority the growing stage in composed of filaments of hyphae (Fig. 1). The hyphae interweave to form a mat or mycelium (Fig. 2). Thus the vegetative stage of most fungi is a myceliated structure. In short, most fungi are molds.[4]

The vegetative stage of a far smaller number of fungi, known as yeasts or yeastlike forms, consists of a single, generally ovoid cell (Fig. 3). Some authors prefer to restrict the use of the term "yeast" to a specific fungal group, the "true" yeasts (hemiascomycete).[4] The members of this group are similar, not only in their vegetative morphology, but also in their biochemical, physiologic, and other characteristics. In contrast, the term "yeast-

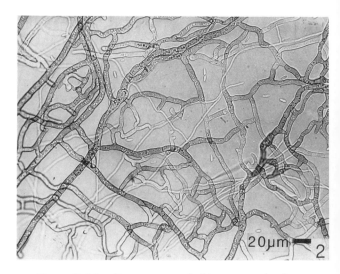

Figure 2. Mycelium composed of interwoven hyphae.

like" is used only as a morphologic definition, i.e., to designate a fungus similar to a "true" yeast in its unicellular vegetative morphology. However, we shall use the terms interchangeably in this general discussion.

The vegetative morphology of a very restricted number of fungi may be either moldlike or yeastlike, depending upon specific environmental conditions. Fungi with such environmentally mutable body forms are called dimorphic. These organisms are usually moldlike when grown at room temperature (25°C) and yeastlike at a higher temperature (37°C).

Several zoopathogenic fungi, including *Histoplasma capsulatum*, *Blastomyces dermatitidis*, and *Sporothrix*

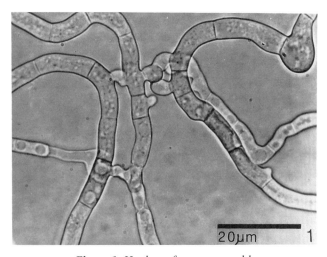

Figure 1. Hyphae of common mold.

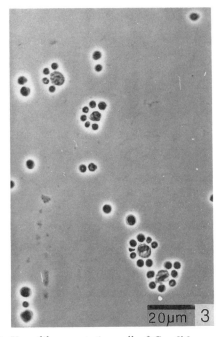

Figure 3. Yeastlike vegetative cell of **Candida** sp. asexually reproducing by budding.

schenckii, are dimorphic in that they are normally moldlike when grown *in vitro* and yeastlike *in vivo*.

The growing body of any fungus, regardless of its morphology, is surrounded by a multilayered, rigid, inflexible wall. While the chemical composition of the wall is quite variable, one can generally identify chitin, glucans, and mannans, along with lipids and proteins, within it. The differential staining properties of this wall permit the identification of fungi as such, either in direct examination of clinical specimens or in paraffin-embedded tissue sections. In addition, the antigenic properties of the wall help to enable serologic diagnosis of several fungal infections.

In addition to the vegetative phase, the fungal life cycle contains asexual and/or sexual reproductive stages in which the population insures its survival through the formation of spores. When discussing general concepts applicable to all fungi we will use the term spore in its most broad sense to refer to any fungal dispersive reproductive or resting propagule. In contrast, in describing specific reproductive structures we will utilize their technical mycologic references such as conidia, ascospores, sporangiospores, etc.

Most fungi form reproductive structures through an asexual mechanism, i.e., mitotic nuclear division. Since there is no fusion of gametes or nuclei and since only mitotic division occurs, asexual propagules are genetically identical to each other and to the parent cell on which or in which they are formed.

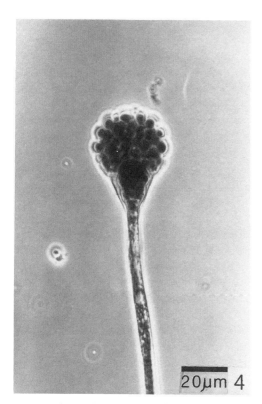

Figure 4. *Sporangia of Absidia.*

In yeasts asexual reproduction generally takes the form of budding. This process involves mitotic division of the vegetative nucleus and then a migration of one of the daughter nuclei into a newly formed expansion of the vegetative cell (Fig. 3). This "ballooned-out" section (bud) of the yeast cell enlarges and eventually seals itself off and separates from the parent cell.[4]

In primitive molds asexual reproduction occurs within a saclike structure called a sporangium (Fig. 4), which generally is situated at the end of a specialized or nonspecialized hypha. The first stage in asexual reproduction is mitotic division of all nuclei within the sporangium. This is followed by cleavage of the sporangial cytoplasm to form uninucleate, motile (zoospores) or nonmotile (sporangiospores) propagules.[4]

In more advanced molds asexual reproduction generally consists of mitotic division of nuclei within hyphae and the "packaging" of each daughter nucleus and its associated cytoplasm within a wall to form a nonmotile, deciduous propagule or conidium. The methods by which the conidia are formed, as well as their shape, size, color, etc., are quite variable.

Since the morphology of viruses is not observable with a light microscope and the morphologic diversity of bacteria is quite limited, sophisticated biochemical and physiologic procedures have been developed for their identification. In contrast, fungi show a wide range of morphologic diversity in their vegetative development and asexual reproduction. Therefore morphologic rather than physiologic characters are mainly used in fungal identification. While for yeasts a limited number of physiologic techniques, such as carbohydrate assimilation and fermentation tests, have been devised, morphology remains critical for their identification.[5] Sporangial morphology, the method of conidial formation, and the morphologic features of sporangiospores and conidia are essential characters required in the identification of molds.[6-8]

Sexual reproduction, i.e., reproduction by meiotic division of a zygotic or fused nucleus, is found in the developmental cycle of many, but not all, fungi. The reproductive process consists of three events: (i) union of two specialized or nonspecialized structures, each housing a genetically different nucleus, or plasmogamy; (ii) fusion of these two nuclei, or karyogamy; and (iii) meiotic division of the fused or zygotic nucleus. Each resulting daughter nucleus is enveloped in cytoplasm and contained within a wall. Since the nuclei within the spores are the product of meiotic division of fused, genetically dissimilar nuclei, the spores will be genetically different from each other and from the parent mycelium on which they were formed.

Mycologists use the different sexual reproductive mechanisms of fungi as a means of broadly classifying them into relatively homogenous groups. Unfortunately no one fungal taxonomic system has been ac-

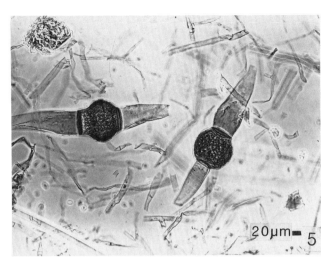

Figure 5. Zygospore of **Rhizopus** sp.

cepted by all mycologists. We shall discuss the classification scheme proposed by Ainsworth.[9] In this system all fungi are incorporated within the division Eumycota, which in turn is divided into five subdivisions:

Mastigomycotina—fungi which form motile reproductive cells (zoospores) most of which are not airborne.

Zygomycotina—molds in which sexual reproduction results in the formation of zygospores (Fig. 5), e.g., *Mucor*, *Absidia*, and *Rhizopus*.

Ascomycotina—advanced fungi in which the sexually formed spore (ascospore) is borne within a sac (ascus, Fig. 6), e.g., *Chaetomium* and *Daldinia*. In addition to a moldlike vegetative phase (commonly observed in the laboratory on artificial media), members of this group form macroscopic structures called fruiting bodies or ascomas which house the asci (commonly observed under natural conditions but rarely found in the laboratory).

Basidiomycotina—advanced fungi in which sexual reproduction results in the formation of spores (basidiospores) situated on the outside of a club-shaped structure (basidium, Fig. 7). The basidia of most basidiomycetes are housed in a complex fruiting body, the most familiar of which are mushrooms. While the basidiospores of some genera will germinate and form a moldlike vegetative phase on artificial media, very rarely will basidiomycetes form basidia, basidiospores, or fruiting bodies under laboratory conditions.

Deuteromycotina (Fungi Imperfecti)—fungi in which there is no known means of sexual reproduction, e.g., *Cladosporium*, and *Alternaria*.

What physical factors affect the development of fungi? While most species develop optimally at a slightly acidic pH (pH = 6.5 to 6.7), other species can grow under conditions which range from strongly acidic (pH = 3.0) to slightly alkaline (pH = 8.0). Similarly, although most fungi grow best at room temperature (20–25°C), some grow at temperatures as low as −8°C or at 50°C or higher. Although most fungi are strict aerobes, several groups, e.g., many yeasts, are facultative anaerobes. A high relative humidity (95%) is generally the most favorable. However, the wall surrounding the asexual or sexual spore inhibits desiccation and permits fungi to survive extreme or prolonged droughts. In short, various fungi are capable of surviving and

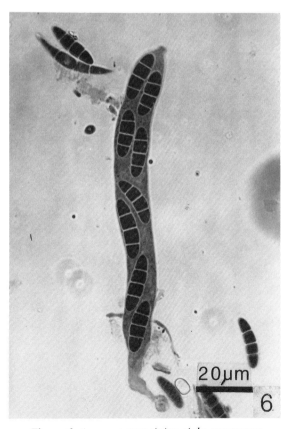

Figure 6. An ascus containing eight ascopsores.

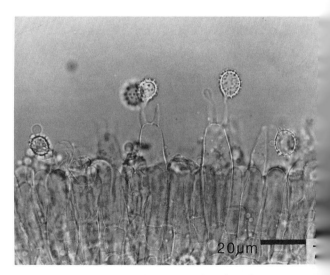

Figure 7. Basidiospores forming on basidia of **Russula** sp., mushroom.

developing under virtually any set of physical conditions.[10]

Since fungi develop over a wide range of physical conditions, we are able to find them exploiting diverse and bizarre habitats. A case of hypersensitivity pneumonitis was attributed to fungus-contaminated buckets used to transport water in a home sauna.[11] Two recent cases of rhinocerebral mucormycosis in poorly controlled diabetics were ascribed to *Rhizopus oryzae* developing in the air conditioner in the physician's office.[12] Fungal contamination of an air conditioner in another case caused hypersensitivity pneumonitis.[13] A cluster of eight cases of aspergillosis in a cancer-treatment facility was caused by development of the mold in the cellulose-based fireproofing material used to coat steel girders.[14]

What techniques are used to determine the presence of fungi in a particular habitat? We shall limit our discussion to techniques of particular relevance to allergists, i.e., sampling for airborne spores.

To evaluate airborne fungi qualitatively in an indoor or outdoor environment, one can use culture and/or slide-sampling procedures. The culture technique consists of exposing a 100-mm petri dish containing Sabouraud dextrose or rose-bengal agar to the air for 15 minutes, incubating the plate right-side up at room temperature, and examining it every other day for a minimum of 7 days. This technique is one of the easiest to use, as the spores deposited from the air onto the agar medium become readily observable as developing colonies. One can even tentatively identify the fungi on the basis of their colony morphologies. However, spores of different sizes are not deposited equally on the agar surface (large or heavy spores fall from the air far more readily than small or light spores); nonviable spores may go undetected; and many fungi will fail to grow or form characteristic structures on an artificial nutrient medium.

The slide-sampling technique consists of exposing a coated (e.g., with Vaseline) microscope slide to the air for up to 24 hours, adding a cover slip, and examining the slide. The major advantages of this procedure are that the sample can be observed immediately, no culturing facilities are required, and the sample will include both viable and nonviable spores. However, it is quite difficult to identify a fungus on the basis of spore morphology alone. While a few, such as those illustrated in this article, can be readily identified, many are nearly impossible to identify by this technique.[15]

Neither of these procedures provides a quantitative evaluation of airborne spores. While the rotorod sampler is a simple and effective means of obtaining quantitative air samples, they must be microscopically examined on a thick transparent rod. While the loss of resolution due to this glass rod is acceptable for the identification of pollens, it is less than acceptable when working with small fungal spores. Several other instruments, e.g., Hirst and Burkard, are available for the quantitative assessment of airborne spores without significant compromise in optical quality.[16] However, the labor required for their operation and their large size make them impractical for use in clinical situations.

When sampling for spores it is important to remember that the propagules become airborne through a number of mechanisms, which respond to different environmental conditions. Wind, rain, light, and changes in relative humidity trigger the release of different spores.[17] In an outdoor environment there are two daily peaks in spore discharge: at 3–6 a.m., when the relative humidity is highest, and at 3–6 p.m., the driest, windiest part of the day. Many known fungal allergens are found during these daytime peaks.[18] There are also seasonal variations. Many spores reach peak concentrations in the air during late summer and fall.[19]

What procedures are used to identify fungi observed in cultures? Here we shall discuss only the basic procedures for identifying the more common fungi of interest to the allergist.

For molds and morphologic features of the spores are the most critical characters, and the simplest method for observing spore development is a slide culture. A block of nutrient agar, 1–2 cm on each side and 2–3 mm deep, is placed on a sterile glass slide, which is supported on a bent glass rod within a sterile petri dish. A small portion of the unknown mold is inoculated at the midpoint of the upper edge of each side of the block. A sterile cover slip is placed over the upper surface, and water is added to the petri dish to maintain moist conditions. The slide can be removed at intervals for direct observation of the development and morphologic features of the conidia, under a compound microscope.

IDENTIFICATION

The air we breathe is the transport medium for spores of tens of thousands of fungal species, and it is impossible to identify all of them. However, the most common airborne spores are also the most likely to elicit allergic responses. Constant contact with these common spores may be a major factor in their allergenicity or, alternatively, being the most common they may simply have been those most investigated. The authors believe the explanation lies between these two poles.

We will discuss both common and uncommon airborne spores that are known to cause allergic reactions. Spore identification is still best accomplished by making a visual impression of the structures and comparing them to photographs of spores of known identity. For each spore illustrated we will describe its stable, salient, morphologic identifying characteristics, as well as those features that are genetically or environmentally variable. References for further information and descriptions are included with each entry.

Alternaria (Fig. 8)—This important allergenic member of the Deuteromycotina forms one of the three most common airborne spores. While its conidia are quite distinctive and permit easy recognition of the genus, they are of little value in species identification due to their inherent morphologic variability and the importance of host specificity in differentiating species.

Identifying characters: Conidia most often 30–50 µm long, born in chains, with a narrow beak at the upper end and a darkened pore at the apex. They are transversely and longitudinally septated, olive to golden brown, and the outer surface is often covered by minute, dark projections. When old, dry, or observed in a nonaqueous medium, the conidia may appear shriveled. Members of the genus grow readily in culture on artificial media as white to gray, downy colonies.

References: 8, 20, 21, 22, 42.

The conidia of *Alternaria* spp. may be distinguished from those of *Pleospora* by the presence of the beak and pore and from *Pithomyces* by the beak and the less regular placement of septa.

While *Alternaria* spp. may be easily grown in culture, they tend to lose their ability to form conidia on artificial media. Since members of the genus are generally found as plant saprobes or parasites, *Alternaria* conidia are among the most common fungal structures comprising the outdoor air spora. However, some species, such as the most common member of the genus *A. alternata,* also may be found indoors growing on moist wood, paper, cloth, evaporative coolers, or air conditioners. While the genus is cosmopolitan in distribution, its conidia may not be the most abundant in some regions. For example, in the Pacific Northwest of the United States, the conidia of *Alternaria* are far less prevalent than those of *Cladosporium.* Because the conidium is comparatively large and ease to identify even low-power microscopic examination, there is a danger of overestimating the relative importance of *Alternaria* in the air spora.

Conidial liberation in *Alternaria* is initiated during times of decreasing relative humidity. As a consequence, the peak level of conidia in the air is usually found during the day when the relative humidity is lowest, temperatures highest, and air movement greatest. While its conidia seldom are absent from air samples, they are most prevalent in the fall and least common in the winter.

Aspergillus—Due to the large number and physiologic diversity of the species which comprise this deuteromycete genus, we have chosen to discuss two of its more common and clinically important species rather than attempting to describe, in general terms, the entire genus.

Identifying characters: Identification of all *Aspergillus* spp. should be based on colony and microscopic characteristics as found on Czapek-Dox agar culture. It is impossible on the basis of isolated conidia to identify *Aspergillus* spp. or to differentiate them from members of such other genera as *Penicillium, Trichoderma,* and *Verticillium.* Conidia of *A. fumigatus* are 2–3.5 µm in diameter, spherical or very slightly elongate, smooth-walled or bearing very minute spines, light green to blue green, and borne in long chains (short chains may occasionally be found in air samples). It grows rapidly on artificial media and may be distinguished from other members of the genus by its long (0.4 mm), unbranched chains of conidia borne on flask-shaped structures (phialides) arranged in a single layer on the upper one-third of a swollen vesicle at the apex of an elongate stalk.

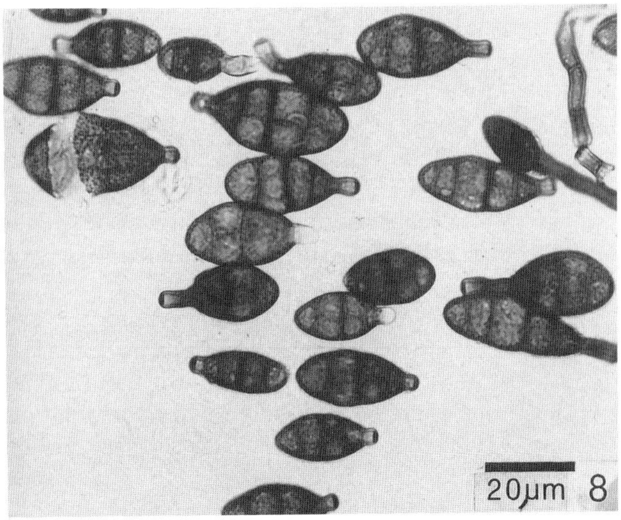

Figure 8. Conidia of Alternaria sp.

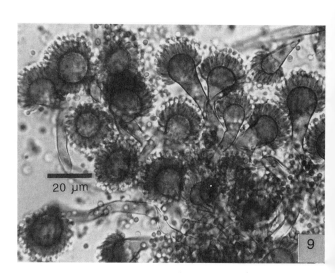

Figure 9. Conidial heads of Aspergillus fumigatus.

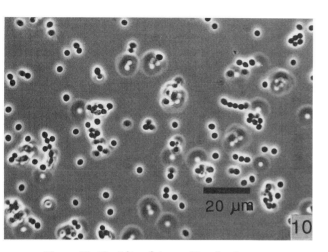

*Figure 10. Conidia of **Aspergillus fumigatus**.*

References: 22, 23.

A. fumigatus (Figs. 9, 10) is probably the most well-known fungal allergen due to its role in allergic bronchopulmonary aspergillosis. The small size of its conidia permits their deep penetration into the respiratory system. In nature, the organism is found in soil and on plant debris, growing over a wide range of temperatures (near freezing to over 45°C[23]). It is well adapted to both man-made and natural habitats such as spoiled food, wet leather, compost, sewerage, tobacco and hay storage barns, and humidifiers. Its conidia are dislodged by air movement and their concentration, in both indoor and outdoor environments, is probably today more correlated to human activities than to natural factors.[24]

Aspergillus niger (Fig. 11).—Identifying characters: Conidia are 3.5–5.0 μm in diameter, spherical, brown (black *en masse*), bearing an irregular wall pattern of short ridges, and borne in long chains (short segments of which are often found in air samples). It grows so readily on artificial media that its white colonies (which become black with the development of conidia) are

frequent laboratory contaminants. It may be readily differentiated from *A. fumigatus* by colony and conidial pigmentation and the formation of conidia in long chains on phialides situated on one to several stalks (metulae) attached over the entire surface of a 40–100 μm vesicle. When viewed with a compound microscope, the conidial forming region appears like a double halo surrounded by chains and clumps of spheres. In addition, the conidia of *A. niger*, unlike *A. fumigatus*, are too large to penetrate into the alveoli and cannot survive over as wide a temperature range.

References: 23, 25.

A. niger is one of if not the most common species of *Aspergillus*. It is worldwide in distribution and may be as common in such natural habitats as soil or on decaying vegetation as in the indoor environment on cotton fabric, leather, spoiled food, evaporation coolers.[21] The ease with which it may be isolated and identified in culture could cause an overestimation of its role as an airborne allergen.

Aureobasidium (Pullularis) pullulans (Fig. 12)—This ubiquitous, black, allergenic deuteromycete is a relatively common constituent of the air spora. It may be isolated at any time of year[26] from a wide range of outdoor (soil, decaying vegetation) and indoor (latex paint, laboratory stock bottles) habitats.

Identifying characters: Two types of conidia generally are found; (1) small, 4–6 $\times$ 2–3 μm, colorless, thin walled, one-celled blastoconidia and (2) large, 12 $\times$ 6 μm, darkly pigmented, thick walled, occasionally 2 or more celled chlamydoconidia.[8] The blastoconidia generally are dispersed by water drops and consequently may be found in highest concentration in the air during wet weather. In culture the colonies are mucoid to pasty, convoluted, white to black in color.

References: 8, 22, 42.

Cladosporium (Figs. 13 & 14)—The most prevalent

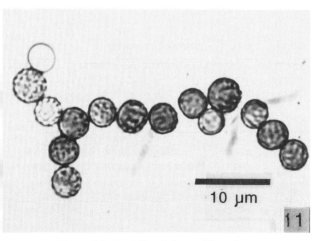

*Figure 11. Conidia of **Aspergillus niger**.*

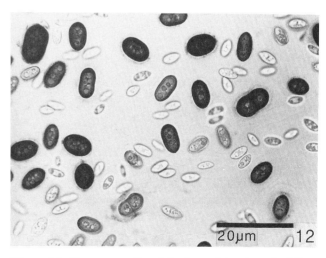

*Figure 12. Two types of conidia formed by **Aureobasidium pullulans**.*

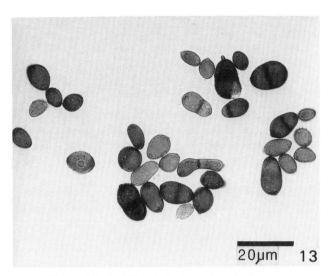

Figure 13. Conidia of **Cladosporium herbarum**.

Members of the genus may be found in nature as plant saprobes or parasites and may be isolated in an indoor environment from textiles, spoiled food, paper, and even damp painted surfaces. The conidia in the outdoor air have a diurnal periodicity being most prevalent in the early afternoon when the relative humidity is lowest, temperatures the highest, and air movement the greatest. Consequently, as one would expect, they are common members of the dry air spora and less frequently recovered in rainy periods. While present in the outdoor air spora all year, they are most commonly found in air samples during the summer and fall.[27,28] In addition, during these periods mowing or harvesting may cause extremely high concentrations of conidia.

Since the conidia of *Cladosporium* sp. are frequently dispersed in long chains, allergists must be able to determine the extent of such chains in the air spora to evaluate their potential to elicit allergic reactions and to estimate their possible penetration into the respiratory system. A Hirst or rotorod air sampler would permit a more accurate analysis of the spora composition than would culturing.

Coprinus comatus (Fig. 15)—This mushroom, commonly known as "shaggy mane," bears basidiospores that commonly are recovered in air samples and are, as those of other mushrooms, known to elicit allergic responses in sensitive individuals.[29] However, the basidiospores of this and other basidiomycetes are not often included in mold surveys because they fail to grow spores in culture on artificial media.[29]

Identifying characters: Basidiospores are 11–15 × 6.5–8.5 μm, smooth, smokey gray to black, with a light-colored pore at one end and an off-center apiculus (projection) at the other. They are found only as part of the outdoor air spora, reaching peak concentration in air samples after midnight and their lowest level at mid-day. The fruiting body, and consequently, its basidiospores most commonly are found in spring and fall on lawns and along roadsides. The basidiospores are often found concentrated in the inky liquid formed

airborne fungal spores in many areas of the Northeast and worldwide, and among the most allergenic, are members of this deuteromycete genus.

Identifying characters: The conidia of members of this genus are distinctive in bearing dark, slightly protruding, ringlike scars at each end. They are pale- or olive-brown, usually elongate, and borne in branched chains with the largest and oldest conidia at the base. The conidia at the branch points have 2 or more scars at one end. Colonies readily develop on artificial media and are velvety to woolly in texture and gray-green to olive-green in color. The two most common members of the genus are *C. herbarum* with 5–15 × 4–6 μm, olive brown, finely warted, single-septate conidia (Fig. 13) and *C. cladosporioides*, which forms 3–7 × 2–4 μm, pale brown, smooth or very finely ornamented, nonseptate conidia (Fig. 14).

References: 8, 20, 22, 42.

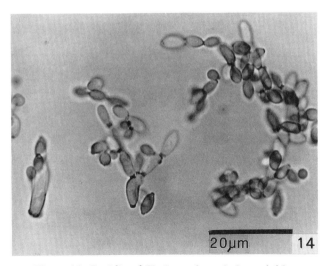

Figure 14. Conidia of **Cladosporium cladosporioides**.

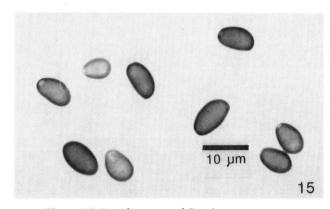

Figure 15. Basidiospores of **Coprinus comatus**.

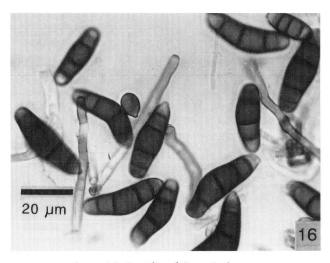

Figure 16. Conidia of *Curvularia sp.*

but a few species, e.g., *C. lunata*, may be isolated from a number of different substrates including soil and painted surfaces. Conidia reach peak concentration in dry, daytime air, and while they may be recovered year around, they have seasonal peaks in the summer and fall.

Daldinia concentrica (Fig. 17)—The ascospores of this fungus are abundant in outdoor air during the spring and fall. However, this fungus will not form fruiting bodies and ascospores in culture on artificial media and consequently, little is known about the allergenic properties of the ascospores.

Identifying characters: Ascospores 12–17 × 6–9 μm, elliptical, slightly inequilateral, black, with a lighter-colored slit on one side. The presence or absence of an internal vacuole is dependent on the mounting medium used to examine the ascospores. The characteristics of the fruiting body, which resembles a small lump of charcoal, are to be found in popular field handbooks on fungi.

References 30, 31.

Daldinia is a common member of the ascomycete family Xylariaceae, genera of which all have similar appearing ascospores. As with most ascomycetes, the ascospores of *Daldinia* are primarily released during daylight, especially after a rain.[28] Since the fruiting body is found growing on rotting wood, generally during Summer and Fall, the ascospores may only be recovered from the outdoor air.

Fusarium (Fig. 18)—The conidia of *Fusarium* are encountered in both indoor and outdoor air.

Identifying characters: Conidia range from 15 to 200 μm in length, are unpigmented, multiseptate, sickle-shaped, and bear a small, off-center, birth-scar near one end which gives them a dog-legged appearance. They readily germinate on artificial media to form white,

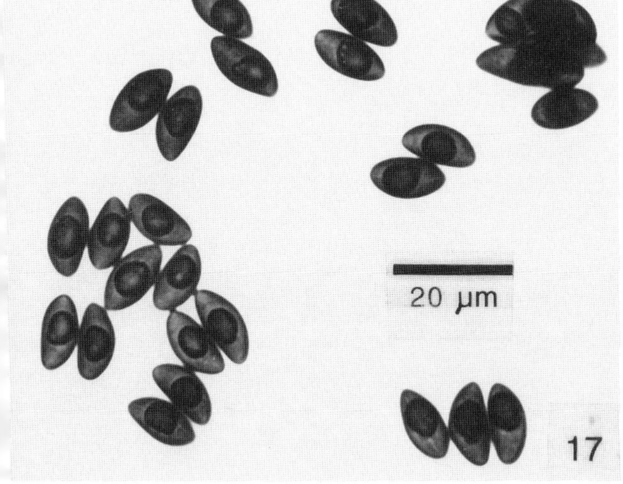

when the tissues of the mushroom break down and may be present, unlike those associated with other common mushrooms, as part of the air spora long after the fruit bodies have disappeared for the season. For a description of the fruit body refer to popular mushroom guides such as Lincoff.[30]

Curvularia (Fig. 16)—While not as common as *Alternaria* and *Cladosporium*, the conidia of this deuteromycetous mold are still a major component of the air spora.

Identifying characters: Conidia are 17 to more than 50 μm long, multiseptate, brown, ellipsoidal or club-shaped, and smooth walled. They are distinguished from other elongate conidia of the air spora by the unequal expansion of one of the middle cells causing the conidia to have a bent or curves shape.

References: 8, 20, 42.

Members of this genus are primarily plant saprobes

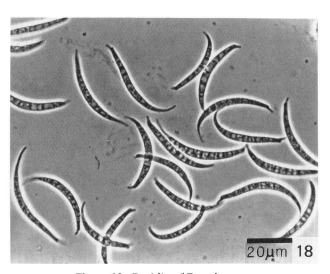

Figure 17. *Ascospores of **Daldinia concentrica**.*

Figure 18. *Conidia of **Fusarium** sp.*

cottony colonies that develop a diffusible, pink pigment.

References: 32, 33.

The genus *Fusarium* forms the asexual portion of the life cycle of ascomycetes in the order Hypocreales. Since members of the genus are common soil fungi and economically important plant pathogens, the conidia comprise a portion of the outdoor air spora. However, the fungus also may be recovered from the indoor environment growing on damp paper and cloth. The conidia are formed in a slime matrix and are discharged in nature by water drops.[28] Therefore, the conidia are most commonly airborne during rainy periods.

Recently, the genus has taken on greater importance as the source of some of the most potent mycotoxins and as opportunistic human pathogens.

Ganoderma (Fig. 19)—This basidiomycete produces basidiospores that are among the most abundant components of the air spora in forest areas. Although an increasing interest is being paid to mushrooms and other basidiomycetes as allergens,[29,34] the fact that *Ganoderma* spp. never form fruiting bodies on artificial media and can only be recognized by their basidiospores contributes to an underestimation of the importance of their basidiospores as an allergenic source.

Identifying characters: Basidiospores are 6.5–9.5 × 5–7 μm, ovoid, straw colored (brown *en masse*), double-walled with minute pores over the surface of the outer wall layer. A large pore surrounded by the outer wall is located at one end and the apiculus is found off-center at the other end. Since the fruiting structures are found only in nature attached to hardwood trees, the basidiospores form part of the outdoor air spora.

References: 30, 43.

Ganoderma applanatum is the most common of several species of this fungus distributed throughout the temperature regions of the world. However, a closely related genus, *Amauroderma*, with morphologically similar basidiospores, is abundant in the tropics.

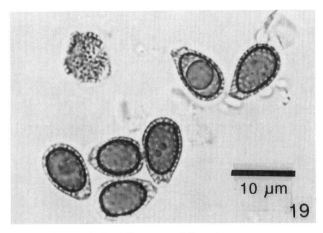

Figure 19. *Basidiospores of* **Ganoderma tsugae.**

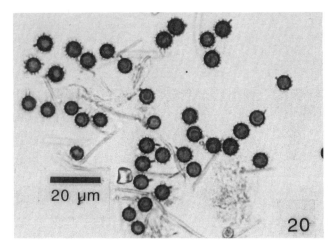

Figure 20. *Basidiospores of* **Lycoperdon** *sp.*

Fruiting structures of *Ganoderma* spp. are perennial, producing a new spore-bearing layer each year for up to 20 years and may become several feel across. They start producing basidiospores in late spring and at peak season, in late summer or early fall, may produce millions of basidiospores each day in a diurnal rhythm with a nighttime peak after midnight. *Ganoderma* is one of the most prolific spore-producing fungi.

Lycoperdon (Fig. 20)—This fungus is one of a group of basidiomycetes that form fruiting structures known as "puffballs". While its basidiospore are not a major component of the air spora and rarely have been implicated in allergic reactions, the inhalation of large numbers of the basidiospores as can occur when handling the fruiting bodies may trigger allergic responses in sensitive individuals. Antigen preparations from several species have been reported as eliciting positive skin test reactions.

References: 29, 34, 35

Identifying characters: Basidiospores are 3–7 μm, spherical, light brown, with smooth or ornamented walls and a single, fine, cylindrical, tubelike projection. While this fungus generally does not grow in culture, its paper-sac-like, pear-shaped, fruiting body (2–9 cm across) can be commonly found in the fall in forests and along the roadside.

References: 30, 31.

There are more than a dozen common basidiomycete species that form puff-balls and similar structures in the Northeastern United States. People are attracted to these fruiting bodies as they are natural dispenser of clouds of basidiospores when agitated or squeezed. Literally millions of the tiny basidiospores are sent into the air (and possibly deep into the respiratory system with a single puff of the sac. There is a long history of the use of puffballs in folk medicine as, for example the apparent dangerous practice of treating nosebleeds by inhaling clouds of the basidiospores. Although thi

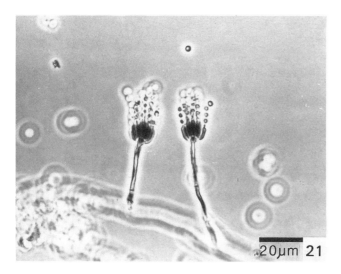

Figure 21. Conidia of **Penicillium** sp. forming on broom-shaped heads.

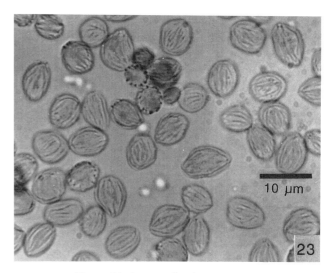

Figure 23. Spores of **Rhizopus oryzae**.

may be very efficacious as the basidiospores would form a matrix for clotting, it could lead to a pulmonary condition described as lycoperdonosis.[35] It is the personal experience of one of us (JHH) that of the fungal specimens within the New York State Mycological Herbarium eliciting the greatest allergic reactions among the workers are those of another puffball-forming basidiomycete, *Bovista pila*.

Penicillium (Fig. 21)—The conidia of this deuteromycete are among the most common in indoor air and its species are among the most difficult to identify.

Conidia are 2.5–4 μm spherical to oblong, smooth-walled or bearing fine ornamentation, with minute collars linking them together in long chains. The conidia are impossible to distinguish from those of numerous other deuteromycetes, e.g., *Aspergillus*, *Phoma*, *Trichoderma*, and *Verticillium*. The mold readily grows on artificial media and is a frequent laboratory contaminant. It may be distinguished by the blue to blue-green color of its colonies and the branched conidia bearing structures resembling broom heads.[36]

Pithomyces chartarum (Fig. 22)—This deuteromycete forms distinctive conidia which, although usually less abundant in the air spora, are morphologically similar to those of *Alternaria*. The mold is found in the same environmental habitats as *Alternaria*, growing on vegetative debris. It grows readily on artificial media in culture.

Identifying characters: Conidia are 18–29 × 10–17 μm, brown, with a finely warty wall ornamentation and usually bearing 3 regular transverse and several longitudinal septa. There is a tiny darkened scar at only one end of the conidium. Colonies are relatively rapid growing, flat, cottony in texture, gray-white to olivaceous in color.

References: 8, 42.

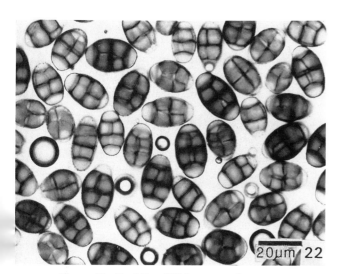

Figure 22. Conidia of **Pithomyces chartarum**.

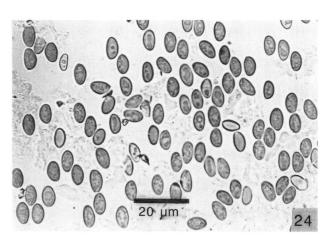

Figure 24. Basidiospores of **Serpula lacrimans**.

Rhizopus oryzae (Fig. 23)—This zygomycete is an extremely common, rapid-growing mold, readily recovered from both outdoor habitats (soil) and indoor sources (spoiled foot, pet fecal matter, and bedding materials along with house dust mites[38]). While it may produce profuse numbers of sporangiospores in less than 3 days, it will all but disappear when its nutrient source is exhausted.

Identifying characters: Sporangiospores are 7–10 μm, ovoid, light smokey gray, with irregular longitudinal ridges on the walls. Since they are formed within a large sac-like structure (sporangium) through random cleavage of the cytoplasm, the sporangiospores bear no pores or other attachment structures. Colonies are cottony and dense, at first white but becoming brown- to black-gray in color and growing rapidly to completely cover a 100-mm petri plate within 48–72 hours.

Reference: 37.

Serpula (Merulinus) lacrimans (Fig. 24)—This allergenic basidiomycete is rare in nature but common in old houses in Northern Europe and increasingly in New England.[39] The fungus is primarily known as the cause of dry rot in wooden structures and has, as such, become a problem in old buildings that have been rehabilitated through the addition of vapor barriers and insulation. Its development is further encouraged by the present fuel conservation programs in which room temperatures are maintained below 70°F.

Identifying characters: Basidiospores 8–12 μm long, nearly oval, ochre yellow when examined microscopically, slightly flattened at one end and bearing the off-center apiculus at the other end. While it is difficult to identify in culture on artificial media, expansive growths of fleshy, wafflelike fruiting structures are readily formed in homes with dry rot.

Reference 30.

The basidiospores may be produced in sufficient quantities to cover shelves and floors with a visible rust-

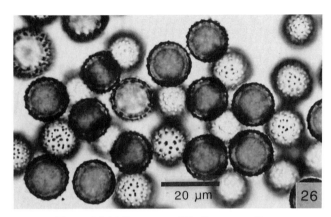

Figure 26. *Teliospores of* **Ustilago maydis.**

brown dust, and it may be found year-round in buildings whenever there is sufficient moisture for its growth.

Stemonitis (Fig. 25)—While technically a Myxomycete (slime mold) and not a fungus, this organism produces large quantities of airborne spores. At least one member of the slime molds has been shown to elicit an allergic response in sensitive individuals.[34]

Identifying characters: Spores 7–10 μm, spherical, relatively thin-walled, with raised, reticulate wall ornamentation, and borne on tiny bottle-brush like structures. The spores may be distinguished from morphologically similar smut (Ustilaginales) spores by their thinner walls.

Reference: 40.

Because the spores of Myxomycetes are difficult to distinguish from one another and from those of smuts and inasmuch Myxomycetes do not readily grow in culture, slime mold spores have been largely ignored as allergens.

Ustilago maydis (Fig. 26)—While the spores of this basidiomycete have been found to cause allergic reactions in some rhinitics,[34] it is more important as a phytopathogen causing corn blight.

Identifying characters: Teliospores (resting spores) are 7–10 μm in diameter, spherical, with walls evenly ornamented with prominent spines but lacking spores, scars, or evidence of other attachment structures.

Reference: 41.

Although it is a basidiomycete, *U. maydis* forms spherical teliospores more abundantly than basidiospores. Further, there is no nocturnal periodicity in teliospore formation as seen in the release of basidiospores. While it is difficult to identify this fungus to species on the basis of the appearance of its teliospores, it is unmistakable when seen on blackened ears of corn in the field. It does not produce fruiting bodies on artificial media nor on indoor substrates. The spores are a major part of the outdoor air spora in late Summer and early Fall, in corn growing regions of the U.S.

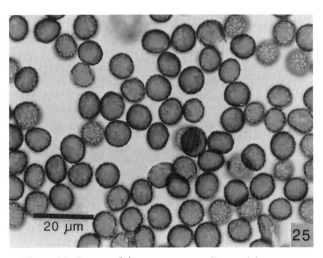

Figure 25. *Spores of the myxomycete* **Stemonitis natans.**

REFERENCES

1. Haeckel EHPA. The Wonders of Life. New York: Harper, 1904.
2. Whittaker RH. New concepts of kingdoms or organisms. Evolutionary relations are better represented by new classifications than by the traditional two kingdoms. Science 163:150–160, 1969.
3. Ross IK. Biology of the Fungi. New York: McGraw-Hill, 1979.
4. Alexopoulos CJ, Mims CW. Introductory Mycology. New York: John Wiley & Sons, 1979.
5. Lodder J (Ed.). The Yeast. A Taxonomic Study. 2nd ed. Amsterdam: North Holland Publishing Co, 1970.
6. von Arx JA. The Genera of Fungi Sporulating in Pure Culture. Lehre: J Cramer, 1974.
7. Baron GL. The Genera of Hyphomycetes from Soil. Baltimore: Williams & Wilkins Co, 1968.
8. Ellis MB. Dematiaceous Hyphomycetes. Kew: CMI Publ, 1971.
9. Ainsworth GC. Introductions and keys to higher taxa. Ch. 1. In: The Fungi, an Advanced Treatise, vol. 4A. Ainsworth GC, Sparrow FK, Sussman AS. (Eds.). Academic Press, 1973, pp. 1–7.
10. Ainsworth GC, Sussman AD (Eds.). The Fungi, An Advanced Treatise, Vol. 3. New York: Academic Press, 1969.
11. Metzger WJ, Patterson R, Fink J, Semerdjian R, Roberts M. Sauna-takers disease. Hypersensitivity pneumonitis due to contaminated water in a home sauna. J Am Med Assoc 236:2209–2211, 1976.
12. England AC, Weinstein M, Ellner JJ, Ajello L. Two cases of rhinocerebral zygomycosis (mucormycosis) with common epidemiologic and environmental features. Am Rev Respir Dis 124:497–498, 1981.
13. Banaszak EF, Thiede WH, Fink JN. Hypersensitivity pneumonitis due to contamination of an air conditioner. N Engl J Med 283:271–276, 1970.
14. Aisner J, Schimpff SC, Bennett JE, Young VM, Wiernik PH. Aspergillus infection in cancer patients. J Am Med Assoc 235:411–412, 1976.
15. Southworth D. Introduction to the biology of airborne fungal spores. Ann Allergy 32:1–22, 1974.
16. Ogden EC, Raynor GS, Hayes JV, Lewis DM, Haines JH. Manual for Sampling Airborne Pollen. New York: Hafner Press, 1974.
17. Meredith DS. Significance of spore release and dispersal mechanisms in plant disease epidemiology. Ann Rev Phytopathol 11:313–342, 1973.
18. Lewis WH, Imber WE, Maniotis J. Allergy epidemiology in the St. Louis, Missouri area. I. Fungi. Ann Allergy 34:374–384, 1975.
19. Ogden EC, Lewis DM. Airborne Pollen and Fungus Spores of New York State. Bull #378. Albany: New York State Museum and Science Service, 1960.
20. Smith EG. Sampling and Identifying Allergenic Pollens and Molds, Vol. II. An Illustrated Identification Manual for Air Samples. San Antonio: Blewstone Press, 1986.
21. Al-Doory Y, Domson JF. Mould Allergy. Philadelphia: Lea & Febiger, 1984.
22. Solomon WR, Mathews KP. Aerobiology and inhalant allergens. Ch. 50. In: Allergy, Principles and Practice, vol. 2. Middleton E, Reed CE, Ellis EF (eds.). CB Mosby, 1983, pp. 1143–1188.
23. Raper KB, Fennell DI. The Genus Aspergillus. Baltimore: Williams & Wilkins Co, 1965.
24. Milner PD, Marsh PB, Snowden RB, Parr JF. Occurrence of Aspergillus fumigatus during composting of sewage sludge. Appl Environ Microbiol 34:765–772, 1977.
25. Al-Musallam A. Revision of the Black Aspergillus Species. Utrecht: Drukkerij Elinkwijk BV, 1980.
26. Al-Doory Y, Domson JF, Howard WA, Sly RM. Airborne fungi and pollens of the Washington DC metropolitan area. Ann Allergy 45:360–367, 1980.
27. Kramer CL, Pady SM, Rogerson CT. Kansas aerobiology III: Cladosporium. Trans Kansas Acad Sci 62:200–207, 1959.
28. Ingold CT. Fungus Spores: Their Liberation and Dispersal. Oxford: Clarendon Press, 1971.
29. Lehrer SB, Lopez M, Butcher BT, Olson J, Reed M, Salvaggio JE. Basidiomycete mycelia and spore-allergen extracts: skin test reactivity in adults with symptoms of respiratory allergy. J Allergy Clin Immunol 78:478–485, 1986.
30. Lincoff GH. The Audubon Society Field Guide to North American Mushrooms. Oxford: Alfred A Knopf, 1981.
31. Smith HW, Smith AH. How to Know the Non-Gilled Fleshy Fungi. Dubuque: Wm C Brown Co, 1973.
32. Booth C. The Genus Fusarium. Kew: CMI Publ, 1971.
33. Joffe AZ. Fusarium Species. Their Biology and Toxicology. New York: John Wiley & Sons, 1986.
34. Santilli J, Rockwell WJ, Collins RP. The significance of the spores of the basidiomycetes (mushrooms and their allies) in bronchial asthma and allergic rhinitis. Ann Allergy 55:469–471, 1985.
35. Strand RD, Neuhauser BD, Sornberger CF. Lycoperdonosis. N Engl J Med 277:89–91, 1967.
36. Raper KB, Thom C. A Manual of the Penicillia. Baltimore: Williams & Wilkins, 1949.
37. Zycha H, Siepmann R, Linnemann G. Mucorales. Lehre: J Cramer, 1969.
38. Andersen A. Microfungi in beds and their relation to house-dust mites. Grana 24;55–59, 1985.
39. O'Brien IM, Bull J, Creamer B, Sepulveda R, Harris M, Burge PS, Pepys J. Asthma and extrinsic allergic alveolitis due to Merulius lacrymans. Clin Allergy 8:535–542, 1978.
40. Martin GW, Alexopoulos CJ. The Myxomycetes. Iowa City: Univ of Iowa Press, 1969.
41. Fischer GW. Manual of the North American Smut Fungi. New York: Ronald Press, 1953.
42. Ellis MB, Ellis JP. Microfungi on Land Plants. An Identification Handbook. New York: Macmillan Publishing, 1985.
43. Gilbertson, RL, Ryvarden L. North American Polypores. Oslo: Fungiflora, 1987.

ANATOMY
AND PHYSIOLOGY

Chapter VIII
Nasal Anatomy and Physiology

Nathan A. Geurkink, M.D.

ABSTRACT

An understanding of the normal anatomy and physiology of the nose is essential to understanding the pathophysiology of various disorders of the nose and paranasal sinuses. Despite the fact that the great majority of people have some serious concerns about dissatisfaction with the shape of their external nose, its internal anatomy and physiological activity are of greater curiosity. Since Proetz' classic monogram in the early 1950s on applied physiology of the nose was published,[1] more and more interest has been given to the understanding of this unique structure.

Not in the least is the anatomy.

REVIEW OF ANATOMY

Structure of the Nasal Cavity:

The gross anatomical structures of the interior of the nose begins with the description of the vestibule. A series of baffles are apparent when looking into the vestibule as well as vibrissae which help to filtrate the air that is breathed. Deeper in the nose one encounters turbinates covered with a mucous membrane having the unusual ability to change humidity, temperature, and air flow capacity. The blood suppy comes primarily from the external carotid artery branches into the anterior and

Associate Professor of Surgery, Section of Otolaryngology and Head & Neck Surgery/Audiology, Dartmouth Medical School, Hanover, New Hampshire 03755. Presented at the Spring 1982 Meeting of the New England Society of Allergy.

posterior portions of the nose. The terminal branch of the maxillary artery supplies the sphenopalatine artery which in turn supply both the lateral and medical wall of the nasal chamber. The anterior and posterior ethmoid branches, which are branches of the ophthalmic artery, supply the superior aspect of the lateral and medial wall of the nose as well as the olfactory cleft with its neuroepithelial membrane.

Nearly all of the functions of the nose, with the exception of olfaction, are related to the vascular system that is under autonomic nervous system control. The parasympathetic innervation of the mucous membrane of the nose arises in the superior salivatory nucleus of the brainstem. Fibers of this nucleus unite with the fibers of the facial nerve and join the postganglionic sympathetic fibers of the superior cervical ganglion after leaving the geniculate ganglion to form the nerve of the vidian canal. This enters the sphenopalatine ganglion. The parasympathetic fibers synapse at this ganglion, and their postganglionic fibers are distributed to the nose, the nasopharynx, and the upper pharynx.

The fibers of the sympathetic nervous system arise from the first and second thoracic segments of the spinal cord in the lateral horn cells. They leave the spinal cord with the anterior nerve roots and synapse in the superior cervical ganglion of the neck. The postganglionic fibers form a network around the internal carotid artery, and these form what is called the deep petrosal nerve. These fibers join the parasympathetic nerve fibers that have come from the seventh cranial nerve and help to form the vidian canal nerve. They are distributed with the parasympathetic nerve fibers as branches of the sphenopalatine nerve.

The histology of the mucous membrane of the nose is rather specialized. The thickness and thermal properties of this lining are regulated by the parasympathetic and sympathetic fibers. There are both superficial and deep layers of arterioles supplying this mucous membrane. Between the capillaries and the venules are numerous sinuses or venous lakes which are connected to both rows of arterioles by the capillaries. At the distal end of the venous lakes are muscle bundles which act as sphincters, and their contraction produces engorgement of the sinuses very similar to erectile tissue in the male reproductive organ. This vascular pattern is most marked in the inferior turbinate area but is present also in the middle turbinate and the septum.

The olfactory epithelium is located in the superior portion of the nasal cavity on both the lateral wall of the nose as well as the adjacent roof and septum. It covers a portion of the superior turbinate and extends over an area between one to three square centimeters. It is more yellowish in color than the pink nasal mucosa. A pseudostratified columnar epithelium consists of specialized olfactory cells, supporting cells, and serous and mucous glands. The olfactory cells are bipolar neurons that act as both peripheral receptors and first order ganglion cells. Ten to twenty million of these cells are in each nasal fossa. Cilium-like rods penetrate into the mucous blanket from these cells, and approximately 1000 filaments on the rods of each cell greatly increase the surface area of the cell itself. The axons of these olfactory cells congregate into bundles to pass through the cribiform plate as olfactory nerves. There are about twenty nerves in each nasal fossa.

FUNCTIONS OF THE NOSE

A review of the functions of the nose would consider the following classifications:

1. respiratory airway
2. conditioning of the air by temperature and
3. humidity control
4. filtration of the inspired air and the associated mechanisms of ciliary action
5. olfaction
6. the contribution of vocal resonance and the initiation of nasal reflex activity

Respiratory Airway:

Because the cross sectional diameter of the anterior nares is smaller than the posterior choana, the air currents which transverse the nasal chambers are different. Inspiratory air currents are directed upward across the superior surface of the inferior turbinate and the middle turbinate into the nasopharynx. This is governed somewhat by the downward direction of the anterior nares and the smooth anterior ends and surfaces of the turbinates which tend to create minimal resistance to the inflow of air. The cartilaginous framework of the nasal alae pre-

vents the collapse of these structures during the negative pressure of inspiration, which varies from a minus 6 mm of water in normal inspiration to approximately minus 200 mm of water in maximum inspiratory effort.

The expiratory airway enters the posterior choana from the nasopharynx and follows a similar route through the nose, but because of the relative constriction of the anterior portion of the nose, a large central eddy or whirling back through the inferior meatus to join the mainstream from the nasopharynx occurs. This action conserves the heat control of the expired air. Deviations of the septum, polyps, or hyperplasia of the mucous membrane would obviously obstruct and disrupt air currents through the nose.

The tidal air drawn in during inspiration meets resistance to airflow. This is partly due to the molecules of the inspired air and partly due to the mass of air coming into contact with the inspiratory passages. The nasal component to the airflow resistance is calculated at approximately 30% of the total resistance to inspiration.

Air Conditioning:

One of the better known functions of the nose is that of providing a rather exact conditioning of the air for the tracheobronchial tree. Both heating and humidification of the inspired air attest to the efficiency of this organ. The specialized vascular nasal mucosa is very important in maintaining the constancy of temperature of the inspired air. The uneven walls of the lateral nasal chamber increase the radiating surface to help warm the air. Ambient air at a temperature of 25° C will be heated to approximately 37° C during its passage from the anterior portion of the nose to the superior aspect of the larynx. External air temperatures from 25° C down to 0° C produce less than a 1° C change in the temperature of air that is at the level of the laryngeal inlet.

Simultaneous with heating of inspired air is its humidification. The physical process of transudation of fluid through the mucosal epithelium is the main supply for moisture that humidifies the inspired air. Secretions of the glands and some of the goblet cells in the nasal mucous membrane provide a smaller volume. The parasympathetic nerve supply to this part of the nose is both secretomotor and vasodilatory. Stimulation would result in secretion of mucous and serous glands and dilatation of blood vessels. This is an efficient process. Air will become between 75% and 95% saturated in the nose alone. The exact volume of fluid necessary to create this percent saturation will vary depending upon the temperature and the relative humidity of the ambient air. It has been calculated that the daily volume of secretions and transudate from the nose is about 1000 cc's. Three-fourths of this is used to saturate the inspired air and the remainder is used in the ciliary mechanisms of cleaning and purifying the inspired air.

Protective:

Filtration of the inspired air begins at the anterior nares. The vibrissae in the nose are responsible for removing particles larger than 15μ in size. Those smaller are removed by the mucous membrane and the mucous blanket in the nose. Only 5% of 1μ particles are removed by the mucous membrane.

Mucociliary Mechanism:

The mucous blanket is probably the most important factor in the protective function of the nose. A film of mucus covers the entire nasal mucosa. It consists of two layers. There is an outer layer that is relatively viscous and rests upon a very thin layer of serous fluid which facilitates the action of the underlying cilia. However, the ends of the cilia are in contact with the overlying film of mucous. The fine particulate matter that enters with the inspired air is filtered out by adhering to this mucous film. This occurs by two separate mechanisms: one is impaction of the particles on the surface of the mucous membrane, and the other is an electrostatic surface charge. This function is so efficient that the posterior choana contains very few bacteria and the sinuses themselves are normally sterile. Two constituents of this mucous blanket are muramidase, formerly known as lysozyme, and immunoglobulin or secretory immunoglobulin. These protein substances are not peculiar to respiratory mucus. The exact site of the production of muramidase is not known but is thought to be inhibitory to bacteria.

Ciliary activity has been studied rather exhaustively. In the front part of the nose, there is a paucity of cilia and the movement of mucous is slow. In this area, it moves only 1-2 mm per hour. However, in the posterior aspect of the nose, the mucous may be propagated 10 mm each minute, and the mucous blanket in the posterior two-thirds of the nose will reconstitute itself approximately every 10 to 15 minutes. This propulsive energy is carried out by the cilia. Each ciliated cell has from 12 to 20 cilia which project from the luminal surface of the cell into the mucus. The beat of the cilia is quick and forceful in a forward propulsive stroke that is followed by a slower recovery stoke. This cycle is repeated hundreds of times each minute. The beating appears to pass from one region to an adjacent posterior one in a metachronous fashion.

There are three ciliary "streams." A relatively small stream from the superior meatus joins with one from the area of the sphenoid sinus. These two intersect with the main antral stream which passes from beneath the middle turbinate to flow anterior to the pharyngeal ostium of the torus tubarius. This continues down the throat just posterior to the posterior tonsillar pillar.

Since the protection afforded by the respiratory epithelium is inherent in its ciliary activity, anything that affects ciliary function is of clinical importance. Drying of the nasal mucous membrane causes cessation of ciliary activity, while prompt moistening will restore its normal activity. If the drying continues for a few minutes, this may lead to disruption and destruction of the cilia. The optimal temperature range for ciliary activity is 28-30°C. Hypotonic saline solutions will inhibit ciliary activity. Hypertonic saline solutions will cause ciliary motions to cease. The cilia are paralyzed by acid solutions. If the pH is reduced to 6.4 or less, the action is arrested. Adrenaline and cocaine will ultimately cause irreversible inhibition of ciliated cells if exposed to them for sufficient time. Ephedrine sulfate apparently has very little effect on ciliary activity.

Olfaction:

The olfactory area in the human nose is confined to the roof of the nasal cavity, the superior part of each superior turbinate in the lateral wall of the nose, and approximately the upper one-third of the nasal septum on each side. The histology of this membrane is a thick, pseudostratified columnar, nonciliated epithelium. It has three types of cells: basal cells, supporting cells, and olfactory receptor cells. These receptor cells are situated among the supporting cells. There are between ten and twenty million olfactory cells. They act as both peripheral sensory receptors and neuron cell bodies with processes.

They are oval in shape. The central end of each olfactory cell is elongated. It acts as a continuous strand or thick axon that is enveloped by the basal cells. These filaments pierce the basement membrane and become directly continuous as a nerve axon of unmyelinated nature. These axons group together to form the fibers of the olfactory nerve which ultimately terminate in the glomeruli of the olfactory bulbs.

Olfactory Stimulation:

The exact mechanism of stimulation to the olfactory system is still unclear. What is clear is that the odor must reach the olfactory area or more specifically, the olfactory mucosa. If air cannot reach this area, there can be no sense of smell. Normal breathing does not necessarily bring the air current into that area of the nasal chamber. Sniffing diverts the air so that it is directed more superiorly to come in direct apposition with the olfactory membrane. Some of the more common theories of smell that have been proposed include inhibition of enzyme mechanisms, hydrogen binding, alterations in the membrane potentials of the cell, an undulating theory, specific molecular receptor sites, and a selective type of adsorption.

The olfactory effect of any substance that is perceived depends on a number of aspects, including whether or not it is volatile, its concentration in inspired air, the exact volume of air that reaches the mucosa of the olfactory region, and the force in which it strikes the mucosa. In addition, the lipid water solubility and the state of the olfactory mucosa are important. Obviously, the integrity of the olfactory nervous pathway and cortical centers for perception are also important.

Olfactory Sensitivity:

Sensitivity of the perception of smell may vary from one day to the next and may be influenced by local conditions in the nose, particularly by smoking. The sensitivity in man is not as acute as it is in other animals.

Olfactory Discrimination:

The exact mechanism to appreciate and distinguish odors is also not clear. However, the human nose can differentiate up to approximately 4000 different odors. Electrophysiological studies tend to support the concept of some degree of selective sensitivity of individual olfactory receptors.

Even though the olfactory mechanism can detect many different odors in high dilutions, its ability to separate small differences in intensity of a given odor is rather poorly developed.

Olfactory Fatigue:

Olfactory fatigue is thought to be a physiological phenomenon located in the central areas of perception of smell. It does not appear to be due to adaptation of the peripheral olfactory receptor.

Speech:

Vocal resonance is another function of the nose. It is obvious that a person's voice is changed with nasal obstruction by whatever cause. The quality of the voice with nasal obstruction is related to the diminution in the normal nasal resonance and has been termed rhinolalia clausa. Rhinolalia aperta results when the vibrating air column passes from the larynx through the pharynx, mouth and into the nose. This occurs in the individual with a cleft palate. Only the nasal consonants, M, N, and NG are made by the vibrating column of air passing from the larynx directly through the nose.

Nasal Reflex Functions:

Reflex functions of the nose can be divided into two primary groups: those that originate from the olfactory area, and those that are initiated at the trigeminal area. The olfactory group of reflexes are those that are related primarily to the digestive actions. Salivary, gastric, and pancreatic glands are reflexly stimulated by the olfactory centers.

The fifth nerve reflexes would include changes in the laryngeal and bronchial musculature, changes in the heart rate, changes in pulmonary ventilation, and reflex sneezing.

Factors Affecting Nasal Blood Flow:

The vasomotor reaction of the nose is affected by many different factors, both local and general. Local factors include temperature, humidity, vasoactive drugs, compression of large veins of the neck, trauma, and inflammation. Changes in both the temperature and the humidity of the air that is inspired will result in either vasodilatation or vasoconstriction depending on the temperature of the air and its humidity. The mucous membrane of the nose reacts to maintain the homeostatic mechanism in the nasopharynx and tracheobronchial airway.

Sympathomimetic drugs applied locally to the nasal mucosa will produce rapid shrinkage with blanching. This may persist for a period of one to three hours, depending upon the drug used. Adrenaline and neosynephrine hydrochloride both have a very vigorous vasoconstrictor effect. Ephedrine is less active but tends to be more prolonged.

Parasympathomimetic drugs will produce congestion of the nasal mucous membrane and will increase the volume of the nasal secretions.

Atropine will cause constriction of the capillaries and contraction of the cavernous tissue in the nose. Cocaine produces a rather marked contraction of these erectile spaces.

If the large veins and arteries in the neck are compressed, congestion of the nasal mucosa will occur. This may be one of the reasons for postural nasal obstruction when a person is horizontal.

Local trauma or inflammation occuring in the mucous membrane will lead to vascular changes characteristic of erythema, congestion, and increased production of nasal secretions.

General factors that affect nasal blood flow are also very interesting. Holmes, Goodell, Wolf, and Wolff in their monogram on the nose[2] have described the emotional factors that are characteristic of nasal symptoms. Fear tends to create a "sympathetic" type of response of the nasal mucous membrane whereas frustration, humiliation, and anxiety tend to engorge the mucous membrane and cause a "parasympathetic" type of response. These effects were demonstrated by biopsying the inferior turbinate mucosa during different periods of emotional conflict in individuals.

General vasomotor reflexes are also present. The nasal vessels may react to other sympathetic vasomotor responses of the body. Auditory stimuli, deep breathing, breath holding, and cold presser tests will produce vasoconstriction in the nasal mucosa. Painful stimulation may also cause marked nasal vasoconstriction. Overventilation may produce dilatation in the nasal vessels.

SUMMARY

The nose in man has a variety of functions which are variously related to its unique anatomy and the vascular tone of the mucous membrane. In addition, it houses the receptor site of the first cranial nerve. Although this nerve tends to be very primitive in man and less effective in monitoring his environment than that found in other animals, it is still a most useful receptor. The nose functions mostly as a guard or watchdog for the lungs. The air is conditioned to a specific range of temperature and humidification. Protective filtration and ciliary mechanisms are abundant. Nasal reflex functions affect pulmonary functions as well. And not the least, the nose may respond to emotional situations to such an intense degree in some people that it too may become quite symptomatic.

A working understanding of the peculiar anatomy of the nasal structures and its functions are important in understanding the pathophysiology of nasal diseases.

REFERENCES

1. Proetz AW. Essays on the Applied Physiology of the Nose. 2nd Ed. St. Louis Annals Publishing Co., 1953, pp. 153.

2. Holmes TH, Goodell H, Wolf S, Wolff HG. The Nose. Springfield, Illinois, Thomas and Company, 1950.

3. English GM. Ch. 28. In: Otolaryngology. Hagerstown, Maryland, Harper & Row, 1976.

4. Ballantyne J, Groves J, (Eds.) Ch. 5. In: Scott Brown's Diseases of the Ear, Nose and Throat. Vol. I 1971, Butterworth and Lippencott Company, Ltd, 1979.

5. Abramson M, Harker LA. Physiology of the nose. Otolaryngol Clin North Am 6:3 Philadelphia, Penn., W.B. Saunders Co., 1973. □

Chapter IX

Airway and Dentofacial Development

George M. Meredith, M.D.

ABSTRACT

All physicians and dentists who evaluate the upper airway and dentofacial skeleton in the growing child should be aware of the wealth of pediatric dental and, especially, orthodontic literature that has been published over the past century as it pertains to airway and dentofacial development. The child who has a genetic predisposition toward the dolichocephalic (narrow) facial skeleton, a neuromuscular deficit, and structural upper airway compromise is particularly at risk for development of the long-face syndrome. Furthermore, the child who has a genetic tendency toward mandibular prognathism, tonsillar and tongue hypertrophy, and who is a chronic mouth-breather, is at particular risk for developing advanced mandibular prognathism. Unfortunately, there is little physician exposure to these concepts during medical school years and even during residency training programs. It behooves each specialty to be aware of the diagnostic and therapeutic modalities and concerns of interrelated specialties. The beneficiaries of this sharing of knowledge will be tomorrow's leaders.

The orthodontic literature contains over 140 articles concerning upper airway compromise as it relates to aberrant dentofacial development.[1-3] It is reasoned that upper airway compromise, especially in the dolichocephalic (narrow-faced) child, as well as in the neuromuscularly deficient child, produces chronic mouth-breathing (Fig. 1). Chronic mouth-breathing calls forth the recruitment of perioral and suprahyoid musculature. The increased tonicity and increased rhythmicity of these muscle groups often produces a negative effect on dentofacial form and function. Often the long-face syndrome develops as a result.

Assistant Clinical Professor of Otolarynagolgy, Eastern Virginia Medical School, Norfolk, VA

The long-face syndrome is characterized by increased anterior vertical height in the lower half of the dentofacial skeleton, excess dentoalveolar height, gummy smile (Fig. 2), posterior crossbite (Fig. 3), high-arched

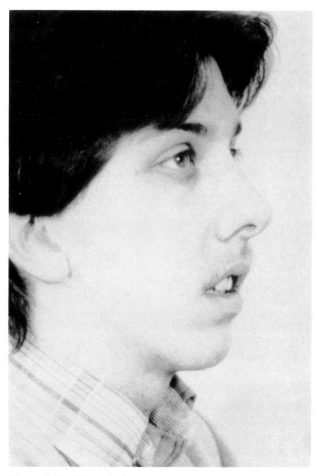

Figure 1. *Dolichocephalic patient with the long-face syndrome, demonstrating the chronic lip apart posture.*

85

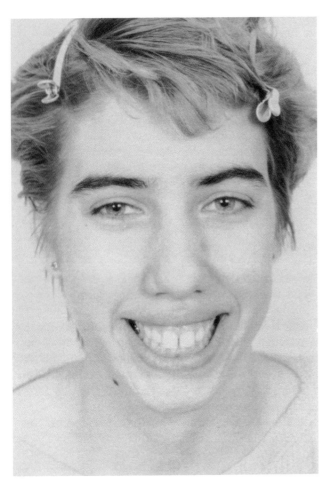

Figure 2. Patient with the long-face syndrome demonstrating excess anterior vertical dentofacial height and gummy smile.

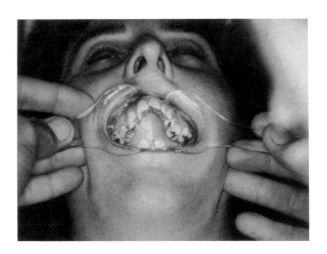

Figure 4. Narrow upper dental arch. Intermolar distance (UM₁) is measured from the lingual cusp of the first maxillary molar to the same point on the opposite side. Timms[37] and others have established normal values here.

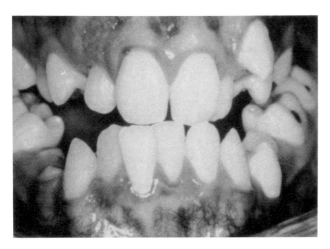

Figure 3. Posterior crossbite.

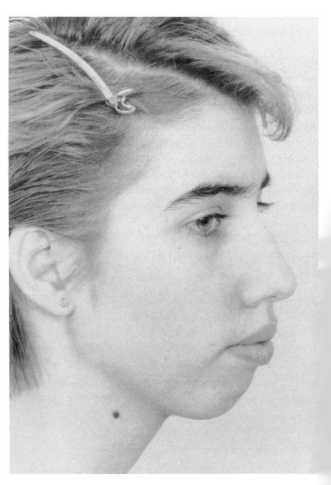

Figure 5. This same patient demonstrates a steep mandibular plane and a Class II (mandibular retrognathic) malocclusion.

palate, narrow upper dental arch (Fig. 4), steep mandibular plane, nasal obstruction, and a Class II (mandibular retrognathic) occlusal relationship (Fig. 5). Harvold, Vargervik, Miller, et al.[4–11] used soft, hollow silicone rubber cones to experimentally produce nasal

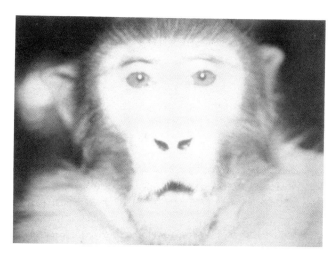

Figure 6. *Young growing rhesus monkey demonstrating the thin, veil-like upper lip, malar flattening, high narrow palatal vault and chronic lip apart posture after experimental production of nasal obstruction.*

obstruction in young growing rhesus monkeys. These rhesus monkeys exhibited significant neuromuscular adaptation. They became chronic mouth-breathers over the next three years. Most of these monkeys developed the long-face syndrome (Fig. 6). When the silicone rubber cones were removed from the nasal vaults of these rhesus monkeys, their dentofacial skeletons returned to normal.

Otolaryngologists, pediatricians, family practitioners, allergists, and general dentists should be aware that orthodontists and some pediatric dentists have the radiographic ability to assess dentofacial development, in a longitudinal fashion, through the use of cephalometric analyses (Figs. 7 and 8). The lateral headplate, or cephalometric radiograph, provides valuable information not only about the size of the adenoidal pad, but also, in high-quality films, information about tonsil size and about the relative size of the posterior end of the inferior turbinate. In the cephalometric analysis, the orthodontist can trace the mandibular plane angle and can determine the anterior vertical height of the upper and lower half of the anterior dentofacial skeleton. Anterior overjet (Class II malocclusion) as well as developing Class III malocclusion (Figs. 9 and 10) can be accurately documented in the carefully done cephalometric radiograph.

Children with macroglossia and marked tonsillar hypertrophy have a tendency to develop Class III (mandibular prognathic) malocclusion because of tongue pressure on the lingual aspect of the lower dental arch. Often, the Class III malocclusion represents a combination of maxillary retrognathia and mandibular prognathism. The Petit Face Mask (Fig. 11) can be used to model the maxilla forward. The Petit Face Mask, at the

same time, slows excessive mandibular growth. Correction of macroglossia (Fig. 12), tonsillar hypertrophy, nasal obstruction and/or the use of the Petit Face Mask can often be used to intercept the developing Class III malocclusion. In addition nasal obstruction seems to adversely affect dentofacial development in this group.

Although there is not unanimity in the orthodontic and pediatric dental literature, the majority of these reports support these interrelationships.[11-23] In contrast, detracting papers have often been based on emotion and obscure anecdotes.[3] One series of detracting papers comes from Vig, Warren, et al.[2,24] as well as from Howard.[25] The patients in the Warren-Vig series consisted of a group of cleft lip-palate patients. Unfortu-

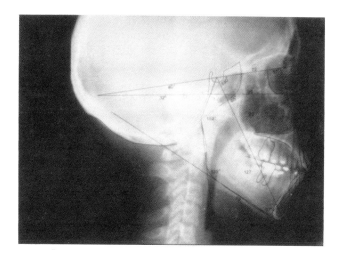

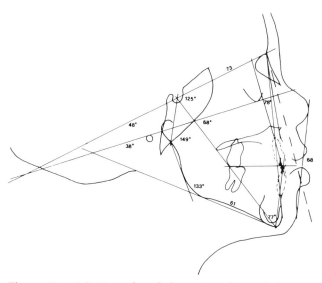

Figures 7 and 8. *Lateral cephalometric radiograph (Fig. 7, top) and accompanying tracing (Fig. 8, bottom) from a patient with the long-face syndrome. Note the steep mandibular plane extending well into the occiput. Also note that the usual 45/55 mid-face (nasion to anterior nasal spine)/lower face (anterior nasal spine to menton) ratio is perverted.*

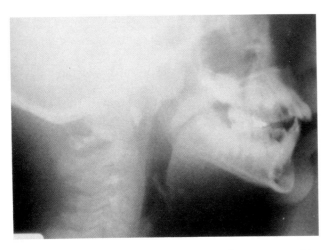

Figure 9. *Class II malocclusion sometimes known as overbite deformity.*

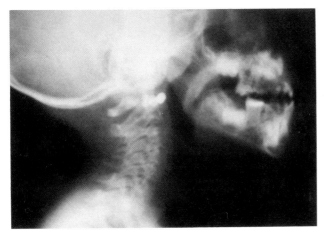

Figure 10. *Class II malocclusion. Mandibular prognathism. Maxillary retrognathia. Underbite deformity.*

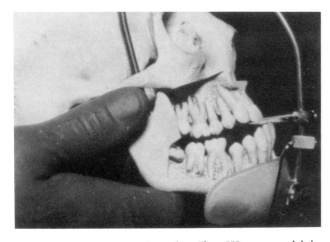

Figure 11. *Petit Face Mask used in Class III cases model the maxilla forward and slow excessive mandibular growth.*

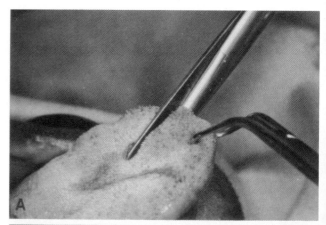

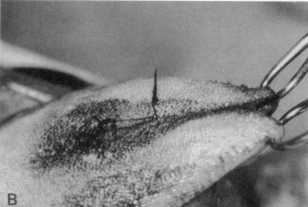

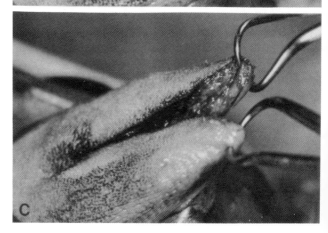

Figure 12. *Anterior tongue wedge resection used to reduce macroglossia in advanced Class III pronounced malocclusions.*

nately, such patients invariably have had numerous nasal/maxillary/palatal procedures, have extensive scarring, and do not represent the typical patient with upper airway compromise. Furthermore, Warren, Vig. et al. failed to present the entire symptom complex that these patients were exhibiting and did not present pertinent items in the upper airway examination. These authors, instead, based their findings on computed tomography scan analysis of formalin-preserved cadaver nasal vaults and on rhinomanometric studies of acrylic nasal vault/oropharyngeal models and on rhinomanometric studies of cleft palate patients who were primarily being evaluated for speech problems.

Hannuksela[21] and Shapiro and Shapiro[22] have demonstrated that children with allergic hypertrophy of the faucial tonsils, adenoidal pad and, later, the inferior turbinates, will often go on to develop the long-face syndrome. Conversely, the child with a normal upper airway is much less likely to develop the long-face syndrome. Children with a genetic proclivity for dolichocephalic dentofacial development are at higher risk. Children with neuromuscular dysfunction are at higher risk. Therefore, the child with upper airway allergy and a dolichocephalic face is particularly at risk (Fig. 13). Allergic hypertrophy of the tonsils, adenoidal pad, and inferior turbinates, when combined with neuromuscular dysfunction and a genetic predisposition for the dolichocephalic face, places that child in the highest risk group of all.

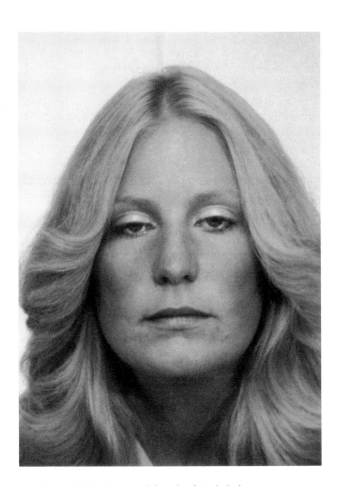

Figure 14. Patient with brachy facial skeleton.

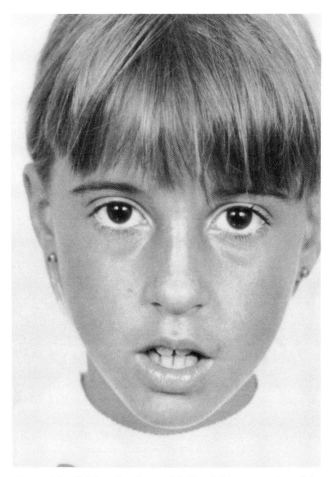

Figure 13. Child with advanced "allergic" hypertrophy of the tonsils, adenoidal pad, and inferior turbinates demonstrating many of the stigmata of the developing long-face syndrome.

Conversely, the brachyfacial (wide maxilla and wide mandible) patient (Fig. 14) is at much lower risk for development of the long face syndrome.

If there are major dentofacial development, as well as quality of life, considerations, in the presence of marked adenotonsillar hypertrophy, a constricted maxillary dental arch, and allergic inferior turbinate hypertrophy, then, adenotonsillectomy, rapid maxillary expansion, and/or partial resection of the inferior turbinates is indicated. Major quality of life considerations associated with marked adenotonsillar hypertrophy include obstructive sleep apnea, enuresis secondary to upper airway compromise, dysphagia for fibrous foods, hyponasality, retarded (obstructive) migration of the nasal mucous blanket, hyposmia, hot potato voice, loud snoring, EDS (excessive daytime sleepiness), poor athletic and scholastic performance, and chronic mouth breathing. Almost invariably, these quality of life considerations return to normal within 6 weeks following adenotonsillectomy, rapid maxillary expansion and/or partial resection of the inferior turbinates. However, even after successful surgery, it may take as long as 1–2 years for patients to unlearn the chronic mouth-breathing mode. Orbicularis oris exercises (Fig. 15) can reduce this time to less than 4 months. Children do unlearn the chronic mouth-breathing habit if upper airway problems have been properly diagnosed and correctly managed. Parents should be so advised.

It is not uncommon for nasal obstruction to recur months or years after adenotonsillectomy. Often pediatricians and allergists incorrectly diagnose this as regrowth of the adenoids. Unless an inadequate adenoidectomy was performed initially, adenoidal tissue generally does not "regrow." The problem, instead, is that of the allergic target organ shifting from the faucial tonsils and adenoidal pad to the inferior turbinates. There are a number of adult studies that clearly demonstrate that the symptom complex associated with allergic, as well as nonallergic (vasomotor rhinitis), inferior turbinate hypertrophy is significantly improved following partial resection of the inferior turbinates.[26–31] In my own relatively small pediatric series of partial resection of the inferior turbinate patients,[32] I was able to produce success rates (86% had relief of nasal obstruction) comparable to those achieved in the larger adult series. Others[33–36] have achieved good results in

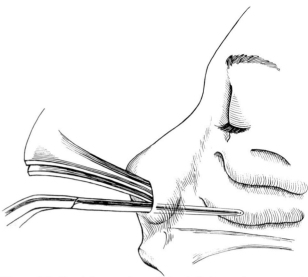

Figure 16. *Partial resection of the inferior turbinate. Light Knight scissors and inferior turbinate (lower one-third) specimen.*

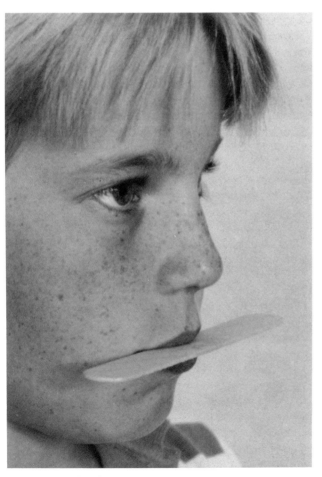

Figure 15. *Orbicularis oris exercises. Ten minutes twice a day. Exercises should be done standing erect, while expanding the chest and using the diaphragm.*

the pediatric group of nasally obstructed patients through the use of electrocautery to reduce the size of offending inferior turbinates. Unfortunately, in my experience, the incidence of recurrent inferior turbinate hypertrophy is higher months or years after electrocautery.[34] Partial resection of the inferior turbinate tends to produce long lasting relief of nasal obstruction. Care must be exercised, however, not to over-resect the inferior turbinate. Over-resection can produce an overly patent airway, which may cause a paradoxical sensation of nasal blockage because of loss of normal intranasal pressure. In addition, over-resection of the inferior turbinate can adversely affect the migration of the nasal mucous blanket. Use of the Gruenwald forceps, as advocated by Sheen,[28] significantly lessens the possibility of overreaction of the inferior turbinate (Fig. 16). Use of heavy electrofulguration to obtain hemostasis after partial resection of the inferior turbinate, especially in the posterior third, is likewise ill-advised. Use of local and topical anesthesia with epinephrine, in approved concentrations,[37–39] can circumvent the need for heavy electrocautery for hemostasis.

Rapid maxillary expansion (RME), also known as rapid palatal expansion, is an inexpensive, nonsurgical method of improving the cross-sectional area of the nasal vault[40,41] (Figs. 17 and 18 a,b). Nonoperative RME can be accomplished in about 3 weeks in the patient aged 3–20 years. Nonoperative RME can be repeated in a year or so[42,43] if upper arch dental crowding and persistent nasal blockade so dictate (Fig. 19). After age 20, if nonoperative RME does not open the mid-palatal suture, operative RME can be performed by the oral or maxillofacial surgeon.

It has been my experience that RME improves nasal obstruction, but not to the degree that one would wish to achieve in advanced situations. In the more advanced cases, partial resection of the inferior turbinate can be used to complement the airway improvement that RME produces. Conversely, in borderline cases of nasal obstruction, RME may be all that is necessary. It must be remembered that many orthodontists feel that RME is contraindicated as a modality for correcting nasal obstruction and upper dental arch crowding if the patient is in neutrocclusion (i.e., no posterior buccal crossbite). Nevertheless, slow expansion of the mandibular dental arch via the use of a lip bumper (Fig. 18b). A Swartz applicance can be used in conjunction with RME if both the maxillary and mandibular arches are constricted and yet the patient has no posterior buccal crossbite.

In the growing patient, who is in the process of developing a Class III (mandibular prognathic) malocclusion (Fig. 11), tonsillar hypertrophy and macroglossia can both play a significant role in the development of this aberrant dentofacial form.[42, 44] Again, it seems that a genetic predisposition toward mandibular prognathism when combined with upper airway problems can be additive. Therefore, it is essential that each physician and dentist who evaluates the child who is in the process of developing a Class III malocclusion be aware of this interrelationship. There are quantitative techniques for evaluating both tonsil as well as tongue size.[44–48] It must be remembered that both tonsil and tongue sizes are relative measurements. The space in which these structures reside, the oropharynx and the "tongue box," should be taken into consideration. A small boy who has a small pharynx and 3+ tonsils, for example, is at greater risk than an average size child with a normal pharynx and 3+ tonsils. The same applies to tongue size. Children with Down's syndrome often

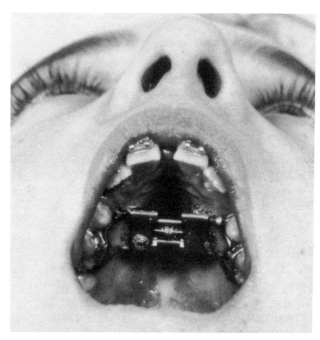

Figure 18a. *Three weeks after beginning RME, the central incisors separate in the midline as the midpalatal suture opens. During the next 3 months, the central incisors come back together, the nasal airway is improved, and the teeth of the upper dental arch are no longer crowded (cf. Fig. 3).*

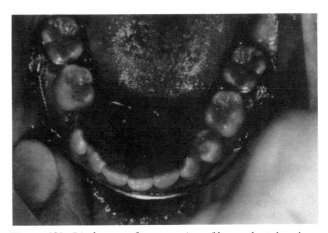

Figure 18b. *Lip bumper for expansion of lower dental arch.*

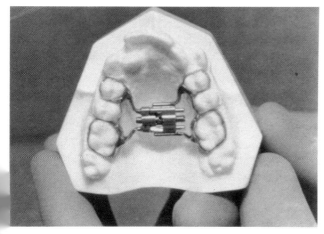

Figure 17. Rapid maxillary expansion appliance. Mother turns the jack screw with a key, twice a day for 3 weeks.

have both neuromuscular deficits and relative macroglossia. The otolaryngologist should be aware that there are techniques for mapping tongue size.[44–48] Wedge resections, based on tongue mapping, can be used to reduce relative macroglossia (Fig. 12).

All modes of upper airway therapy, as well as watchful waiting, have to be evaluated in a longitudinal fashion. The rhinomanometric analysis of the growing child's nasal airway, as was precisely demonstrated by Principato and Wolf[35] should serve as a baseline. As the child's maxilla grows and the cross-sectional area of the nasal vault expands with growth, nasal resistance decreases. Therefore, whether hyposensitization, sur-

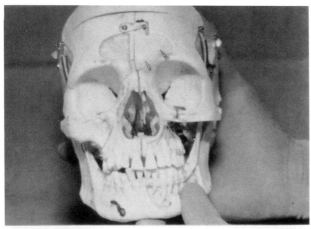

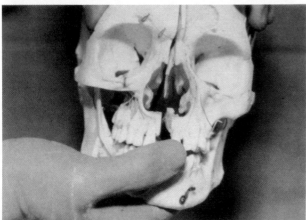

Figure 19. By opening the mid-palatal suture, rapid maxillary expansion not only provides more room for the teeth of the crowded upper dental arch, but it also serves to improve the cross-sectional area of the nasal vault, thus improving nasal respiration.

gical correction, functional appliances, orthopedic appliances (RME), or nontherapy avenues are taken, the results may be assessed in an objective, thorough, meaningful manner. A detailed history and physical examination should be complemented by serial cephalometric x-rays, posteranterior polytomograms or CAT scans of the nasal vault (three pertinent cuts in appropriate cases), rhinomanometric studies and, in selected cases, sleep laboratory studies.

SUMMARY

All physicians and dentists who evaluate the upper airway and dentofacial skeleton in the growing child should be aware of the wealth of pediatric dental and, especially, orthodontic literature that has been published over the past century as it pertains to airway and dentofacial development. The child who has a genetic predisposition toward the dolichocephalic (narrow) facial skeleton, a neuromuscular deficit, and structural upper airway compromise is particularly at risk for development of the long-face syndrome. Furthermore, the child who has a genetic tendency toward mandibular prognathism, tonsillar and tongue hypertrophy, and who is a chronic mouth-breather, is at particular risk for developing advanced mandibular prognathism. Unfortunately, there is little physician exposure to these concepts during medical school years and even during residency training programs. It behooves each specialty to be aware of the diagnostic and therapeutic modalities and concerns of interrelated specialties. The beneficiaries of this sharing of knowledge will be tomorrow's leaders.

REFERENCES

1. Rubin RM. Effects of nasal airway obstruction on facial growth. Ear Nose Throat J 66(5):44–53, 1987.
2. Vig PS, Johnson L Jr. New Vistas in Orthodontics. Philadelphia: Lea and Febiger, 1985.
3. O'Ryan FS, Gallagher DM, LaBanc JP, Epker BN. The relation between naso-respiratory function and dentofacial morphology: A review. Am J Orthod 82:403–410, 1982.
4. Harvold EP. The role of function in the etiology and treatment of malocclusion. Am J Orthod 54:883–898, 1972.
5. Harvold EP, Vargervik K, Chierici G. Primate experiments on oral sensation and dental malocclusion. Am J Orthod 63:494–508, 1973.
6. Miller AJ, Vargervik K. Neuromuscular changes during long-term adaptation of the Rhesus monkey to oral respiration. In McNamara JA Jr. (ed). Naso-respiratory Function and Craniofacial Growth. Monograph 9, Craniofacial Growth Series. Ann Arbor: University of Michigan 1979, pp 1–26.
7. Harvold EP. Neuromuscular and morphological adaptations in experimentally induced oral respiration. In McNamara JA Jr. (ed). Naso-respiratory Function and Craniofacial Growth. Monograph 9, Craniofacial Growth Series. Ann Arbor: University of Michigan, 1979, pp 149–164.
8. Harvold EP, Tomer B, Vargervik K et al. Primate experiments on oral respiration. Am J Orthod 79:359–372, 1981.
9. Vargervik K, Miller AJ, Chierici G et al. Morphologic response to changes in neuromuscular patterns experimentally induced by altered modes of respiration. Am J Orthod 85:115–124, 1984.
10. Miller A, Vargervik K, Chierici G. Experimentally induced neuromuscular changes during and after nasal airway obstruction. Am J Orthod 85:385–392, 1984.
11. Harvold EP, Chierici G, Vargervik K. Experiments on the development of dental malocclusions. Am J Orthod 61:38–44, 1972.
12. Tomes CS. The bearing of the development of the jaws on irregularities. Dent Cosmos 15:292–296, 1873.
13. Ketcham AH. Treatment by the orthodontist supplementing that by the rhinologist. Laryngoscope 22:1286–1299, 1912.
14. Hawkins AC. Mouth-breathing as the cause of malocclusion and other facial abnormalities. Texas Dent J 83:10–15, 1965.
15. Subtelny JD. The significance of adenoid tissue in orthodontia. Angle Orthod 24:59–69, 1954.
16. Linder-Aronson S, Woodside D. The channelization of upper and lower anterior face heights compared to population standards in males between ages 6 to 20 years. Eur J Orthod 1:25–40, 1979.
17. Quinn GW. Airway interference and its effect upon the growth and development of the face, jaws, dentition and

associated parts. NC Dent J 60:28–31, 1978.

18. Rubin RM. Mode of respiration and facial growth. Am J Orthod 78:504–510, 1980.

19. McNamara JA Jr. Influence of respiratory pattern on craniofacial growth. Angle Orthod 51:269–299, 1981.

20. Bushey RS. Alterations in certain anatomical relations accompanying the change from oral to nasal breathing. MS Thesis. Chicago: University of Illinois, 1965.

21. Hannuksela A. The effect of moderate and severe atopy on the facial skeleton. Eur J Orthod 3:187–193, 1981.

22. Shapiro GC, Shapiro PA. Nasal airway obstruction and facial development. Clin Rev Allergy 2:225–235, 1984.

23. Long RE, McNamara JA. Facial growth following pharyngeal flap surgery: Skeletal assessment on serial lateral cephalometric radiographs. Am J Orthod 87:187–196, 1985.

24. Vig PS, Sarver DM, Hall DJ, Warren DW. Quantitative evaluation of nasal airflow in relation to facial morphology. Am J Orthod 79:263–272, 1981.

25. Howard C. Inherent growth and its influence on malocclusion. J Am Dent Assoc 19:642–651, 1932.

26. Hannuksela A. The effect of moderate and severe atopy on the facial skeleton. Eur J Orthod 3:187–193, 1981.

27. Fry HJH. Judicious turbinectomy for nasal obstruction. Aust NZ J Surg 42:291–294, 1973.

28. Sheen JH. Aesthetic Rhinoplasty. St. Louis: C. V. Mosby, 1978, pp. 184–194.

29. Courtiss EH. Resection of obstructing inferior nasal turbinates. Plast Reconstr Surg 62:249–257, 1978.

30. Spector M. Partial resection of the inferior turbinates. Ear Nose Throat J 61 (April):28–32, 1982.

31. Pollock R, Rohring RJ. Inferior turbinate surgery. Plast Reconstr Surg 74:227–236, 1984.

32. Meredith GM. Surgical reduction of hypertrophied inferior turbinates: a comparison of electrocoagulation versus partial resection. J Plast Reconstr Surg, in press.

33. Goode RL. Surgery of the turbinates. J Otolaryngol 7:262–268, 1978.

34. Saunders WH. Surgery of the inferior nasal turbinates. Ann Otol Rhinol Laryngol 91(4, Pt. 1):445–447, 1982.

35. Principato JJ, Wolf P. Pediatric nasal resistance. Laryngoscope 95:1067–1069, 1985.

36. Richter H. Personal communication.

37. Devgan BK, Leach W. Submucosal diathermy of inferior turbinates. Eye Ear Nose Throat Mon 55(5):156–158, 1976.

38. Beck JC. Pathology of intramural electrocoagulation of the inferior turbinate. Ann Otol Rhinol Laryngol 39:349–363, 1930.

39. Katz RL, Matteo RS, Papper EM. The injection of epinephrine during general anesthesia. Anesthesiology 23:597–560, 1962.

40. Eirew HL. Rapid maxillary expansion. Dent Update 3:251, 1976.

41. Gray LP. Rapid maxillary expansion. J Laryngol Otol 89:601–614, 1975.

42. Timms DJ. Some medical aspects of rapid maxillary expansion. Br J Orthod 1:127–132, 1974.

43. Timms DJ. Rapid Maxillary Expansion. Amador City, CA: Quintessence Publishing Company, 1982.

44. Meredith GM, Weimert TA, Vargervik K, et al. The airway and dentofacial development. Ear Nose Throat 66: Nos. 5 and 6, 1987.

45. Petit HP. Macroglossia. J Pediatr Dent 10:199–210, 1986.

46. Austermann KH, Machtens E. The influence of tongue asymmetries on development of jaws and the position of teeth. Int J Oral Surg 3:261–265, 1974.

47. Olow-Nordenram M, Mordenram A. Partial tongue excision in the treatment of apertognathia. Oral Surg Oral Pathol 35:152–159, 1973.

48. Simard S. Effect of experimental microglossia on craniofacial growth. Am J Orthod 70:304–315, 1976.

Chapter X

Olfaction: Physiology and Pathology

John J. Ballenger, M.S., M.D.

ABSTRACT

Belatedly the study of the physiology of olfaction has received a great deal of interest. This manuscript is a review of this subject and suggested treatment of its disorders.

Although odors play a less important part in the life of humans than they do in that of animals, they do influence the choice of food, are of some importance socially, and may on occasion warn of toxic gases and contaminated goods. Doty[1] has suggested that certain human body external secretions (pheromones) influence behavior in a manner similar to that demonstrable in animals and insects. The greater ability of the human female to detect musk-like odors during ovulations and a decreased ability during menstruation is thought to be such an instance and is considered a likely pheromonal effect. Androsterone sulfate, found in the sweat and urine of men, has been proposed as a pheromone sexually attractive to women.[1,2] Clearly the nuisance caused by environmental odors is becoming an increasingly frequent problem. In Sweden 13% of the public has reported annoying environmental odors and in the United States 25–59% of the complaints made to air pollution control agents were related to odors.[3]

The human olfactory neuroepithelium is located above the supreme turbinate or superior in the vault of the nose and occupies about 2 cm² (1 cm on each side) or 1½% of the total nasal mucosa. By comparison the rabbit olfactory area occupies about 900 mm². The olfactory mucosa is constantly being renewed—perhaps in a cycle of about 30–40 days.[4–6] In the older human adult there frequently is a more or less widespread replacement of the olfactory mucosa with respiratory epithelium, likely as a result of aging or as a result of environmental (including infections) insults. The olfac-

Associate Professor: Northwestern University Medical School and Chief, Emeritus, Division Otolaryngology/Head and Neck Surgery. Evanston Hospital, Evanston, IL 60201

tory neuroepithelium is unique in being the only neuroepithelium that is exposed directly to the outside environment.

In considering olfaction in man, note must be made of three organs of olfaction that at one time in the past were of functional significance and anatomically are still represented. It is also important to recognize that olfaction and taste are perceptively interwoven. The physiology of taste is not covered in this article.

In 1811 Jacobson described a structure, tubular in nature, on the septum of some mammals whose efferent nerves projected to a portion of the olfactory bulb. This became known as Jacobson's or the vomeronasal organ. In the human, a remnant is found in the anterior-inferior part of the nasal septum, but its functional significance is not clear. *Best and Taylor's Physiological Basis of Medical Practice*[7] states that the walls of the vomeronasal organ are lined with a neuroepithelium similar to that of olfactory epithelium itself and the receptor cells contain microvilli but no cilia. It further states that the vomeronasal organ in animals is concerned with pheromonal or sexual detection and that this is not a function of the olfactory mucosa. The terminal nerve,[7] although found in mammals as a plexus of fine branching nerve bundles on the nasal septum, also is of little or no functional significance. Masera's septal organ, described in 1943,[8] contains bipolar neurons and sends discrete nerve bundles toward the olfactory bulb. The true functional significance is not known.

OLFACTORY EPITHELIUM

There is no true olfactory submucosa. The lamina propria of the olfactory area contains the branched tubuloalveolar glands of Bowman which produce a thin mucous covering of the olfactory mucosa. The composition of this mucus is unknown, but it is relatively different from that covering the respiratory area of the nose and likely is a solvent for the odor particles. The olfactory mucus is not propelled by underlying cilia in the same sense as that of the respiratory mucus, but possibly it is "drawn" across the olfactory mucosa by the traction from nearby respiratory (motile) cilia (see olfactory cilia discussed below). The lamina propria also contains blood vessels, connective tissue, and the axons of the ciliated olfactory receptors. The axons of the olfactory neurons coalesce into large bundles and, proceeding centrally, pass through the cribriform platae as fila olfactoria en route to synapse with second order neurons in the glomeruli of the olfactory bulb (Fig. 1).

The olfactory epithelium is usually described as consisting of three types of cells: the supporting (or sustentacular), the basal, and the olfactory. In recent years a fourth type, the microvillar cell, has been described.[9,10] The pseudostratified neuroepithelium is slightly thicker than the respiratory epithelium and is unique because of the exposure of nerve cells directly to the outside environment. Jafek[10] reports that the neurons number approximately $30,000/mm^2$, which is far fewer than those possessed by lower animals and justifies the description of the human as microsmatic.

The supporting (sustentacular) cell is a tall, slender cell with an apically located nucleus. Numerous branched microvilli extend from the free surface of the cell to form a network entangled with the olfactory cilia and microvilli from adjacent cells. The supporting cells themselves possess no cilia or basal bodies. Adjacent to supporting cells are usually olfactory cells with which

there is an intimate contact and which relationship may facilitate intercellular or metabolic transfer. The supporting cells appear to envelop the olfactory axons and dendrites.[10]

Beneath the free surface, the supporting cell contains many organelles, including mitochondria, free ribosomes, and membrane-lined vesicular inclusions. The cytoplasm basal to the nucleus is organelle-poor. The organelles produce a secretion into the overlying mucous layer.

The ultimate function of the supporting cell is not clear. They probably are not involved in fluid transport as nonciliated cells of the respiratory mucosa may be. It is possible that they participate in the olfactory response by releasing their secretion in response to at least some odorants.[11] It is clear that the numerous microvilli greatly increase the surface area. These cells also may have a phagocytic roll in removing the odorant molecules from the mucus after the stimulus. And finally, as mentioned above, the supporting cells may provide protection for the bipolar olfactory cells by investment and isolation.

The basal cells are stem cells and are the source of the receptor neurons and supporting cells which are lost during normal turnover or after injury. They are located just above the lamina propria, are 4–5 μm in diameter, and have a centrally located nucleus.

The olfactory cell is a bipolar neuron that very likely is the smell receptor.[10] Unlike all other neurosensory cells in the body, the olfactory receptor is exposed to the external environment. The neurons are continually being renewed in a cycle of about 30–40 days.[4–6] At its apical end is a modified dendrite which extends to the mucosal surface and thickens into a club-shaped form, the olfactory knob or vesicle, and from which the cilia project. The surface of the olfactory vesicle also contains microvilli whose function is unknown but seem at least to increase the surface area exposed to the odorant.

Radiating from the vesicle and bathed by the mucus are 10–30 olfactory cilia of some 50–200 μm in length. They usually display, on cross-section near the basal part of the cilium where the diameter is about 250 nm, the "9 plus 2" pattern characteristic of respiratory cilia. Occasionally 9 plus 0, 9 plus 4, megacilia, etc., are noted and the significance in regard to olfactory acuity is not known. The tubule pairs in general do not possess dynein arms which is an obvious difference from respiratory cilia and presumably the reason the mature cilia are most probably nonmotile. It is not likely that ciliary motility is necessary for the smell receptor function.[10] In the upper part of the cilium, singlets rather than doublets are found on cross-section. The cilia arise from basal bodies located distally in the cell and are provided with rootlets oriented parallel to the long axis of the cell bodies. The odorous particles are believed to

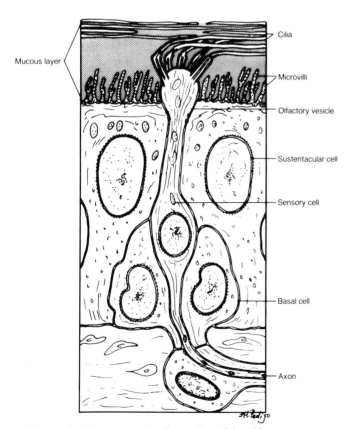

Figure 1. *Diagrammatic illustration of the olfactory mucosa.*

Mucous layer

Cilia

Microvilli

Olfactory vesicle

Sustentacular cell

Sensory cell

Basal cell

Axon

be adsorbed onto intramembranous particles on the free surface of the cell or the cilia.[9,10] Three types of cilia can be identified, two of which may be motile and contain adenosine triphosphate as the energy source. The motile cilia are found early in the replacement cycle and before synapse with the olfactory bulb is made. Their activity may be related to odorant removal. The nonmotile ciliated cell is "mature" and has synapsed with bulb.

The flask-shaped microvillar cells are the most superficially located in the olfactory mucosa. The cell body tapers upward to a narrow neck at the apex where it gives rise to 75–100 microvilli which project into the mucous blanket. Neither cilia nor basal bodies are present. The microvillar cell at its neck is intimately attached to the neighboring supporting cells or the bipolar neurons. At the lower end of the cell body a long slender cytoplasmic process extends toward the basement membrane which can be said to resemble an axon. The function of the microvillar cell is unknown, but it may be a chemoreceptor. Similar cells are found in the vomeronasal organ of lower mammals.[4,9]

Theories of Olfaction

According to the stereochemical theory of olfaction each of the seven primary odors or modalities of the sense of smell possesses an electrophilic nature. The olfactory neuroepithelium is then presumed to possess receptor sites that are receptive to different shapes and dimensions so that a particular odor molecule is attracted to a particular receptor in a lock and key type of chemical recognition. The primary odors, according to this scheme, are: ethereal, camphoraceous, musky, floral, pepperminty, pungent, and putrid. Additional odors, including the almond odor, are supposed to be complex combinations caused by the molecule fitting two or more primary receptor sites. Another mechanism suggested is the adsorption of the odorant onto the cilia, resulting in a molecular transformation such that a nerve action potential is initiated by the flow of Na^+ or K^+ across the membrane.

Still another theory of olfaction involves the basic assumption that the molecular quality perceived as odor lies in certain vibrational movements of the odor molecules. Some sort of interaction occurs between this vibration and the receptor organ.[13] Each primary odor (perhaps as many as 25, according to Wright) would correspond to a small range of frequencies. The fact is, however, that the method of odor identification and coding is largely unknown and will have to await further investigation.

It is likely, whatever the actual details are, that the first event in the initiation of an impulse in the olfactory nerve is the excitation of the olfactory vesicles or cilia, perhaps by way of a solution of the odorous particle in the mucus. Intramembranous particles presumably representing receptor sites have been found both on the free mucosal surface (microvilli) and on the cilia in freeze-dried preparations. Pinocytotic vacuoles often are found in association with the vesicles. Upon stimulation of the receptor cells, a change in electric potential is produced that causes an impulse to travel to the olfactory bulb where the mitral and tufted cells are stimulated. The change in membrane potential, the electro-olfactogram, can be measured. The amplitude varies in different regions of the olfactory epithelium, and the shape, duration, and latency intervals are related to the intensity of the stimulus. It seems more likely that different odorant molecules adsorb differentially in time and space across the olfactory epithelium, rather akin to that seen in a chromatographic column.[14] The olfactory bulb displays a continuous background of electric activity and is interrupted by brief or long bursts of increased activity during olfactory stimulation. The olfactory mucosal pattern of stimulation is reflected in the bulb. Quality may depend upon the pattern of excitation of the receptor cells. Olfactory fatigue occurs within seconds during continuous stimulation and recovery follows promptly upon cessation of the stimulus.[11]

The proximal end of the olfactory cell tapers into a filament less than 1 μm thick, the axon. As an unmyelinated fiber it extends below the basal lamina to join with axons from adjacent cells to form fascicles which become invested by Schwann cells and penetrate the cribriform plate. The joined fascicles become the grossly visible fila olfactoria which lead to the olfactory bulbs lying on the cribriform plate where synapse is made with second-order neurons. The synapse is made with tufted and mitral cells which are found in spherical tangles of nerve fibers or neuropils, called olfactory glomeruli.

The olfactory neuroepithelium is also provided with myelinated fibers from the trigeminal nerve. The distal fibers of the trigeminal nerve arborize between the supporting cells under the epithelial surface, and here they are unmyelinated. Presumably they respond to sensory (but not odorous) stimuli.

After leaving the olfactory bulbs, the second order neurons form the olfactory tract which passes along the base of the frontal lobe to enter in a complex pattern in the pyriform cortex, the anterior commissure, the caudate nucleus, the olfactory tubercle, and the anterior limbus of the internal capsule with secondary connections.

Animals can be divided into microsmatic and macrosmatic classes, depending on the acuteness of the sense of smell. In the former, to which humans belong, the olfactory sense is poorly developed and is not of importance to the safety of the animal or its ability to procure food. In the latter group the sense of smell is well developed and is of great importance to the animal.

There apparently is no "disuse atrophy" of the olfactory mucosa after laryngectomy. When the proper connections are made so that an adequate airflow through the nose occurs, the olfactory mechanism can be shown to be intact.[15]

Taxonomy

Various terms have been used to describe alterations in acuteness of the perceived sense of smell. Commonly anosmia suggests the total loss of smell and Table I lists many of the contributing causes to a partial or complete loss. Partial loss or hyposmia suggests a reduced sensitivity to all or most odorants and specific anosmia reduced sensitivity to one or a very few odorants. Parosmia or hyperosmia implies an increased sensitivity to all or many odorants. Dysosmia suggests a distortion of the perceived odor or the perception of an odor that does not exist.

OLFACTORY DISORDERS

The accurate clinical evaluation of olfactory function is considerably compromised by the virtual impossibility of separating responses of cranial nerve V from I and the perceptual interweaving of odor and taste. Added to these are the confusions introduced by the aging process[4,20,21] of the replacement of olfactory epithelium with a squamous or respiratory type and also by the loss of bulb neurons. There is no pure olfactory stimulant although freshly ground coffee is closer than most. Doty[22] reviewed the subject of these disorders.

The initial evaluation of olfactory dysfunction (see Table I) should be done carefully and systematically and the explanation may be forthcoming at that point.[23] The accurate, quantitative testing of olfaction leaves much to be desired. Cain et al.[24] have described a monorhinic method to measure odor threshold by use of various concentrations of butanol presented in an ascending sequence. Odor identification makes use of common odorous items (e.g., baby powder and coffee grounds) and pungent items (e.g., ammonia) to separate the function of cranial nerve V from I. A list of odor names is shown to the patient so that word-finding difficulties are overcome. Doty and others[17,22,25,26] have developed a birhinic, self-administered, test which is available by mail for home or office use and is called the University of Pennsylvania Smell Identification Test (UPSIT). Forty microencapsulated odorants are released by scratching the leaves of standardized odor-impregnated test booklets. Each odorant is accompanied by four choices from which the subject must make a selection. Doty believes the test "... reliably reflects subtle aspects of smell function" and separates out malingerers. An attempt to identify normosmotics also has been made by others.[27] Snow[28] is investigating a scheme of evaluating olfaction by the intravascular route.

TABLE I

Causes of Smell Impairment

I. Intranasal odorant airway obstruction
  A. Trauma
  B. Edema
    1. Allergic, including polyps and vasomotor rhinitis
    2. Inflammatory edema
  C. Exudates
  D. Neoplasms
II. Intranasal mucosal destruction
  A. Atrophic rhinitis
  B. Aging mucosal replacement
  C. Viral infections
    1. The "common cold"
    2. Influenza-like upper respiratory infections
  D. Toxic chemicals and drugs, e.g., cocaine, formaldehyde, tyrothricin,[16] sulfuric acid mist, sulfur dioxide, chemotherapeutic agents and others[17,18]
III. Head trauma
  A. Fracture of the cribriform plate
  B. Shearing laceration of the olfactory nerves
  C. Hemorrhage causing interference with the frontal lobes, olfactory bulbs or tracts
IV. Intracranial lesions
  A. Tumors both neoplastic, benign, or vascular, usually bilateral involving the undersurface of the frontal lobes and cribriform plate
  B. Ischemia of the olfactory apparatus
  C. Infection
V. Endocrine
  A. Kallman's syndrome
  B. Turner's syndrome
  C. Others[19]
VI. Psychiatric problems and malingering

Congenital Dysosmia

Amoore[29] and Berglund and Lindvall[30] suggest that a phenomenon of odor blindness loosely akin to color blindness occurs. Kallman's syndrome, the most widely recognized congenital clinical problem involving olfaction, is usually associated with hypogonadism and may also involve agenesis of the olfactory bulbs and stalks and faulty development of the hypothalmus. Deafness and other symptoms may be present. In this affliction trigeminal response to strong stimulants is retained. Korsakoff's disease or syndrome is often associated with a depression of olfaction, perhaps on the basis of malnutrition, but it is possible that an alcoholic aphasia makes the testing unreliable.

Endocrine Olfactory Problems

The best recognized of these is Turner's syndrome in which the gonadal excretion is at fault. Individuals suffering from Addison's disease, low thyroid function, diabetes mellitus, and other endocrine problems also may complain of related dysosmia.

Mechanical Airway Obstruction

The odorous particle may mechanically be prevented from reaching the mucosa (e.g., growths, extreme turgescence of the mucosa, etc.) and thus no stimulation occurs. A deviated nasal septum is unlikely to offer enough of an impediment to compromise olfaction.

Virus Infections

The influenza virus, rhinovirus, herpes simplex virus and others are associated with destruction of the respiratory nasal mucous membrane and cilia and perhaps destruction of the olfactory receptor cells also occurs.[34] The physiological correlate of destruction of the olfactory mucous membrane is hyposmia. Decrease in the olfactory sense was found by Henkin and Smith[31] in viral hepatitis. Multiple sclerosis and Parkinson's disease (although of questionable pathogenesis) may affect olfaction.

Trauma

Doty[22] states that physical trauma to the head results in depression of the olfactory sense in perhaps 5–10% of such situations, being more frequent when the trauma is more severe. Injuries that tear the bulbs from the cribriform plate or fracture the plate itself result frequently in anosmia with significant recovery in perhaps 30% of cases. Injudicious surgery in the region of the cribriform plate may injure the olfactory filia.

Intracranial Tumors and Lesions

The olfactory tract and bulbs are relatively sensitive to pressure so that transmitted pressure from nearby tumors, benign or malignant, can depress olfactory function. These include meningiomas, pituitary growths, tumors inside or on the floor of the third ventricle and tumors of the frontal lobes. Displacement or traction by a more distant lesion (e.g., hydrocephalus) can result in olfactory depression. Temporal lobe tumors disturb the central connections. Irradiation can depress the sensitivity of the olfactory mucosa. Temporal lobe epilepsy is associated with olfactory depression.

Air Pollutants, Drugs, and Toxic Chemicals

Perhaps the best example of the topical application of a drug injuring the olfactory mucosa is zinc sulfate[30] although Henkin and others[18,31,32] believe that low body zinc levels are associated with low olfactory acuity. Antineoplastic drugs can result in hyposmia, perhaps by depressing the normal turnover of the bipolar olfactory neurons. The list of toxic drugs reported to deleteriously affect the sense of smell includes ethanol, topical cocaine, formaldehyde, organic solvents, SO_2, tyrothricin (topical), and many others. However, Doty et al.[33] using the UPSIT test found no olfactory deficit in the employees of a chemical plant.

Treatment

Alternatives for treatment of olfactory disturbances are discouragingly few in number unless there is a specific abnormality such as allergy, benign nasal growths, hypothyroidism, etc., to correct. Too often there has been a destructive olfactory epithelial process with replacement by squamous or respiratory epithelium from aging, trauma, the environment, or disease and little can be done. Reduction in the intensity of inflammation in post-viral or post-traumatic situations by use of corticosteroids may be of value early and probably after a 10-day per os course of such medication the benefit has been secured. Zinc to correct a deficiency has been tried in the past for individuals with olfactory disorders but has not yielded much success. Dietary supplementation with vitamins likewise has yielded little benefit.

REFERENCES

1. Doty RI. Olfactory communication in humans. Chem Senses 6:351–376, 1981.
2. Engen T. The human uses of olfaction. Am J Otolaryngol 4:250–251, 1983.
3. U.S. National Research Council. Odors from stationary and mobile sources. Board of Toxicology and Environmental Health Hazards. Washington, D.C.: National Academy of Sciences, 1979.
4. Graziadei PPP. In: Muller-Schwarze D, Mozell M, eds. Chemical Signals in Vertebrates. New York: Plenum Press, 1976, pp. 435–454.
5. Nakashima T, Kimmelman CP, Snow JB. Structure of human fetal and adult olfactory neurepithelium. Arch Ortolaryngol 110:641–646, 1984.
6. Nakashima T, Kimmelman CP, Snow JB Jr. Immunohistopathology of human olfactory epithelium, nerve and bulb. Laryngoscope 95:391–396, 1985.
7. Olfaction and taste. In: West JB, ed. Best and Taylor's Physiological Basis of Medical Practice, 11th ed. Baltimore: Williams & Wilkins, 1985, chap. 65.
8. Masera R. Sul'esistenze di un particolare organo olfattivo nel setto nasale cavia e di altri roditori. Arch Ital Anat Embriol 48:157–212, 1943.
9. Moran DT, Rowley JC III, et al. The fine structure of the olfactory mucosa in man. J Neurocytol 11:721–746, 1982.
10. Jafek BW. Ultrastructure of human nasal mucosa. Laryngoscope 93:1576–1599, 1983.
11. Hornung DE, Mozell MM. Smell: human physiology. In: Meiselman HL, Rivlin RS, eds. Clinical Measurement of Taste and Smell. New York: Macmillan Publishing Co., 1986, chap. 2.
12. Proctor DF, Andersen IB, eds. The Nose. New York: Elsevier Biomedical Press, 1982, p. 281.

13. Moulton DG, Beidler LM. Structure and function in the peripheral olfactory system. Physiol Rev 47:1–52, 1967.

14. Mozell MM, Hornung DE, et al. Initial mechanisms basic to olfactory perception. Am J Otolaryngol 4:238–245, 1983.

15. Tatchell RH, Lerman JW, Watt J. Olfactory ability as a function of nasal air flow volume in laryngectomies. Am J Otolaryngol 6:426–432, 1985.

16. Seydell EM, McKnight WP. Disturbances of olfaction resulting from intranasal use of tyrothricin. Clinical report of 7 cases. Arch Otolaryngol 47:465–470, 1948.

17. Smith DV. Taste, smell and psychophysical measurement. In: Meiselman HL, Rivlin RS, eds. Clinical Measurement of Taste and Smell. New York: The Macmillan Publishing Co., 1986, pp. 1–18.

18. Cancalon P. Degeneration and regeneration of olfactory cells induced by $ZnSO_4$ and other chemicals. Tissue Cell 14:717–733, 1982.

19. Schiffman SS. Taste and smell in disease. N Engl J Med 308:1275–1279, 1337–1343, 1983.

20. Doty RL, Shaman P, et al. Smell identification ability: changes with age. Science 226:1441–1443, 1984.

21. Smith CG. Age incidence of atrophy in olfactory nerves in man. J Comp Anat 77:589–595, 1942.

22. Doty RL. A review of olfactory dysfunctions in man. Am J Otolaryngol 1:57–79, 1979.

23. Feldman JI, Wright HN, Leopold DA. The Initial evaluation of dysosmia. Am J Otolaryngol 7:431–444, 1986.

24. Cain WS, Gent J, et al. Clinical evaluation of olfaction. Am J Otolaryngol 4:252–256, 1983.

25. Doty RL, Shaman P, et al. University of Pennsylvania Smell Identification Test—a rapid quantitative olfactory function test for the clinic. Laryngoscope 94:176–178, 1984.

26. Doty RL, Shaman P, Dann M. Development of the University of Pennsylvania Smell Identification Test: a standardized microencapsulated test of olfactory function. Physiol Behav 32:489–502, 1984.

27. Heywood PG, Costanzo RM. Identifying normosmotics. A comparison of two populations. Am J Otolaryngol 7:194–199, 1986.

28. Snow JB. Clinical problems in chemosensory disturbances. Am J Otolaryngol 4:224–227, 1983.

29. Amoore JE. Specific anosmia: a clue to the olfactory code. Nature 214:1095–1098, 1967.

30. Berglund B, Lindvall T. In: Proctor DF, Andersen IB, eds. The Nose. New York: Elsevier Biomedical Press, 1982, chap. 11.

31. Henkin RL, Smith FR. Hyposmia in acute viral hepatitis. Lancet 1:823–826, 1971.

32. English GM, ed. Otolaryngology. Philadelphia: J. B. Lippincott, 1986, vol. 2, chap. 5.

33. Doty RL, Gregor T, et al. Quantitative assessment of olfactory function in an industrial setting. J Occup Med 28:457–460, 1986.

34. Jafek BW, Hartman D, et al. Postviral olfactory dysfunction. Am J Rhinology 4:91–99, 1990. □

Chapter XI

Rhinomanometry and Experimental Nasal Challenges

James A. McLean, M.D.

ABSTRACT

This brief review covers several features of rhinomanometry and experimental nasal challenges. The experimental studies outlined include the collaborative work of many individuals, have been published previously, and are only summarized here. For a broader discussion and specific details, the references are suggested.

In one of the early reviews of nasal challenge results in allergic patients, Holman et al.[1] reviewed the previous attempts and pointed to the pioneer work of Kirkman, who developed hay fever after sniffing sweet vernal grass in 1835. Blackley, the father of clinical allergy, tested himself in 1873 with pollen instillations on the conjunctival, nasal, and parabuccal mucosae. Even after the introduction of allergen skin tests, clinicians continued to use nasal challenge in difficult cases, although certainly not as much as skin tests, which became the diagnostic tool in establishing etiologic relationships.

Over the ensuing years, attempts to reproduce natural outdoor exposures resulted in the use of whole pollen grains, which could be sniffed, dropped into the nose from a toothpick, or inhaled from stirred suspensions. Later, defatted pollen grains and allergy extracts were dripped from a glass rod or pipette, aerosolized from nebulizers, atomizers, and compressors, and injected directly into the nasal mucosa or placed on felt or paper discs inserted onto the nasal mucosa. Recently, some

investigations have utilized the "turbo-inhaler" for delivering whole pollen grains in nasal challenge studies.

Various methods of assessment have also been used in the past to determine if the results of nasal challenge were positive or negative: grading the severity of various hay fever symptoms with a numerical rating, counting the amount of medication used to control symptoms, and the "sneeze-drip" index, i.e., spontaneous sneezes are counted and the number of "drips" of nasal secretions collected and counted per unit of time. In 1958, Aschan and Drettner[2] added the semiquantitative measurement of nasal airway resistance as a parameter of assessment. They used pollen grains, pollen extracts, and histamine for nasal challenge with allergic and control individuals and studied the effects of an antihistamine, of phenylephrine, and of immunotherapy.

ANATOMY AND PHYSIOLOGY OF THE NOSE

A brief review of some anatomic and physiologic components of the nose is important because the response of the nasal mucosa to challenge is greatly influenced by differences from the bronchial mucosa and airway when describing pulmonary challenge and responses. The nasal mucus blanket follows a narrow and tortuous passage posteriorly and mainly inferiorly to the nasopharynx. The nasal mucosa, containing many goblet cells and glands contributes to this mucus flow and traps some of the small particle (>3 μm) able to enter the nose and pass through the tortuous passages. Passage of aerosols of larger size with nasal challenges are influenced by the speed of delivery with the larger particles impacting on the mucosa surface.

The nasal mucosal structure is physiologically important in modulating the air conditioning and olfactory functions of the nose. These functions are aug-

Professor Emeritus Internal Medicine, University of Michigan Medicine Center

mented by the variable airway dimensions that are anatomically fixed in some areas[3] (narrowest at the internal ostium just inside the vestibule) and reversible in others, the latter (mucosal responsiveness) being the basic indicator of nasal reactivity in nasal challenges. When nasal secretions do not vary, nasal patency is mainly a function of vascular filling and the content of fluid within the nasal mucosa. Anatomically the mucosa allows for rapid fluid shifts and rapid vascular uptake of agents applied to the mucosa. Aiding these functions are the open endothelial cell junctions in the submucosa, the multiple transcellular fenestrae, and the exceedingly porous basement membrane of small vessels. Additionally, nasal mucosal and submucosal consistency and consequent nasal patency are influenced greatly by the unique structure of the nasal vasculature. Arterioles run parallel to the surface just below the mucosal surface and are "resistance" vessels for heat and moisture exchange and foster rapid gas and solid absorption. Deeper in the mucosa in the "capacitance" system lie thin-walled veins and venous lakes capable of marked volume changes similar to erectile tissue. In addition, arteriovenous shunts, controlling sphincters, and connecting capillaries link arterial and venous segments and further modify their responses.

This highly responsive vascular system is under humoral and autonomic control with sympathetic stimulation producing primarily a decrease in mucosal flow with an increase in nasal patency manifest as a decrease in nasal airway resistance (NAR); parasympathetic stimulation (cholinergic) results in an increased glandular secretion rate and increased mucosal blood flow with a decrease in nasal patency (with an increase in NAR). In experiments with volunteer research subjects, aerosolized atropine inhibits the increased NAR induced by cholinergic (aerosolized methacholine) challenge, i.e., inhibition of parasympathetic tone,[4] although it does not do so in the cat. Other rhinometry studies confirm that adrenergic agents cause vasoconstriction in humans,[5] and the nasal vasculature is said to be more responsive to adrenaline than is the heart.[6] Histamine challenge responses are blocked by premedication with H1 and H2 antagonists indicating that corresponding receptors occur in the nose.[7]

Beside the state of the nasal airway itself and its autonomic regulation, associated factors must not be overlooked when nasal challenge experiments are carried out. Inflammation, including allergic rhinitis, heightens nasal responsiveness as do priming, cooling the extremities, and recumbency (see below). Painful stimuli to the nasal vestibule, upper lip, and infraorbital structures, as well as emotions, exercise, endocrine factors, and changes in position also modify nasal responsiveness and consequently nasal response parameters (see below). Another factor influencing nasal responsiveness is spontaneous periods of reciprocating nasal

patency, named the "nasal cycle." These alternating changes in patency occur at 1.5-6 hour intervals in the majority of human subjects.[8, 9] While these opposing nasal patency fluctuations are measurably followed and recorded, the total nasal resistance remains constant. But single airway measurements need to recognize these phasic variations. Stellate ganglion block has been shown to counteract this recurring cycle.

ASSESSMENT OF NASAL PATENCY

In assessing nasal patency, the resistance to airflow provides a useful index of mucosal response. However, it is recognized by many workers in this field that mild to moderate symptoms may be experienced with little or no change in NAR.

In normal tidal breathing, resistive forces are opposed by a driving pressure gradient since the nasal airway acts as a rigid conduit. Also, nasal airflow is turbulent, even at low flow (or quiet breathing), because the nasal passages are narrow and tortuous. Rohrer's formula appears to best describe these nasal pressure-flow relationships:

$$Pressure = K_1 \cdot flow^2 + K_2 \cdot flow + K_3$$

where K_1 and K_2 are constants for a given nasal airway at given condition of patency and K_3 is usually negligible under most circumstances. Some workers believe that K_1 reflects NAR more accurately than do the other indices.

Pressure and flow change throughout the nasal respiratory cycle; Figure 1 emphasizes that relationship. Each is dependent on the other, and the measurement of one alone is insufficient; thus, nasal airway resistance is the pressure drop associated with a specific rate of flow. It may be expressed as the slope of the nasal pressure-flow curve at the flow point considered. Since NAR varies throughout the respiratory cycle, comparison of NAR data should relate to a single (reference) flow rate examined at each phase of testing.[10] Efforts to use a fixed pressure drop as a common reference are not as satisfactory theoretically but have been utilized by some.

Peak expiratory flow rates (nasal) have been described as a parameter of airway patency. Unfortunately this method is very effort dependent and therefore less reproducible. Nasal airway resistance measurements are made during quiet breathing. Two basic approaches are used for acquiring flow and pressure drop data. (For a description of anterior and posterior rhinomanometry techniques, see Reference 11). Anterior rhinomanometry is carried out more easily by almost all adults and most children.[12, 13] Some workers believe posterior rhinomanometry reveals higher resistance than anterior measurements.[13] The difficulties of anterior rhinomanometry due to the variability in breath to breath measurement, the effect of under- or overbreathing, and some subjects' inability to produce a smooth transition

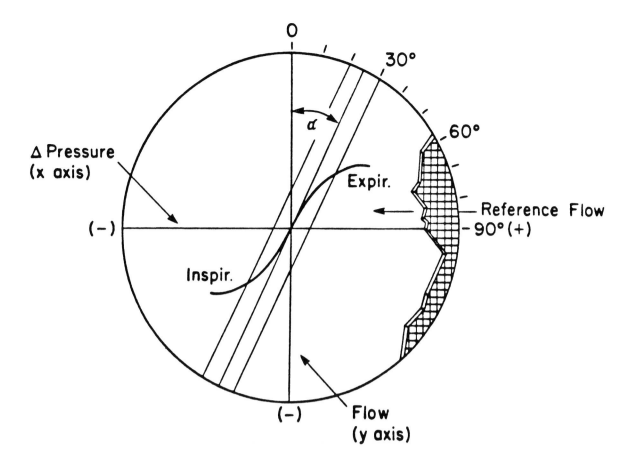

Figure 1. *The flattened, S=shaped Δ P=V curve, characteristic of nasal respiration by normal subjects, as displayed on the axes of an oscilloscope. Flow and pressure connections are made to project the inspiratory segment in the lower left and the expiratory segment in the upper right quadrant of the display. The early and late phases of inspiration and those of expiration, respectively, are shown superimposed. A ruled overlay (shown) assists measurement of the curve's slope [or the pressure value corresponding to the reference flow (arrow)]. The axes are pre-calibrated to permit NAR to be read directly from the value of angle ∝ in degrees, as shown at the upper right. (Modified with permission from J Allergy 36:65, 1965.)*

between inspiration and expiration while measurements are being made has been noted; these workers believe more consistency can be obtained with the addition of a BBC microcomputer.[14] Posterior rhinomanometry does not require instrumentation of the nares and is superior in this respect; however, some 15–30% of subjects cannot tolerate the required flexible tube in their mouths. Posterior rhinomanometry shows less scatter and greater consistency with compared to anterior rhinomanometry.[15] The two methods seem to produce similar results in children and subjects with only mild or moderate airway obstruction. Total airway resistance may be measured also by body plethysmography and nasal and pulmonary resistance calculated separately.

NAR measurements can be compared in the same subject at different times and among different subjects only if a common reference measurement point is selected, e.g., an index flow rate. Unfortunately this is not always done. Investigators should remember that the absolute change in resistance for a given change in nasal patency will vary with the initial level of resistance.

Nebulized solutions, in general, produce particle droplets small enough to pass through the nose. Therefore, atomizers producing larger droplets have been favored, and studies have shown that they deliver a more constant amount with fairly even distribution and deeper penetration than squeeze-bottle plastic nebulizers (see below).

After suitable acclimatization to room temperature and humidity, baseline measurements are first obtained, and then the "nonspecific" nasal reactivity is determined using the diluent control as the challenge material. The rise from baseline values for NAR measured over 15 minutes has averaged 22.5, 26, and 20.5% with three separate investigators using a single physiologic buffered saline (PBS) challenge. Intrasubject differences are definite, however, and this control challenge should be carried out after baseline NAR determination is made with every experiment. Because provocative protocols may require serial challenges, we carried out serial PBS challenges at 15-minute intervals (for six challenges). With this repetitive "control" challenge, it was found that approximately half the subjects' NAR values increased 50% or more over the baseline, but in only 15% did the NAR increase over 100%. While variability in response to control challenge was present when subjects were tested on two or more occasions, it appears that repeated nasal challenge in a manner analogous to bronchial challenge testing is feasible.

In general, most workers measure NAR for 15 minutes after each challenge since the major response has occurred during that interval, and NAR readings often have returned to or near the baseline by that time. However, this sequence will not allow the investigator to determine if late-phase responses occur.[16]

If response to the PBS challenge does not exceed the baseline by 30%, the experiment is continued. Responses to challenges with allergens and pharmacologic agents are not considered significant unless the baseline and PBS challenge NAR values are relatively low, i.e., less than 50% increase in NAR with the active agent producing an increase in NAR over 100%. While this results in a decrease in sensitivity, it increases the probability that NAR results will be specific and reproducible.

RESULTS OF NASAL CHALLENGE

Initial experiments were designed to determine if atopic subjects reacted differently than normal or nonatopic subjects to the buffered saline (1) used as diluent and (2) used as the nonspecific challenge to assess nonspecific nasal reactivity following the establishment of the baseline NAR for each experiment.[4] A single PBS aerosol challenge was carried out in 102 subjects: 32 nonatopic, 36 asymptomatic atopic (out of season), and 34 symptomatic atopics (during the grass or ragweed pollen seasons). The mean baseline NAR before PBS aerosol challenge did not differ significantly between the three groups (Figure 2). Although the nonatopic subjects on average showed less responsiveness to PBS than did the other two groups, the differences among the groups were not statistically significant. Nineteen atopic subjects were studied both in and out of their season. The mean increase in NAR after PBS challenge was higher when the subjects were symptomatic but the difference between symptomatic and asymptomatic periods again was not significant. In addition, the maximal percent increase in NAR after PBS showed no correlation with the individuals' baseline NAR.

The modest increase in NAR usually obtained with PBS stimulation appears to be due to reflex parasympathetic stimulation was demonstrated by aerosolized atropine almost completely inhibited the PBS-induced NAR increases.

Others have shown similar challenge results by rhi-

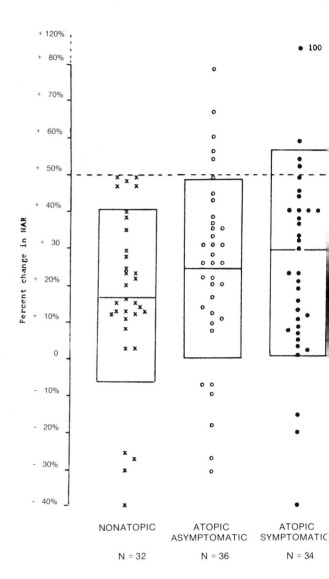

Figure 2. Peak change in NAR after a single challenge with 0. ml buffered saline. Enclosed areas show 1 SD about the mean (From J Allergy Clin Immunol 58:565, 1976; with permission

nomanometry between allergic and nonallergic individuals.[17, 18] Recent studies show that titrating histamin challenges may differentiate between controls and non allergic rhinitis if smaller changes in NAR are monitored[19] (and also suggested that both nasal cavities should be challenged and that the histamine respons was independent of the baseline NAR value). Utilizin a positive or negative histamine challenge response b this method will differentiate between normal and symptomatic subjects, again suggesting nasal hyper reactivity to histamine in allergic rhinitis exists in similar manner to bronchial hyperreactivity in asth matics.[20]

Since isoproterenol produces bronchodilation i asthmatic subjects, its effect on the nose was studied i asthmatic as well as hay fever subjects.[21] NAR increase more than 100% in 30 of the 53 subjects, and there wa no significant difference in the response of the atopi and nonatopic groups. The 11 asymptomatic hay fever subjects who had asthma did not differ from the other groups. The same was true of the subgroup of symptomatic hay fever subjects with a history of asthma. In addition, isoproterenol failed to lower NAR in symptomatic hay fever subjects. In the group of subjects experiencing an increase in NAR with isoproterenol, 2.0 mg of intranasal propranolol (0.1 ml of 1% solution in each nostril) completely inhibited this rise in NAR.

Thus, the effects of isoproterenol on the patency of the nose are opposite to those in the bronchial airways. The smooth muscle dilator response in the bronchi is probably the same as the effect on the nasal vasculature, i.e., some vasodilation. Since the effect of isoproterenol could be blocked by propranolol, b-adrenergic receptors were most likely involved. The effects of isoproterenol on allergen-induced increases in NAR theoretically pit the direct effect on the vasculature against the inhibition of mediator release. The vascular effect seems to predominate.

Because of the clinical knowledge that allergic triggers are only one source of exposure for hay fever patients, the nasal effect of an irritant was investigated.[22] To establish a suitable dosage range for NH_3 required to produce a greater than 100% increase in NAR, several concentrations were tested, 1.44 mM NH^3 with a 20-second exposure in each nostril provided subjective nasal irritation that was only transient in duration. Twenty-seven subjects were studied: 12 nonatopic control subjects, 9 allergic rhinitis subjects without asthma, and 6 allergic rhinitis subjects with asthma. There was no significant difference in the NAR changes in any group to the four levels of exposure to NH_3, and within the atopic group there was no significant difference between allergic rhinitis subjects with and without asthma. The mean percent NAR increase following 20 seconds of exposure to compressed air was similar to that evoked by a PBS control and was comparable for the atopic and nonatopic groups.

Atropine and chlorpheniramine were used as pharmacologic blocking agents to study their effect on the nasal response to NH_3. Each subject's baseline NAR was determined, then a PBS challenge, then NH_3 (which produced a significant rise in NAR), then either 1 mg/ml of atropine aerosolized or 3 mg/ml of chlorpheniramine aerosolized intranasally, and finally a repeat challenge with NH_3. The NAR response to the second NH_3 exposure after aerosolized atropine was markedly attenuated; the mean percent inhibition was 89% (Figure 3). Additional control subjects who received PBS instead of atropine prior to the second NH_3 exposure showed the usual response, i.e., a significant increase in NAR. Data also indicated that atropine inhibited the NH_3 response in both nonatopic and atopic subjects.

Aerosolized chlorpheniramine, 3 mg/ml, in place of atropine tended to produce a small direct increase in

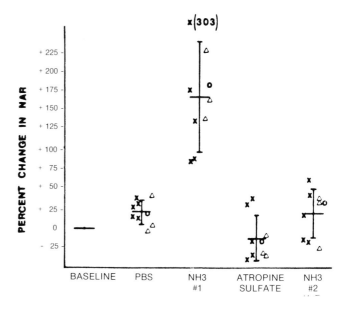

Figure 3. *Inhibition of NH_3-induced changes in NAR by atropine. X — Nonatopic subjects; 0 — Allergic rhinitis subjects without asthma; Δ — Allergic rhinitis subjects with a history of asthma. (From Ann Otol Rhinol Laryngol 88: 228, 1979; with permission.)*

NAR, but this had returned to near baseline levels before the following challenge with NH_3. In no instance, with either atopic or nonatopic subjects, did the antihistamine produce substantial inhibition of NH_3-induced increase in NAR (Figure 4).

The increased NAR produced by NH_3 is most likely due to vascular dilatation in the nasal mucosa and/or edema resulting from increased vessel permeability, although excess nasal secretion also could be playing a role. The failure of an antihistamine, chlorpheniramine, to inhibit the effects of NH_3 on NAR reduces the likelihood that mast cell histamine release is an important mechanism in this process. On the other hand, the pronounced inhibition obtained with atropine suggests that the effect of NH_3 is largely mediated by parasympathetic reflex effects on the nasal vasculature.

In 1968, Connell[23] showed a priming effect on the nasal mucosa when he demonstrated that the nasal mucosa becomes hyperresponsive during antigen challenge on consecutive days. This appeared relevant to such clinical problems as symptoms occurring with low pollen counts at the end of the pollen season, intolerance to irritants during active hay fever symptoms, difficulties in assessing patterns of symptoms with multiple sensitivities, and the trend toward intranasal challenge testing and the use of intranasal immunotherapy (see below).

Experiments were designed to determine if priming could be elicited with an irritant and whether priming with an allergen simultaneously heightens responsiveness to an irritant.[24] Atopic subjects received progressively larger ragweed aerosol challenges until a dose was

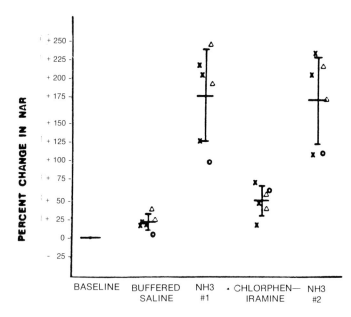

Figure 4. *Attempted inhibition of NH₃-induced changes in NAR by chlorpheniramine. See legend to Fig. 3. (From Ann Otol Rhinol Laryngol 88:228, 1979; with permission.)*

established that increased NAR by at least 200%. That dose was then repeated on day 2, 3, 4, 8, and 15. Subjects experienced increased NAR responsiveness that was statistically significant by day 3 or 4 and also experienced hay fever symptoms. This priming was reproducible and also transient, becoming less by days 8 and 15. One month later, these same subjects were challenged with NH₃ on days 1, 2, 3, 4, and 8. They had an increased responsiveness in their NAR, but the rise was short of statistical significance. One year later the same subjects received an NH₃ challenge one week prior to ragweed aerosol challenges on day 1, 2, 3, and 4. Again there was a significant increase in NAR and symptoms developed. NH₃ challenge was repeated on day 5 and then again one week later on day 12. There was no priming by ragweed to the irritant NH₃ on days 8 and 12. However, NH₃ and ragweed were aerosolized on different days in this experiment, while during the pollen season, ragweed and irritants are inhaled simultaneously and produce an increase in symptoms. Work by Schumacker and Pain[25] during the grass pollen season also suggests that priming is short-lived. However, in a trial of intranasal immunotherapy (see below) there appeared to be increased nasal reactivity following preseasonal intranasal immunotherapy. More recent challenge testing reveals that histamine and methacholine do not exert a priming effect,[26] although increased reactivity to histamine and methacholine occurs after antigen exposure.[27, 28]

In an attempt to better understand the distribution and clearance of solutions applied to the nasal mucosa, buffered saline was tagged with technetium (⁹⁹ᵐTc)

pertechnetate and delivered by various techniques to the nose in the same manner as for nasal challenge testing.[29] A No. 251 DeVilbiss atomizer was compared to a No. 114 and a No. 127 DeVilbiss atomizer, a pipette, a commercial squeeze bottle, and a spray bottle. There was considerable intrasubject variation with reproducibility in four identical experiments. All subjects gave a 26.4% mean coefficient of variation. Pipetting produced a rapid passage through the nose with radioactivity already present in the oropharynx within the first minute. With all the delivery methods, a major portion of the radioactive materials could be seen to travel posteriorly through the inferior portion of the nose into the nasopharynx and pharynx, although a significant amount also remained far anteriorly in the nose. None of the methods used for intranasal administration of ⁹⁹ᵐTc pertechnetate resulted in a widespread distribution of the tracer throughout much of the nasal cavity.

To determine whether residual radioactivity remaining on the nasal mucosa at 20 minutes after delivery was on the mucosal surface itself or absorbed into the submucosa, clearance (disappearance of) the radioactive material was determined after nasal washes with saline. After washing at 1 minute, clearance was 96% and at 29 minutes was 92%. This indicates that the ⁹⁹ᵐTc pertechnetate remaining at 20 minutes, largely located far anteriorly, is not substantially bound to or within the mucosa at the time. Mygind and Versterhauge[30] produced a cast of the human nose and found that the amount and distribution of aerosolized material from a squeeze type plastic bottle nebulizer was broader and shorter than the pressurized aerosols delivered. However, a recent report found similar nasal distribution between a metered-dose aerosol unit and a metering pump deliver unit.[31] Deposition is mostly in the anterior third of the nose if a nasal spray pump is used.[32]

There are three components to the deposition and clearance of materials introduced into the human nose. The first is a very rapid "water shed" or run-through occurring largely within the first minute and seen especially well following administration of solutions by pipette. The second component relates to the progressive movement of material toward the nasopharynx within about 15–30 minutes and is probably due to mucociliary clearance. The third phase consists of a very slow disappearance, over a number of hours, of material initially retained far anteriorly in the nose. These second and third phases of nasal clearance observed by us are in agreement with the observations of Aoki and Crowley[33] and Proctor et al.[34]

Several workers in the past have used NAR measurements as one parameter in evaluating the results of nasal immunotherapy. Our first double-blind study[35] compared the efficacy of preseasonal short ragweed extract intranasal immunotherapy with a dilute histamine placebo control. During the next ragweed season a more prolonged treatment with a larger dose of intranasal polymerized ragweed was evaluated in a similar manner. Although others reported limited success with this therapy, we were unable to show any significant effect as assessed by daily symptom diaries and examination in season. In early August of the first year, the ragweed-treated group showed a mean decrease in the log protein N concentration of ragweed extract required to produce a greater than 150% increase in NAR (i.e., heightened reactivity). This differed significantly from the mean increase observed in the placebo-treated group. This may well have represented a "priming effect" since the tests were carried out soon after a recent treatment with ragweed, and there was no significant difference between the groups when retested in October. Work by others on the attenuation of tissue changes during the early phases of immunotherapy reveal no difference in nasal peak flow or nasal airway resistance, amount of nasal secretions, sneezing counts or skin test sensitivity diminution with ragweed treatment at 8 weeks (1/4 maintenance dose of grass extract)[36] and at 1-3-6 months (1/2 maintenance dose of ragweed).[37]

With recent attention to aspirin's role in producing asthma and the apparent beneficial effect on the severity of asthma after aspirin "desensitization," we studied the effects of intranasal aspirin administration. Intranasal aerosolized aspirin administration in concentrations up to 22.3 mg/day did not increase NAR more than did buffer. Also this dose did not prevent the increase in NAR produced by histamine and methacholine challenges. These studies were carried out in a single-blind fashion. Then in a double-blind experiment oral aspirin (1200 mg), sodium salicylate (1200 mg), or placebo was given 45 minutes prior to an aerosol ragweed challenge. Oral indomethacin (75 mg) was used in a single-blind fashion: tripling doses of aerosol ragweed were sprayed into each nostril until NAR was increased by more than 150%.[38] A comparison of the percent NAR increase with and without antecedent nasal aspirin administration showed significant decreased response to ragweed aerosol challenge. Sodium salicylate and indomethacin also significantly decreased the NAR response to aerosol ragweed challenge. However, other workers report an increase in nasal resistance as measured by anterior rhinomanometry 45 minutes after ingestion of 900 mg of aspirin.[39]

The effects of environmental pollution (indoors and outside) has been investigated in allergic asthmatics breathing altered air with 0.5 ppm SO_2 by face mask (or nasal challenge) and exercising; statistically significant reductions occurred in FEV_1 and an increase in nasal work of breathing was shown via posterior rhinomanometry.[40]

APPLICATIONS OF NASAL CHALLENGES

Nasal provocation, with NAR measurements as semiquantitative assessment, has been used for many types of investigative procedures.[11] Pharmacologic agents have been used in nasal challenge to study normal and abnormal upper airway physiology. Histamine, methacholine, isoproterenol, propranolol, atropine, chlorpheniramine, phenylephrine, polymyxin B, aspirin, arachidonic acid derivatives, bradykinin, serotonin,[41] cromolyn, clemastine and ketotifen,[42] and substance P,[43] have been used in challenge and to investigate "blocking" conditions. NH_3 and SO_2 have been used to produce nasal obstruction and helium air mixtures, hypercapnia, oxygen-rich mixtures, distilled water,[44] a hyperosmolar aerosol,[45] and carbon black have been used as challenge material in studying nasal physiologic responses. Various physiologic experiments have been carried out including the effects of temperature, position, and pressure. Recumbency decreases nasal patency[46, 47] as does cooling the trunk and extremities[47–49] and axillary pressure.[50] NAR measurements reveal increased ipsilateral and decreased contralateral resistance responses to lateral recumbency.[51] In humans monitored by posterior rhinomanometry afferent reflexes (sneezing induced by allergen challenge and skin cooling producing nasal vasoconstriction) have been demonstrated.[47, 49, 52] Exercise produces a decrease in NAR proportional to the amount of work[53, 54] and is probably related to an increased sympathetic discharge.[55] Nasal mucus velocity and nasal mucociliary clearance have been observed. Nasal challenge of stable asthmatic subjects followed by NAR and pulmonary function testing has been carried out in studies of the pathogenesis of allergen-induced asthma.[56]

The immunologic aspects of rhinitis have been investigated using "specific" aeroallergens in nasal challenges: pollens of grasses, ragweed, birch, Japanese cedar, sorrel; green algae; dog, cat, and human "danders"; mites, house dust, and fungi. Nasal challenge with allergens provides a fairly controllable model for evaluating the protective ability of various therapeutic agents. Some investigators have utilized a "titration" approach, i.e., several incremental challenge doses are used, and the response to treatment is measured by a change in threshold reactivity. Another approach is the establishment initially of a suprathreshold allergen-challenging dose, which is then used as the dose for subsequent challenges with the treatment medication being varied.[57] An interesting physiologic study on the response of the nose to bronchial provocation (ultrasonic nebulized distilled water) revealed an increase in NAR in patients with allergic rhinitis as well as asthmatic subjects with rhinitis symptoms.[58] The reverse, nasal challenge with histamine produced the predicted increase in NAR in subjects with hayfever and asthma

107

plus a drop in FEV_1 in 8/12 subjects.[59] Cellular changes in samples before and after challenge with specific antigen, e.g., birch pollen (collected by plastic strips on the nasal mucosa and brush samples) reveal an immediate increase in eosinophils that is maintained and correlates with the degree of nasal symptomatology and increase in nasal peak flow; an increase in mast cells after days 4–5 of nasal challenge; and nasal lavage analysis showing a decrease in histamine content/mast cell, i.e., apparently reflecting a release into secretions.[60] Other workers have found an immediate cellular response to specific allergen challenge (correlated with assessment of nasopharyngeal - nostril- pressure gradient) of eosinophils within 30 minutes (if count preceding challenge is considered),[61] while there is an increase in neutrophils and eosinophils preceding the late phase response with a subsequent drop and then an increase in epithelial cells and goblet cells.[62] Polymyxin B, a direct histamine liberator, has been used to probe mast cell reactivity in allergic and "vasomotor" rhinitis patients; symptomatic hay fever subjects showed the greater NAR response to aerosolized polymyxin B, but could still respond with further histamine provoked increases in NAR.[63] Pathophysiologic studies on the mediators involved in the immunologic response to specific antigen challenge initially involved rhinomanometric studies (which proved to be too variable after nasal washings) as well as secretion analysis revealing histamine, TAME-esterase, and PGD_2 present.[52] Following specific challenges (cat, mite, grass), increases in NAR, histamine, sulfidopeptide leukotrienes, total cell count, neutrophils, and eosinophils have been demonstrated by other workers.[44] Histamine, LTD_4, PGD_2, and PAF have been used as challenging agents, and the mediators histamine and LTD_4 appear to have the most important roles in increasing NAR and producing symptoms.[64]

Nasal provocation results have been used as one of the criteria in determining patients suitable for immunotherapy. NAR measurements also have been used to help assess treatment results of immunotherapy. Nasal provocation and NAR indices have been used to evaluate H_1 and H_2 blockers, cromolyn, fenoterol (a B_2-adrenergic agonist), and beclomethasone. NAR measurements also have been used in evaluating many other medications, e.g., phenylephrine, pseudoephedrine, ephedrine, phenylpropanolamine, cocaine, and some proprietary agents. Treatment results with Beconase (beclomethasone) on perennial nonatopic rhinitis subjects have been monitored by symptom scoring and active anterior rhinomanometry.[65]

NAR values have been helpful in assessing patients for corrective dentofacial or nasal surgery. The surgical effects of stellate ganglion block and vidian nerve resections have been monitored by pre- and postoperative NAR determinations, as well as assessment of reduction of nasal obstruction by nasal septoplasty, turbinate reduction, and rhinoplasty.[66] Adenoidectomy selection in children has been assessed by comparing preoperative radiology and rhinomanometry.[67]

Attempts to correlate nasal challenge results by rhinomanometry with other immunologic parameters have been carried out. Correlations among clinical evaluation, skin test reactions, conjunctival reactions, nasal challenge results, in vitro histamine release data, serum IgE, IgG, IgA, and IgM levels, or IgG antibodies to the challenge antigen levels, and specific radioallergosorbent test values have been evaluated by many workers in various combinations often with divergent results.[11] Unfortunately, the different methods used for testing, the various concentrations used for challenge, the manner of determining nasal airway patency, and the criteria for a "positive" challenge make the results difficult to compare between investigators even when these other response indicators also are included in the research protocol.

Nasal challenge, using methods of assessment other than NAR measurements, have been used in "rhinitis" patients to better understand the basic pathophysiology of nasal reactivity. In these instances, investigators have monitored various parameters to assess the effects of nasal challenge: light microscopic evaluation of basophils and mast cells from nasal scrapings of allergic individuals in and out of season, i.e., natural challenge[68]; other studies monitoring the natural pollen season reveal symptoms and the quantitative increase in TAME-estrase levels,[69] electron microscopy examination of cellular changes following radiolabeled allergen nasal challenge in nasal epithelial cells and the mucus layer.[70] The physical characteristics of nasal secretion have been investigated following provocation studies: allergen challenges, out of season, reveal an increase in viscosity measured by a viscosimeter and spinability; similar changes in magnitude were obtained with histamine challenges, although lesser ones occurred with methacholine.[71] The therapeutic effect of various medications in protecting against symptoms produced by nasal challenge, e.g., cromolyn, H_1 and H_2 blocker antihistamines individually and in combination, antihistamine decongestant mixtures and aerosol steroids; measurement of mucus flow and mucociliary action[72] including utilizing eosinophilic extracts (major basic protein) for provocation;[73] quantitation of eustachian tube obstruction by tympanometry[74, 75]; monitoring of mediator release and subsequent identification followed in some studies by blockage with medications[76]; and measuring of changes in nasal blood flow by hydrogen gas clearance or via laser Doppler velocimetry,[77] an apparently more accurate and reproducible method. Physiologic studies on nasal reflexes with unilateral histamine challenge produce secretions from both sides of the nose,[78] i.e., a reflex-mediated glandular secretion, as demonstrated by the reduction in secretion on the side of the unilateral vidian neurectomy.[79] Analyses of unilateral histamine-induced secretion in atopic and nonatopic subjects reveal increased albumin and nonsecretory IgA on the ipsilateral (stimulated) side and increased glandular protein secretory IgA contralaterally confirming a direct effect on the vascular bed and a reflexly mediated contralateral secretion, which is a glandular response.[80]

Arachidonic acid metabolites have been studied in patients with nasal symptoms as well as asthma. Their role in early antigen challenge was evaluated in allergic subjects with and without premedication with aspirin; the early increase in levels of PGE, PGD_2, PGF_2 alpha, and thrombaxane were significantly inhibited but not the level of histamine, TAME-esterase activity, leukotrienes, or the amount of sneezing.[81] Pretreatment of allergic subjects with systemic steroids did not affect the early antigen provocation results probably related to mast cell activation and mediator release but did reduce mediator release during the late-phase response and the rechallenge 11 hours later (again the immediate response occurred); the responses being monitored by mediator analysis and cellular inflammatory cell influx (basophils, eosinophils, neutrophils) and sneezing.[82] In contrast, topical steroid pretreatment blocks the early, late, and rechallenge responses as monitored by the same parameters.[83] Increased mediator release (histamine, TAME-esterase, kinens PGD_2) in nasal washings has been demonstrated with a concomitant increase in symptomatology after priming exposure of ragweed sensitive patients, although other mechanisms also may be involved.[84] Even a single out-of-season laboratory exposure followed by a specific challenge 11 hours later results in an increased mediator secretion in nasal washings and was attributed to the priming effect.[85]

In planning nasal provocation experiments, both the form of nasal challenge and the type of response assessment are governed by the primary intent and design of the experiment. In addition, experimental nasal challenges must be conducted so that the subject selection, delivery system, and response assessment have adequate controls.

Valid nasal testing and measurement methods are now available. Research workers and clinicians should work to standardize methods in order to better interpret their results and thereby, further aid practicing physicians and their patients.

SUMMARY

Nasal anatomic and physiologic components that influence both nasal challenge procedures and nasal airway resistance measurements are briefly described. The importance of obtaining physiologic baseline NAR measurements and minimal changes with physiologic buffered saline prior to each nasal challenge experiments is emphasized so that meaningful and reproducible challenge NAR values can be obtained. Our own results of nasal challenge in normal and atopic subjects are described for the following agents: ragweed pollen, histamine, methacholine, the irritant gas NH_3, polymyxin B, and isoproterenol. The blocking effects of atropine, chlorpheniramine, aspirin, indomethacin, and sodium salicylate on the ragweed and NH_3-induced increase in NAR are described. Mention is made of the numerous other investigative and clinical applications of nasal challenges and rhinomanometry.

REFERENCES

1. Halpern SR, Holman J, Whittaker C. The correlation between skin and respiratory mucous membrane tests with molds in allergic rhinitis. Ann Allergy 19:1407–1414, 1961.
2. Aschan G, Drettner B. Nasal obstruction in provocation experiments in patients with hay-fever. Acta Otolaryngol (Suppl) (Stockh) 140:91–99, 1958.
3. Bridger GP, Proctor DF. Maximum nasal inspiratory flow and nasal resistance. Ann Otol Rhinol Laryngol 79:481–488, 1970.
4. McLean JA, Mathews KP, Ciarkowski AA. The effects of topical saline and isoproterenol on nasal airway resistance. J Allergy Clin Immunol 58:563–574, 1976.
5. McLaurin JW, Shipman WF, Rosedale R Jr. Oral decongestants. Laryngoscope 71:54, 1961.
6. Malcolmson KG. The vasomotor activities of the nasal mucus membrane. J Laryngol Otol 73:73, 1959.
7. Secher C, Kirkegaard J, Burum P, Maansson A, Osterhammel P, Mygind N. Significance of H_1 and H_2 receptors in the human nose. Rationale for topical use of combined antihistamine preparations. J Allergy Clin Immunol 70:73, 1959.
8. Eccler R. Cyclic changes in human nasal resistance to airflow. J Physiol 272:75P, 1977.
9. Hasegawa M, Kern EB. The human nasal cycle. Mayo Clin Proc 52:28, 1977.
10. Hamilton LH. Nasal airway resistance, its measurement and regulation. Physiologist 22:43–49, 1979.
11. Solomon WR, McLean JA. Nasal provocative testing. In: Spector SL, ed. Provocative Challenge Procedures: Background and Methodology. Mount Kisco, NY: Futura Publishing Company, Inc. pp. 569–625, 1989.
12. Georgitis JA. The applicability of rhinomanometry in nonatopic children: Comparison of three techniques. J Allergy Clin Immunol 75:614, 1985.
13. Ghaem A, Martineaud JP. Determination of nasal resistance in healthy subjects using 2 technics of rhinomanometry. Bull Eur Physiopathol Respir 21:11, 1985.
14. Stevens JC, Jones AS, Lancer J, Beckingham E. A microcomputer-based procedure for carrying out rhinomanometry. J Med Eng Technol 11:278, 1987.
15. Dvoracek JE, Hillis A, Rossing RG. Comparison of sequential anterior and posterior rhinomanometry. J Allergy Clin Immunol 76:577–582, 1985.
16. Dvoracek JE, Yuninger JW, Kern EB, Hyatt RE, Gleich GJ. Induction of nasal late-phase reactions by insufflation of ragweed-pollen extract. J Allergy Clin Immunol 73:363–368, 1984.
17. Borum P, Gronborg H, Brofeldt S, Mygind N. Nasal reactivity in rhinitis. Eur J Respir Dis 64 (Suppl 128):65, 1983.
18. Gerth Van Wijk R, Dieges PH. Comparison of nasal responsiveness to histamine, methacholine in allergic rhinitis patients and controls. Clin Allergy 17:563, 1987.

19. Van De Heyning PH, Haesendonck J, Creten W, De Saegher D, Claes J. Histamine nasal provocation test. An evaluation of active anterior rhinomanometry and of threshold criteria of provocative dose. Allergy 44:482, 1989.

20. Mullins RJ, Olson LG, Sutherland DC. Nasal histamine challenges in symptomatic allergic rhinitis. J Allergy Clin Immunol 83:955, 1989.

21. McLean JA, Mathews KP, Solomon WR, et al. Effect of histamine and methacholine on nasal airway resistances in atopic and nonatopic subjects. Comparison with bronchial challenges and skin test responses. J Allergy Clin Immunol 59:165, 1977.

22. McLean JA, Mathews KP, Solomon WR, Brayton PR, Bayne NK. Effect of ammonia on nasal resistance in atopic and nonatopic subjects. Ann Otol Rhinol Laryngol 88:228–234, 1979.

23. Connell JT. Quantitative intranasal pollen challenge. II. Effect of daily pollen challenge, environmental pollen exposure and placebo challenge on the nasal membrane. J Allergy 41:123–139, 1968.

24. Bacon JR, McLean JA, Mathews KP, Banas JM. Priming of the nasal mucosa by ragweed extract or by an irritant (ammonia). J Allergy Clin Immunol 67:111–116, 1981.

25. Schumacher MJ, Pain MCF. Nasal challenge testing in grass pollen hay fever. J Allergy Clin Immunol 64:202–208, 1979.

26. Gronberg H, Borum P, Mygind N. Histamine and methacholine do not increase nasal reactivity. Clin Allergy 16:597, 1986.

27. Borum P. Nasal methacholine challenge: A test for the measurement of nasal reactivity. J Allergy Clin Immunol 63:253, 1979.

28. Konno A, Togawa K, Nishihira S. Seasonal variation of sensitivity of nasal mucosa in pollinosis. Arch Otorhinolaryngol 232:253, 1981.

29. McLean JA, Bacon JR, Mathews KP, Thrall JH, Banas JM, Hedden J and Bayne NK. Distribution and clearance of radioactive aerosol on the nasal mucosa. Rhinology 22:65–75, 1984.

30. Mygind N, Vesterhauge S. Aerosol distribution in the nose. Rhinology 16:79–88, 1978.

31. Hallworth GW, Padfield JM. A comparison of the regional deposition in a model nose of a drug discharged from metered aerosol and metered-pump nasal delivery systems. J Allergy Clin Immunol 77:348–353, 1986.

32. Newman SP, Moren F, Clarke SW. Deposition pattern from a nasal pump spray. Rhinology 25:77, 1987.

33. Aoki FY, Crowley JCW. Distribution and removal of human serum albumin-technetium 99m instilled intranasally. Br J Clin Pharmacol 3:869–878, 1976.

34. Proctor DF, Anderson I, Lundqvist G. Clearance of inhaled particles from the human nose. Arch Intern Med 131:132–139, 1973.

35. Mathews KP, Bayne NK, Banas JM, McLean JA, Bacon J. Controlled studies of intranasal immunotherapy for ragweed pollenosis. Int Arch Appl Immunol 66:218–224, 1981.

36. Osterballe O. Nasal and skin sensitivity during immunotherapy with two major allergens 19, 25 and partially purified extract of timothy grass pollen. Allergy 37:169, 1982.

37. Dantzler BS, Tipton WR, Nelson H, Osart P. Tissue threshold changes during first months of immunotherapy. Ann Allergy 45:213, 1980.

38. McLean JA, Bacon JR, Mathews KP, Banas J, Capati D, Bayne NS. Effects of aspirin on nasal responses in atopic subjects. J Allergy Clin Immunol 72:187–192, 1983.

39. Jones AS, Lancer JM, Moir AA, Stevens JC. Effect of aspirin on nasal resistance to airflow. Br Med J 290:1171–1173, 1985.

40. Kuenic JQ, Morgan MS, Horike M, Pierson WE. The effects of sulfur oxides on nasal and lung function in adolescents with extrinsic asthma. J Allergy Clin Immunol 96:813, 1985.

41. Tonnesen P, Schaffalitzky de Muckdell OB, Mygind N. Nasal challenge with serotonin in asymptomatic hayfever patients. Allergy 42:447, 1987.

42. Corrado OJ, Ollier S, Phillips MJ, Thomas JM, Davies RJ. Histamine and allergen induced changes in nasal airway resistance measured by anterior rhinomanometry: Reproductivity of the technique and the effect of topically administered antihistaminic and antiallergic drugs. Br J Clin Pharmacol 24:783, 1987.

43. Devillier P, Dessanges JF, Rakoshianaka F, Ghaem A, Boushey HA, Lockhart A, Marsac J. Nasal response to substance P and methacholine in subjects with and without allergic rhinitis. Eur Respir J 1:356, 1988.

44. Meslier N, Braunstein G, Lacroque J et al. Local cellular and humoral responses to antigenic and distilled water challenges in subjects with allergic rhinitis. Am Rev Respir Dis 137:617, 1988.

45. Silber G, Proud D, Warner J et al. In vivo release of inflammatory mediators by hyperosmolar solutions. Am Rev Respir Dis 137:606, 1988.

46. Hasegawa M, Saito Y. Postural variations in nasal resistance and symptomalogy in allergic rhinitis. Acta Otolaryngol (Stockh) 88:268, 1979.

47. Solomon WR. Comparative effects of transient body surface cooling, recumbency and induced obstruction in allergic rhinitis and control subjects. J Allergy 37:216, 1966.

48. Kortekangas AE. Effect of testing technique on nasal pressure variation. Acta Otolaryngol (Stockh) 75:249, 1973.

49. Drettner B. Vascular reactions of the human nasal mucosa on exposure to cold. Acta Otolaryngol (Suppl) (Stockh) 166:1, 1961.

50. Davies AM, Eccles R. Reciprocal changes in nasal resistance to airflow caused by pressure applied to the axilla. Acta Otolaryngol (Stockh) 99:154, 1985.

51. Cole P, Haight JSJ. Posture and nasal patency. Am Rev Respir Dis 129:351, 1984.

52. Naclerio RM, Meijer HL, Kagey-Sobotka A, Adkinson NF Jr, Meyers DA, Norman PS, Lichtenstein LM. Mediator release after nasal airway challenge with allergen. Am Rev Respir Dis 128:597, 1983.

53. Forsyth RD, Cole P, Shephard RJ. Exercise and nasal patency. J Appl Physiol 55:860, 1983.

54. Syabblo NC, Bundgaard A, Widdicome JG. Effects of exercise in nasal airflow resistance in breathing subjects and in patients with asthma and rhinitis. Bull Eur Physiopathol Respir 21:507, 1985.

55. Olson LG, Strohl KP. The response of the nasal airway to exercise. Am Rev Respir Dis 135:356, 1987.

56. Schumacher MJ, Cota KA, Taussig LM. Pulmonary response to nasal-challenge testing of atopic subjects with stable asthma. J Allergy Clin Immunol 78:30–35, 1986.

57. Brooks CD, Nelson A, Parzyck R, Maile MH. Protective effect of hydroxyzine and phenylpropranolamine in the challenged allergic nose. Ann Allergy 47:316, 1981.

58. Gherson G, Moscato G, Yidi I, Salvaterra A, Candura F. Non-specific nasal reactivity: A proposed method of study. Eur J Respir Dis 69:24, 1986.

59. Yan K, Salome C. The response of the airways to nasal stimulation in asthmatics with rhinitis. Eur J Respir Dis 64(Suppl 128):105, 1983.

60. Pipkorn U, Karlsson G, Enerback L. Nasal mucosal response to repeated challenges of pollen allergen. Am Rev Respir Dis 140:729, 1989.

61. Pelican Z. The changes in the nasal secretions of eosinophils during the immediate nasal response to allergen challenge. J

Allergy Clin Immunol 72:657, 1983.

62. Pelican Z, Pelikan-Filipek M. Cytologic changes in the nasal secretions during the late nasal response. J Allergy Clin Immunol 83:1068, 1989.

63. McLean JA, Mathews KP, Brayton PR et al. intranasal effects of pharmacologic agents in hay fever and vasomotor rhinitis (Abstract). J Allergy Clin Immunol 61:191, 1978.

64. Okuda M, Watase T, Mezawa A, Liu C. The role of leukotriene D_4 in allergic rhinitis. Ann Allergy 60:537, 1988.

65. Jones NS, Kenyon GS. Topical nasal steroids in non-atopic perennial rhinitis, subjective symptom scores and objective measurement and nasal resistance by active anterior rhinomanometry. J Laryngol Otol 102:1085, 1988.

66. Gordon ASD, McCaffrey TV, Kern EB, Pallanch JF. Rhinomanometry for pre-operative and post-operative assessment of nasal obstruction. Otolaryngol Head Neck Surg 101:20, 1989.

67. Parker AJ, Maw AR, Powell JE. Rhinomanometry in the selection for adenoidectomy and its relationship to preoperative radiology. Int J Pediatr Otorhinolaryngol 17:155, 1989.

68. Hastie R, Heroy JH III, Levy DA. Basophil leukocytes and mast cells in human nasal secretions and scrapings studied by light microscopy. Lab Invest 40:554–561, 1979.

69. Andersson M, Svensson C, Andersson P, Pipkorn U. Objective monitoring of the allergic inflammatory response of the nasal mucous in patients with hayfever during natural allergen exposure. Am Rev Respir Dis 139:911, 1989.

70. Watanabe K, Watanabe I. Changes of nasal epithelial cells and mucus layer after challenge of allergen. Ann Otol Rhinol Laryngol 90:204–209, 1981.

71. Brofeldt S, Mygind N. Viscosity and spinability of nasal secretions induced by different provocation tests. Am Rev Respir Dis 136:353–6, 1987.

72. Greenstone M, Cooper P, Warner J, Cole PJ. Effect of acute antigenic challenge on nasal ciliary beat frequency. Eur J Respir Dis (Suppl)128:449–450, 1983.

73. Liu C, Okuda M. Injurious effect of eosinophil extract on the human nasal mucosa. Rhinology 26:121, 1988.

74. Friedman RA, Doyle WJ, Casselbrant ML, Bluestone O, Fireman P. Immunologic-mediated eustachian tube obstruction: A double-blind crossover study. J Allergy Clin Immunol 71:442–447, 1983.

75. Skoner DP, Doyle WJ, Fireman P. Eustachian tube obstruction (FTO) after histamine nasal provocation: A double-blind dose response study. J Allergy Clin Immunol 79:27, 1987.

76. Togias AG, Naclerio RM, Warner J, Proud D, Kagey-Sobotka A, Nimmagadda I, Norman PS, Lichtenstein LM. Demonstration of inhibition of mediator release from human mast cells by azatadine base. In vivo and in vitro evaluation. JAMA 255:225–229, 1986.

77. Druce HM, Bonner RF, Patow C, Choo P, Summers R, Kaliner MA. Response of nasal blood flow to neurohormone as measured by laser-Doppler velocimetry. J Appl Physiol 57:1276–1283, 1984.

78. Konno A, Terada N, Okamato Y, Togawa K. The role of the chemical mediators and mucosal hyperreactivity in nasal allergy. J Allergy Clin Immunol 79:620, 1987.

79. Kunno A, Togawa K. Role of the vidian nerve in nasal allergy. Ann Otol 88:258, 1979.

80. Raphael GD, Meredity SC, Baraniuk JN, Druce HM, Banks SM, Kaliner MA. The pathophysiology of rhinitis. II. Assessment of sources of protein in histamine-induced nasal secretions. Am Rev Respir Dis 139:791, 1989.

81. Brown MS, Peters SP, Adkinson NF Jr, Proud D, Kagey-Sobotka A, Norman PS, Lichtenstein LM, Naclerio RM. Arachidone acid metabolites during nasal challenge. Arch Otolaryngol Head Neck Surg 113:179, 1987.

82. Pipkorn U, Proud D, Lichtenstein LM et al. Effect of short term systemic glucocorticoid treatment of human nasal mediator release after antigen challenge. J Clin Invest 80:957, 1987.

83. Pipkorn U, Proud D, Lichtenstein LM et al. Topical steroid pretreatment inhibits mediator release in vivo. N Engl J Med 316:1506, 1987.

84. Wachs M, Proud D, Lichtenstein LM, Kagey-Sobota A, Norman PS, Naclerio RM. Observations on the pathogenesis of nasal priming. J Allergy Clin Immunol 84:942, 1989.

85. Naclerio RM, Proud D, Tobias A, Adkinson NF Jr, Meyers DA, Kagey-Sobotka A, Plaut M, Norman PS, Lichtenstein LM. Inflammatory mediators in antigen-induced rhinitis. N Engl J Med 313:65, 1985.

RECENT RELATED REVIEWS

Druce HM. Nasal provocation challenge-strategies for experimental design. Ann Allergy 60:191, 1988.

Pierson WE. Objective measurements of nasal airway testing. J Allergy Clin Immunol 81(pt 2):949, 1988.

Raphael GD, Meredith SD, Baraniuk JN, Kaliner MA. Nasal reflexes. Am J Rhinol 2:109, 1988.

Schumacher MJ. Rhinomanometry. J Allergy Clin Immunol 83:711, 1989.

Chapter XII

The Upper Airways: Interface between the Lungs and the Ambient Air

Donald F. Proctor, M.D.

ABSTRACT

The upper airways provide access for ambient air to the lungs, and the nasal passages carry out physiologic functions both different from and supplemental to those of the lower conducting airways. They are the first target of and the first line of defense against airborne disease. For their protection, it is important to understand those environmental factors that may lead to their injury.

Under most circumstances, the nasal passages are interposed between the ambient air and the lungs and, in this position, they provide the first line of defense against airborne hazards.[1-3] Under some circumstances (heavy exercise or nasal obstruction), the lips are parted and inspired air flows through both the nasal and oropharyngeal airways. In this paper, I will describe some of the modifications in the ambient air that may be expected during inspiration through the nose and speculate upon the alternative situation when oronasal breathing occurs.[4-6]

In discussing nasal physiology, two considerations are of importance: the capacity of the nose to modify those physical characteristics in the ambient air which might adversely affect the tracheobronchial airways or

Emeritus Professor of Environmental Health Sciences, Otolaryngology, Anesthesiology. The Johns Hopkins Medical Institutions, The Johns Hopkins School of Hygiene and Public Health, Baltimore, MD

the lung periphery, and the possibility that some of those factors might have a transitory or lasting injurious effect upon the nose. Anatomically, the nasal airway offers a sharp contrast to the trachea. Whereas the trachea is a simple, wide, low resistance passage, the nose is a complex, convoluted passage with a high resistance to airflow.[7,8] About one-half of the total airflow resistance from nostrils to alveoli is accounted for by the nose.[9-12]

NASAL CAPACITY FOR AIR MODIFICATION

As indicated in Figure 1, the total nasal passage undergoes two bends, one at the nasal valve anteriorly and the other at the nasopharynx. Air enters the nostrils in an upward direction, passes through the nasal valve, bends to follow the middle and inferior meatuses to the nasopharynx, and then bends downward. Although there is, in the main passage, a large total cross-section and surface area, the width of the passage is everywhere quite narrow (Fig. 2). Of special importance is the very small cross-section through the nasal valve. These anatomical characteristics, combined with the nature of the nasal mucosa with its mucociliary system, are responsible for the nasal capacity for air modification.[13] The high linear velocity necessary for air to pass through the nasal valve and the bend in the passage just beyond that point results in impaction of inhaled particles. The large cross-section and surface area in the main passage, plus the close proximity of the air to mucosal surfaces, assure effective exchange of temperature and water vapor and absorption of foreign gases.[14-18]

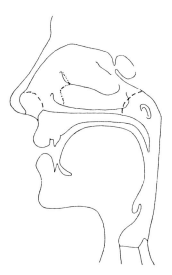

Figure 1. *Lateral view of upper airways. Dashed line to left marks the beginning of the nasal valve. Dashed line to right marks the end of the nasal septum and beginning of the nasopharynx. Dotted line indicates region where mucociliary clearance moves forward. Note proximity of tongue to palate, characteristic of most oronasal breathing. (Reprinted with permission from Proctor and Andersen.[11])*

Inhaled particles with an aerodynamic equivalent diameter of 10 μm or more are essentially fully removed during nasal passage. The great majority of particles between 5 and 10 μm aerodynamic equivalent diameter are also removed, and a significant proportion of smaller particles (including submicronic) are likewise prevented from reaching the lower airways.[19-21] The temperature of inspired air, from very cold to very warm ambient, is adjusted toward that of the body. In the nasopharynx, inspired air is usually at about 32–37°C. The capacity of the nasal humidification system is such that even the most dry inspired air is saturated with water vapor well before it reaches the nasopharynx.[15,17,18] At the same time, water-soluble foreign gases (such as sulfur dioxide and formaldehyde) are absorbed in the nasal secretions, and even the very insoluble gas ozone is about 40% removed during nasal passage.[22]

The effectiveness of the nose in accomplishing these important defenses of the lungs is dependent upon the rich vascularity of the mucosa and submucosa, and the function of the mucociliary system.[23-34] The capacity of both the vascular and secretory systems for adjustment to changes in the ambient air enables the nose to withstand sudden or severe atmospheric variations. These we encounter not only in connection with weather, climate, and rapid travel, but also in going in and out of heated or cooled buildings. The complex, erectile vascular network and the secretory glands[23] are under the control of the autonomic nervous system,[24,30]

but the exact reflex arcs involved are not yet fully understood.

The delicate mucosa of the paranasal sinuses is not as rich in either vasculature or secretory cells, and it does not appear to react to the same degree to reflex stimuli. Still, the secretions lining their extensive surfaces are continually swept into the nasal passages all along the major lines of inspiratory airflow. This may be the main physiologic usefulness of these troublesome cavities, although they also act to prevent injury to the base of the brain associated with blows to the face.

Our concept of airway secretions has undergone significant change, especially in the past decade.[14,30] We now know that they do not consist of a simple continuous "carpet" of homogeneous mucus. In the peripheral airways of the lungs, there are no cells capable of secreting mucus. Such cells (goblet) make their appearance about the 12th generation of bronchi, and submucous glands somewhat higher up. Both goblet cells and glands are in copious numbers in the nose.[11] Thus, mucus per se, as secreted by these cells, is normally absent in the small airways of the lungs, sparse in the small bronchi, and may exist in a nearly continuous coat in the trachea and the nose. A layer of periciliary fluid underlies mucus and also lines the small airways of the lungs. It is in this thin serous fluid that cilia beat, perhaps touching overlying mucus at the full extent of their length in their forward beat. The presence of this fluid in a sufficient depth to bathe beating cilia, but not so deep as to prevent proximity of mucus to cilia

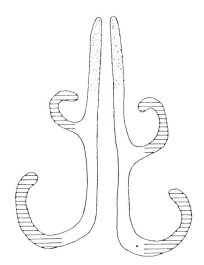

Figure 2. *Section through the main nasal airway. The stippled area shows the olfactory region, and the meatuses are indicated by the horizontal lines. The clear areas are the region through which most inspired air passes. Note that the airway is everywhere quite narrow. (Reprinted with permission from Proctor and Andersen.[11])*

tips, is essential to clearance. Obviously, it is an important constituent of airway secretions and yet we know relatively little of its sources and control. It seems likely that any influence limiting its secretion or transudation or resulting in its appearance in excess quantity could seriously impair airway defenses.

Just as the major bronchi and trachea can be cleared of excess secretions by coughing, the nasal passages can be cleared by sniffing, sneezing, nose blowing, or, in the case of the anterior region of the nose, by manual cleaning. But these actions are only effective when there is an excess of secretions. Those fluids normally lining the nasal passages to a depth of only a few microns above the epithelial surfaces (as is also the case for the tracheobronchial airways) are dependent upon ciliary activity for their clearance. Over anterior portions of both inferior and middle turbinates, where most inhaled dusts are deposited, that clearance is forward (Fig. 1). Through the remainder of the nasal passages, mucociliary clearance is toward the nasopharynx. Fluids are prevented from accumulating there through the action of the soft palate on swallowing.

ENVIRONMENTAL FACTORS AFFECTING THE NOSE

Since the mucociliary clearance of mucosal surfaces is essential to maintenance of nasal defenses, it is important to be able to measure it under ordinary circumstances and when adversely affected. We have found the placement of a small tagged particle in the anterior nose and tracing of its transit by external detection of radiation to be most effective.[33-36] When that technique is not available or desirable, a useful substitute is the similar placement of a small particle of saccharine.[11] The time that passes until the taste of sweet is noted, divided by the distance traveled, yields clearance rates which compare well with the radioactive particle method.

In normal human volunteers, the average nasal clearance rate is some 5–7 mm/min, but the range, even in young healthy adults, is from under 1 to over 20 mm/min.[10] The reason for such a wide variation is not understood, but we have postulated the possibility that epithelial trauma associated with recurrent childhood infections or exposure to polluted air may be responsible for those with such low clearance rates. Viral infections are associated with desquamation of respiratory epithelium. Ordinarily, normal mucociliary function is restored in 2 to 6 weeks,[39,40] but the possibility exists that restoration of a fully normal epithelium may be incomplete.

In addition to viral infections, what other factors may result in a transitory or lasting injury to nasal defense mechanisms? Neither the humidity nor temperature of ambient air seems to exert any adverse effect, but sudden extreme changes in temperature remain to be studied. We do know that normal subjects are not harmed by dry air,[17] and there is no evidence that those suffering from respiratory disease suffer injury from dry air. Indeed, we have long recommended dry climates for patients with chronic respiratory disease. Certainly humidifiers are not free from hazard. The house dust mite and molds thrive in damp rooms, and the water sources for humidifiers serve as excellent culture media for a number of pathogenic microorganisms.

Unpublished studies indicate that those living in extreme cold climates may have average clearance rates below those living in hot, humid, dry or temperate climates. Allergy per se, does not seriously impede mucociliary clearance,[33,34,41-43] but in allergic rhinitis, nasal congestion and rhinorrhea may interfere with nasal airflow, and in some circumstances, the slow-reacting substance of anaphylaxis may exert an adverse influence. Sulfur dioxide and formaldehyde in sufficient concentration can impair clearance.[11,16,37] Exposure to hardwood dust, as in the furniture or boot industry, can impair clearance, and long-term exposure can be followed by squamous metaplasia and adenocarcinoma of the sinuses.[44,45] Formaldehyde[22] has resulted in nasal cancer in rodents,[46] but there is as yet no evidence of carcinogenesis in humans related to formaldehyde. Ozone increases nasal airflow resistance. Hypothyroidism is associated with a sort of vasomotor rhinitis,[47] and emotional stress may result in a variety of nasal symptoms.[48] Far more research will be necessary before we can state what other influences adversely affect nasal function. We especially need to have more investigations of the effects of drugs commonly used systemically or topically in the treatment of nasal disease.[36]

The potential of the nose as a portal of entry for systemic drugs is just being recognized.[38] There can be little doubt that this will grow rapidly into an increasingly important and widely used therapeutic modality, but the otolaryngologist and the allergist must be aware that drugs administered in that manner may produce both signs and symptoms of rhinitis.

While considering factors that may adversely affect the nose (as well as injuring the lungs if they pass through upper airways into them), it is important to realize that problems of indoor air pollution have been relatively neglected. We do spend the great majority of our time indoors, and pollution there is grossly different from that outdoors. Sulfur dioxide is readily absorbed on interior surfaces and its level indoors is generally well below that in community air. On the contrary, nitrogen dioxide may be found, in homes in which cooking is done with gas, in concentrations well above that outdoors. Formaldehyde is a special problem indoors, especially in mobile homes where walls are often of chipboard or plywood, and in other homes where urea formaldehyde foam has been used for insulation. A multitude of other pollutants are found in workplaces, and occupational exposure must be considered in patients with respiratory symptoms.

Under some circumstances, demands for pulmonary ventilation exceed that possible through the nose. The nasal valve is a collapsible airway, and when, on inspiration, the pressure there falls about 10 cm H_2O below ambient, no further increase in airflow is possible.[7] It is then necessary to supplement the nasal breathing with the parallel oropharyngeal airway, oronasal breathing.[4] When this occurs, usually at ventilation volumes in excess of 30–40 liters/min, air flows through both of these parallel passages. The oropharyngeal airway can be very wide when the tongue is depressed and drawn forward and the palate is raised, as in yawning. In most circumstances, that sort of airway is not employed. Rather, the tongue and palate remain in close proximity and inspired air passing through the mouth may be modified nearly as effectively as that passing through the nose.[11] It is well to remember that oronasal breathing also occurs in connection with conversation, not merely with exercise.

During the past decade research on the problem of obstructive sleep apnea has led to a better understanding of the physiology of airflow through the upper airways. In contrast to the tracheobronchial tree where expiratory flow limitation has long been recognized, the upper airways consist of a series of inspiratory flow-limiting segments. Normally a number of the muscles surrounding the upper airways undergo an increase in tone with each inspiration, thus bracing the nasopharyngeal airways against the negative inspiratory pressure within them. In the face of any reduction in the efficacy of this system (as seen in sleep apnea) any increase in nasal airway resistance, as in rhinitis, is of special importance.[5,49-51]

UPPER AIRWAY DEFENSE MECHANISMS

I would be remiss if, in this very brief review, I did not mention other relevant points in connection with upper airway defense mechanisms:

1. During the past decade, it has become increasingly clear that certain persons suffer from dyskinetic (often called immotile) cilia.[52-54] In such persons, mucociliary clearance is either absent or severely impaired, and there is marked susceptibility to respiratory disease as in Kartagener's syndrome.

2. The permeability of airway secretions to materials deposited on or absorbed in their surfaces is an important factor in determining whether noxious substances reach and injure the epithelium.[55] Very little is known of what factors influence this.

3. Living cells exist in airway secretions, among which are mast cells.[56-58] Whether allergic reactions may originate in surface contact of allergen with these cells, without permeation to and through the mucosa is not yet clear.

4. The tonsils and adenoids play an active role in the development of immunity, especially in childhood.[59] Their surgical extirpation is unjustified except when intrinsic disease far outweighs the value of their preservation.

5. There are important nasopulmonary reflexes which may result in bronchoconstriction.[60]

6. Finally, any physician interested in the upper airways should keep in mind the multiplicity of functions in which they are involved: breathing, deglutition, phonation, wind instrument playing, sneezing, coughing, sucking, straining, nose blowing, etc. One of our important research needs is to seek the nervous pathways involved in appropriate action to fit each function and to determine how such functions may be affected by such a common affliction as rhinitis.

Much more remains to be learned about the normal physiology of the upper airways. A better understanding of those influences that may impair their role in respiratory defenses[1,61] will be important in our efforts in preventive medicine.

REFERENCES

1. Brain JD, Proctor DF, Reid L, eds. Respiratory Defense Mechanisms. New York, Marcel Dekker, 1977.
2. Mygind N, Rasmussen FV, Mølgaard F, eds. Cellular and Neurogenic Mechanisms in Nose and Bronchi. Eur J Respir Dis 64 (suppl 128), 1983.
3. Proctor DF. The upper airways and larynx. In Macklem PT, Mead J, eds. Handbook of Physiology, The Respiratory System, Part 1. Bethesda, MD, American Physiological Society, 1986, chap. 6, pp. 63–74.
4. Niinamaa V, Cole P, Mintz S, Shephard RJ. Oronasal airflow. Respir Physiol 43:69–75, 1981.
5. Proctor DF. The naso-oro-pharyngo-laryngeal airways. Eur J Respir Dis 64 (suppl 128):89–96, 1983.
6. Rodenstein DO, Stanescu DC. State of art: the soft palate and breathing. Am Rev Respir Dis 134:311–325, 1986.
7. Bridger GP, Proctor DF. Maximum nasal inspiratory flow and nasal resistance. Ann Otol Rhinol Laryngol 79:481–489, 1970.
8. Hamilton LH. Nasal airway resistance: its measurement and regulation. Physiologist 22:43–49, 1979.
9. Cole P. Upper respiratory airflow. Chapter 7. In Proctor DF, Andersen I, eds. The Nose, Upper Airway Physiology and the Atmospheric Environment. Amsterdam, Elsevier, 1982.
10. McLean JA, Mathews KP, Solomon WR, Brayton PR, Ciarkowski AA. Effect of histamine and methacholine on nasal airway resistance in atopic and non-atopic subjects. J Allergy Clin Immunol 59:165–170, 1972.
11. Proctor DF, Andersen I, eds. The Nose, Upper Airway Phys-

iology and the Atmospheric Environment. Amsterdam, Elsevier, 1982.

12. Cole P, Haight JSJ. Posture and nasal patency. Am Rev Respir Dis 129:351–354, 1984.

13. Cole P. Modification of inspired air. In Proctor DF, Andersen I, eds. The Nose, Upper Airway Physiology and the Atmospheric Environment. Amsterdam, Elsevier, 1982, chap. 14.

14. Aharonson EF, Ben-David A, Klingberg MA. Air Pollution and the Lung. Jerusalem, Israel Universities Press, 1976.

15. Andersen I, Lundqvist G, Proctor DF. Human nasal mucosal function under four controlled humidities. Am Rev Respir Dis 106:438–449, 1972.

16. Andersen L, Lundqvist G, Jensen PL, et al. Human response to controlled levels of sulfur dioxide. Arch Environ Health 28:31–39, 1974.

17. Andersen I, Lundqvist G, Jensen PL, Proctor DF. Human response to 78 hours exposure to dry air. Arch Environ Health 29:319–324, 1974.

18. Proctor DF, Andersen I, Lundqvist G. Human nasal mucosal function at controlled temperatures. Respir Physiol 30:109–124, 1977.

19. Brain JD, Valberg PA. Deposition of aerosol in the respiratory tract. Am Rev Respir Dis 120:1325–1373, 1979.

20. Proctor DF. The upper airways I. Nasal physiology and defense of the lungs. Am Rev Respir Dis 115:97–130, 1977.

21. Wolfsdorf J, Swift DL, Avery ME. Mist therapy reconsidered: an evaluation of the respiratory deposition of labelled water aerosol produced by jet and ultrasonic nebulizers. Pediatrics 43:799–808, 1969.

22. Brain JD. The uptake of inhaled gases by the nose. Ann Otol 79:529–539, 1970.

23. Cauna N. Blood and nerve supply of the nasal lining. In Proctor DF, Andersen I, eds. The Nose, Upper Airway Physiology and the Atmospheric Environment. Amsterdam, Elsevier, 1982, chap. 3.

24. Eccles R. Neurological and pharmacological considerations. In Proctor DF, Andersen I, eds. The Nose, Upper Airway Physiology and the Atmospheric Environment. Amsterdam, Elsevier, 1982, chap. 8.

25. Foster WM, Bergofsky EH, Bohning DE, et al. Effect of adrenergic agents and their mode of action on mucociliary clearance in man. J Appl Physiol 41:146–152, 1976.

26. Jackson RT, Burson JH, Effect of inflammatory mediators on nasal mucosa. Arch Otolaryngol 103:441–444, 1977.

27. Malm L. Sympathetic influence on the nasal mucosa. Acta Otolaryngol 83:20–21, 1977.

28. Mygind N, Pedersen M, Nielsen MH. Morphology of the upper respiratory epithelium. In Proctor DF, Andersen I, eds. The Nose, Upper Airway Physiology and the Atmospheric Environment. Amsterdam, Elsevier, 1982, chap. 4.

29. Porter R, Rivers J, O'Connor M, eds. Respiratory Tract Mucus. Ciba Foundation Symposium No. 54 (new series). Amsterdam, Elsevier, 1978.

30. Proctor DF, Adams GK. Physiology and pharmacology of nasal function and mucus secretion. Pharmacol Ther B 2:493–509, 1976.

31. Brofeldt S, Mygind N, Sørensen CH, Readman AS, Marriott C. Biochemical analysis of nasal secretions induced by methacholine, histamine, and allergen provocations. Am Rev Respir Dis 133:1138–1142, 1986.

32. Kaliner M, Shelhamer JH, Borson B, Nadel J, Patow C, Maram Z. Human respiratory mucus. Am Rev Respir Dis 134:612–621, 1986.

33. Wanner A. Clinical aspects of mucociliary transport. Am Rev Respir Dis 116:73–125, 1977.

34. Andersen I, Proctor DF. Measurement of nasal mucociliary clearance. Eur J Respir Dis 64 (suppl 128):37–40, 1983.

35. Andersen I, Lundqvist G, Mølhave L. Indoor air pollution due to chipboard used as a construction material. Atmos Environ 9:1121–1127, 1972.

36. Saketkhoo K, Yergin BM, Januszkiewicz A, Kovitz K, Sackner MA. The effect of nasal decongestants on nasal mucous velocity. Am Rev Respir Dis 118:251–254, 1978.

37. Proctor DF. The inspiratory path to the lungs. In Frank et al., eds. Inhalation Toxicology of Air Pollution: Clinical Research Considerations. Philadelphia, American Society for Testing Materials, 1985, pp. 39–42.

38. Proctor DF. Nasal physiology in intranasal drug-administration. In Chien YW, ed. Transnasal Systemic Medication. Amsterdam, Elsevier 1985, pp. 101–106.

39. Sakakura Y, Sasaki Y, Hornick RB, Togo Y, Schwartz AR, Wagner HN Jr, Proctor DF. Mucociliary function during experimentally induced rhinovirus infection in man. Ann Otol 82:203–212, 1973.

40. Winternitz MC, Wason IM, McNamara FP. The Pathology of Influenza. New Haven, CT, Yale University Press, 1920.

41. Ahmed T, Greenblatt DW, Birch S, Marchette B, Wanner A. Abnormal mucociliary transport in allergic patients with antigen-induced bronchospasm: role of slow reacting substance of anaphylaxis. Am Rev Respir Dis 124:110–114, 1981.

42. Mygind N. Nasal Allergy. Oxford, Blackwell, 1978.

43. Wihl J-A, Mygind N. Studies on the allergen-challenged human nasal mucosa. Acta Otolaryngol 84:281–286, 1977.

44. Andersen HC, Andersen I, Solgaard J. Nasal cancer, symptoms and upper airway function in woodworkers. Br J Industr Med 34:201–207, 1977.

45. Black A, Evans JC, Hadfield EH, et al. Impairment of nasal mucociliary clearance in woodworkers in the furniture industry. Br J Industr Med 31:10–17, 1974.

46. Swenberg JA, Kerns WD, Mitchell RI, Gralla EJ, Pavkoa KL. Induction of squamous cell carcinoma of the rat nasal cavity by inhalation exposure to formaldehyde-vapor. Cancer Res 40:3398–3402, 1980.

47. Proetz AW. Further observations on the effects of thyroid insufficiency on the nasal mucosa. Laryngoscope 60:627–633, 1950.

48. Holmes TH, Goodell H, Wolf S, Wolff HG. The Nose. Springfield, IL, Charles C Thomas, 1950.

49. Cole P, Haight JSJ. Mechanisms of nasal obstruction in sleep. Laryngoscope 94:1557–1559, 1984.

50. Collett PW, Brancatisano AP, Engel LA. Upper airway dimensions and movements in bronchial asthma. Am Rev Respir Dis 133:1143–1149, 1986.

51. Strohl KP, Redline S. Nasal CPAP therapy, upper airway activation, and obstructive sleep apnea. Am Rev Respir Dis 134:555–558, 1986.

52. Corkey CWB, Levison H, Turner JAP. The immotile cilia syndrome: a longitudinal survey. Am Rev Respir Dis 124:544–548, 1981.

53. Mygind N, Nielsen MH, Pedersen M, eds. Kartagener's syndrome and abnormal cilia. Eur J Respir Dis 64 (suppl 127):1–167, 1983.

54. Rossman CM, Lee RMKW, Forrest JB, Newhouse MT. Nasal ciliary ultrastructure and function in patients with primary ciliary dyskinesia compared with that in normal subjects with various respiratory diseases. Am Rev Respir Dis 129:161–167, 1984.

55. Kontou-Karakitsos K, Salvaggio JE, Mathews KP. Compar-

ative nasal absorption of allergens in atopic and non-atopic subjects. J Allergy Clin Invest 55:241–248, 1975.

56. Hastie R, Heroy JH, Levy DA. Basophil leukocytes and mast cells in human nasal secretions and scrapings studies by light microscopy. Lab Invest 40:554–561, 1979.

57. Otsuka H, Dolovich J, Befus D, Bienenstock J, Denburg J. Peripheral blood basophils, basophil progenitors and nasal metachromatic cells in allergic rhinitis. Am Rev Respir Dis 133:757–762, 1986.

58. Togias AG, Naclerio RM, Peters SP, Nimmagadda I, Proud D, Kagey-Sobotka A, Adkinson NF Jr, Norman PS, Lichtenstein LM. Local generation of sulfidopeptide leukotrienes uopn nasal provocation with cold, dry air. Am Rev Respir Dis 133:1133–1137, 1986.

59. Korsrud FR, Brandtzaeg P. Immune systems of human nasopharyngeal and palatine tonsils. Clin Exp Immunol 39:361–370, 1980.

60. Kaufman J, Chen JC, Wright GW. The effect of trigeminal resection on reflex bronchoconstriction after nasal and nasopharyngeal irritation in man. Am Rev Respir Dis 101:768–769, 1970.

61. Quinlan MF, Salman SD, Swift DL, et al. Measurement of mucociliary function in man. Am Rev Respir Dis 99:13–23, 1969. □

Chapter XIII

Lung Function in Allergic Rhinitis

Sidney S. Braman, M.D.

ABSTRACT

Allergic rhinitis and asthma are traditionally viewed as distinctly different diseases. Allergic rhinitis affects the upper respiratory tract while asthma is a disorder of the lower respiratory tract. Evidence is presented to show that the characteristic features of bronchial asthma, such as reversible airflow obstruction and bronchial hyperresponsiveness, are present in many patients with allergic rhinitis despite the absence of bronchial symptoms. One of these features, bronchial hyperresponsiveness, may be useful in predicting which group of patients with allergic rhinitis are at greatest risk of developing asthma.

LUNG FUNCTION IN ALLERGIC RHINITIS

Allergic rhinitis is a disorder of the upper respiratory tract (nasal passages) causing symptoms of rhinorrhea, sneezing, and nasal obstruction. Asthma is a disease of the lower respiratory tract (bronchi, bronchioles) with lower respiratory tract symptoms of wheezing, dyspnea, and cough. Despite obvious clinical differences, these two apparently disparate disorders are commonly grouped together and may be different manifestations of the same disease. Striking pathologic and pathophysiologic similarities and strong epidemiologic associations have led to this conclusion. Both conditions are included as diseases of an inherited allergic diathesis (atopy) mediated by the immediate IgE dependent hypersensitivity reaction. Immediate skin test reactivity to a variety of antigens is characteristic, and provocation of symptoms by the same aeroallergens that cause these positive skin tests will occur. For example, the inhalation of ragweed, both naturally occurring and in the laboratory, can cause symptoms of rhinitis and asthma simultaneously in a susceptible individual. Following exposure, both nasal and bronchial mucosa show mucosal edema and an eosinophilic inflammatory reaction with hypertrophy of mucus glands.

The frequent coexistence of allergic rhinitis and asthma in the general population is well established. In one survey of 1,125 allergic patients, Smith and Knowler[1] found that 78% of patients with allergic asthma reported nasal symptoms while 38% of patients with allergic rhinitis had symptoms of asthma. In a 20-year followup study of atopic children, Rackemann[2] found that 20 of 86 patients (23%) with allergic rhinitis and no prior asthma, subsequently developed asthma during the study period. Similarly, Hagy and Settipane[3] found that 6% of college students with allergic rhinitis developed bronchial asthma over a 7-year period, compared to 1.3% of students without allergic rhinitis. In addition to these well studied epidemiologic associations between asthma and allergic rhinitis, there are similarly important genetic factors contributing to this association since both conditions are frequently transmitted within families.

In an attempt to further define the relationship between asthma and allergic rhinitis, evidence for lower

Professor of Medicine, Brown University Program in Medicine, and Director, Division of Pulmonary and Critical Care Medicine, Rhode Island Hospital, Providence, R.I.

respiratory tract (asthmatic-type) dysfunction in patients with allergic rhinitis and no prior history of asthma will be examined. While a consensus on the definition of asthma has not been reached, three characteristic features of asthma have been agreed upon by an American Thoracic Society/American College of Chest Physicians Joint Committee[4] and the Allergy Foundation of America:[5] 1) increased resistance to air flow manifested by slowing of forced expiration; 2) reversibility of airflow obstruction either spontaneously or as a result of therapy; 3) hyperresponsiveness of the airways to a variety of stimuli resulting in further reduction in expiratory flow.

Evidence suggesting that these abnormalities exist in patients with allergic rhinitis will be reviewed.

ASSESSMENT OF AIRFLOW OBSTRUCTION

During an acute attack of asthma, airflow obstruction occurs in both large, (i.e. central airways) and more peripheral airways (less than 2 mm in diameter). Asthmatics in remission show airflow abnormalities predominantly in smaller airways. During the acute asthmatic attack, all parameters of airflow obstruction measured will be markedly abnormal: airway resistance (R_{AW}) by body plethysmograph, and expiratory flow rates from the timed vital capacity maneuver (FEV_1, $FEV_{1\%}$ and FEF_{25-75}), and the maximal expiratory flow volume (MEFV) curve (FEF_{50}, FEF_{25}). To the contrary, when airflow obstruction is limited to the peripheral small airways, these conventional measurements of airflow obstruction (R_{AW}, FEV_1, $FEV_{1\%}$) may be normal. This is because the small airways contribute only 10–20% of the total airway resistance and considerable obstruction to flow can occur in these airways before conventional physiologic tests become abnormal making the peripheral airways the lung's "quiet zone". However, since small airways contribute a greater percentage to the total airway resistance at lower lung volumes than at higher lung volumes, assessment of flow rates at low lung volumes (FEF_{25-75} and FEF_{50}) may detect obstruction limited to small airways. Newer physiologic tests of lung function have been developed to assess this "quiet zone" of the lung. One such test, the closing volume, (CV), determines the volume (measured as a % of vital capacity) at which peripheral airways begin to close during a maximal expiration. Either loss of elastic recoil (emphysema) or bronchial obstruction (asthma) cause premature closure of airways and elevate the closing volume. Another test which attempts to differentiate between large and small airway abnormalities utilizes the density dependence characteristics of airflow from MEFV curves. Airflow in large airways is density dependent due to convective forces and turbulence of flow. Breathing a low density gas mixture of 80% helium, 20% oxygen causes an increase in expired flow when compared to air if the major site of obstruction is in the large airways. In contrast, flow in peripheral airways is laminar and no density dependent, and He-O_2 MEFV curves may no show significant improvement in expiratory flow i airway obstruction is primarily in the small airways. A very low lung volumes, near end-expiration, flow n longer remains density dependent in most normal subjects indicating that small airways play a role in flow limitation. The point where the curves are superimposed is called the volume of isoflow ($V_{iso}\dot{V}$) and i expressed as a percentage of vital capacity. Obstruction to flow in small airways increases the $V_{iso}\dot{V}$. One additional test of small airway dysfunction is the assessmen of lung compliance at increasing frequencies of respiration. A drop in dynamic compliance with increasing respiratory frequency reflects maldistribution of ventilation to peripheral lung units. Therefore, obstruction at the level of small airways may cause "frequency dependence of lung compliance."

EVIDENCE FOR AIRFLOW OBSTRUCTION IN ALLERGIC RHINITIS

While evidence for the exact site of airflow obstruction in allergic rhinitis is conflicting, most studies however agree that abnormalities in airway function do exist in patients with allergic rhinitis despite the absence of lower respiratory tract symptoms. Brown et al[6] demonstrated (as far back as 1946) that patients with allergic rhinitis and no history of asthma frequently show a reduction in vital capacity during pollen season. More recently, Doggett et al[7] found that the majority o patients with allergic rhinitis have an elevated airway resistance as well as a reduction in FEF_{25-75} and $\dot{V}_{iso}\dot{V}$ leading them to conclude that both large and smal airway obstruction occurs in subjects with allergic rhinitis. Further observations by the same group showed that the prevalence of airway abnormalities out o pollen season was considerably less and were more likely in large airways since only airway resistance wa abnormal.[8,9] Morgan and Hall[10] evaluated 20 subject with asymptomatic allergic rhinitis for evidence of airway abnormalities. Frequency dependence of compliance was present in 40% of these patients and wa interpreted as showing evidence of obstruction in smal airways. In that study,[10] FEV_1, closing capacity (a sum of closing volume and residual volume), FEF_{25-75} and FEF_{50} were less sensitive in detecting these abnormalities. Fairshter et al.[11] did extensive pulmonary function testing on 16 asymptomatic patients with allergic rhinitis as compared to 31 controls. Tests reflecting smal airway obstruction such as FEF_{25-75}, FEF_{50} and FEF_2 and CV were indistinguishable between the two groups Airway resistance and its reciprocal conductance, dic show statistically significant differences between the two groups. They concluded that the site of airway obstruction in their subjects with allergic rhinitis was in the central airways. However, the mean values for airway resistance in the study remained within the normal range and in only 3 subjects with rhinitis, were both R_{AW} and G_{AW} abnormal. These investigators extended their studies to include tests for density dependence of flow.[12] Similar conclusions were reached in this second study. The results of Lidington et al.[13] are similar to results of a group of patients that we have studied.[14] We studied the pulmonary function of 23 nonsmoking patients with ragweed sensitive-allergic rhinitis during the winter months when all were asymptomatic. Twenty non-atopic controls were similarly tested. We could find no difference in specific conductance and $FEV_{1\%}$ between our rhinitis patients and controls while a significant difference was found in the percent predicted: FEF_{50} (75.5% vs 94.5%) and $V_{iso}.\dot{V}.$ (14.1% vs 8.7%) ($P < .01$, $P < .05$). We concluded that asymptomatic allergic rhinitis patients, as a group, demonstrated airflow obstruction in small airways when compared to nonatopic controls.

In summary, several studies have described abnormal lung function in patients with allergic rhinitis and no prior history of asthma. Evidence for airflow obstruction in both central and peripheral airways, similar to bronchial asthma have been found. Why some patients with allergic rhinitis manifest these changes is not clear. The relationship of these airflow abnormalities to the future development of asthma has not been studied.

ARE LUNG FUNCTION CHANGES IN ALLERGIC RHINITIS REVERSIBLE?

A hallmark of asthma is reversibility of airflow obstruction. This may be demonstrated in the laboratory following the standard inhalation of a bronchodilator. Several studies have addressed the question of reversibility of pulmonary function abnormalities in allergic rhinitis. Fairshter et al[11] found complete reversibility of the large airway obstruction in their patients with allergic rhinitis following the inhalation of isoproterenol. Since normal subjects show large increases in conductance following an inhaled bronchodilator[11] that is indistinguishable from asthmatics, the significance of this large airway response in allergic rhinitis is unclear. Further studies by Fairshter et al.[12] evaluating density dependence of MEFV curves, before and after inhalation of isoproterenol, showed differences in the site of isoproterenol-induced bronchodilatation in normal and rhinitis patients. Normal subjects showed bronchodilatation in small upstream airways while patients with allergic rhinitis showed dilatation in central airways. The different response in allergic rhinitis patients was thought to be due to the relative increase in the resting tone of their large airways. An alternative hypothesis, supported by studies by Lidington et al.[13] is that the inhaled bronchodilators dilate normal central airways and unmask obstruction of peripheral airways not readily reversed by these medications.

Several studies have looked for spontaneous resolution of airway abnormalities in allergic rhinitis patients from the symptomatic spring (grass pollen) or fall (ragweed) season to the asymptomatic winter months. Fairshter[12] was unable to document fluctuations in airway resistance that correlated with variations of symptomatology during seasons. Others[8-10] have documented seasonal variations of lung function in patients with allergic rhinitis. For example, Morgan and Hall[10] showed a seasonal reversibility of small airway abnormalities (frequency dependence of compliance) in 6 of 20 patients studied. In two additional patients, persistent small airways dysfunction beyond the rhinitis season correlated with persistent symptoms, unlike the patients with reversible abnormalities.

It thus appears from the studies discussed that the airflow obstruction seen in some patients with allergic rhinitis is reversible. As with asthma, this reversibility may be spontaneous and seasonal or may follow an inhaled bronchodilator. However, unlike asthma, the abnormalities in allergic rhinitis are mild and not of the magnitude that causes lower respiratory tract symptoms.

BRONCHOPROVOCATION TESTING FOR ASTHMA

The airways of patients with asthma are 100–1000 times more sensitive to a variety of inhaled bronchoconstricting agents than are normal subjects. They demonstrate a decrease in expiratory flow rates or an increase in R_{AW} at much lower inhaled concentrations of these agents than a normal population. Bronchoprovocation testing with cholinergic agents such as methacholine and carbachol, histamine, cold air, and a variety of aeroallergens has been used to improve our understanding of the pathogenesis of obstructive airway diseases. In addition, bronchial challenge tests can uncover the presence of bronchial hyperreactivity in patients with atypical presentations of asthma or patients in remission at the time of testing. Since exercise-induced bronchoconstriction is common in patients with asthma, exercise challenge can also be used as a bronchoprovocation test.

Bronchial hyperreactivity has been documented in a number of conditions associated with acute (e.g. postviral) or chronic (e.g. smokers) bronchial inflammation and is therefore not specific for asthma. However, the degree of bronchial sensitivity seen in patients with asthma and its persistence for years after relief of symptoms distinguishes it from other conditions. Hyperresponsiveness of the airways is a constant feature of asthma and is important in the pathogenesis of lower respiratory tract symptoms.

The most commonly used tests to assess the degree of bronchial hyperresponsiveness following bronchial challenge are the change in FEV_1 and SG_{aw} from baseline values. The provocation dose (PD) of bronchoconstrictor to cause a 20% reduction in FEV_1 (PD_{20}) or a 35% reduction in SG_{aw} (PD_{35}) is often established for comparative studies.

HYPERRESPONSIVENESS OF AIRWAYS IN ALLERGIC RHINITIS

Several studies[14-18] have shown that the airways of some patients with allergic rhinitis are more responsive to bronchoconstricting agents than are normal subjects. The prevalence of this finding varied since the nature of the provoking agent, the doses administered, and the populations evaluated have differed. Elsewhere in this book, Townley describes his experience with methacholine inhalation challenge in a large number of patients with atopic diseases. It is clear from the bronchial challenge studies that up to 50% of patients with allergic rhinitis will demonstrate bronchial hyperresponsiveness. Although, as a group, patients with allergic rhinitis are considerably less responsive to methacholine or histamine than asthmatics, there is considerable overlap between the two groups. A recent refinement in bronchial challenge[19] by cold air inhalation was able to separate the two groups from each other and from normals. Exercise challenge[20] used for bronchoprovocation has also shown differences between asthmatics, rhinitis patients and normals. Rhinitis patients with past history of episodic wheezing are more likely to show bronchial hyperresponsiveness than those without this history. We evaluated other clinical features that may predict a positive bronchial challenge in 23 patients with seasonal ragweed allergic rhinitis.[14] There were no significant differences in the age of onset of allergic rhinitis, the severity of rhinitis, frequency of family history of asthma, or presence of bronchial symptoms following viral respiratory infections between those patients with and without heightened bronchial reactivity.

Whether the airway response to nonspecific (pharmacologic) agents correlates with the response to specific (antigen) bronchial challenge is a subject of considerable interest. Permutt and colleagues[21] could show no correlation between the response to a cholinergic agent and reactivity to inhaled ragweed in ragweed sensitive patients with allergic rhinitis. Furthermore, when response to both agents was compared in patients with rhinitis or asthma, bronchial responses to inhaled antigen in ragweed sensitive allergic rhinitis and asthma patients showed little or no differences. However, significant differences in bronchial responsiveness to methacholine were noted in these two groups. Ahmed and his colleagues have similarly shown that ragweed-sensitive patients with allergic rhinitis and those with bronchial asthma have qualitatively and quantitatively comparable airway responses during antigen challenge.[22] Other studies using house dust mite and grass pollen for bronchoprovocation have also shown similar bronchial responses among allergic asthmatic and rhinitis patients, while histamine inhalation showed more marked reaction in the asthmatics.

It is clear, therefore, that a significant number of patients with allergic rhinitis and no lower respiratory tract symptoms show the asthmatic feature of heightened bronchial responsiveness when compared to normals. These patients demonstrate bronchial hyperresponsiveness to specific antigens as well as nonspecific (i.e., pharmacologic) agents. While lower airway responses to inhaled antigen may be similar to those of asthmatics, distinct differences between the groups have been shown: (1) A deep inspiration may transiently improve bronchoconstriction in rhinitis subjects while the same maneuver has little effect in asthmatics.[23] (2) The degree of nonspecific bronchial hyperresponsiveness is considered greater in asthmatics, although some overlap does occur. (3) Some bronchoprovocation tests such as exercise testing and cold air challenge may not demonstrate bronchial hyperresponsiveness in patients with allergic rhinitis.[19,24]

MECHANISMS OF LOWER AIRWAY DYSFUNCTION IN ALLERGIC RHINITIS

Considerable evidence is accumulating that demonstrates the distinguishing physiologic features of asthma: (1) increased resistance to airflow, (2) reversibility of airflow obstruction, and (3) hyperresponsiveness of airways is present in some patients with allergic rhinitis who have no asthmatic symptoms. The cause of these abnormalities is, to date, unknown. One speculation is that the presence of diseased nasal passages prevents normal conditioning of inspired air and as a result "an unaccustomed burden would be cast on the lower airways."[25] Another possibility postulated by Townley et al.[26] is that patients with allergic rhinitis have partial beta adrenergic blockade, similar to that seen in asthma. The demonstration[27] of autoantibodies to beta adrenergic receptors in a patient with allergic rhinitis and two patients with asthma has provided a potential mechanism for receptor blockade and a cause for beta adrenergic hyporesponsiveness in both conditions.

There is growing evidence that the expression of asthma in certain patients with allergic rhinitis is due to the interaction of two factors: (1) the presence of nonspecific bronchial hyperresponsiveness and (2) the intensity of the allergic response and its subsequent cascade of inflammatory reactions. Nonspecific bronchial hyperresponsiveness may be genetically determined; acquired or altered by environmental factors such as respiratory viruses, air pollution, or cigarette smoke; and further modified by the allergic response.

Several studies have shown increases in nonspecific bronchial responsiveness in rhinitis subjects during the pollen season.[28,29] These results are consistent with laboratory studies that have shown enhancement of bronchial reactivity following inhalation challenges with pollens.[30,31] Busse and Swenson[32] have shown that the intensity of bronchoconstriction to an inhaled antigen correlates with (1) the baseline histamine inhalation challenge, a manifestation of nonspecific bronchial responsiveness, and (2) the plasma histamine level, a manifestation of the intensity of the allergic response.

Nonspecific bronchial hyperresponsiveness in patients with allergic rhinitis is likely the most important link to bronchial asthma. If bronchial responsiveness is normal or mildly increased, lower airway function will remain normal unless an intense antigen challenge occurs in the lower airways. On the other hand, rhinitis patients with marked bronchial hyperresponsiveness may show asthmatic responses to cold air and may demonstrate diurnal variability of peak flow rates.[33] This may occur in the absence of lower airway symptoms and without an antecedent antigen challenge. We have shown that this latter group of allergic rhinitis patients are also more likely to develop overt asthma when compared to those without bronchial hyperresponsiveness.[34] We prospectively studied 40 ragweed-sensitive patients over a four- to five-year period. Nineteen percent of those who were initially hyperresponsive to methacholine developed asthma, while none of those with normal airway responses developed lower airway symptoms. Why only some patients with allergic rhinitis and hyperresponsiveness airways develop asthma is not understood and should be the subject of future studies.

REFERENCES

1. Smith JM, Knowler L. Epidemiology of asthma and allergic rhinitis. I. In a rural area. II. In a university-centered community. Am Rev Respir Dis 92:31–8, 1965.
2. Rackemann F, Edwards MC. Asthma in children: A follow-up of 688 patients after an interval of twenty years. N Engl J Med 246:815, 1952.
3. Hagy GW, Settipane GA. Risk factors for developing asthma and allergic rhinitis. J Allergy Clin Immunol 58:330–336, 1976.
4. ACCP-ATS. Joint Committee on Pulmonary Nomenclature: Pulmonary terms and symbols. Chest 67:383, 1975.
5. Norman PS. In vivo methods of the study of allergy. Ch. 16. In: Middleton E, Reed CE, Ellis EF (eds). Allergy Principles and Practice. St. Louis, MO: C V Mosby Co, 1978, pp 256–264.
6. Brown EA, Nobili C, Sannella T, Wadsworth GP. Dyspnea and diminished vital capacity as a symptom and a sign in hay fever. Dis Chest 12:205, 1946.
7. Doggett WE, Chester EH, Belman MJ, Schwartz HJ. Prevalence of airway obstruction in allergic rhinitis. Am Rev Respir Dis 113(Part 2):158, 1976.
8. Howard DW, Doggett WE, Gerblich AA, Chester EH, Schwartz HJ, Belman MJ. Seasonal variation of thoracic airway obstruction in allergic rhinitis. Chest 70:429, 1976.
9. Gerblich AA, Schwartz HJ, Chester EH. Seasonal variation of airway function in allergic rhinitis. J Allergy Clin Immunol 77:676–81, 1986.
10. Morgan EJ, Hall DR. Abnormalities of lung function in hay fever. Thorax 31:80, 1976.
11. Fairshter RD, Chiu JT, Wilson AF, Novey HS. Large airway constriction in allergic rhinitis. J Allergy Clin Immunol 59:243, 1977.
12. Fairshter RD, Novey HS, Marchioli LE, Wilson AF. Large airway constriction in allergic rhinitis: Response to inhalation of helium-oxygen. J Allergy Clin Immunol 63:39, 1979.
13. Lidington RE, Cotton DJ, Graham BL, Dosman JA. Peripheral airway obstruction in patients with rhinitis. Ann Allergy 42:28, 1979.
14. DeCotiis BA, Braman SS, Corrao WM. Pulmonary function studies and the prevalence of bronchial hyperreactivity in patients with allergic rhinitis. Am Rev Respir Dis 117:64, 1980.
15. Townley RG, Dennis M, Itkin IH. Comparative action of acetyl-beta-methacholine histamine and pollen antigens in subjects with hay fever and patients with bronchial asthma. J Allergy 36:121, 1965.
16. Townley RG, Ryo UY, Kolotkin BM, Kang B. Bronchial sensitivity to methacholine in current and former asthmatic and allergic rhinitis patients and control subjects. J Allergy Clin Immunol 56:429, 1975.
17. Stevens WJ, Vermeire PA. Bronchial responsiveness to histamine, an allergen in patients with asthma, rhinitis and cough. Eur J Respir Dis 61:203, 1980.
18. Cockcroft DW, Killian DN, Mellon JJ, Hargreave FE. Bronchial reactivity to inhaled histamine: A method and clinical survey. Clin Allergy 7:235, 1977.
19. Deal EC Jr, McFadden ER Jr, Ingram RH Jr, Breslin FJ, Jaeger JJ. Airway responsiveness to cold air and hyperpnea in normal subjects and in those with hay fever and asthma. Am Rev Respir Dis 121:621, 1980.
20. Schofield NM, Green M, Davies RJ. Response of the lung airway to exercise testing in asthma and rhinitis. Br J Dis Chest 74:155, 1980.
21. Permutt S, Rosenthal RR, Norman PS, Menkes HA. Bronchial challenge in ragweed-sensitive patients. In: Lichtenstein LM, Austen KF (eds). Asthma, Physiology, Immunopharmacology and Treatment. San Diego, CA: Academic Press Inc, 1973.
22. Ahmed T, Fernandez RJ, Wanner A. Airway responses to antigen challenge in allergic rhinitis and allergic asthma. J Allergy Clin Immunol 67:135–145, 1981.
23. Fish JE, Ankin MG, Kelly JF, Peterman VI. Comparison of responses to pollen extract in subjects with allergic asthma and nonasthmatic subjects with allergic rhinitis. J Allergy Clinical Immunol 65:154–161, 1980.
24. Schofield NM, Green M, Davies RJ. Response of the lung airway to exercise testing in asthma and rhinitis. Br J Dis Chest 74:155–163, 1980.
25. Proctor DF. The upper airways. I. Nasal physiology and defense of the lungs. Am Rev Respir Dis 115:97, 1977.
26. Townley RG, McGeady S, Bewtra A. The effect of beta-adrenergic blockade on bronchial sensitivity to acetyl-beta-methacholine in normal and allergic rhinitis subjects. J Allergy Clin Immunol 57:358, 1976.
27. Venter JC, Frazer CM, Harrison LC. Autoantibodies to B$_2$-adrenergic receptors: A possible cause of adrenergic hyporesponsiveness in allergic rhinitis and asthma. Science 207:1361, 1980.
28. Madonini E, Briatico-Vangosa G, Pappacoda A, Maccagni G,

Cardani A, Saporiti F. Seasonal increase of bronchial reactivity in allergic rhinitis. J Allergy Clin Immunol 79:358–363, 1987.

29. Boulet LP, Morin D, Milot J, Turcotte H. Bronchial responsiveness increases after seasonal antigen exposure in non-asthmatic subjects with pollen-induced rhinitis. Ann Allergy 63:114–119, 1989.

30. Boulet LP, Cartier A, Thomson NC, Roberts RS, Dolovich J, Hargreave FE. Asthma and increases in nonallergic bronchial responsiveness from seasonal pollen exposure. J Allergy Clin Immunol 71:399–406, 1983.

31. Bar-Sela S, Schlueter DP, Kitt SR, Sosman AJ, Fink JN. Antigen-induced enhancement of bronchial reactivity. Chest 88:114–116, 1985.

32. Busse WW, Swenson CA. The relationship between plasma histamine concentrations and bronchial obstruction to antigen challenge in allergic rhinitis. J Allergy Clin Immunol 84:658–666, 1989.

33. Ramsdale EH, Morris MM, Roberts RS, Hargreave FE. Asymptomatic bronchial hyperresponsiveness in rhinitis. J Allergy Clin Immunol 75:573–577, 1985.

34. Braman SS, Barrows AA, DeCotiis BA, Settipane GA, Corrao WM. Airway hyperresponsiveness in allergic rhinitis. A risk factor for asthma. Chest 91:671–674, 1987.

Chapter XIV

Allergic Rhinitis and Airway Reactivity to Mediators

Robert G. Townley, M.D.

ABSTRACT

Why some members of the family develop allergic rhinitis and others develop asthma has puzzled allergists for many years. We have reviewed our experience with bronchoprovocation and airway reactivity to methacholine in subjects with allergic rhinitis, bronchial asthma and normal controls. All current asthmatics and only about 10% of normal subjects with a negative family history for atopy respond to methacholine after 200 breath units or less. Although about 50% of allergic rhinitis subjects may show >20% decrease in FEV_1 with 800 breath units or less of methacholine, many of these subjects reach a "plateau" i.e. increasing the dose of methacholine does not result in a further decrease in FEV_1. Only about 5% show a high positive response without a plateau phenomena. These subjects respond to 50 breath units or less, and the FEV_1 shows a further decrease with increasing concentrations of methacholine. These subjects are at greater risk for developing bronchial asthma.

BACKGROUND

A number of studies more than 30 years ago have shown that patients with bronchial asthma are exquisitely sensitive to histamine and acetylcholine, as indicated by a decrease in vital capacity and forced expiratory volume in the first second (FEV_1).[1,2,3,4] Spe-

Professor of Medicine & Assoc. Prof. Microbiology, Creighton University, Omaha, NE 68178.

cific allergens to which they are sensitive produce the same response. There is less agreement concerning the bronchial reactivity of patients with hay fever. Curry[1] reported that parenteral administration of histamine produced a sizeable reduction in vital capacity in eight of nine subjects with active asthma, whereas it produced no significant change in vital capacity in two control groups of normal individuals and patients with hay fever. In a subsequent article[2] on the effects of methacholine and histamine in eleven patients with allergic rhinitis, the reported maximum decrease in the vital capacity produced by either of these chemical mediators was 10%, which cannot be considered significant. Brown and his co-workers[5] have shown that patients with hay fever (without history of bronchial asthma) may frequently show diminished vital capacity during the pollen season.

In 1965, Parker, Bilbo, and Reed,[6] using a simplified provocative methacholine aerosol test (25 mg/ml), confirmed that the diagnosis of asthma could be made in asthmatic persons during their symptom-free intervals. In the same year, Townley, Dennis, and Itkin,[7] using methacholine aerosol (10 mg/ml), demonstrated marked sensitivity of all asthmatics and lesser sensitivity of approximately one-half of fourteen hay fever subjects to this cholinergic agent.

Eight of these fourteen hay fever subjects had their first episode of wheezing following an aerosol inhalation of pollen extract. Sputum examinations confirmed the presence of many eosinophils within minutes after specific allergen challenge. The appearance of eosinophils in the sputum, the fall in FEV_1, with cough, tightness, and wheezing after specific allergen, and the subsequent response to bronchodilators indicate that these were

Table I — Bronchial Sensitivity in Hay Fever, Asthma and Nonatopic Subjects

Subjects	Methacholine (10 mg/ml)		Histamine base 1 (mg/ml)		Allergen 10,000 PNU/ml	
	No. inhalations	No. pos.* responses	No. inhalations	No. pos. responses	No. inhalations	No. pos. responses
Hay fever – 14 adults						
Average	77	8	81	6	40	11
Range	15-150		30-150		3-75	
Asthma –25 adults						
Average	2.8	25	24	25	9.5	22
Range	1-12		3-100		1-75	
Nonatopic – 8 adults						
Average	>150	0	>150	0		
Range						

*Positive response=15% decrease in FEV_1

indeed allergic changes simulating asthma in hay fever subjects.

Eight hay fever subjects showed a significant decrease in FEV_1 after methacholine and six after histamine inhalations. These results are summarized in Table I.

When the amounts of methacholine and histamine are compared milligram for milligram of base, they are of approximately equal potency in producing bronchial obstruction in asthmatic individuals. However, of the fourteen hay fever subjects, there were only six with positive histamine challenges, compared with eleven who had positive allergen challenges.

All of the twenty-five asthma patients tested and none of the eight nonatopic controls showed a significant decrease in FEV_1 following methacholine and histamine challenge in the doses employed.

In terms of bronchial sensitivity to the number of inhalations of the preparations used, the asthma patients were approximately 27 times as sensitive to methacholine as the hay fever group, but only four times as sensitive to pollen inhalation.

With allergen challenge, cough was often very productive, up to 15 or 20 ml of viscid sputum, loaded with eosinophils. The coughing and collecting of sputum were under direct observation of the authors to avoid the possibility of nasal secretions being obtained.

This is in agreement with Kallos[8] findings upon chal-lenging guinea pigs with specific antigens and with histamine and methacholine. Although histamine and methacholine would produce bronchospasm, they would not produce the characteristic histologic pattern. When antigen was inhaled by the guinea pigs, a large number of eosinophils were found in the bronchi, whereas after histamine and methacholine only a few eosinophils appeared.

Although a group of fourteen allergic rhinitis subjects is perhaps too small for making a strict comparative analysis, the fact that eight of the fourteen demonstrated wheezing for the first time seems significant. Although the asthma patients were on average 27 times as sensitive to methacholine as the allergic rhinitis group, it has been shown that they are 200 to 1,000 times as sensitive as nonatopic persons.

More recently, a large group of subjects were studied to compare the bronchial sensitivity to methacholine in current and former asthmatic and allergic rhinitis patients and control subjects. Ninety-eight subjects underwent methacholine aerosol challenge at a concentration of 5 mg/ml. All atopic groups differed significantly in their bronchial response to methacholine compared to nonatopic control subjects. Nineteen normal subjects had a mean decrease of 11.4% in forced expiratory volume in one second (FEV_1) with 128 methacholine inhalations, and only two decreased by greater than 20%, Table II.

Table II — Responses to FEV$_1$ After Methacholine (5 mg/ml) Inhalations*

Subjects (Na)	Mean No. Methacholine Inhalations (range)	P Values Compared To Controls	% Decrease In FEV$_1$ (range)	P Values Compared To Controls	No. of Positive Methacholine Responses
Normal controls (19)	128.4 (20-160)	—	11.4% (1-26%)	—	2
Allergic rhinitis (27)	92.2 (4-160)	<0.10 NS	19% (1-41%)	<0.01	15
Former asthmatics (34)	47.8 (1-160)	<0.001	22.4% (0-43%)	<0.001	28
Current asthmatics (18)	4.5 (1-40)	<0.001	32.6% (20-64%)	<0.001	18

Per cent decrease in FEV$_1$ represents the mean of the first positive response (i.e., FEV$_1$ decreased=20%) obtained when methacholine was given in the sequential manner outlined. Mean methacholine inhalations calculated from the lowest number of inhalations needed to elicit the positive response. When no positive response occurred, values at 160 inhalations were used.

Four of these responders developed greater diminuation in FEV$_1$ response with additional methacholine inhalations in a manner similar to that seen in the asthmatic patients. Eighteen current asthmatics showed the greatest bronchial sensitivity to methacholine with a mean 32.6% decrease in FEV$_1$ at 4.5 inhalations. One hundred per cent of current asthmatics and 82% (28 of 34) of former asthmatics (free of asthma symptoms for 1 to 20 yr.) showed a positive response to methacholine. A 20% decrease in FEV$_1$ with a total of 40 inhalations of 5.0 mg/ml (200 breath units) or less is consistent with a diagnosis of "current asthma." Twenty of 34 former asthmatics responded in this manner. The methacholine aerosol test can be useful in the diagnosis of previous and current asthma and may be of value in predicting the future of asthma in hay fever patients.[9]

All former asthmatics had symptoms for a mean of 7.5 yr. (range, 1 to 20) and were free of asthma for a mean of 8.5 yr. (range, 1 to 30). Current asthmatics had their symptoms for a mean of 11.1 yr. (range, 1 to 28) and were free of asthma for an average of 4 months prior to the experiment (range, 1 wk to 12 mo). All groups were comparable with regard to age of subjects, baseline FEV$_1$, and predicted FVC and FEV$_1$ except for the current asthmatic group who had lower pulmonary functions.

Using the minimum amount of methacholine inhalations resulting in a 20% or greater decrease in FEV$_1$, the responses of patients in the various groups are shown in Table II. It should be noted that for all atopic groups the decrease in FEV$_1$ following methacholine was statistically significant compared to the control group (asthmatics, $p<0.001$; allergic rhinitis, $p<0.01$).

The response of patients with allergic rhinitis almost parallel the results obtained in control patients with the exceptions that:

1. The responses of four patients overlaps those seen in the asthmatic group. Two of the four patients began to manifest symptoms of asthma during their subsequent hay fever season.

2. Four additional allergic rhinitis patients had positive reactions to methacholine under 40 inhalations. However, unlike the asthmatic group, additional inhalation of methacholine did not result in a further decrease of FEV$_1$ but rather a "plateau phenomenon" occurred. That significant bronchoconstriction has occurred in these patients is evidenced by their rapid reversal to baseline FEV$_1$ values following the administration of isoproterenol.

Only 6 of 34 former asthmatics who allegedly had asthma early in childhood, had less than 20% decrease in FEV$_1$. In some former asthmatics, a plateau response following 20 or 40 inhalations was noted.

Figure 1 represents the total accumulative minimum number of methacholine inhalations resulting in a positive FEV$_1$ response. This demonstrates the exquisite sensitivity of the current asthmatics to methacholine inhalation. Seventeen of 18 such patients needed 10 or less inhalations before marked bronchoconstriction

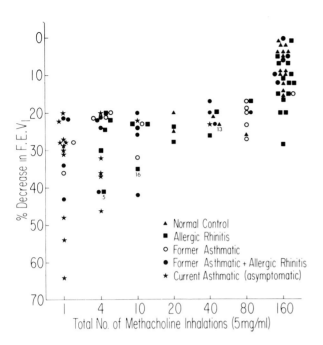

Figure 1. *Minimum number of methacholine inhalations resulting in a positive FEV$_1$ response (i.e., 20% or greater decrease in FEV$_1$). For patients never achieving a positive response, the FEV$_1$ at 160 breaths was plotted. Current asthmatics showed the greatest sensitivity with positive response at 10 or less methacholine inhalations. Numbers refer to patients discussed in the text. Abscissa refers to total number of methacholine inhalations accumulated.*

occurred. All former asthmatics had positive responses to inhalations of methacholine with the exception of 6 patients previously discussed.

An increase in the percentage of positive responses in former asthmatics might have been obtained if a higher concentration of methacholine aerosol had been used.

In contrast to Parker and co-workers,[6] where hay fever patients did not differ from controls in response to methacholine, our previous study[7] showed that 8 of 14 hayfever patients (57%) had positive methacholine response. Similarly, in this study, allergic rhinitis subjects had a significant decrease in FEV$_1$ compared to normals (p<0.01), with 15 out of 27 (56%) having 20% or greater decrease in FEV$_1$.

In our previous report,[7] bronchial sensitivity to methacholine showed no overlap among patients with hay fever and asthma. However, in our more recent study, we found 4 allergic rhinitis patients with marked responses that were in the range seen in asthmatics, and 2 of these subsequently developed asthma. Although from previous work, [6,7,10,11] we expected all our normal controls to be unresponsive to methacholine (at least until a large

number of inhalations had been taken), positive responses were seen in two apparently normal subjects who denied having an acute respiratory infection or a personal or family history of hay fever, asthma, or bronchitis. Both patients received intradermal skin tests for inhalants and had reactions of 7 x 8 mm weals, with 30 x 35 mm erythema to house dust and feathers only. Such apparently normal persons could very well be latent asthmatics and should be followed for development of asthma. Studies evaluating large groups of asthmatics and their families as well as control populations for methacholine sensitivity are currently underway in an effort to discover "potential asthmatics" and to determine if methacholine sensitivity can be a genetic marker for asthma. We found no positive correlation between duration of asthma and methacholine sensitivity. Furthermore, three asthmatics, following their first attack of asthma, were challenged with methacholine aerosol and developed marked bronchoconstriction,[12] thus, indicating that hypersensitivity to cholinergic aerosol was already present. However, among former asthmatics, the degree of bronchoconstriction experienced with methacholine was related to the severity of past asthma symptoms.

The methacholine inhalation test is a safe and simple procedure with good reproducibility and may be of value in screening subjects with allergic rhinitis and siblings of asthmatics and controls for latent asthma. The effects of methacholine are short-lived (20-30 min), and bronchoconstriction can be easily reversed with inhalation of isoproterenol or injection of epinephrine. Furthermore, in patients with a history of recent dyspnea of uncertain etiology, the diagnosis of asthma can be excluded by a negative response to 40 inhalations of 5 mg/ml of methacholine.

We have found that a number of individuals with allergic rhinitis, and some former asthmatics, demonstrate a dose-response curve with a plateau phenomenon. These individuals show an initial decrease in FEV$_1$ of greater than 20% but with additional inhalations show no further decrease and in some cases an increase in FEV$_1$. This suggests a feedback mechanism between the beta adrenergic and the cholinergic systems. We interpret these findings as indicating that these individuals have sufficient intact beta adrenergic receptors to overcome the effects of additional methacholine inhalations. In contrast, current asthmatics show a progressive fall in FEV$_1$ with additional methacholine inhalations which may be due to insufficient beta adrenergic receptors.

METHODOLOGY

The methacholine responsiveness may be determined by one of two methods: (1) by determining dose-response curves to increasing concentrations of methacholine while keeping the number of breaths and the volume of methacholine inhaled constant,[13] and (2) by determining dose-response curves by keeping the concentration constant while increasing the number of inhalations of methacholine.[7] The first method is more widely used and has been recommended by the American Academy of Allergy to provide a standard and uniform method. It is described in detail elsewhere.[13] The second method has been used since 1962 and has been the basis for a number of short-term and long-term studies. We recently compared both of these methods to determine the short-term reliability of each method. The dose-response curves and thus the degree of bronchial sensitivity were determined in 19 subjects in a randomized 4-way crossover study. Each subject was challenged twice by each method at 1-week intervals. The short-term reproducibility for both methods was good (r=0.934 and 0.942 respectively). The correlation between methods was also significant (r=0.953).[14]

The detailed methodology has been described in detail in recent publications.[13,14,15,16] These articles describe the methods of aerosol administration, effect on particle size, various mediators and antigens that can be used and also the exact methodology for the dilution and delivery of the agents. The types of pulmonary function tests after bronchial provocation challenges are also described.

These publications also describe the method of expression of data by determining the cumulative provocation dose (PC_{20}) for FEV_1 and PD_{35} or PC_{35} for SGaw. The measurement of the PD_{20} is of great help and importance in research protocols. The measure provides a basis for comparison of the effect of drugs on bronchial reactivity and also to determine the reproducibility of the test. Although any of the parameters including FVC, FEV_1, SGaw, FEF_{25-27}, PEFR can be measured, FEV_1 is the most convenient. A drop greater than 20% to any standard concentration of methacholine is considered a positive test.

CHARACTERIZATION OF METHACHOLINE INHALATION RESPONSES

Plateau Phenomenon

As previously stated, we found a subgroup of allergic rhinitis patients who had a decrease of 20% or greater in FEV_1 but with increasing doses of methacholine demonstrated a plateau phenomenon[9,17,18] as shown in Figure 2. Some of the patients[9] actually showed an improvement in their pulmonary function tests with higher doses of methacholine. According to this criteria, they would have been classified as having high- or medium-positive reactions. To avoid this false high-positive classification, we found that the area under the dose-response curve is more reliable in defining the degree of sensitivity.[17,18,19]

Area is calculated by integrating the best-fit parabola of the methacholine dose-response curve, Figure 3. The est cutoff point is either a 35% drop in FEV_1 or 160

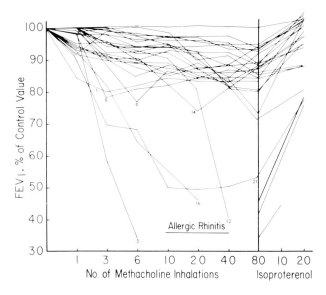

Figure 2. *Dose-response curves of allergic rhinitis patients to sequential methacholine inhalations. Response to number of inhalations of isoproterenol following bronchoconstriction. Numbers refer to patients. Some allergic rhinitis patients demonstrated hypersensitivity to the bronchoconstrictive effect of methacholine.*

METHACHOLINE(5mg/ml) CHALLENGE

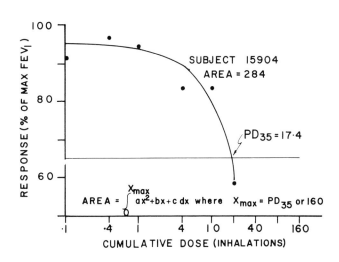

Figure 3. *A least-squares fitted, parabolic dose-response curve. Provocative dose at 35% (PD_{35}) is the right-hand limit (Xmax) of the integral. The X axis has been logarithmically transformed for ease of presentation.*

inhalations of methacholine. Area values that correspond to the previously defined response categories are shown in Table III.

Using these parameters, an analysis of the methacholine challenge responses in 371 subjects was made.[18] All results were subdivided in terms of high, medium, low, or negative inhalation responses. Of current asthmatics,

Table III — Characterization of Methacholine Inhalation Responses

Category	% Drop in FEV$_1$	Total No. of breaths	% Drop in FEV$_1$ Ratio=No. of breaths	Area under the curve
High	≥20%	0.1-10	>2.00	0-306.25
Medium	≥20%	11-40	0.05-1.99	306.25-1,225
Low	≥20%	41-160	0.13-0.49	1,225-4,000
Negative	<20%	160	<0.125	4,000-5,600

We consider persons with areas of less than 306 to be high-positive responders. Areas from 306 to 1,225 are classed as medium-positive. 1,225 to 4,000 as low-positive, and 4,000-5,600 as negative. These classes were obtained from traditional single-point estimates of response, i.e., HIGH=fall in FEV$_1$ greater than 20% after 10 cumulative inhalations of methacholine aerosol at 5 mg/ml. MEDIUM=greater than 20% after 40 cumulative inhalations. LOW=greater than 20% after 160 cumulative inhalations, and NEGATIVE=less than 20% fall after 160 cumulative inhalations.

95% fall into the high or medium category of methacholine sensitivity. Many nonasthmatics show an initial (I) positive methacholine response (fall in FEV$_1$≥20%) that would remain stable in spite of additional methacholine inhalations (i.e., a plateau phenomenon). To delineate between a true positive methacholine response and a plateau response, we developed a computer program to calculate the area (A) under the dose-response curve. Results are shown in Table IV.

This plateau phenomenon occurred least frequently in current asthmatics and most frequently in the allergic rhinitis subjects. Current asthmatics are the most sensitive and members of nonatopic families the least sensitive. The plateau phenomenon may be due to sufficient intact beta adrenergic receptors to counteract additional inhalation of methacholine without a further fall in FEV$_1$.

Airway Reactivity in Atopic Families

To evaluate the familial nature of asthma and the methacholine responsiveness, we studied 47 atopic and 26 nonatopic families. Atopic families had at least one child with current asthma. There were 648 members in these families. In 26 nonatopic families, 237 members had no reported history of asthma, hayfever, or atopic eczema for at least three generations of first- and second-degree relatives. The proband with asthma, his or her siblings, parents, and grandparents made up the study group. All probands were excluded for genetic analysis.[14]

These studies have demonstrated that:

1) Over 90% of asthmatics have high- or medium-positive responsiveness to methacholine, Figure 4. Only three individuals' responses were negative, and they were former asthmatics who had been completely free of symptoms for several years.

2) Less than 5% of individuals with hay fever or nonatopic normal subjects (normals) show a high-positive methacholine response. These subjects may well be at risk for developing asthma.

3) Twenty-seven percent of subjects with allergic rhinitis and 49% of normal subjects had a completely negative methacholine response.

4) Thirty percent of subjects with allergic rhinitis, 18% of normal individuals from families with a history of asthma and 8% of normal individuals from normal (nonatopic) families were medium-positive to methacholine.

5) The rest of the subjects were low-positive to methacholine, i.e. they had 20% decrease in FEV$_1$ but only after inhalation of >200 cumulative breath units of methacholine. (One breath unit=one inhalation of 1 mg/ml).

Chi-square analysis of our data in Figure 4 showed that:

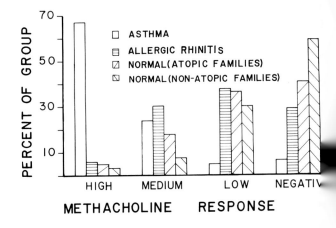

Figure 4. *Response as defined in Table III.*

Table IV — Dose Response Curve

	Asthma Families						Nonatopic Families	
	Current Asthma, 63 pts.		Allergic Rhinitis, 68 pts.		Nonatopic, 155 pts.		Nonatopic, 85 pts.	
Methacholine response	I*	A	I	A	I	A	I	A
Negative	1	1	37	44	50	53	54	68
Low-positive	3	11	19	32	16	31	22	23
Medium-positive	16	13	28	16	21	12	13	9
High	79	75	16	7	13	6	11	0

*Percent with initial reaction based on $FEV_1 \geq 20\%$ (I), or area under dose-response curve (A).

1. Normals from asthma families were significantly different from normals from control families ($p < 0.01$).

2. Hay fever patients were not significantly different from normals from atopic families ($p > 0.05$).

3. Asthmatics were different from all other groups.

4. Hay fever patients were different from normals of nonatopic families only.

When frequency of positive responses for the methacholine challenge in the normals from atopic and nonatopic families was determined, two peaks of subpopulations were obtained in the atopic (asthmatic) families (Figure 5).

In contrast, the normals from nonatopic families have a single uniform distribution with no corresponding subpopulation of the methacholine responders. The individuals with a peak in the positive test range may be potential asthmatics, and this bimodal distribution in the atopic families suggests a single biochemical or physical characteristic associated with airway reactivity.

Natural History of Airway Reactivity and Atopic Disease Status

Five families (56 subjects) were evaluated repeatedly over a period of four to seven years. Ten common aller-

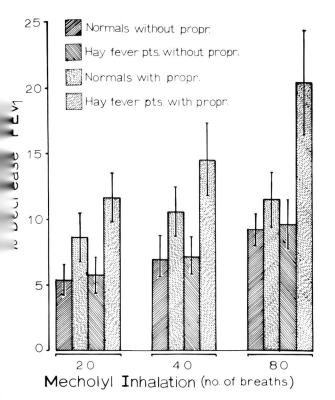

Figure 5. Comparison of the effect of propranolol on the bronchial response to methacholine in normal and allergic rhinitis subjects. Vertical bars represent mean % decrease in $FEV_1 \pm$ the standard error of the mean.

Table V — Correlation Coefficient, for Symptom Score, IgE and MICR.

	Symptom Score	IgE	MICR
Skin test score	0.419	0.410	0.344
MICR	0.744	0.417	—
IgE	0.489	—	—

(all p values < 0.01, df=49)

MICR = methacholine inhalation challenge response.

gens were used for the skin testing using both prick and intradermal methods. The skin test score is the sum of ten coded responses. Methacholine inhalation challenge response (MICR) was determined by measuring the area under the dose-response curve. IgE levels were determined by PRIST method (Pharmacia). There were 166 evaluations performed (range 1-8 evaluations/subject, average three evaluations/subject) over a period of four to seven years. The three objective measures of atopy (MICR, skin test, IgE) are significantly correlated among themselves and with a symptom score for asthma derived from the questionnaire. Correlation coefficients (r) for the various comparisons are shown in Table V.

However, the methacholine challenge response correlated best with the symptom score (r = .744).

In four young subjects, we have observed the onset of asthma during the follow-up period. In these subjects, MICR (and in one subject serum IgE) became abnormal before the onset of symptoms. These findings suggest that in family members at high risk for asthma, a positive MICR and/or an elevated serum IgE may predict the subsequent development of clinical asthma.

Altounyan[19] reported an increase in airway responsiveness to histamine during the grass pollen season in grass pollen sensitive subjects. Cockroft et al[20] observed an increased response to histamine and methacholine in subjects with allergen-induced late asthmatic response. This group of investigators also reported that isolated early asthmatic responses with falls in FEV$_1$ of 20–40%, virtually never observed increased responsiveness to histamine.[21]

Furthermore, the increase in histamine response, following an allergen-induced late asthmatic response, may persist for one or more days up to several weeks and the degree of increased non-allergic responsiveness correlates with the severity of the late asthmatic response. The relationship to the late asthmatic responses suggests that mechanisms involved in their production are also important to the development of nonallergic hyperreactivity and the induction of asthma. The reason for the difference in tendency among subjects to develop late asthmatic responses is not known. One possible mechanism we intend to explore is that the resultant increased nonallergic hyperreactivity to methacholine, whether it be induced by allergen exposure or viral respiratory infection, is associated with an altered alpha and beta adrenergic receptor density and responsiveness. This could be reflected by a change in the beta and alpha adrenergic receptors in their peripheral mononuclear leukocytes and platelets respectively. In this regard, we have reported the converse of the above to be true; that is, if we alter the adrenergic receptor responses either by blocking beta receptors alone or simultaneously stimulating alpha receptors, we increase responsiveness to histamine, meth-

acholine, serotonin or antigen in mice and guinea pigs,[22,23] and to methacholine in persons with asthma[24] and allergic rhinitis subjects who have never had asthma.[24]

The Effect of Beta Adrenergic Blockade on Bronchial Sensitivity to Methacholine in Normal and Allergic Rhinitis Subjects

We studied the effect of propranolol by inhalation on the sensitivity to methacholine inhalation in normal and allergic rhinitis subjects in order to determine if beta adrenergic blockade alters the sensitivity to mediators in nonasthmatic atopic individuals. The two groups were matched in terms of their initial unresponsiveness to methacholine. A second group of five allergic rhinitis subjects who also have never experienced any asthma symptoms but showed a positive response to methacholine was studied separately.

Under these conditions of aerosol administration for both propranolol and methacholine, we obtained mean decreases in FEV$_1$ of 11% and 20.6% in the normal subjects and the allergic rhinitis patients, respectively (Figure 5). This decrease for the allergic rhinitis patients was statistically significant as compared to that of the normal subjects (p<0.05). This decrease in FEV$_1$ following propranolol in 6 of 14 allergic rhinitis patients was associated with clinical symptoms of asthma, i.e., wheezing, coughing, and tightness in the chest for the first time in their lives. That these symptoms were reversed with isoproterenol could suggest a partial beta adrenergic blockade as being instrumental in asthma.

The second group of five allergic rhinitis patients who were sensitive to methacholine even before propranolol developed an even more marked sensitivity to methacholine following propranolol, and all five experienced the symptoms of asthma for the first time in their lives. We have also tried to explain the difference in response between normal subjects and allergic rhinitis patients on the basis of a dose-effect curve of beta blockade involving airway smooth muscle and mast cells. It could be speculated that the mast cells in the airways of allergic rhinitis subjects may be more susceptible to the effects of beta adrenergic blockade.

The autonomic nervous system abnormalities in allergy has recently been reviewed by Kaliner et al.[26] They measured alpha and beta adrenergic and cholinergic responsiveness in allergic subjects and normal controls. Subjects with allergic rhinitis had beta adrenergic hyporesponsiveness and cholinergic hyperresponsiveness whereas allergic asthma was also association with excessive alpha adrenergic responsiveness.

Further studies of the autonomic abnormalities among allergic rhinitis, asthmatic and normal subjects should help to characterize the mechanism of airway reactivity. In the meantime, the reason why some individuals in certain families develop allergic rhinitis and others develop asthma remains unanswered. Although both diseases are familial and have the same allergic, immunologic and eosinophilic characteristics, the overriding characteristic that separates these two diseases is the airway reactivity that is the *sine qua non* of asthma.

REFERENCES

1. Curry JJ. The action of histamine on the respiratory tract in normal and asthmatic subjects. J Clin Invest 25:785, 1946.
2. Curry JJ. Comparative action of acetyl-beta-methacholine and histamine on the respiratory tract in normals, patients with hay fever, and subjects with bronchial asthmna. J Clin Invest 26:430, 1947.
3. Crews SJ, Herxheimer H. The protective influence of graded doses of promethazine on induced asthmatic attacks of graded intensity. Internat Arch Allergy 3:329, 1952.
4. Schiller IW, Lowell FC. Effect of drugs in modifying response of asthmatic subjects to inhalation of pollen extracts as determined by vital capacity measurements. Ann Allergy 5:564, 1947.
5. Brown EA, Nobili C, Sannella T, Wadsworth GP. Dyspnea and diminished vital capacity as a symptom and sign in hay fever. Dis Chest 12:205, 1946.
6. Parker CD, Bilbo RE, Reed CE. Methacholine aerosol as test for bronchial asthma. Arch Intern Med 115:452, 1965.
7. Townley RG, Dennis M, Itkin IH. Comparative action of acetyl-beta-methacholine, histamine, and pollen antigens in subjects with hay fever and patients with bronchial asthma. J Allergy 36:121, 1965.
8. Kallos P, Pagel W. Experimentelle untersuchungen uber asthma bronchale. Acta med Scandinav 91:292, 1937.
9. Townley RG, Ryo UY, Kolotkin BM, Kang B. Bronchial sensitivity to methacholine in current and former asthmatic and allergic rhinitis patients and control subjects. J Allergy Clin Immunol 56:429, 1975.
10. Itkin IH. Bronchial hypersensitivity to mecholyl and histamine in asthma subjects. J Allergy 40:245, 1967.
11. Felarca AB, Itkin IH. Studies with the quantitative inhalation challenge technique. I. Curve of dose response to acetyl-beta-methacholine in patients with asthma of known and unknown origin, hay fever subjects and nonatopic volunteers. J Allergy 37:223, 1966.
12. Cookson DU, Reed CE. A comparison of the effects of isoproterenol in the normal and asthmatic subject. Am Rev Respir Dis 88:636, 1963.
13. Chai H, Farr RS, Froehlich LA, et al. Standardization of inhalation challenge procedures. J Allergy Clin Immunol 56:323, 1975.
14. Townley RG, Bewtra AK, Nair NM, Brodkey FD, Watt GD, Burke KM. Methacholine inhalation challenge studies. J Allergy Clin Immunol 64:569, 1979.
15. Hargreave FE, Ryan G, Thomson NC, O'Byrne PM, Latimer K, Juniper EF, Dolovich J. Bronchial responsiveness to histamine or methacholine in asthma: measurement and clinical significance. J Allergy Clin Immunol 68:347, 1981.
16. Thomson NC, Roberts R, Bandouvakis J, Newball H, Hargreave FE. Comparison of bronchial response to prostaglandin F_{2a} and methacholine. J Allergy Clin Immunol 68:392, 1981.
17. Reed CE, Townley RG. Asthma: Classification and pathogenesis. In: Allergy – Principles and Practice. Middleton E, Reed CE, Ellis EF. (Eds.) St. Louis, The C.V. Mosby Company, 1978, pp. 659-677.
18. Townley RG, Guirgis HA, Villacorte GV, et al. Methacholine dose response curves in atopic and nonatopic individuals. J Allergy Clin Immunol 55:92, 1975.
19. Altounyan REC. Changes in histamine and atropine responsiveness as a guide to diagnosis and evaluation of therapy and obstructive airways disease. In: Sodium Cromoglycate in Allergic Airways Disease. Pepys J, Frankland AW. (Eds.) London: Butterworths, 1970, pp.47-53.
20. Cockroft DW, Ruffin RE, Dolovich J, Hargreave FE. Allergen-induced increase in nonallergic bronchial reactivity. Clin Allergy 7:503, 1977.
21. Cartier A, Frith PA, Dolovich MB, Morris M, Morse JCL, Newhouse MT, Hargreave FE. Allergen-induced increase in nonallergic airway responsiveness to histamine. J Allergy Clin Immunol 65:207, 1980.
22. Townley RG, Trapani IL, Szentivanyi A. Sensitization to anaphylaxis and to some of its pharmacological mediators by blockade of the beta adrenergic receptors. J Allergy 39:177, 1967.
23. Townley RG, Daley D, Selenke W. The effect of agents used in the treatment of bronchial asthma on carbohydrate metabolism and histamine sensitivity after beta-adrenergic blockade. J Allergy 45:71, 1970.
24. Ryo UY, Townley RG. Comparison of respiratory and cardiovascular effects of isoproterenol, propranolol and practolol in asthmatics and normal subjects. J Allergy Clin Immunol 57:12, 1976.
25. Townley RG, McGeady S, Bewtra A. The effect of beta-adrenergic blockade on bronchial sensitivity to acetyl-beta-methacholine in normal and allergic rhinitis subjects. J Allergy Clin Immunol 57:358, 1976.
26. Kaliner M, Shelhamer JH, Davis PB, Smith LJ, Venter JC. Autonomic nervous system abnormalities and allergy. Ann Int Med 96:349, 1982. □

Chapter XV

Nasal Reflexes

Gordon D. Raphael, M.D., Scott D. Meredith, M.D., James N. Baraniuk, M.D., and Michael A. Kaliner, M.D.

ABSTRACT

Nasal reflexes are neurally mediated reactions which arise either through direct stimulation of the nasal mucosa or through stimulation of pathways elsewhere in the body which indirectly involve the nose. The neural pathways involved in these reactions are complex, and the exact nature of the stimuli which trigger these reflexes has not been completely detailed. This review presents a discussion on the innervation of the nose, updates the current understanding about nasal neuropeptides, and then summarizes information about several different types of nasal reflexes.

Physicians are frequently asked to evaluate patients who complain of perplexing nasal symptoms. A clear understanding of the neural regulation of the nose, as well as an appreciation of normal nasal reflexes, may help the physician determine whether or not a nasal pathologic condition exists. The array of potential nasal responses is surprisingly complex and involves nervous pathways which utilize both classical neurotransmitters and neuropeptides. These responses are regulated by nasal reflexes, many of which are initiated within the nose and may involve not only the nasal mucosa but also organs elsewhere in the body. Conversely, reflexes originating from organs outside of the nose may also affect nasal function. The purpose of this review is to summarize the current understanding of nasal reflexes, the innervation of the nose, and the growing body of information regarding nasal neuropeptides.

INNERVATION OF THE NOSE

The innervation of the nasal mucosa regulates nasal blood flow, controls glandular secretion, and serves to protect the lower airways against irritants.[1] The

Allergic Disease Section, Laboratory of Clinical Investigation, National Institute of Allergy and Infectious Diseases, National Institutes of Health, Bethesda, MD

nervous supply can be conceptually divided into sensory nerves, which include the olfactory nerve and branches of the trigeminal nerve, and autonomic nerves, which regulate vasomotor function and secretion. Neuropeptides such as substance P (SP) and vasoactive intestinal peptide (VIP) are present in these nerves and may play important roles in normal nasal function.

The olfactory nerve (CN I) supplies the special sense of smell. Superficial processes from this nerve innervate the olfactory or Schneiderian membrane in the superior nasal cavity. Central projections extend from this membrane to the olfactory bulbs at the base of the frontal lobes and then to the brainstem. Another nerve, the nervus terminalis, runs parallel to each olfactory tract, and sends terminal branches into the superior nasal cavity along with fibers of the olfactory nerve. This nerve, sometimes referred to as the 13th cranial nerve, is thought to possess olfactory function in some animal species, and may serve as a possible afferent pathway mediating the sneeze reflex in man.[1,2]

The tactile, mechanical, and nociceptive sensory supply of the nasal mucosa is derived from the ophthalmic (V_1) and maxillary (V_2) divisions of the trigeminal nerve. The ophthalmic division arises in the trigeminal ganglion and travels through the cavernous sinus where it is joined by postganglionic sympathetic nerve fibers. The ophthalmic nerve continues into the orbit and then branches to form the nasociliary nerve. This nerve further branches to form the anterior and posterior ethmoidal nerves which provide both sensory and sympathetic innervation to the superior and lateral nasal cavity (Fig. 1).

The maxillary division of the trigeminal nerve also originates in the trigeminal ganglion and travels to the pterygopalatine fossa, where two branches pass inferiorly to the sphenopalatine ganglion. These fibers merge with postganglionic sympathetic and parasympathetic

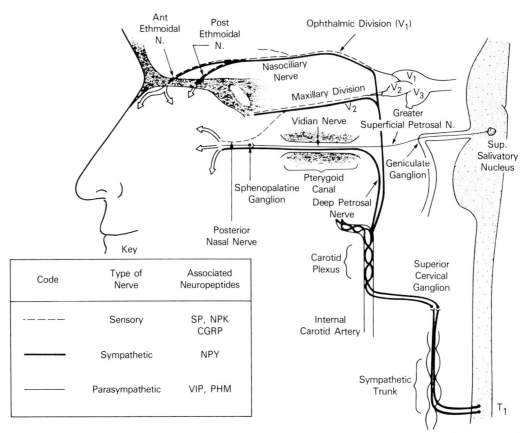

Code	Type of Nerve	Associated Neuropeptides
– – – – –	Sensory	SP, NPK CGRP
——	Sympathetic	NPY
——	Parasympathetic	VIP, PHM

Figure 1. *The innervation of the human nasal mucosa involves sensory nerves, sympathetic nerves, and parasympathetic nerves. Both classical neurotransmitters and neuropeptides have been identified in these nerves (see text for details).*

fibers and then enter the nasal cavity as the posterior nasal nerve. This nerve provides the majority of sensory afferent nerve fibers to the nasal mucosa.

Autonomic innervation of the nasal mucosa is supplied by nerves from both the sympathetic and parasympathetic nervous systems. Together these systems regulate the secretory and vasomotor activity of the submucosal glands and blood vessels and thus play important roles in humidification and thermoregulation of inspired air and in regulation of nasal airway patency.

Sympathetic fibers originate in the thoracic spinal cord and ascend via the sympathetic trunk to synapse in the superior cervical ganglion (Fig. 1). Postganglionic fibers exit from this ganglion and ascend as a plexus along the internal carotid artery. Some of the fibers leave this plexus to form the deep petrosal nerve, while other fibers are believed to reach the nasal mucosa by traveling along the ethmoidal and infraorbital branches of the trigeminal nerve.[1] The deep petrosal nerve is then joined by parasympathetic fibers from the greater superficial petrosal nerve and together they enter the pterygoid canal as the Vidian nerve. The Vidian nerve exits the canal into the pterygopalatine fossa to form the sphenopalatine ganglion. Postganglionic sympathetic fibers pass through the sphenopalatine ganglion

without synapsing, enter the nasal cavity as part of the posterior nasal nerve, and are distributed to mucosal blood vessels with branches of V_2 (Fig. 1).

Parasympathetic fibers originate in the superior salivatory nucleus of the brainstem and join the facial nerve (CN VII) as the nervus intermedius. These fibers continue with the facial nerve to the geniculate ganglion where they branch to form the greater superficial petrosal nerve. These fibers then merge with fibers of the deep petrosal nerve to form the Vidian nerve. Parasympathetic fibers synapse in the sphenopalatine ganglion. Postganglionic fibers are distributed to glands and blood vessels in the nasal mucosa with branches of V_2.

In summary, the majority of sensory nerves in the nasal mucosa are supplied by branches of the trigeminal nerve. Consequently, many nasal reflexes which originate from the nose involve this afferent pathway. The autonomic nervous supply, in contrast, is anatomically complex and regulates both secretory and vasomotor activities of the nose. Together these nervous systems provide the afferent and efferent limbs of nasal reflexes.

NEUROPEPTIDES IN THE NOSE

The classical neurotransmitters of the postganglionic autonomic nerves are acetylcholine (ACh) and norepinephrine (NE). However, stimulation of these nerves after pretreatment with cholinergic and adrenergic antagonists still produces significant physiologic changes. The observation that exogenous administration of neuropeptides mimics parasympathetic and sympathetic nerve stimulation led to the hypothesis that neuropeptide-containing nerves may participate in the regulation of nasal blood flow, glandular secretion, and physiologic responses in both health and disease.[3] At least six neuropeptides have been identified in nasal nerves (Table I). Unique combinations of neuropeptides are present in sensory, parasympathetic, and sympathetic nerves.[4–7]

The concept that several neuropeptides can coexist with classical transmitters in one nerve has wide ranging implications for better understanding of neural physiology and pathophysiology. A single neuron may release one transmitter under one set of conditions and several transmitters under different conditions.[8,9] Release of both a classical neurotransmitter and one or more neuropeptides leads to complex pre- and postsynaptic interactions, which may "fine tune" neurologic response.[7,8]

Neuropeptides are contained within varicosities, which are bulb-like thickenings that are strung like beads along the neural axon. Once released from these varicosities, neuropeptides diffuse locally to interact with available receptors on target cells. The stimulation produced by neuropeptides is slower in onset but longer in duration than that from classic neurotransmitters. Neuropeptides have no mechanisms for neuronal reuptake and therefore continue to interact with their receptors until displaced or degraded by cell membrane-associated proteolytic enzymes which are widely distributed throughout the body. Inhibition of neuropeptide-degrading enzymes could prolong the survival of neuropeptides and amplify their effects.[11]

Sensory peptidergic nerves are predominantly small, nonmyelinated C-fibers.[12,13] Bare terminal endings are present in the epithelium of the nasal mucosa. These nerves branch extensively and extend to vessels, glands, and, in other tissues, to smooth muscle. The cell bodies of these nerves are located in the trigeminal ganglion. These sensory fibers can be immunohistochemically identified by the presence of tachykinins and calcitonin gene-related polypeptide (CGRP).[5] Tachykinins are a group of structurally and functionally related peptides.[14] In humans, SP, neuropeptide K (NPK), and neurokinin A (NKA) are the tachykinins which have been identified and characterized. Related tachykinins in other species include neurokinin B (NKB), eledoisin, eledoisin-related peptide, physallaemin, and kassinin. CGRP is a neuropeptide which is structurally unrelated to the tachykinins.

Sensory fibers depolarize and release their transmitters in response to a broad range of irritant and pharmacologic stimuli including: capsaicin (the active agent in red peppers), bradykinin, histamine (via H_1 receptors), serotonin, prostaglandins, leukotrienes, complement-derived anaphylatoxins, VIP, formaldehyde, cigarette smoke, high doses of nicotine, and antidromic stimulation.[3,5,15] Depolarization can be blocked by opiates, clonidine, and local anesthetics.

The depolarization of a single intraepithelial or subepithelial nerve ending leads to depolarization of an entire, widely branched C-fiber. Neuropeptides released from these C-fibers depolarize adjacent nerves, triggering an axon reflex which can rapidly initiate a widespread injury response and produce changes in blood flow and glandular secretion. Since mast cells are frequently located near subepithelial neurons, axon reflex-induced mast cell degranulation could serve as a potent amplifier of irritant stimulation.[14]

Sensory nerves innervate both resistance and capacitance vessels. CGRP produces a potent relaxation of arterial smooth muscle but has no effect on venous tissue.[16] SP can also produce arterial vasodilation, but appears to require the concomitant presence of an endothelium-derived relaxation factor.[17] SP has a greater effect on capacitance vessels (postcapillary venules and veins), where it produces venodilation and increases vascular permeability.[3] NKA has a relatively weak effect on venous tissue.

Neuropeptides may have an important role in control of glandular secretion. Coles et al.[18] demonstrated that SP induces a rapid release of preformed mucus from

TABLE I

Effects of Neuropeptides Found in Peptidergic Nerves

Type of Nerve	Arterial Vessels	Venous Vessels	Vascular Permeability
Sensory			
CGRP	Dilates	—	*
SP	Dilates	Dilates	Increases
NKA	—	—	*
Parasympathetic			
VIP	Dilates	Dilates	*
PHM	Dilates	Dilates	ND
Sympathetic			
NPY	Constricts	—	—

—, No effect; ND, Not done; *, Induces small wheals after intradermal injection, which may reflect changes in vascular permeability; CGRP, calcitonin gene-related peptide; SP, substance P; NKA, neurokinin A; VIP, vasoactive intestinal peptide; PHM, polypeptide with histidine at the N-terminal and methionine at the C-terminal; NPY, neuropeptide Y.

tracheal glands without stimulating active acinar cell secretion. SP may also increase nasal secretion by an axon reflex-mediated stimulation of parasympathetic nerves.[3] NKA may act synergistically with SP, as this combination augments the production of a watery parotid secretion in the rat.[19] CGRP does not directly stimulate secretion, but produces local arterial vasodilation which results in an increased fluid flux and an indirect increase in secretion. It is apparent from these and other studies that SP, NKA, and CGRP can produce varied effects. Since all three neuropeptides have been found to coexist in the same neuron and may be released simultaneously, the response may be determined by the availability and distribution of specific receptors.

Postganglionic parasympathetic nerves contain ACh, VIP, and polypeptide with histidine at the N-terminal and methionine at the C-terminal (PHM).[20-22] VIP induces arterial and arteriolar vasodilation.[4] When combined with PHM, VIP induces vasodilation of capacitance vessels. ACh, VIP, and PHM also increase glandular secretion, but the details of this putative role are poorly defined. In salivary glands, VIP augments ACh-induced secretion, induces atropine-resistant vasodilation and glandular secretion, increases transepithelial water and ion transport producing a watery discharge, and inhibits the release of macromolecules.[23,24] In contrast, VIP in tracheal glands appears to decrease mucus release,[18] an action opposite to that of SP. These preliminary findings suggest that VIP has no direct effect on secretory cells, but potentiates glandular secretion by increasing blood flow, which in turn increases transepithelial fluid flux.

The release of ACh, VIP, and PHM is dependent upon the frequency of electrical impulses in the neuron.[8] At low frequencies, only ACh is released, while at higher frequencies, all three are released. Since VIP and PHM have no reuptake mechanism, they remain in the postsynaptic region until degraded, producing a prolonged effect. In this manner, a graded tissue response can be attained that is dependent upon the intensity of nerve stimulation.

The sympathetic nervous system controls vasoconstriction and nasal patency. Sympathetic nerves in the superior cervical ganglion have been shown to contain both NE and neuropeptide Y (NPY), a neuropeptide which is similar to pancreatic polypeptide. Lundberg et al.[25] suggested that NPY-NE fibers may counter the effects of vasodilatory VIP-ACh fibers and thus serve as important vasoconstrictors of arteriolar resistance vessels. In contrast, sympathetic fibers containing only NE (without NPY) produce vasoconstriction of capacitance vessels.[4,9] NE fibers are also found near glands where they exert relatively mild effects.

Although the details of neuropeptide effects in the human nasal passage are still being defined, they may play important roles in the control of vasodilation, tissue vascular permeability, and glandular secretion. Their wide distribution and their coexistence in autonomic nerves suggest that they may participate in the maintenance of nasal homeostasis and may also contribute to nasal reflexes.

NASAL REFLEXES

Nasal reflexes can be broadly divided into two categories: reflexes which arise from stimulation of nasal mucosa, paranasal sinuses, and nasopharynx; and those which reflexively involve the nose (Table II). Reflexes which arise from nasal stimulation include the rhinosinobronchial reflex, the sneeze reflex, the nasonasal reflex, the sniff reflex, the nasopharyngeal reflex, the nasolaryngeal reflex, and the nasosalivary reflex. Reflexes which arise from elsewhere and reflexively involve the nose include the posture reflex, the crutch reflex, the exercise reflex, the cold reflex, the heat reflex, the light reflex, and the bronchonasal reflex. The neurologic pathways of most of these reflexes have not been completely elucidated and the names used here have been chosen to reflect the origin and tissues involved.

Reflexes which Arise from Nasal Stimulation

The best known nasal reflex is the rhinosinobronchial reflex, often referred to as the diving reflex. In its classic form, the diving reflex involves the immersion of the head into cold water, producing an immediate suppression of respiration (apnea), bronchoconstriction, closure of the larynx, bradycardia, decreased cardiac output, and vasoconstriction of vessels supplying

---

TABLE II

Nasal Reflexes

Reflexes which arise from the nose
  Rhinosinobronchial reflex
  Sneeze reflex
  Nasonasal reflex
  Nasopharyngeal reflex
  Nasolaryngeal reflex
  Nasosalivary reflex
Reflexes arising elsewhere and involving the nose
  Posture reflex
  Crutch reflex
  Exercise reflex
  Cold reflex
  Heat reflex
  Light reflex
  Bronchonasal reflex

---

the skin, muscle, splanchnic bed, and renal circulation, but not the carotid artery.[2,26,27] These reflex responses prevent water from entering the lung, decrease oxygen demands, and maintain cerebral circulation, thereby permitting a prolonged underwater dive.[28] The two major effector organs in this reflex are the lung (nasobronchial reflex) and the cardiovascular system (nasocardiac reflex).

The nasobronchial reflex is generally triggered by the inhalation of dust, smoke, strong odors (e.g., ammonia, perfume) gases (e.g., sulfur dioxide), aerosolized chemicals, and other irritants. Nasal stimulation reflexively produces an immediate bronchoconstriction with cessation of respiration in the expiratory phase (apnea) due to relaxation of the inspiratory muscles.

Several investigators have studied this reflex using different experimental models. In a rabbit model, chronic unilateral nasal obstruction produced hypoinflation of the ipsilateral lung with the development of a subsequent thoracic deformity.[29] In a human model, air blown directly into one nostril of a laryngectomized patient produced hyperinflation of the ipsilateral thorax. Pretreatment with locally applied anesthesia or atropine inhibited this hyperinflation on subsequent challenge.[27,29] These data suggest that nasal stimulation with air produces bronchodilatation.

In contrast, nasal stimulation with irritants can produce bronchoconstriction rather than bronchodilation. Yan and Salome[30] sprayed histamine into the noses of 12 subjects with allergic rhinitis and asthma. All 12 developed marked nasal congestion with a 6-fold increase in nasal airway resistance (NAR). Although the histamine did not enter the lower airways, 8 of the 12 subjects experienced decreases in their pulmonary function (FEV$_1$) which lasted for up to 30 minutes after nasal histamine stimulation. Crystalline silica particles insufflated into the noses of humans[31] or granulated charcoal dust blown into the noses of cats[32] produced bronchoconstriction (increased pulmonary airway resistance). Local atropine treatment or cooling of the vagus nerve prior to provocation prevented respiratory symptoms in humans and blocked the bronchoconstrictive response. These studies suggest that nasal irritation produces bronchoconstriction rather than bronchodilation and that the vagus nerve is involved in the efferent pathway of the reflex.

The trigeminal nerve has been shown to be involved in the afferent pathways of these reflexes. In one study, five subjects with tic douloureux who had undergone unilateral transection of the second branch of the trigeminal nerve for symptomatic relief of this disease were challenged with intranasal crystalline silica dust, and pulmonary airway resistance was measured.[33] Challenge of the "intact" side of the nose produced nasal mucosal burning and lacrimation in all subjects and

caused a statistically significant increase in pulmonary airway resistance. Nasal challenge of the denervated side failed to produce either local symptoms or pulmonary airway resistance changes. Studies by Allen[34] further defined the afferent neural circuit in this reflex. He found that the inhalation of strong odors produced apnea by stimulation of the maxillary nerve (V$_2$) and not through stimulation of either the ethmoidal nerve or the olfactory nerve. One concludes from these studies that the trigeminal nerve is the major afferent pathway in this reflex.

The nasocardiac reflex is another important component of the rhinosinobronchial reflex. Nasal stimulation produces bradycardia, a decrease in cardiac output, and vasoconstriction of the blood vessels supplying the skin, muscle, splanchnic bed, and renal circulation.[2,26,35,36] Vasoconstriction does not occur, however, in the carotid circulation, thus preserving the blood flow to the brain. Electrical stimulation of the trigeminal nerve can reproduce this reflex, while pretreatment with either intravenous atropine or transection of the maxillary nerve and/or ethmoidal nerve blocks both the bradycardia and the fall in blood pressure accompanying electrical stimulation.[26]

Extreme responses to the nasocardiac reflex have resulted in dangerous arrhythmias and even death. This reflex is presumed to be responsible for the "sudden sniffing death" which has occurred in some people who sniff glue to cleaning fluid. Cardiopulmonary collapse has been precipitated by the insertion of nasogastric tubes in some patients. Reflex cardiopulmonary arrests have occasionally followed inhalation of water into the upper respiratory tract.[37] In addition, this reflex may account for a few cases of crib death, where mucus regurgitation has been proposed as the cause of cardiac arrest in these babies.[35] Thus, stimulation of the rhinosinobronchial reflex may produce dramatic, systemic, and even lethal consequences.

A common reflex experienced by virtually everyone is the sneeze reflex. This reflex has not been studied as extensively as the rhinosinobronchial reflex. A typical sneeze involves a coordinated sequence of responses following an appropriate stimulus.[2] First, an initial paresthetic nasal sensation develops, followed by a deep inspiration and then a forceful expiration against a closed glottis. Characteristic behaviors include blinking the eyes, contracting facial and nasal muscles, and occasionally performing violent head and body movements. Frequently there is an associated rhinorrhea and lacrimation. Many of the following stimuli are capable of producing a sneeze: nasal histamine instillation; allergen challenge; inhalation of the same chemical irritants previously discussed; electrical stimulation of afferent neural pathways through the ethmoidal nerve, or efferent pathways through the Vidian nerve or greater superficial petrosal nerve; exposure to bright lights; and cooling of the skin over several portions of the body.[2]

The nasonasal reflex describes the phenomenon where stimulation of one side of the nose produces reflexive changes on the opposite side. A typical example involves allergic reactions where an allergen interacts with the nasal mucosa on one side of the nose and induces nasal secretions from both sides. Konno and Togawa[38] performed unilateral nasal provocation with histamine and collected nasal secretions from both sides. They then repeated these challenges after performing ipsilateral Vidian neurectomies and/or anesthetizing the nasal mucosa with topical cocaine.[38] Unilateral histamine challenge produced bilateral nasal secretion, with a contralateral secretory response of about 60% of the challenge side. Histamine stimulation after ipsilateral Vidian neurectomy abolished the ipsilateral secretory response, but preserved the contralateral response. Histamine stimulation after both ipsilateral Vidian neurectomy and topical anesthesia blocked secretion from both sides. This elegant experiment showed that the Vidian nerve accounts for most of the efferent glandular response to unilateral nasal stimulation, whereas sensory nerves (i.e., the trigeminal nerve) are responsible for the afferent arm of the reflex.

The remaining reflexes which arise from nasal stimulation have not been well defined. The sniff reflex describes the response in anesthetized animals when exposed to strong odors. The nasopharyngeal reflex (also called the aspiration reflex) describes a similar observation where nasal stimulation triggers a rapid, repetitive series of inspiratory efforts which draw foreign bodies back into the nasopharynx where they can either be coughed up or swallowed. Both the sniff reflex and the nasopharyngeal reflex can clear the nose of mucus or other foreign material. The nasolaryngeal reflex describes the laryngeal constriction which develops after nasal or nasopharyngeal stimulation.[28] This reflex is similar to the rhinosinobronchial reflex in that it helps to protect the lung from noxious stimuli. The rhinosalivary reflex[39] is analogous to the canine Pavlovian reflex and describes the increased salivation which occurs in response to certain inhaled stimuli.

Reflexes Arising Elsewhere and Involving the Nose

One of the most common nasal reflexes, the posture reflex, defines the nasal obstruction which develops when a person lies down. Upon assuming the lateral recumbent position, there is an increase in ipsilateral NAR and a decrease in contralateral NAR. This response to body position is independent of head position. In a study by Cole and Haight,[40] subjects lying on their backs (dorsal recumbency) rotated their bodies to the lateral recumbent position while maintaining their heads facing upwards. The NAR increased ipsilaterally

and decreased contralaterally depending on which side was dependent, despite the fact that the head position did not change. Horizontal rotation of the head from side to side while sitting or standing produced no change in NAR.

Reflex nasal congestion can also be produced by applying unilateral pressure to the trunk and/or limbs.[41] Subjects were placed in the dorsal recumbent position while a mattress supported only one side of their bodies.[40] The NAR increased on the mattress side of the body and decreased on the unsupported side, suggesting that unilateral pressure applied by the mattress to the trunk caused reflexive changes in NAR.

A similar reaction is seen in the crutch reflex, where as crutch applied against the axilla produces ipsilateral nasal congestion. Davies and Eccles[42] studied 29 subjects who, while seated, applied a crutch firmly against one axilla for 15 minutes. In more than 80% of the cases, the NAR increased on the side ipsilateral to the crutch and decreased on the contralateral side. The authors proposed that sensory receptors in the skin were stimulated by pressure and caused an ipsilateral change in sympathetic activity which increased the NAR.

In the exercise reflex, the performance of vigorous exercise produces an immediate drop in total NAR. The decrease in NAR begins within 30 seconds, reaches a nadir in about 5 minutes, and then persists for up to 30 minutes after completion of exercise.[43,44] The magnitude of the decrease in NAR varies proportionally with the amount of work, decreasing by 39% at a workload of 75 watts and by 49% at workload of 100 watts.[43] The rapid initial drop in NAR mirrors the general circulatory response to exercise and appears to result from vasoconstriction secondary to increased sympathetic discharge.[45] This reflex reliably occurs in normal subjects and in most, but not all, subjects with allergic rhinitis,[43,46] perhaps reflecting differences in baseline nasal resistance.

In the exercise reflex, the amount of work and not the body position determines the response. Assessments of NAR taken from subjects performing equal amounts of work in either the erect or dorsal recumbent position, or measured when they breathed through either their noses or their mouths, indicated that no differences in NAR were produced. In contrast, isocapneic hyperventilation without exercise failed to alter the baseline NAR.[45] Thus the decrease in NAR was strictly dependent on the work of exercise.

Several reflexes have been elicited by cold temperature. The inhalation of cold air has been shown to cause bronchospasm in asthmatics. Exposure to the cold for prolonged periods may cause rhinorrhea in many people. Nasal provocation with cold, dry air was found to produce rhinorrhea and nasal congestion associated with the release of inflammatory mediators into nasal washings. Previous studies by Anderson et al.[47] showed that dry air does not, by itself, significantly alter nasal mucus production. Therefore Togias et al.[48] proposed that cold air challenge increased nasal mucosal osmolarity, producing a nonimmunologic release of inflammatory mediators and causing nasal secretion and congestion. However, the pathogenesis of cold air-induced rhinorrhea remains controversial, and Ostberg et al.[49] recently proposed that the etiology involves a cholinergic reflex, resulting in an ipratropium-inhibitable glandular hypersecretion. Probably both mechanisms contribute to cold-induced rhinorrhea.

Cooling of the extremities also affects nasal function. Inserting a foot into a bucket of cold water produces a reflexive increase in NAR due to a decrease in nasal blood flow and an increase in mucosal congestion.[27] This effect may last for hours after removing the foot from the cold water.

Cold stimulation may also affect the lower airways. When a cold stimulus is placed on the face and/or nose (over areas of trigeminal nerve innervation), bronchoconstriction develops. In a study by Josenhans et al.[50] plastic bags containing ice water or room temperature water were placed over the side of the face (ears, cheeks, and nose) while the subjects performed pulmonary function tests. Water at 23° C produced no pulmonary function changes, whereas water at 4° C produced a 14% drop in airway conductance. Furthermore, in the rhinosinobronchial reflex, it has been suggested that cold receptors may be more important in triggering the reflex bronchoconstriction than the actual immersion of the face into water.[51]

In contrast to cold stimulation of the face, cold stimulation of the trunk produces an increase in respiration. Keatinge and Nadel[52] measured respiratory responses in subjects exposed to cold water showers. Ice-cold water produced initial gasps followed by an increase in respiration. There was an inverse relationship between water temperature and level of respiration which was independent of pain perception.

Heat and light have also been implicated in producing reflexes involving the nose. Infrared light rays from dull red or dark sources applied to the skin of the face or trunk produce nasal congestion.[1] Details of this heat reflex are unknown. A light reflex has also been described in which exposure to bright light from the outdoors or from an ophthalmoscope causes an immediate sneeze response.[53] This response occurs only after a period of relative darkness and only upon the initial exposure. Male Caucasians most frequently manifest this reflex, and it appears to bear no relationship to atopic status.

The final reflex which will be mentioned is the bronchonasal reflex. Gherson et al.[54] performed bronchial provocation with ultrasonic nebulized distilled water and noted that NAR increased in 19 of 23 allergic rhinitis subjects and in 2 of 12 normal subjects, without causing any sneezing or rhinorrhea. In asthmatic subjects, NAR increased after ultrasonic nebulized distilled water challenge only in those subjects who also complained of rhinitis. The mechanism of this reflex is unclear, but does not appear to involve parasympathetic efferent nerves since there is no secretory response to ultrasonic nebulized distilled water challenge.

REFERENCES

1. Eccles R. Neurological and pharmacological considerations. In: Proctor DF, Anderson IB, (eds). The Nose: Upper Airway Physiology and the Atmospheric Environment. Amsterdam: Elsevier Biomedical Press, 1982, pp 191–214.
2. Widdicombe JG. Reflexes from the upper respiratory tract. In: Fishman AP, Cherniak NS, Widdicombe JG, Geiger SR, (eds). Handbook of Physiology. Section 3. The Respiratory System. Volume II, Control of Breathing, Part 1. Washington, DC: American Physiological Society, 1986. pp 363–394.
3. Hua X-Y. Tachykinins and calcitonin gene-related peptide in relation to peripheral functions of capsaicin-sensitive sensory nerves. Acta Physiol Scand 127(suppl 5511):1–45, 1986.
4. Änggård A, Lundberg JM, Lundblad L. Nasal autonomic innervation with special reference to peptidergic nerves. Eur J Respir Dis 64(suppl 128):143–148, 1983.
5. Lundblad L. Protective reflexes and vascular effects in the nasal mucosa elicited by activation of capsaicin-sensitive substance P-immunoreactive trigeminal neurons. Acta Physiol Scand Suppl 529:1–42, 1984.
6. Dale H. Pharmacology and nerve endings. Proc R Soc Med 28:319–332, 1934.
7. Eccles JC. Clinical transmission and Dale's principle. Prog Brain Res 68:3–13, 1986.
8. Iversen LL. Chemical signaling in the nervous system. Prog Brain Res 68:15–21, 1986.
9. Lundberg JM, Hökfelt T. Multiple co-existence of peptides and classical transmitters in peripheral, autonomic and sensory neurons: functional and pharmacological implications. Prog Brain Res 68:241–262, 1986.
10. Stimler-Gerard NP. Neutral endopeptidase-like enzyme controls the contractile activity of substance P in guinea pig lung. J Clin Invest 79:1819–1825, 1987.
11. Borson DB, Corrales R, Varsano S, Gold M, Viro N, Caughey G, Ramachandran J, Nadel JA. Enkephalinase inhibitors potentiate substance P-induced secretion of $^{35}SO_4$-macromolecules from ferret trachea. Exp Lung Res 12:21–36, 1987.
12. Cauna N. Blood and nerve supply in nasal lining. In: Proctor DF, Anderson IB, eds. The Nose: Upper Airway Physiology and Atmospheric Environment. Amsterdam: Elsevier Biomedical Press, 1982, pp 45–69.
13. Uddman R, Malm L, Sundler F. Substance-P-containing nerve fibers in the nasal mucosa. Arch Otorhinolaryngol 238:9–16, 1983.
14. Foreman JC. Neuropeptides and the pathogenesis of allergy. Allergy 42:1–11, 1987.
15. Foreman JC, Jordan CC. Neurogenic inflammation. Trends Pharmacol Sci 5:116–119, 1984.
16. Hanko J, Hardebo JE, Kåhrström J, Owman C, Sundler F. Calcitonin knee-related peptide is present in mammalian cerebrovascular nerve fibers and dilates pial and peripheral arteries. Neurosci Lett 57:91–95, 1985.
17. Furchgott RF. Role of the endothelium in responses of vas-

cular smooth muscle. Circ Res 53:557–573, 1983.

18. Coles SJ, Bhaskar KR, O'Sullivan DD, Neill KH, Reid LM. Airway mucus: composition and regulation of its secretion by neuropeptides in vitro. In: Mucus and Mucosa, Ciba Foundation Symposium 109. London: Pitman, 1980, pp 40–60.

19. Ekström J. Neuropeptide and secretion. J Dent Res 66:524–530, 1987.

20. Lundberg JM, Fahrenkrug J, Larson O, Änggård A. Corelease of vasoactive intestinal polypeptide and peptide histidine isoleucine in relation to atropine-resistant vasodilation in cat submandibular salivary gland. Neurosci Lett 52:37–42, 1984.

21. Uddman R, Alumets J, Densert O, Håkanson R, Sundler F. Occurrence and distribution of VIP nerves in the nasal mucosa and tracheobronchial wall. Acta Otolaryngol (Stockh) 86:443–448, 1978.

22. Uddman R, Sundler F. Vasoactive intestinal polypeptide nerves in human upper respiratory tract. ORL 41:221–226, 1979.

23. Said SI. Vasoactive intestinal peptide: Isolation, distribution, biological actions, structure-function relationships and possible functions. In: Glass GBJ, ed. Gastrointestinal Hormones, New York, Raven Press, 1980, pp 245–273.

24. Uddman R, Malm L, Fahrenkrug J, Sundler F. VIP increases in nasal blood during stimulation of the Vidian nerve. Acta Otolaryngol 91:135–138, 1981.

25. Lundberg JM, Änggård A, Hökfelt T, Kimmel J. Avian pancreatic polypeptide (APP) inhibits atropine resistant vasodilation in cat submandibular salivary gland and nasal mucosa: possible interaction with VIP. Acta Physiol Scand 110:199–201, 1980.

26. Patow CA, Kaliner MA. Nasal and cardiopulmonary reflexes. ENT J 63:78–81, 1984.

27. Mygind N. Non-immunological factors. In: Mygind N, ed. Nasal Allergy. Oxford: Blackwell Scientific, 1978, pp 140–154.

28. Widdicombe JG. Defensive mechanisms of the respiratory system. In: Widdicombe JG, ed. International Review of Physiology, Vol 14, Respiratory Physiology II. Baltimore: University Park Press, 1977, pp 291–315.

29. Drettner B. Pathophysiologic relationship between the upper and lower airways. Ann Otol Rhinol Laryngol 79:499–505, 1970.

30. Yan K, Salome C. The response of the airways to nasal stimulation in asthmatics with rhinitis. Eur J Resp Dis 64(suppl 128):105–108, 1983.

31. Kautman J, Wright GW. The effect of nasal and nasopharyngeal irritation on airway resistance in man. Am Rev Respir Dis 100:626–630, 1969.

32. Widdicombe JG, Kent DC, Nadel JA. Mechanism of bronchoconstriction during inhalation of dust. J Appl Physiol 17:613–616, 1962.

33. Kaufman J, Chen JC, Wright GW. The effect of trigeminal resection on reflex bronchoconstriction after nasal and nasopharyngeal irritation in man. Am Rev Respir Dis 101:768–769, 1970.

34. Allen WF. Effect of various inhaled vapors on respiration and blood pressure in anesthetized, unanesthetized, sleeping, and anosmic subjects. Am J Physiol 88:620–632, 1929.

35. Allison DJ. Reflexes from the nose. N Engl J Med 299:1468, 1978.

36. James JEA, Daly MdeB. Reflex respiratory and cardiovascular effects of stimulation of receptors in the nose of the dog. J Physiol 220:673–696, 1972.

37. James JEA, Daly MdeB. Nasal reflexes. Proc Soc Med 62:1287–1293, 1969.

38. Konno A, Togawa K. Role of the Vidian nerve in nasal allergy. Ann Otol Rhinol Laryngol 88:258–266, 1979.

39. Settipane G. Rhino-sino-bronchial reflex. Immunol Allergy Prac 7:498–501, 1985.

40. Cole P, Haight JSJ. Posture and nasal patency. Am Rev Respir Dis 129:351–354, 1984.

41. Konno A. Bilateral rhinometry. Jpn J Otolaryngol 72:49–65, 1969.

42. Davies AM, Eccles R. Reciprocal changes in nasal resistance to airflow caused by pressure applied to the axilla. Acta Otolaryngol (Stockh) 99:154–159, 1985.

43. Forsyth RD, Cole P, Shephard RJ. Exercise and nasal patency. J Appl Physiol 55:860–865, 1983.

44. Syabbalo NC, Bundgaard A, Widdicombe JG. Effects of exercise on nasal airflow resistance in healthy subjects and in patients with asthma and rhinitis. Bull Eur Physiopathol Respir 21:507–513, 1985.

45. Olson LG, Strohl KP. The response of the nasal airway to exercise. Am Rev Respir Dis 135:356–359, 1987.

46. McFadden ER Jr. Nasal-sinus-pulmonary reflexes and bronchial asthma. J Allergy Clin Immunol 78:1–3, 1986.

47. Anderson IB, Lundqvist GR, Proctor DF. Human nasal mucosal function under four controlled humidities. Am Rev Respir Dis 106:438–449, 1972.

48. Togias AG, Naclerio RM, Proud D, Fish JE, Adkinson NF Jr, Kagey-Sobotka A, Norman PS, Lichtenstein LM, Nasal challenge with cold, dry air results in release of inflammatory mediators. Possible mast cell involvement. J Clin Invest 76:1375–1381, 1985.

49. Østberg B, Winther B, Mygind N. Cold air-induced rhinorrhea and high-dose ipratropium. Arch Otolaryngol Head Neck Surg 113:160–162, 1987.

50. Josenhans WT, Melville GN, Ulmer WT. The effect of facial cold stimulation on airway conductance in healthy man. Can J Physiol Pharmacol 47:453–457, 1969.

51. Kawakami Y, Natelson BH, DuBois AB, Cardiovascular effects of face immersion and factors affecting diving reflex in man. J Appl Physiol 23:964–970, 1967.

52. Keatinge WR, Nadel JA. Immediate respiratory response to sudden cooling of the skin. J Appl Physiol 20:65–69, 1965.

53. Everett HC. Sneezing in response to light. Neurology 14:483–490, 1964.

54. Gherson G, Moscato G, Vidi I, Salvaterra A, Candura F. Non-specific nasal reactivity: a proposed method of study. Eur J Respir Dis 69:24–28, 1986.

Chapter XVI

Sleep Apnea and Nasal Patency

Richard P. Millman, M.D.

ABSTRACT

Clinical investigations over the last decade have revealed that sleep may not be the benign rejuvenating state it was once considered. Sleep apnea is now frequently recognized, and it is clear that patency of the nasal passages and the nasopharynx is crucial for successful treatment of the syndrome. Furthermore, partial or complete nasal obstruction even in normal subjects can cause sleep disruption, hypopneas, and apneas. This may partially explain some of the daytime drowsiness seen in patients with conditions such as allergic rhinitis.

Obstructive sleep apnea was first described in 1965. In the last 12 years there has been a marked burgeoning of knowledge about the syndrome. In a recent call for research grants the National Institutes of Health suggested that 2–4% of the population may suffer from this condition. As will be discussed below, patency of the nasal passages and the nasopharynx has been shown to be a major factor in the pathogenesis of this disorder.

AN INTRODUCTION TO BASIC SLEEP PHYSIOLOGY

In order to fully understand the role of the nose in obstructive sleep apnea, it is important to understand some rudimentary sleep physiology. Sleep can be divided into five stages. Nonrapid eye movement (NREM) sleep consists of stages 1 and 2 of "light sleep," and stages 3 and 4 which are typically referred to as "deep sleep" or "delta sleep." Rapid eye movement (REM) sleep is the fifth stage and is classically thought of as the state associated with dreaming. In point of fact, dreaming occurs throughout sleep, although the dreams associated with REM sleep are typically con-

crete and more easily recalled. REM sleep is furthermore characterized by an active cortex, generalized hypotonia of the body, and rapid eye movements associated with electrical discharges from the pontine-geniculate-occipital region of the brain. There are usually three or four NREM-REM cycles in the course of a typical night sleep with each lasting 90–120 minutes. A greater proportion of deep sleep occurs in the first half of the night, with more REM sleep in the latter half of the night.

Even in subjects without sleep apnea there are differences in breathing pattern in the different stages of sleep. Stages 1–2 sleep is characterized by periodic breathing, while breathing becomes very regular in Stages 3–4 sleep.[1] Breathing in REM sleep has classically been described as irregular. Part of this irregularity appears to be related to an inhibition of ventilation which occurs in association with the phasic rapid eye movement activity.[2] The variability in the measurement of ventilation in REM sleep may be dependent on the degree of phasic activity in any given REM period. REM sleep can potentially be dangerous for patients with certain medical conditions, such as chronic obstructive lung disease. Air trapping and hyperinflation lead to flattening of the diaphragm in a patient with chronic obstructive lung disease. The diaphragm is thus at a mechanical disadvantage, and the patient has to rely on the intercostal muscles to maintain normal ventilation. During REM sleep these intercostal muscles become hypotonic, the functional residual capacity of the lung decreases, and the patient can become profoundly hypoxic.[3]

OBSTRUCTIVE SLEEP APNEA

Obstructive sleep apnea is a syndrome characterized by recurrent collapse of the pharynx during sleep. By arbitrary definition an obstructive apnea lasts for at least 10 seconds; respiratory effort continues despite a total absence of nasal and oral airflow.[4] Typically the resumption of airflow is heralded by an arousal seen on the electroencephalograph (EEG) to a lighter stage of

Division of Pulmonary and Critical Care Medicine, Rhode Island Hospital, and the Department of Medicine, Program in Biology and Medicine, Brown University, Providence, RI

sleep or to the awake state. Sometimes the airway is not totally obstructed and there is a partial decrease in airflow; this is called an obstructive hypopnea. The literature is very confusing about the definition of a hypopnea. In our laboratory we define a hypopnea as a decrease in nasal and oral airflow lasting at least 10 seconds and associated with at least a 2% fall in oxygen saturation and a subsequent arousal. Other laboratories require a 4% fall in oxygen saturation. Patients with obstructive sleep apnea can also be observed to have central apneas during which ventilatory drive is totally turned off for at least 10 seconds. Sleep apnea has been arbitrarily defined as greater than five apneas and hypopneas per hour sleep or greater than 30 episodes per night.[4] This definition has recently been criticized since frequent apneas and hypopneas are now observed in healthy elderly subjects with minimal clinical sequelae.[5] A practical working definition of the obstructive sleep apnea syndrome is the finding of frequency apneas and hyponeas during sleep in association with the typical complex of symptoms.[6]

It is felt that the oropharynx and nasopharynx collapse during an obstructive apnea when the negative pressure that develops in the hypopharynx during inspiration is greater than the force generated by contraction of the pharyngeal musculature responsible for keeping the airway patent.[7] In the awake state these muscles are actively contracting with resultant dilatation of the upper airway. When one goes to sleep the pharyngeal muscles relax and the airway loses tone. If the airway narrows sufficiently, airflow will become turbulent, leading to vibration of the uvula, soft palate, and posterior faucial pillars, and to snoring. An obstructive apnea occurs if the airway totally collapses.

During the obstructive event the patient struggles to breathe, negative intrathoracic pressure increases, and further suction is applied to the pharynx. Hypoxia, acidemia, and hypercapnia result with subsequent profound physiological consequences. These have been recently reviewed,[8] but in brief there is systemic vasoconstriction, pulmonary vasoconstriction, and increased vagal tone. Rises in systemic and pulmonary pressure are observed,[9] as well as slowing of the heart rate.[10] With the eventual resumption of airflow there is a further rise in blood pressure as the heart rate increases.[11] With a reduction in oxygen saturation to below 60%, ventricular arrhythmias may occur.[12] It is not clear which of these changes actually trigger the EEG arousal. Once an arousal occurs the patient wakes up, the pharyngeal musculature contracts, the airway opens, and a very loud snoring sound is produced as air rushes through a narrow orifice under pressure. The patient may be observed to move around in bed prior to drifting back to sleep. Once the patient is asleep, the throat again collapses and the process starts once more.

The vast majority of these events are unrecognized by the patient, and it is frequently the spouse that bring the problem to medical attention.

Sleep obviously becomes extremely fragmented and in moderate to severe cases the patient is unable to get into deep restorative stages 3 and 4 sleep. Variable but significant daytime sequelae can occur including hypersomnolence, irritability, impairments in memory, attention, concentration, and the ability to solve complex problems, and clinical depression. Sustained systemic hypertension is very common.[11] Furthermore, recent studies have demonstrated that 30% of patients with essential hypertension actually have obstructive sleep apnea, which is either a cause or a contributing factor to the high blood pressure.[13,14] A small percentage of patients develop sustained pulmonary hypertension, cor pulmonale, polycythemia, and daytime hypoxia and hypercapnia consistent with the Pickwickian syndrome.

RISK FACTORS IN THE DEVELOPMENT OF OBSTRUCTIVE SLEEP APNEA

Various factors that play a role in the pathogenesis of obstructive sleep apnea are shown in Table I. It is intuitively obvious that a narrow throat will tend to collapse more easily during sleep than an open one. Thus, narrowing of the oropharynx or the nasopharynx by macroglossia (myxedema, acromegaly), adenotonsillar hypertrophy, or retrognathia has been associated with obstructive sleep apnea. Obesity is also a significant risk factor. The exact mechanism is unknown, but it has been speculated that the pharynx is extrinsically narrowed in these patients by excess adipose tissue. In other patients the only abnormality may be a deep set palate and long uvula, thus compromising the pharynx.

Experimental studies have shown that the pharynx of a patient with obstructive sleep apnea, besides being narrower, is also more collapsible[15] and that the point

---

TABLE I

Risk Factors for the Development of Obstructive Sleep Apnea

Male sex
Postmenopausal state
Obesity
Adenotonsillar hypertrophy
Retrognathia
Nasal obstruction
Evening alcohol ingestion
Macroglossia
Hypothyroidism
Acromegaly

---

of collapse is located in the oropharynx.[16] The degree of collapsibility is variable; alcohol consumption in the evening can induce snoring and obstructive apneas in susceptible individuals by causing selective relaxation of the pharyngeal musculature without compromising diaphragmatic function.[17] This means that the pharynx will be relatively more hypotonic and thus will be collapsed easily by negative inspiratory hypopharyngeal pressure.

Men are at a greater risk of developing sleep apnea than women. Unless they have significant abnormalities of the pharynx, women tend not to develop apneas until after they have gone through menopause. It is felt that menstruating women are somehow protected by circulating progesterone, which is a known ventilatory stimulant.[18]

NASAL OBSTRUCTION AND THE DEVELOPMENT OF SLEEP APNEA

While it is well recognized that enlarged tonsils and adenoids can lead to obstructive sleep apnea, there is now substantial evidence that partial and complete obstruction of the nasal passages can also cause apneas and hypopneas associated with microarousals and subsequent sleep disruption. This was first noted by early polysomnographic studies of patients with complete nasal obstruction from nasal packing[19] and with partial nasal obstruction from a deviated nasal septum[20] or allergic rhinitis.[21] In the latter study the predominant findings were frequent microarousals associated with only mild changes in breathing pattern.

Allergic rhinitis provides one of the best models of reversible nasal obstruction. McNicholas and his colleagues[22] examined seven patients during an attack of allergic rhinitis and 6–8 weeks later after their symptoms had resolved. During the attack the subjects had more frequent and longer obstructive apneas than when their symptoms had resolved, although none of the subjects had enough events to meet the arbitrary criteria for the diagnosis of the obstructive sleep apnea syndrome. In male patients there was a direct relationship between the increase in nasal resistance during the allergic rhinitis season and the corresponding increase in obstructive apneas. Four of the patients complained of daytime sleepiness during the attack. This raises some interesting speculation about whether the daytime drowsiness seen in hayfever sufferers is purely due to the sedative effects of the oral antihistamines that they are taking or is in fact at least partly due to disrupted sleep.

In a patient with a slightly decreased pharyngeal cross-sectional area (as measured by acoustic reflection), occupational exposure to guar gum dust produced reversible obstructive sleep apnea syndrome with loud snoring, observed nocturnal apneas, and daytime sleep-

iness.[23] Guar gum powder is used in the food industry as an additive and the patient was exposed to substantial quantities of this substance in the plant where he worked. Along with the the sleep complaints he noted irritated eyes, nasal congestion, and rhinorrhea, which were worse when he was at work. At the height of his symptoms, polysomnography revealed 14 obstructive apneas per hour sleep and his nasal resistance was elevated (3.2 cm H_2O/L/sec). Seventeen days after leaving the work environment his symptoms had resolved and the nasal resistance had decreased by 50% to 1.6 cm H_2O/L/sec. A repeat sleep study showed only 1 apnea per hour. One could postulate that he developed the full-blown sleep apnea syndrome, because his pharynx was narrowed.

Complete experimental occlusion of both nasal passages during sleep has also been shown to result in recurrent apneas and hypopneas with subsequent sleep disruption even in normal subjects.[24-26] The first of

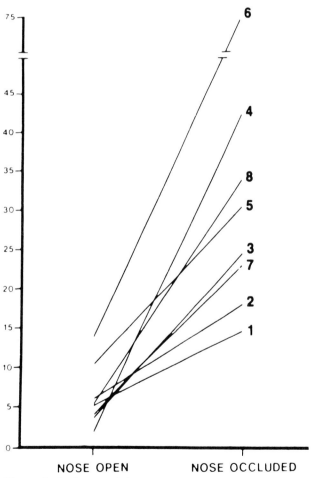

Figure 1. *Occlusion of the nose produces an increase in obstructive apneas and hypopneas during sleep. (From Suratt PM, Turner BL, Wilhoit SC. Effect of intranasal obstruction on breathing during sleep. Chest 90:324–328, 1986, with permission.)*

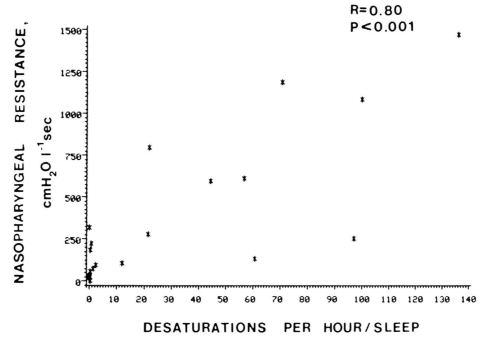

Figure 2. *The relationship between the number of episodes per hour sleep of oxyhemoglobin desaturations of at least 4% and awake nasopharyngeal resistance. (From Suratt PM, McTier RF, Wilhoit SC. Collapsibility of the nasopharyngeal airway in obstructive sleep apnea. Am Rev Respir Dis 132:967–971, 1985, with permission.)*

these studies demonstrated a predominance of central apneas, suggesting that obstruction of the nose caused a generalized decrease in respiratory drive.[24] One could criticize this study, however, for the use of a relatively insensitive respiratory strain gauge to detect respiratory effort. Those studies using an esophageal balloon, which is the most sensitive instrument for detecting changes in intrathoracic pressure, have in fact demonstrated that the apneas and hypopneas that occur with nasal occlusion are obstructive.[25,26] As shown in Figure 1, an otherwise normal subject actually developed over 75 obstructive apneas and hypopneas per hour sleep when his nostrils were blocked.[26]

In patients with known obstructive sleep apnea, the degree of nasal patency has been shown to correlate with the severity of the nocturnal events.[27] Awake nasopharyngeal resistance correlates significantly with the number of apneas and hypopneas per hour sleep, the average oxyhemoglobin desaturation per event, and the number of falls in oxygen saturation of at least 4% per hour sleep (Fig. 2). Although another study has failed to confirm this observation,[28] one could criticize those authors for the use of anterior rhinomanometry to measure awake nasal resistance.

One possible mechanism leading to the collapse of the pharynx with nasal obstruction is that nasal occlusion results in a change in the pressure gradient across the oropharynx promoting its collapse. Olsen and his associates[25] noted that inspiratory intrapleural pressures were consistently greater when the nose was occluded than when it was open. This would imply that oral breathing during sleep is a high rather than a low resistance pathway. Mouth breathing would thus result in an increase in oropharyngeal resistance favoring the collapse of the airway during sleep. It is interesting to note that the nose is the preferred pathway for breathing during sleep in adults,[29] further suggesting that it is the lower resistance pathway for inspiratory airflow.

One would perhaps wonder why mouth breathing does not automatically begin when the nasal passages are partially or completely occluded. The application of subatmospheric pressure to the upper airway of a spontaneously breathing animal leads to a marked increase in inspiratory upper airway muscle airway activity.[30] This reflex is transmitted through the superior laryngeal nerves. In human infants, upper airway occlusion during sleep immediately results in a large increase in phasic genioglossus muscle activity.[31] In sleeping adult humans, however, nasal occlusion in NREM sleep does not produce an immediate increase in inspiratory genioglossal activity as seen in Figure 3.[32] Although there are mild increases in genioglossal activity with each respiratory effort against the blocked nasal passages, a marked increase in genioglossal muscle activity and subsequent mouth breathing does not occur until the subject arouses. In four of the subjects evaluated during this study, genioglossal activity was actually absent during nasal blockade, and it did not resume

146

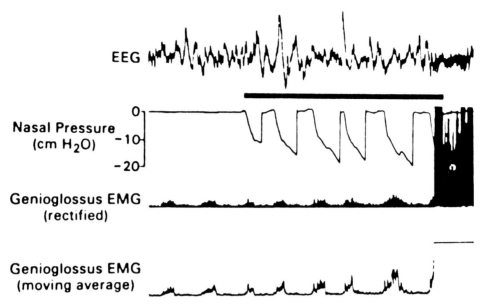

Figure 3. *Nasal airway occlusion during NREM sleep in a subject with phasic genioglossal muscle activity. During occlusion of the nasal passages,——, there is minimal increase in genioglossal electromyogram (EMG) activity until an electroencephalographic (EEG) arousal occurs. (From Kuna ST, Smickley J. Response of genioglossal muscle activity to nasal airway occlusion in normal sleeping adults. J Appl Physiol 64:347–353, 1988, with permission.)*

until an EEG arousal had occurred. During nasal occlusion in REM sleep, mouth breathing could occur with or without a change in sleep state.

Thus, patency of the pharynx during sleep depends on the balance between the forces working to keep the airway open, specifically contraction of the pharyngeal musculature, and the forces working in concert to collapse the pharynx. The latter include the negative suction pressure that develops in the hypopharynx during inspiration as a result of diaphragmatic and intercostal muscle contraction and the resistance of the nasal passages.[7]

THE NOSE AND TREATMENT OF OBSTRUCTIVE SLEEP APNEA SYNDROME

These above observations obviously imply that it is important to ensure that the nasal passages remain open when a patient with obstructive sleep apnea is treated. A failure to deal with significant nasal occlusion can result in a poor response to other treatment modalities, such as the uvulopalatopharyngoplasty which only opens up the oropharynx and nasopharynx. Treatment of nasal obstruction may require surgery and deviated nasal septal repairs have resulted in both subjective and objective improvement in patients with obstructive sleep apnea.[20,33–35] In patients with inflammatory narrowing of the nose, as in allergic rhinitis, topical nasal steroid inhalers or systemic antihistamine-decongestants often prove efficacious. Some patients with mild sleep apnea note a decrease in snoring and a lessening of daytime somnolence with these medica-

tions and do not require an evaluation in the sleep laboratory to confirm the diagnosis.

Another approach to the treatment of sleep apnea is the use of nasal continuous positive airway pressure.[36,37] The patient sleeps with a tight fitting nose mask connected by tubing to a blower. Air is forced down the nose and pharynx, forcing the airway open and thus overcoming the negative inspiratory hypopharyngeal pressure. The airway does not open because of a stimulation of the pharyngeal musculature; the forced air works purely as a pneumatic splint to open the pharynx.[38]

CONCLUSION

Clinical investigations over the last decade have revealed that sleep may not be the benign rejuvenating state it was once considered. Sleep apnea is now frequently recognized, and it is clear that patency of the nasal passages and the nasopharynx is crucial for successful treatment of the syndrome. Furthermore, partial or complete nasal obstruction even in normal subjects can cause sleep disruption, hypopneas and apneas. This may partially explain some of the daytime drowsiness seen in patients with conditions such as allergic rhinitis.

REFERENCES

1. Shore ET, Millman RP, Silage DA, Chung D-CC, Pack AI. Ventilatory and arousal patterns during sleep in normal young and elderly subjects. J Appl Physiol 59:1607–1615, 1985.
2. Millman RP, Knight H, Kline LR, Shore ET, Chung DCC, Pack AI. Changes in compartmental ventilation in association

with eye movements during REM sleep. J Appl Physiol 65:1196–1202, 1988.

3. Fletcher EC, Gray BA, Levin DC. Nonapneic mechanisms of arterial oxygen desaturation during rapid-eye-movement sleep. J Appl Physiol 54:632–639, 1983.

4. Guilleminault C, van den Hoed J, Mitler MM. Clinical overview of the sleep apnea syndromes. In: Guilleminault C, Dement WC, eds. Sleep Apnea Syndromes, New York: Alan R Liss, 1978, pp. 1–12.

5. Knight H, Millman RP, Gur RC, Saykin AJ, Doherty JU, Pack AI. Clinical significance of sleep apnea in the elderly. Am Rev Respir Dis 136:845–850, 1987.

6. Tobin MJ, Cohn MA, Sackner MA. Breathing abnormalities during sleep. Arch Intern Med 143:1221–1228, 1983.

7. Block AJ, Faulkner JA, Hughes RL, Remmers JE, Thach B. Factors influencing upper airway closure. Chest 86:114–122, 1984.

8. Millman RP. Snoring and apnea. Clin Chest Med 8:253–264, 1987.

9. Tilkian AG, Guilleminault C, Schroeder JS, Lehrman KL, Simmons B, Dement WC. Hemodynamics in sleep-induced apnea. Studies during wakefulness and sleep. Arch Intern Med 143:714–719, 1976.

10. Guilleminault C, Connolly S, Winkle R, Melvin K, Tilkian A. Cyclical variation of the heart rate in sleep apnea syndrome. Mechanisms and usefulness of 24 h electrocardiography as a screening technique. Lancet 1:126–131, 1984.

11. Shepard JW. Hemodynamics in obstructive sleep apnea. In: Fletcher EC, Ed. Abnormalities of Respiration during Sleep. Diagnosis, Pathophysiology and Treatment. Orlando, FL: Grune & Stratton, 1986, pp. 39–61.

12. Shepard JW Jr, Garrison MW, Grither BS, Dolan GF. Relationship of ventricular ectopy to oxyhemoglobin desaturation in patients with obstructive sleep apnea. Chest 88:335–340, 1985.

13. Fletcher EC, DeBehnke RD, Lovoi MS, Gorin AB. Undiagnosed sleep apnea in patients with essential hypertension. Ann Intern Med 103:190–195, 1985.

14. Kales A, Bixler EO, Cadieux RJ, Schneck DW, Shaw LC III, Locke TW, Vela-Bueno A, Soldatos CR. Sleep apnoea in a hypertensive population. Lancet 2:1005–1008, 1984.

15. Suratt PM, Wilhoit SC, Cooper K. Induction of airway collapse with subatmospheric pressure in awake patients with sleep apnea. J Appl Physiol 57:140–146, 1984.

16. Smith PL, Wise RA, Gold AR, Schwartz AR, Permutt S. Upper airway pressure-flow relationships in obstructive sleep apnea. J Appl Physiol 64:789–795, 1988.

17. Krol RC, Knuth SL, Bartlett D Jr. Selective reduction of genioglossal muscle activity by alcohol in normal human subjects. Am Rev Respir Dis 129:247–250, 1984.

18. Block AJ, Wynne JW, Boysen PG. Sleep-disordered breathing and nocturnal oxygen desaturation in postmenopausal women. Am J Med 69:75–79, 1980.

19. Taasan V, Wynne JW, Cassisi N, Block AJ. The effect of nasal packing on sleep-disordered breathing and nocturnal oxygen desaturation. Laryngoscope 91:1163–1172, 1981.

20. Lavie P, Zomer J, Eliaschar I, Joachim Z, Halpern E, Rubin A-HE, Alroy G. Excessive daytime sleepiness and insomnia. Association with deviated nasal septum and nocturnal breathing disorders. Arch Otolaryngol 108:373–377, 1982.

21. Lavie P, Gertner R, Zomer J, Podoshin L. Breathing disorders in sleep associated with "microarousals" in patients with allergic rhinitis. Acta Otolaryngol 92:529–533, 1981.

22. McNicholas WT, Tarlo S, Cole P, Zamel N, Rutherford R, Griffin D, Phillipson EA. Obstructive apneas during sleep in patients with seasonal allergic rhinitis. Am Rev Respir Dis 126:625–628, 1982.

23. Leznoff A, Haight JS, Hoffstein V. Reversible obstructive sleep apnea caused by occupational exposure to guar gum dust. Am Rev Respir Dis 133:935–936, 1986.

24. Zwillich CW, Pickett C, Hanson FN, Weil JV. Disturbed sleep and prolonged apnea during nasal obstruction in normal men. Am Rev Respir Dis 124:158–160, 1981.

25. Olsen KD, Kern EB, Westbrook PR. Sleep and breathing disturbance secondary to nasal obstruction. Otolaryngol Head Neck Surg 89:804–810, 1981.

26. Suratt PM, Turner BL, Wilhoit SC. Effect of intranasal obstruction on breathing during sleep. Chest 90:324–329, 1986.

27. Suratt PM, McTier RF, Wilhoit SC. Collapsibility of the nasopharyngeal airway in obstructive sleep apnea. Am Rev Respir Dis 132:967–971, 1985.

28. Blakely BW, Mahowald MW. Nasal resistance and sleep apnea. Laryngoscope 97:752–754, 1987.

29. Gleeson K, Zwillich CW, Braier K, White DP. Breathing route during sleep. Am Rev Respir Dis 134:115–120, 1986.

30. Mathew OP. Upper airway negative pressure effects on respiratory activity of upper airway muscles. J Appl Physiol 56:500–505, 1984.

31. Carlo WA, Miller MJ, Martin RJ. Differential response of respiratory muscles to airway occlusion in infants. J Appl Physiol 59:847–852, 1985.

32. Kuna ST, Smickley J. Response of genioglossus muscle activity to nasal airway occlusion in normal sleeping adults. J Appl Physiol 64:347–353, 1988.

33. Dayal VS, Phillipson EA. Nasal surgery and the management of sleep apnea. Ann Otol Rhinol Laryngol 94:550–554, 1984.

34. Heimer DH, Scharf SM, Lieberman A, Lavie P. Sleep apnea syndrome treated by repair of deviated nasal septum. Chest 84:184–185, 1983.

35. Rubin AHE, Eliaschar I, Joachim Z, Alroy G, Lavie P. Effects of nasal surgery and tonsillectomy on sleep apnea. Bull Eur Physiopathol Respir 19:612–615, 1983.

36. Sanders MH. Nasal CPAP effect on patterns of sleep apnea. Chest 86:839–844, 1984.

37. Sullivan CE, Berthon-Jones M, Issa RQ. Remission of severe obesity-hypoventilation syndrome after short-term treatment during sleep with nasal continuous positive airway pressure. Am Rev Respir Dis 128:177–181, 1983.

38. Strohl KP, Redline S. Nasal CPAP therapy, upper airway activation, and obstructive sleep apnea. Am Rev Respir Dis 134:555–558, 1986. □

CLINICAL DISEASES

Chapter XVII

The Epidemiology of Allergic Rhinitis

J. Montgomery Smith, M.D.

ABSTRACT

Allergic rhinitis belongs to the IgE-mediated family of conditions older allergists called the allergic diathesis. These are atopic eczema, allergic rhinitis, and extrinsic asthma. Whether all asthma of the intrinsic or non-IgE mediated type and the nasal equivalent, hypertrophic sinus disease with nasal polyps, also belong to this group continues to be debated. Weaker epidemiologic connections repeatedly have been found between these conditions and the atopic diseases, but definitions are a frequent difficulty.

Available data do not tell us with certainty whether the different manifestations of atopy represent genetic differences in host susceptibility or effects of environmental factors. Allergen exposure at a critical developmental time or intercurrent viral respiratory infection affecting the host responses have been suggested for this role. What we do know is that there is a tendency for these diseases to take certain forms in certain families. Schwartz[1] demonstrated this nicely many years ago in a careful study of all the living relatives of a large group of asthmatics in Denmark. More recently McKee[2] gave us figures from initial health examinations of people entering a Kaiser Permanente health plan in California. He found that 41% of people with allergic rhinitis had relatives with allergic rhinitis and only 9% had asthmatic relatives. On the other hand, 44% of those with allergic rhinitis and asthma had asthmatic relatives. Eczema also occurs more often in certain allergic families and even nasal polyps and intrinsic asthma are found more often in families where there are others with nasal polyps or intrinsic asthma.[3,4]

+*Department of Internal Medicine, University of Iowa Hospitals, Iowa City, Iowa*

GENERAL INCIDENCE

It is much more difficult to gather epidemiological data about hay fever and allergic rhinitis than about asthma because of difficulties in making the diagnosis by history. In Table I, figures from many countries since 1926 are given. There are some fairly clear indications that asthma has become more common and often more severe than in the first quarter of the century. Allergic rhinitis probably also has become common. It was recognized in antiquity but, as far as one can make out, was less common than in modern "developed" societies. Blakely's works,[5] the best known of nineteenth century studies, cite only 16 patients with hay fever that had come to his notice. However, there are anomalies to be found among the generally lower figures in earlier years so that questions of recognition arise. The much lower number of cases in "underdeveloped" countries is also attributed to difficulties in identifying cases because of language problems, but judging by the lower number of cases of asthma and eczema in the same population it seems likely all these conditions are considerably less common in some relatively isolated tribal groups. There are other groups where the number of cases in village populations approach the experience of Europeans, Australians, and Americans.

Experiences in New Guinea with regard to asthma (with positive skin tests and IgE specific for inhalants) is of particular interest. In the 1970s cases of asthma began to develop in the Fore group of New Guinea village people.[6] Six of the first seven cases recognized at the regional hospital were in people who had worked in the European-influenced community and returned to the villages. Adults were affected rather than children. Since 1976 there has been an increase in cases

TABLE I

Occurrences of Allergic Rhinitis Reported from Various Countries Since 1936

Author	Type Population	Number	Hay Fever
Rehsteiner 1926[46] Switzerland	Rural population	12,600	0.3 0.12–0.2 1.6–4.9
Service 1936[47] Colorado	General urban population	3,143	10.6
Catsch 1943[48] Germany	Mental hospital	1,961	0.9 1.1
Tipps 1954[49]			16.2
Van Arsdal & Motulsky 1959[50] Seattle, WA	U. of Washington		12
Spoujitch 1958[51] Yugoslavia	Farm workers	89,223	4.8
	Civil servants (breakdown not stated)		23.0
Williams 1958[52] Britain	Not stated	36,889	0.44 0.74
Maternowski & Mathews 1962[37] Michigan	U. of Michigan, Ann Arbor		13.4
Van Schnyder 1960[53] Switzerland	General urban population	15,632	4.0–8.6
Broder et al. 1962[16] Michigan	General urban population	1,272	9.7
Sherry & Scott 1968[38] Washington, DC	Howard University		13.9
Giles et al. 1968[54] Australia	Questionnaire and sample exam		6.8
Hagy & Settipane 1969[9] Providence, RI	Brown University		21.1
Varonier 1970[55] Switzerland	School children 5–6	4,781	0.9
	Adolescents	2,451	4.3
Lubs 1971[19]	Twins, 47–86 Questionnaire exam	14,000	14.8
Lebowitz 1975[8] Arizona	General population (in area where many immigrants move for respiratory problems) Tests and interviews	3,850	41
Kjellman 1977[56] Sweden	Questionnaire-medical records School children age 7	1,325	1.5–5.9 (3.8)
Burr et al.[57] Wales	1/8 population over 70	418	7.9
Marks 1978[58] Florida	School children ages 5–16+ Questionnaire, 1/2 returned	3,468	12.1
McQueen et al.[59] New Zealand		2,347	10.4 6.2
Haahtela 1980[60] Finland	Adolescents questionnaire, physical exam. prick tests	708	13–15
Lynch 1984[61] Venezuela	Urban sample	445	19
	Rural sample	336	9.5
Varonier et al. 1984[62] Switzerland	School questionnaire and physician's examination		
	Age 4–6	3,270	1.1
	Age 15	3,500	6.1
Skarpaas 1985[63] Norway	Random sample of school children 6–14 Questionnaire	1,772	5.4

until now 7.3% of adults are affected. Still only 0.6% of the children were asthmatic, and as in countries where asthma is common, most cases were in households with affected adults.

The latest New Guinea study is of another geographic area.[7] There asthma is appearing disproportionately among people who have moved from the vicinity where the disease has become common. If in future an increasing number of cases develop in young children the inevitable conclusion must be that some factor transmitted among adults and then to children has an important role in the development of asthma and possibly atopy. The groups doing this research deserve substantial financial support and further contributions of research personnel thoroughly familiar with the study of both atopy and asthma. For example, armed with knowledge of the pollen and mold seasons it might be possible to identify cases of seasonal nasal allergy despite the language difficulties that have inhibited study of atopic disease other than asthma.

Modern figures for allergic rhinitis usually range from 5% of 20% in both Europe and America, but there is considerable variation reflecting either real differences or definition problems. The very high (41%) rates reported in native-born Arizonians may be the result of the many families who moved to the Southwest to escape the pollens and molds of other parts of the country.[8]

The epidemiology of positive skin tests sometimes has been used as a true measure of the prevalence of atopy because it is an objective test. Hagy and Settipane[9] have shown clearly in their studies of college students that strongly positive skin tests indicate a high risk that respiratory symptoms will develop (see Table II). Less strongly positive tests are much less certainty an indication of atopy. Barbee et al.[10] in the Tuscon studies, graphed an index value derived from the size and number of positive tests against the frequency of respiratory allergy in a large general population and found an ascending curve that reached 93% at their highest skin test score. Yet many asymptomatic people among those with skin tests "2 mm or more" or "greater than control" cannot be classified with certainty as atopic in the sense of having the long-lasting abnormal IgE response characteristic of atopic disease. IgE is a normal antibody response, and a positive test may reflect current or recent exposure. For example, substantial doses of ragweed by injection cause a specific IgE response and positive skin tests in normal subjects,[11] but these responses disappear a few weeks after injections stop.

A good example of a situation where high IgE is maintained by repeated exposure is the case of bee keepers who receive repeated stings.[12] Many of these people lose their high IgE within a few months of giving up their bees. These people fail to show the prolonged high IgE independent of further allergen exposure that characterizes atopy. It is probable that many skin tests slightly or even moderately positive to things people are heavily exposed to, such as house dust, are not indicative of atopy in the sense of disease or abnormal response. Thus, positive skin tests cannot be used as an objective basis for epidemiologic studies of atopy without also considering symptoms and environmental exposure. These problems illustrate the frustration epidemiologists have in defining atopic diseases and comparing data.

Whatever the susceptibility factors for atopy they must be relatively common because of the very high rates of atopic disease in some communities; for example the 21% with hay fever at Brown University and Pembroke College, which draw students from many parts of the USA.[9] The importance of environmental factors also is evidenced by changes in the rate of occurrence of these diseases in various populations moved from low-rate isolated communities in underdeveloped countries to places where these diseases are common.[13-15] There are several clear examples of this

---

TABLE II

Allergic Rhinitis Among College Students (Brown University and Pembroke College)

Number	Asymptomatic Students skin tests (pollen)	Percentage symptomatic 3 yr later	Percentage symptomatic 7 yr later
515	Negative	2	7.7
31	1 +	7	23.3
38	2 +	16	29.4
23	3 +	30	35.0
7	4 +	43	71.4

From Hagy FW, Settipane GA. J Allergy Clin Immunol 58:330, 1976. Of the 65 new cases, 11.6% occurred among previously asymptomatic students.

phenomenon with regard to asthma. Less data exist for rhinitis because rhinitis is less easily diagnosed by history among people who have language barriers and possibly different perceptions of disease.

ALLERGIC RHINITIS SUSCEPTIBILITY FACTORS

Age and family

The most important strong predisposing factors for allergic rhinitis are a positive family history and youth.

Roughly 75% of allergic rhinitis cases begin symptoms by the age of 25, and there is reason to suppose that the great majority of these cases have been sensitized at a very young age. The highest risk time for children born into a household with allergic members is in the first ten years of life. The risk is on the order of 30% for those with a unilateral history and somewhat higher for a bilateral family history in most studies.

Most figures for allergic rhinitis appear to show a later age at onset than for asthma, but it is difficult to differentiate allergic rhinitis symptoms from the recurrent viral colds of young children. At a young age allergic rhinitis is found to be more frequent in boys, while girls catch up in their teens. Typical figures from our studies and those of Broder et al. are shown in Table III.[16–18] The differences between teenaged boys and girls are not large, but the same differences have been found by many authors.

Hagy and Settipane's studies[9] of college students make clear the importance of family history in allergic disease still active in young adults. Most had developed symptoms much earlier, and 64% had allergic first-degree relatives. Nonseasonal allergic rhinitis had developed or been recognized at an average age of 9.1 years and hay fever at 10.6 years.

On the other hand, when hay fever develops for the first time in adults, a positive family history in predecessors is much less common. For example, in our rural study only 4 men and 27 women who had grown up in households with allergic members had developed respiratory allergy after the age of 25. This can be compared with 169 with no family history of allergy who developed symptoms after the age of 25 (approximately 1/5 households had members with respiratory allergy).

In a situation of heavy occupational exposure such as farming or exposure to the enzymes used for laundry products there are many cases of asthma, but with more moderate exposure to outdoor allergens adults usually develop allergic rhinitis rather than asthma (Table IV).[17] A good example of the development of hay fever in adult onset atopy is seen in the study by Ramirez et al.[18a] of military personnel at Brooke Army Medical Center in Texas. The majority of their patients had developed allergic rhinitis rather than asthma after moving to Texas and were allergic only to mountain cedar.

Of 1,084 cases of asthma, hay fever, or dander sensitivity found in the Iowa rural and urban populations studied by us some years ago, 110 subjects with a negative family history had developed symptoms under the age of 20 and another 295 after age 20.[17, 18] One of every four cases had developed in an adult without a known family background of atopy. Heredity in asthma and allergic rhinitis have been assumed to be of major importance because of the family related epidemiology. Certainly the majority of strong and multiple allergies are found in the young of affected households. However, the patients with single allergies, later onset, and a negative family history are certainly also atopic in the sense of a prolonged self-perpetuating IgE mediated allergy.

Studies of twins show greater concordance for atopy in monozygotic pairs. On the other hand, these studies also show that environmental factors also must be important.[19, 20] A study of adult twins in the armed services emphasizes the increasing importance of environment in older onset cases.[21]

Sibbald et al.[22] have been quoted recently for postulating that inheritance for asthma and atopy are genetically separated. They base this view on finding that

TABLE III

Age at Onset of Allergic Rhinitis

Age	Iowa Population Studies				Michigan Studies			
	Male	%	Female	%	Male	%	Female	%
Under 10	171	50	102	36	51	31	37	20
10–19	57	17	75	27	49	30	69	38
Over 20	115	33	104	37	65	39	75	42
Total	343	100	281	100	165	100	181	100

TABLE IV

Onset of Asthma and Hay Fever Over Age 20

	Male	Female	Total
Rural Study (603)			
Allergic Rhinitis	73	46	119
Asthma	47	20	67
TOTAL	120	66	186
City Study (506)			
Allergic Rhinitis	42	58	100
Asthma	14	17	31
TOTAL	56	75	131

skin test negative asthmatic subjects with onset after age 30 have fewer affected relatives than do young asthmatics with positive skin tests. Since late onset but definitely atopic allergic rhinitis patients also have fewer allergic relatives than do those who develop the disease at a young age. The family pattern with respect to age at onset and relatives affected are not very different for asthma and atopy. On the other hand, some allergic families have far more asthma than others. There are no available data that tell us whether we are dealing with several similar diseases affecting the immune system and respiratory system or a single disease whose different presentation depends on age, genetic make up, allergen exposure, and other environmental influences.

ALLERGEN EXPOSURE

It is hard to estimate how many potentially susceptible people fail to become allergic or to manifest an allergy from lack of a suitable allergen exposure. In rural occupations, the ubiquity of allergens both animal and vegetable should ensure that allergens suitable to all comers are available. Yet, several reports suggest a slightly lower occurrence of positive skin tests and symptomatic respiratory allergy in rural areas as compared to nearby urban populations.[23, 24] It can be postulated that this is because affected people leave the farm, but that is not the only possible cause of the phenomenon. In the Iowa rural environment a probable influence of heavy occupational allergen exposure is seen in an excess of men but not women developing asthma in adulthood. On the other hand 1/5 rural families had allergic members compared with 1/4 urban households (Table IV).

If one compares the age at onset for allergic rhinitis in the Iowa and Michigan studies it looks as though the extremely high exposure to pollens and mold in Iowa may have encouraged earlier onset or earlier recognition of allergic rhinitis (Table III).[17] A recent British study notes this same finding. Despite this, most studies comparing urban and rural populations have found atopic disease, if anything, less common in rural areas.

In slums and under the difficult living conditions of various tribal peoples (Canadian Indians,[25] New Guinea hut dwellers,[6] and rural Africans[15]), allergens must be abundant, yet none of these people suffer as much allergic disease as do the more affluent townspeople or university students in the same underdeveloped county.[15] It has been postulated that parasitic diseases with high IgE protect against atopy either by competing for mast cell IgE receptors or by down regulation of the IgE response. This is an unlikely explanation since there are other rural populations where atopic disease and parasitic diseases are common and co-exist.[26]

Allergen avoidance for children born into allergic families who have at least a 30% chance of developing allergies at an early age is logical. Not having house pets in the infant's home and breast feeding to avoid allergens have been recommended. Yet the results of studies of animal avoidance have not been as convincing as our experience in practice seems to be.[27] This is partly because such studies often have been of an effect on the occurrence of atopic disease in general rather than the effect on allergy to animals in particular. Another confounding factor is seen in a Dutch study where dog protein residues were found commonly in carpets where there recently had been no dog.[28] Short

TABLE V

The Prevalence of Ragweed Pollinosis in Foreign and Native Students at a Midwestern University

Native Land	Total No.	No. With Ragweed Pollinosis	No. "Atopic"	No. With Familial Atopy
India and Pakistan	90	5 (6%)	16 (18%)	13 (14%)
China	75	12 (16%)	17 (23%)	12 (16%)
Philippines	40	3 (8%)	7 (17%)	6 (15%)
South America (11 countries)	43	3 (7%)	7 (16%)	8 (16%)
Near East (Turkey, Iran, Iraq)	41	5 (12%)	8 (20%)	7 (17%)
Western Europe	12	3 (25%)	4 (33%)	3 (25%)
Eastern Europe	9	3 (33%)	3 (33%)	2 (22%)
Miscellaneous	12	4 (33%)	6 (50%)	3 (25%)

Maternowski and Mathews (1962).

TABLE VI

Atopic Families Differ in Occurence in Asthma

Subject	Relative's Disease	
	372 Rural Iowa	198 HMO
Allergic	42% Rhinitis	41% Rhinitis
Rhinitis	28% Asthma*	9% Asthma*
	30% Neg	50% Neg
Asthma	24% Rhinitis	25% Rhinitis
	50% Asthma	44% Asthma
	24% Neg	31% Neg

* Modified by environment.

follow-up also may be fault since a study of teenagers found them more likely to be allergic to animals if there was history of household pets early in life.[29]

Breast feeding as a means of allergen avoidance possibly has a role where the infant has been sensitized *in utero* and already at birth has IgE above the normal infant range. Except for that group numerous studies have been almost equally divided in finding protection and no protection against the development of atopy.[30]

There has been a recent flurry of interest in very early exposure to inhalant allergens as a risk factor in the development of allergy. Retrospective studies of month of birth in relationship to pollen allergy suggest among hay fever patients that there may be an excess of births one to two months before pollen seasons. Data have been summarized by David & Beards[31] who conclude that more data are needed before considering the evidence convincing.

There are some industrial exposure situations where the numbers of affected people are definitely increased (i.e., platinum salts[32]). In other situations like the laundry enzyme detergent experience, the number of new cases of respiratory allergy developing per annum is about the same as the number of new cases per annum expected for general populations. More cases of asthma occur but the total number of cases considering both asthma and allergic rhinitis are very similar. (Compare Salvaggio[33] enzyme experience with Broder's Tecumseh, MI experience over a four-year period.[34])

It seems likely that ragweed accounts for higher rates of allergic rhinitis in America than in Europe until one realizes that allergic rhinitis is just as common in those parts of the United States where ragweed is not a problem. One is left with the distinct possibility that failure to meet a suitable antigen is a relatively unimportant determinant of the number of cases of allergic respiratory disease. On the other hand the severity of symptoms, age at onset, and the form the disease takes (whether asthma or rhinitis) may depend strongly on allergens.

RACE AND SOCIAL CLASS

A number of studies suggest that upper social class tends to predispose to allergic rhinitis and atopy (the differences are usually not large). For example, in Rhyne's studies,[35] the well-to-do suburban child had the most frequent positive skin tests. A recent study in Singapore showing less asthma and atopy in Chinese than in Malaysians suggests racial differences and genetic influences.[36] However, location does not necessarily mean that environmental factors are the same, and one would have to know much more about the interplay between the racial groups to guess at the meaning of these findings. The studies of foreign students by Maternowski and Mathews[37] confirm the impression that ragweed hay fever is very common in Chinese students. For many of these students this is a first experience of allergy (Table V). Morrisson Smith looked for allergic disease in the school children of Birmingham, a British industrial city of many races.[13] He found a much greater incidence of atopic problems in children born in England compared to those born elsewhere, primarily in underdeveloped countries. There appears to be so much environmental influence on the occurrence of atopic disease and asthma that no conclusions can be made about racial differences. The only thing one can say is that given the right environment, genetic permissiveness for these diseases must exist in at least 10 to 20% of many very different racial groups.

INFECTION AS A POSSIBLE DETERMINANT IN SENSITIZATION OR MANIFESTATION OF RESPIRATORY ALLERGY

Viral infections appear to have a determining influence on the time of onset of symptoms in at least some cases of asthma. The number of respiratory infections per annum in the two sexes at various ages also parallels the development of new cases of asthma during the first half of life.[16, 34, 38] No such clear parallel appears if one graphs the male and female experience with allergic rhinitis (onsets in each five-year span). Thus, there is no epidemiologic indication of a connection between respiratory infections and allergic rhinitis.[39]

There has been a good deal of interest in viral infections as possible adjuvants in the development of IgE responses to allergens. Frick[40] has reported studies in this area and found a time link or parallel between the development of new antibody responses to viruses and to environmental allergens during the first years of life. We will need to wait for follow-up before we know whether these IgE responses (presumably boosted by the intercurrent viral infections) will have the characteristic duration of atopy. (There seems to be no follow-up, and a number of years have passed.)

The relationship of viral infection and allergy is not at all as clear as the relationship of viruses and asthma. Head colds are so common that a connection between nasal virus infections and allergic rhinitis may never be clearly demonstrated.

There are a number of ways in which viruses could be expected to affect the airways or immune system:

1. Damage and inflammation of epithelial surfaces can make nerve endings vulnerable to irritants.[41]

2. Viruses and some bacteria can affect adrenergic responsiveness (for example pertussus decreases B adrenergic responsiveness).[42]

3. Products of bacteria and of inflammation can affect the release of mast cell mediators.

4. Many viruses and bacteria can act as adjuvants for immune responses and can stimulate formation of specific IgE for the organism.[43]

5. Some viruses are capable of directly infecting cells of the immune system such as lymphocytes and macrophages. They may cause changes in cell products or behavior including prolonging survival in tissue culture.[44]

6. Viruses can change or damage chromasomal material in ways that continue to affect pathology without continued presence of the virus.[45]

Clearly there are many ways in which infections could have a role in the atopic diseases as either primary causes or secondary modifiers localizing or exaggerating effects. However, there are no data to prove any role. The discussion of possible effects is therefore largely speculative, especially with regard to nasal allergy.

PROGNOSIS

Strongly positive skin tests often develop several years before symptoms. In the students studied by Hagy and Settipane[9] markedly positive skin tests were highly predictive of atopic symptoms while less strongly positive tests were considerably less so.

Once symptoms have developed the duration of symptoms is generally a matter of many years but occasionally there is a quite sudden unexplained improvement. In these cases we usually suspect that the environment has changed in some unrecognized way. However, sometimes an allergen such as ragweed seems to have been responsible for symptoms, and yet improvement occurs despite exposure to ragweed.

Asthma seems to have a greater tendency to spontaneously remit than does nasal allergy.

In the past there has been a dictum that hay fever should be treated with allergen injections to prevent the development of asthma. In general population studies, the development of asthma after hay fever has occurred in only about 10% of subjects.[34] Since there is no reliable way of predicting who will develop asthma, treatment for prevention is not warranted. On the other hand there is considerable evidence that far more asthma occurs where there are others in the family with asthma (see Table VI). Since a disproportionate number of family members with more serious disease may appear in an allergy specialty setting, it is possible that differences might appear in that setting and not in general populations. This may account for figures from clinic follow-up studies showing that more untreated than treated children with hay fever develop asthma. Our present state of knowledge is limited enough that hay fever should be treated for its own sake and not on the theory that asthma thus can be prevented.

CONCLUSIONS

Allergic rhinitis is an extremely common disease affecting roughly 10–20% of Americans and probably closer to 10–15% of Northern Europeans. There is a great deal of evidence to suggest it is more common in developed than underdeveloped countries and that environmental factors are important.

Studies of the epidemiology of asthma have been plagued by difficulties of definition. Allergic rhinitis has similar problems made worse by ill-defined similar conditions that are difficult to describe and categorize even in those studies where examination and skin tests have been done. It is very important to have carefully described and carefully chosen populations, and to state definitions of various categories of diagnosis clearly so that the data can be looked at, including and excluding various groups. There are many studies that count numbers of cases (variously defined) but make no effort to look at clustering of cases or sequence of cases as we would with most other diseases of unknown cause. This is at least partly because the family distribution causes us to accept the current theory that these diseases are totally explained by a hereditary defect in IgE responsiveness. The varying epidemiology from country to country, and changes in incidence that occur among people of the same race who change their environment, make it clear that genetic permissiveness for the development of the atopic diseases is very common in most races studied—given the right environment.

Determining the environmental factors that affect the development of atopy should be a prime target area for research. Well-done epidemiological studies that do more than just count cases, are much needed.

REFERENCES

1. Schwartz M. Heredity in bronchial asthma. Acta Allergol 15:3–288, 1952.
2. McKee WD. The incidence and familial occurrence of allergy. J Allergy 38:226–232, 1966.
3. Lockey RF, Rucknagel DL, Vanselow NA. Familial occurrence of asthma, nasal polyps and aspirin intolerance. Ann Intern Med 78:57, 1973.
4. von Maur K, Adkinson NF, Van Metre TE Jr, Marsh DG, Norman PS. Aspirin intolerance in a family. J Allergy Clin Immunol 54:380, 1974.
5. Blakley C. Experimental Researches on the Causes and Nature of Asthma Catarrhus Aestivus. London: Balliere Tindall and Cox, 1873.
6. Woolcock AJ, Dowse GK, Temple K, Stanley H, Alpers MP, Turner KJ. The prevalence of asthma in the South-Fore people of Papua New Guinea. A method for field studies of bronchial reactivity. Eur J Respir Dis 64:571, 1983.
7. Turner KJ, Dowse GK, Stewart GA, Alpers MP, Woolcock AJ. Prevalence of asthma in the South Fore people of the Okapa distrinct of Papua New Guinea. Int Arch Allergy Appl Immunol 77:158, 1985.
8. Lebowitz MD, Knudson RJ, Burrows B. Tucson epidemiologic study of obstructive lung disease. Am J Epidemiol 102:137, 1975.
9. Hagy GW, Settipane GA. Risk factors for the development of asthma and allergic rhinitis: A 7-year follow-up of college students. J Allergy Clin Immunol 58:330–336, 1976.
10. Barbee RA, Lebowitz MD, Thompson HC et al. Immediate skin-test reactivity in a general population sample. Ann Intern Med 84:129–133, 1976.
11. Greenert S, Bernstein IL, Michael JG. Immune responses of nonatopic individuals to prolonged immunization with ragweed extract. Lancet 2:1121–1123, 1971.
12. Reisman RE, Arbesman CE, Lazell M. Observations on the aetiology and natural history of stinging insect sensitivity: Application of measurements of venom-specific IgE. Clin Allergy 9:303, 1979.
13. Smith JM. Studies of the prevalence of asthma in childhood. Allergol Immunopathol 3:127, 1975.
14. Waite DA, Eyles EF, Tonkin SL, O'Donnell TV. Asthma prevalence in Tokelauan children in two environments. Clin Allergy 10:71, 1980.
15. Van Niekerk CH, Weinberg EG, Shore SC et al. Prevalence of asthma: A comparative study of urban and rural Xhosa children. Clin Allergy 9:319, 1979.
16. Broder I, Barlow PP, Horton RJ. The epidemiology of asthma and hay fever in a total community: Tecumseh, Michigan. J Allergy 33:513–524, 1962.
17. Smith JM, Knowler LA. Epidemiology of asthma and allergic rhinitis. I. In a rural area. II. In a university-centered community. Am Rev Respir Dis 92;16, 1965.
18. Schachter J, Higgins MW. Median age at onset of asthma and allergic rhinitis in Tecumseh, Michigan. J Allergy Clin Immunol 57:342, 1976.
18a. Ramirez DA. The natural history of mountain cedar pollinosis. J Allergy Clin Immunol 73:88, 1984.
19. Lubs ML. Allergy in 7000 twin pairs. Acta Allergol 26:249, 1971.
20. Bazaral M, Orgel HA, Hamburger RN. Genetics of IgE and allergy: Serum IgE levels in twins. J Allergy Clin Immunol 54:288–304, 1974.
21. Peat JK, Britton WJ, Salome CM, Woolcock AJ. Bronchial hyperresponsiveness in two populations of Australian schoolchildren. III. Effect of exposure to environmental allergens. Clin Allergy 17:291, 1987.
22. Sibbald B. Extrinsic and intrinsic asthma: Influence of classification on family history of asthma and allergic disease. Clin Allergy 10:313, 1980.
23. Cottin S, Corroller F, LeRest F et al. Frequence et etiologie de l'asthme chez le jeune adulte: Etude systematique dans une population de 190,000 jeune adultes. Poumon Coeur 27:403, 1971.
24. Rodriguez de la Vega A, Tejerio Fernandez A, Gomez Echeverria A et al. investigation of the prevalence and inheritance of bronchial asthma in San Antonio de los Banos, Cuba. Bull Pan Am Health Organ 9:221, 1975.
25. Gerrard JW, Geddes CA, Reggin PL et al. Serum IgE levels in white and métis communities in Saskatchewan. Ann Allergy 37:91, 1976.
26. Lynch NR, Medouze L, DePrisco-Fuenmayor MC, Verde O, Lopez RI, Malave C. Incidence of atopic disease in a tropical environment: Partial independence from intestinal helminthiasis. J Allergy Clin Immunol 73:229, 1984.
27. Luoma R. Environmental allergens and morbidity in atopic and non-atopic families. Acta Paediatr Scand 73:448, 1984.
28. Vanto T, Koivikko A. Dog hypersensitivity in asthmatic children. Acta Paediatr Scand 72;571, 1983.
29. Suoniemi I, Bjorksten F, Haahtela T. Dependence of immediate hypersensitivity in the adolescent period on factors encountered in infancy. Allergy 36:263, 1981.
30. Smith JM. Epidemiology and natural history of asthma, allergic rhinitis, and atopic dermatitis (eczema). In: Middleton E Jr, et al., eds. Allergy: Principles and Practice, 3rd ed. St. Louis: CV Mosby Company, p. 915, 1988.
31. David TJ, Beards SC. Asthma and the month of birth. Clin Allergy 15:391, 1985.
32. Dally MB, Hunter JV, Hughes BG, Stewart M, Taylor AJN. Hypersensitivity to platinum salts population study. Am Rev Respir Dis 123:230, 1981.
33. Salvaggio JE. Occupational asthma. J Allergy Clin Immunol 64:646–649, 1979.
34. Broder I, Higgins MW, Mathews KP, Keller JB. IV. Epidemiology of asthma and allergic rhinitis in a total community: Tecumseh, Michigan. J Allergy Clin Immunol 54:100, 1974.
35. Rhyne MB, Nathanson CA, Mellits D, Rodman AC. Determination of the prevalence and special needs of children with bronchial asthma or atopic dermatitis. Project report to U.S. Department of Health, Education and Welfare, Washington, D.C., U.S. Department of Labor, 1971.
36. Mun CT. Pattern of bronchial asthma in Singapore. Singapore Med J 13:154, 1973.
37. Maternowski CJ, Mathews KP. The prevalence of ragweed pollinosis in foreign and native students at a midwestern university and its implications concerning methods for determining the inheritance of atopy. J Allergy 33:130, 1962.
38. Sherry MN, Scott RB. Prevalence of allergic diseases in freshman college students: a survey based on a predominately Negro population. Ann Allergy 26:335, 1968.

39. Monto AS, Ullman BM. Acute respiratory illness in an American community: The Tecumseh study. JAMA 227:164, 1974.
40. Frick OL, German DF, Mills J. Development of allergy in children. I. Association with virus infections. J Allergy Clin Immunol 63:228, 1979.
41. Hudgel DW, Langston L, Selner JC, McIntosh K. Viral and bacterial infections in adults with chronic asthma. Am Rev Respir Dis 120:393, 1979.
42. Szentivanyi A. The beta adrenergic theory of the atopic abnormality in bronchial asthma. J Allergy 42:203, 1968.
43. Pauwels R, Verschraegen G, Van Der Straeten M. IgE antibodies to bacteria in patients with bronchial asthma. Allergy 157:665, 1980.
44. Bang F. Genetics of resistance of animals to viruses. Adv Virus Res 23:269, 1978.
45. Hupert J, Wild TF. Is the continued presence of virus necessary? Adv Virus Res 31:357, 1986.
46. Rehsteiner R. Beitraege zur Kenntnis der Verbreitung des Heufiebers. Med Diss Zurich, 1926.
47. Service WC. The incidence of major allergic diseases in Colorado Springs. JAMA 112:2034, 1939.
48. Catsch A. Korrelationspathologische Untersuchungen (4). Z menschl Verebungs Konstitutionsl 25:94-127, 1941. Korrelationspathologische Untersuchungen (6). Z menschl Vererbungs Konstitutionsl 26:218–240, 1943.
49. Tips RL. A study of the inheritance of atopic hypersensitivity in man. Am J Hum Genet 6:328, 1954.
50. Van Arsdel PP, Motulsky AG. Frequency and heritability of asthma and allergic rhinitis in college students. Acta Genet 9:101, 1959.
51. Spoujitsch V. L'allergie et son retentissement social dans les differents pays. Yougoslavie III Congress Int Allergol Flammarion, Paris, 1958, p. 881.
52. Williams DA, Leopold JG. Death from bronchial asthma: Discussion. In: Halpern DN, Holtzer A. eds. *Third International Congress of Allergology*, Paris: Flammarion et Cie, 1958, p. 119.
53. Van Schnyder UW. Neurodermatitis asthma-rhinitis. Basel: S Karger, 1960.
54. Giles GG, Gibson HB, Lickiss N, Shaw K. Respiratory symptoms in Tasmanian adolescents: A follow up of the 1961 birth cohort. Aust N Z J Med 14:631, 1984.
55. Varonier HS. Prevalence of allergy among children and adolescents in Geneva, Switzerland. Respiration 27:115, 1970.
56. Kjellman NI. Atopic disease in seven-year-old children. Acta Paediatr Scand 66:465–471, 1977.
57. Burr ML, Charles TJ, Roy K, Seaton A. Asthma in the elderly: An epidemiological survey. Br Med J 1:1041, 1979.
58. Marks MB, Caputo L, Mirmelli P, Zaragoza J. Prevalence of childhood allergy in a subtropical environment. Clin Pediatr 17:613, 1978.
59. McQueen F, Hodaway MD, Sears MR. A study of asthma in Dunedin suburban area. N Z Med J 89:335, 1979.
60. Haahtela T, Jaakonmaki I. Relationship of allergen-specific IgE antibodies, skin prick tests and allergic disorders in unselected adolescents. Allergy 36:251–256, 1981.
61. Lynch NR, Medouze L, di Prisco-Fuenmayor MC, Verde O, Lopez RI, Malave C. Incidence of atopic disease in a tropical environment: Partial independence from intestinal helminthiasis. J Allergy Clin Immunol 73:229, 1984.
62. Varonier HS, De Haller J, Schopfer C. Prevalence de l'allergie chez les enfants et les adolescents. Helv Paediatr Acta 39:129, 1984.
63. Skarpaas IJK, Gulsvik A. Prevalence of bronchial asthma and respiratory symptoms in schoolchildren in Oslo. Allergy 40:295, 1985.

Chapter XVIII
Nasal Disease

John T. Connell, M.D.

ABSTRACT

The nose is exposed to many substances in the external environment, to its own neurogenic system and to various materials (ingested chemicals, foods, hormones, cellular infiltrates, etc.) brought to it via the blood supply. Is it any wonder that nasal diseases arise from a variety of causes of many different pathophysiological forms?

For the clinician, the etiological diagnosis of chronic rhinitis is frustrating. Three possibilities are usually available to him: allergic rhinitis, infectious rhinitis, and vasomotor rhinitis. Vasomotor rhinitis is a term utilized when the findings fit no other category of disease. It is a convenient term to describe disease of unknown etiology. The term often means different things to different physicians, a defect that makes it almost useless.

Twenty years ago I began to do nasal biopsies and studied the histopathology of the nasal mucosa in an attempt to differentiate causes of rhinitis. Since then I have examined over 1500 biopsies. I was initially confused by the marked variation found from patient to patient in the pathology of their mucosa. It eventually became apparent to me that nasal disease can take many forms, thereby explaining the variety of findings. New discoveries in other scientific areas confirm that a variety of heretofore unknown mechanisms could cause the types of nasal pathology I was seeing. Thus, chronic rhinitis is a heterogeneous group of diseases with multiple etiologies.

It is vital that one recognize that nasal disease constitutes a variety of heterogeneous diseases since correct treatment requires a correct diagnosis. In recognizing our deficiencies in this area, more efforts will be made to seek out explanations for the currently perplexing and unexplained findings.

The external surface of the nasal mucosa is columnar epithelium. Some of the columnar cells are ciliated. Others are globular and produce mucus. An acellular basement membrane composed of a complex glycoprotein substance lies immediately beneath the epithelium. This basement membrane may act as a barrier to various chemicals (such as antigens) and possibly even particulate matter such as bacteria and viruses. In this way it may protect the submucosa. The submucosa beneath the basement membrane is a loose network of blood vessels with a supporting structure of collagenous fibriles. Glands are interspersed throughout the mucosa.

Mast cells occur singly in the mucosa at a density of 200 to 400 cells/cu. mm. of tissue. Mast cells are a normal cellular constituent whose most likely function is to control blood vessel diameter and blood flow by controlled release of a number of different mediators. The mast cell mediators also affect itch receptors and can initiate infiltrations of cells such as the eosinophil. Inflammatory cells are probably absent in the mucosa of newborn and normal noses. But, since the nose is bombarded on every breath with a variety of inhalant particulate and gaseous chemicals and infectious organisms, it is quite possible that "normal" noses do not exist in modern society. Thus, a few inflammatory cells may be seen in the so-called

Director, Nasal Diseases Study Center, Holy Name Hospital, Englewood, New Jersey 07631. Presented at the Spring 1982 meeting of the New England Society of Allergy.

161

"normal" mucosa. In this sense inflammatory cells include polymorphonuclears, lymphocytes, plasma cells, monocytes, and eosinophils.

The pathology seen in nasal biopsies by light microscopy may involve the epithelium, the basement membrane, and the lamina propria, or it may consist of an infiltrate of inflammatory cells. Caution must be used in interpreting the pathology, for a biopsy represents the findings at one instant. Pathology may change from time to time, and what is thought of as a unique disease may only be one stage of a disease.

ABNORMALITIES NOT ASSOCIATED WITH THE IMMUNE SYSTEM

1. Neurogenic Disease:

In about 1 per cent of patients with obvious severe nasal symptoms, primarily diffuse rhinorrhea, no histological abnormalities can be found in the mucosa except for edema. The abnormality causing such disease is most likely located in the hypothalamus or the hind brain at the origins of the parasympathetic nervous system, or the parasympathetic nerves themselves. In these patients, surgical resection of the Vidian nerve causes prompt cessation of symptoms. It is interesting to note that some patients so treated have a relapse in one to two years following the procedure. This observation suggests that nerve regeneration has occurred and the abnormal parasympathetic system is once again intact. This disease is probably an abnormality of some part of the parasympathetic system.

2. Epithelial Abnormalities:

Epithelial abnormalities occur in about 20 per cent of patients with chronic rhinitis. The abnormality is usually one in which the ciliated columnar epithelium is replaced by cuboidal cells or even squamous epithelium. In some cases epithelial cells appear swollen and vasculated with enlarged extracellular spaces. The cause of these changes is unknown. Perhaps they will eventually be found to parallel certain skin diseases, for example, contact dermatitis. The nose, because of its exposure to a variety of inhaled chemicals, could theoretically develop a type of contact dermatitis or other abnormalities. *For instance, I have seen a few patients who had active metal dermatitis on wrists, ears, etc. whose primary complaint was nasal congestion. Their nasal mucosa was brownish-red and dry. It is conceivable that they had delayed hypersensitivity of the nose produced by metal elements introduced into the nares on fingers.*

One of the consequences of loss of goblet cells and ciliated epithelium is the loss of the mucus blanket which continuously washes the nasal surface. The mucus blanket moves from the front to the back of the nares, carrying inhaled contaminants posteriorly to eventually

be swallowed. The normal air-conditioning functions of the nose are ablated when the normal epithelium is altered to one of squamous cells.

3. Rhinitis Medicamentosa:

Patients with rhinitis medicamentosa may have a variety of histological mucosal abnormalities, or they may have no histological pathology. The detrimental effect of drugs is apparently a physiological one not associated with infiltrates.

Rhinitis medicamentosa is one clinical entity which is readily recognized by the physician. It may occur following the abuse of topical nasal alpha adrenergic drugs, the oral use of some antihypertensive agents, or at times in women using contraceptive hormones. The pathophysiology of these conditions is suspected but not proven. Abuse of topical adrenergic drugs could produce exhaustion of mediators or metabolites of target cells, causing vasodilatation. Antihypertensive drugs cause medicamentosa by depleting norepinephrine stores, thereby preventing the action of norepinephrine on peripheral sympathetic nerves.[1] Reserpine is known to deplete norepinephrine intragranular pools by blocking active transport of norepinephrine from cytoplasmic to intragranular pools. Guanethidine causes active release of norepinephrine from the intragranular mobile pool, eventually causing depletion of the reserve pool.

The manner in which contraceptive hormones cause medicamentosa is unknown. Nasal mucosa is said to resemble genital tissue in that both are erectile tissues. The erectile response is due to the type of vascular system present and could cause engorgement of the turbinates. In addition, it is possible that hypersecretion in the nose could result from the use of female hormones.

If the subject has no chronic nasal disease but did develop medicamentosa from the drugs mentioned, the expectation is that except for edema, no other histological abnormalities would be found. In my experience about one-third of patients with rhinitis medicamentosa do not have histological abnormalities. The two-thirds who do have abnormalities probably had them prior to the use of the drug. In fact, most patients who abuse topical nasal drugs started to use them because they already had a nasal problem.

The only pertinent physical finding in those who are nose-drop abusers is the intense red color of the mucosa and the turbinate swelling.

4. Rhinitis of Endocrine Origin:

Hypothyroidism is often accompanied by nasal complaints. *In the one case I have seen, the nasal mucosa was extremely boggy with large white turbinates. The only histological finding was intense edema.* The mechanism producing nasal abnormalities in hypothyroidism is unknown but well may be related to intense extracellular edema causing nasal obstruction.

5. Nasal Mastocytosis:

One case that intrigued me when I first began doing nasal biopsies was that of a black 21 year old female who had severe rhinitis all her life. She did not complain of nasal itching. I found 40,000 mast cells/cu. mm. in her nasal mucosal biopsy (normal value for mast cells is 200/cu. mm.) An allergic work-up failed to reveal any indication of allergy. I subsequently found that about 30 per cent of patients with chronic nasal disease had a mast cell count of 2000 or greater. This observation suggested that the mast cell had something to do with the production of nasal symptoms. In 1968, I reported this condition as "nasal mastocytosis."[2]

Many patients who have an elevated mast cell count state that they had no nasal problem until they got a "cold that never went away." It is not known whether they actually had an upper respiratory infection which left them with an elevated mast cell count or whether the so-called "cold" was misinterpreted and was actually the start of the disease. In others, the onset of the disease is insidious. About one in six patients had a history of present or past migraine headaches. This finding is provocative when one recalls that migraine headaches were once thought to be histamine related and that the mast cell secretes histamine. One patient in six recognizes that the ingestion of alcohol causes a marked rhinitis in 5 to 15 minutes. This finding is also similar to that found by Soder et al[3] in systemic mastocytosis where alcohol ingestion frequently causes severe abdominal pain. Many patients with elevated nasal mast cell counts also react with rhinitis to various fumes, such as turpentine, perfumes, etc. There is nothing to suggest that the patients are allergic to alcohol or the various fumes. It seems much more likely that the stimulus for mediator release is through non-allergic mechanisms.

There is no indication that these patients have IgE-mediated disease. They characteristically have low IgE levels and as a group are skin test negative. This finding may be perplexing to some because of the association of IgE molecules fixing to the mast cell. However, it should be recalled that the primary function of mast cells is not related to IgE and many non-IgE mechanisms can cause the mast cell to secrete or release mediators. Selye[4] has called the mast cell the "emergency kit" of the body, meaning that through its mediators it plays a protective role. The mast cell may be thought of as a "microprocessor" whose purpose is to maintain homeostasis through its mediators.

Why do patients with nasal mastocytosis have symptoms? One, and the most plausible explanation, is that the mast cell responds to many stimuli by releasing a variety of or specific mediators depending on the stimulus. It is then easy to see that a diffuse stimulus affects many more mast cells in patients with mastocytosis and causes an excessive but nontheless a physiological response. The fact that the response is excessive leads to symptoms.

Why do mast cells accumulate in large numbers, and why may the condition exist for years? Mast cells are said to increase in tissues affected by an inflammatory response. *I studied nasal mucosa obtained from 100 routine autopsies. Patients who had intranasal catheters (Levin tubes or 0_2 catheters) in place during the last few days of life were the only patients who consistently had increased nasal mast cell counts. This would suggest that irritation in some way was as least one cause for a temporary local increase in mast cells. Why increased numbers of mast cells may persist for years is unknown.*

There are no characteristic findings on physical examination in nasal mastocytosis. The mucosa may appear normal or slightly pale.

Patients with mast cell disease do not respond to antihistamines and do not particularly choose to use oral decongestants. In a small series, some responded to beclomethasone nasal spray.[5] The effect of cromolyn is unknown, although in systemic mastocytosis cromolyn did prevent attacks when given in large doses.

6. Eosinophilic Disease of the Nose:

It is difficult to decide whether eosinophilic infiltrates should be discussed under non-immunological mechanisms or whether they should be included under immunological mechanisms since they are so intimately associated with allergic rhinitis. Vacuoles in blood eosinophils were reported in a large number of patients with eosinophilia.[6] Eosinophils were frequently found in increased numbers in diseases which had no recognized association with IgE mediated conditions. For instance, a slight eosinophilia in the second week was found following myocardial infarction. Furthermore, it is known that the eosinophil infiltrates the infarcted tissue at about this time.

In 1975, I wrote that a non-allergic disease associated with eosinophilic infiltrates occurred in the nose and that breakdown of eosinophils may in fact cause the symptoms.[8] Non-IgE mediated eosinophilic disease of the nose has recently been reported by other laboratories.[9,10] In nasal biopsies this disease is characterized by an intense infiltrate of eosinophils. Many of the eosinophils appear to be ruptured with their granules dispersed in the tissue. This finding does not appear to be an artifact.

Gleich[11] has reported that 40 percent of the contents of the eosinophil consists of major basic protein (MBP). MBP is a harsh chemical. Recent studies utilizing fluorescent-tagged MBP suggest that MBP may cause micro-ulcerations of the bronchial wall.[12] This finding, if verified, is consistent with the hypothesis that MBP could cause tissue damage and symptoms in the nose if released from ruptured eosinophils. Thinning of the basement membrane is found in allergic rhinitis, eosinophilic disease of the nose, and polyposis. The element common to all of these diseases is infiltrates of eosinophils. A unifying theory of basement membrane damage could be that MBP from the eosinophil dissolves the glycoprotein structure of the basement membrane.

There is no explanation for this increased number of eosinophils in the nasal mucosa. The onset of the disease is insidious and can apparently last for years. It occurs in the young but, more often in adults. *The worst case I have ever seen was in a 76 year old man.* Eosinophilic disease is infrequent, occurring in less than 1 per cent of patients with chronic rhinitis.

Symptoms are primarily severe nasal congestion and rhinorrhea. Unlike allergic rhinitis, itching of the nares is absent. By definition, findings of IgE mediated disease are absent. For the present, I believe that eosinophilic disease of the nose should not be diagnosed when polyps are present. More often than not, eosinophils are present in the nasal mucus in great numbers in both conditions. On the other hand, the etiology for both is still unknown. Furthermore, very marked infiltrates of lymphocytes and plasma cells are found in the polyps and nasal mucosa in patients with polyps, whereas, patients with eosinophilic disease only have eosinophils. It seems safer to define them independently until more information is available.

Physical examination is quite helpful in that the nasal mucosa is very pale or even yellowish or white. *In my experience, pale membranes are associated primarily with eosinophilic infiltrates — the paler the membrane, the more eosinophils present.*[13]

The only effective, albeit usually temporary, therapy is large doses of systemic steroids.

NASAL DISEASE CAUSED BY IMMUNOLOGICAL MECHANISMS

1. Allergic Rhinitis:

Allergic rhinitis may occur as a seasonal or perennial disease. Approximately 30 per cent of patients with chronic nasal disease have allergic perennial rhinitis.

Three histopathological findings are common in allergic rhinitis.[13] They are: destruction or loss of the basement membrane, infiltrates of eosinophils, and what appear to be nuclear fragments of destroyed cells. The destroyed cells may be remnants of once intact eosinophils because eosinophilic granules are frequently seen scattered amongst the fragments thought to be degenerating nuclei.

The time the biopsy is obtained in relation to the acuteness of the clinical allergic reaction must be considered in evaluating the histology. An acute short antigen exposure would be expected to produce only infiltrates of eosinophils. Kline et al[14] showed in skin test biopsies that eosinophils appeared about 30 minutes after antigen was injected and were disappearing by 24 hours. On the other hand, if the biopsy is obtained after repeated and prolonged antigen exposure over days or weeks, such as occurs during the ragweed pollinating season, one might expect to find eosinophilic infiltrates, basement membrane damage, and what are believed to be broken and damaged eosinophils. If the biopsy is obtained days after the last allergic exposure, basement membrane damage could be the only finding. Finally, biopsy, weeks or months after the last exposure, may show only a normal mucosa. These findings have not been observed serially in any one individual, but are postulated from isolated biopsies done in numerous patients with allergic rhinitis.[13]

It has been previously indicated that one theoretical function of the basement membrane is to act as a protective barrier by preventing various substances from gaining access to the submucosa. In many patients with active allergic rhinitis of days or weeks duration, the basement membrane is destroyed. This loss could facilitate the entrance of soluble antigens and could be at least one factor causing the "priming effect."[15] Healing of the basement membrane can occur as evidenced by the finding of a normal membrane in allergic individuals when they are free of exposure to antigen for some weeks.

A very thin and fragmented basement membrane is found in the mucosa of almost all cases who have nasal polyps. This strong association is noteworthy, for when we understand why it occurs we may better understand nasal polyposis.

It is interesting that in all other nasal diseases, the basement membrane appears quite normal even though there are extensive other abnormalities. It is quite likely that basement membrane damage will be found to be caused by specific chemicals (mediators? enzymes? other?) released in certain diseases. As stated earlier, MBP released from damaged eosinophils may be a prime suspect.

2. Immune Cell Infiltrates:

About 50 per cent of individuals with chronic rhinitis have an infiltrate of lymphocytes, plasma cells, and eosinophils. In some cases the infiltrate may be a pure one of one cell type only. Do immune cell infiltrates represent a single disease or a series of diseases? For instance, plasma cell myeloma is a unique systemic disease characterized by vast numbers of plasma cells. Various immune deficiency diseases may be characterized histologically by a single cell type. At the other extreme is Hodgkins disease and its various subtypes in which multiple types of immune cell infiltrates may be seen. Obviously, we do not know yet whether there is a series of nasal diseases associated with immune cell infiltrates.

The most common finding in this category is a mixed cellular infiltrate consisting primarily of lymphocytes, some plasma cells, and eosinophils varying from none to marked in number. This finding probably represents a complete immunological response of unknown type.

The next most frequent finding is a pure lymphocytic infiltrate. An interesting speculation is whether these lymphocytes are of one specificity or another, such as all T cells or all B cells or a mixture. Future studies in which enumeration of T and B cells are done in blood or in tissues will be able to elucidate this problem.

One 12 year old patient I saw for severe chronic rhinitis had a dense, pure lymphocytic infiltrate in his nasal mucosa when first biopsied in 1973. In 1981, he developed nasal polyps. Do certain types of immune cell infiltrates signal an immunological defect which will eventually cause nasal polyps?

Intense plasma cell infiltrates are always associated with at least a few lymphocytes. Do severe plasma cell infiltrates suggest a failure in the feedback mechanisms required to slow antibody production, or do they represent a persistent stimulus for formation of antibodies?

Patients with immune cell infiltrates all have nasal symptoms of rhinorrhea primarily, and frequently congestion. Seventy to 80 per cent have normal serum IgE levels. There is nothing in the history to suggest what mix of cells will be found on biopsy. Whereas eosinophilic infiltrates are almost always associated with a very pale mucosa, the mucosa is more often red when infiltrated with lymphocytes or plasma cells. The finding can occur in any age group. Treatment of immune cell infiltrates is unsuccessful except for steroids. The mediators released by lymphocytes are not inhibited by antihistamines nor reversed by decongestants.

3. Nasal Polyposis:

Nasal polyposis is just as great an enigma today as it was in ancient history. The pathology of polyps is not limited to the polyps alone. The nasal mucosa is also affected as shown by its pale color on physical examination and frequent finding of immune cells infiltrating the mucosa.

Nasal polyposis probably represents a number of different diseases, as evidenced by its varient forms. Clinically, some polyps are associated with high IgE levels in the serum and in the polyp fluid while in a significant number of cases IgE levels are normal. Some cases of polyposis are associated with aspirin intolerance and asthma while others are not.[16] There is also a variation in the immune cells comprising the polyp. In most cases, the cells are a mixture consisting of lymphocytes, plasma cells, and eosinophils. In other rarer cases, eosinophils or plasma cells may be absent. Rarely, mast cells may be increased. The stimulus for this production is unknown. It seems clear that the defect is fairly extensive because of the nasal mucosal involvement in addition to the polyps. That the polyp itself is not the basic abnormality is readily apparent because of recurrences after polypectomy.

ANATOMICAL LESIONS

1. Deviated Septum:

A deviated septum is an anatomical deformity which has far greater physiological and pathological implications than is appreciated by most physicians. It is not generally recognized that nasal respiration is primarily through one nostril at a time. One nares rests (congested) while the other works (decongested). This has been shown in various studies demonstrating the cycling phenomenon which occurs naturally[17] or may be hastened in pathological conditions.[18] The cause of cycling is not known. Logically, it would seem to represent the body's prudent attempt to permit a nostril which has functioned for one to three hours to rest. During the resting stage, the nostril could be rehabilitated chemically and physically.

When the septum is deviated and cycling interfered with, one finds turbinate hypertrophy on the most patent side, mucosal atrophy on the obstructed side, and a nasal discharge. The consequences of this lesion, besides the physical discomfort are unknown.

Septal deviation may be a result of a broken nose. The septum is the most commonly fractured bone in the body and septal deviation the most common cause of nasal pathology (with the exception of acute coryza). *In screening approximately 4000 randomly selected subjects for pharmacological experiments over the last 10 years, I found that about 20 per cent had a septal deviation. Of this 20 per cent about one-quarter were severe enough, in my estimation, to require corrective surgical procedures.*

2. Cartilagenous Deformities:

Due to exhuberant surgery, or cartilagenous degeneration caused by age or disease, the lateral cartilages of the nose may be injured. This leads to a collapse of the lateral walls of the nose, compromising the airway and causing difficulties on inspiration. For unknown reasons, this condition is frequently accompanied by a slight but persistent rhinorrhea. It can readily be demonstrated by elevating the lateral walls with Q-tips inserted in the nares. The patient will observe that inspiration is now normal. Treatment is surgical.

3. Atrophy of the Mucosa:

Mucosal atrophy may occur with aging or disease. The patient frequently complains of severe congestion. This complaint is unexplainable since examination of the nares demonstrates a more than adequate airway. Surgical implantation of cartilage to partially obstruct the airway has been successful in some cases. It is unknown why the patient feels congested when the airway is patent and is relieved when the airway is partially obstructed.

4. Tumors of the Nose:

Tumors are merely mentioned for completeness. I would refer the reader to other sources where tumors are discussed in greater detail.

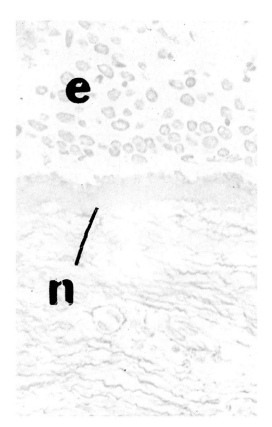

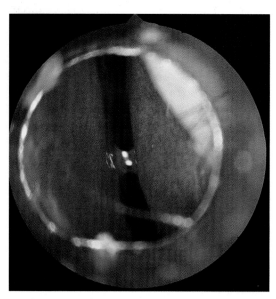

C. Nasal mucosa of patient during ragweed hay fever season showing a pale slightly bluish-tinged membrane. About 50 percent of patients with typical ragweed hay fever have a pale membrane. In others, the color may be pink, red, or white.

A. **Normal basement membrane (n)** shown at 400x magnification reticulum stain. The basement membrane is immediately beneath the epithelium (e). It is an acellular homogeneous band of glycoproteins.

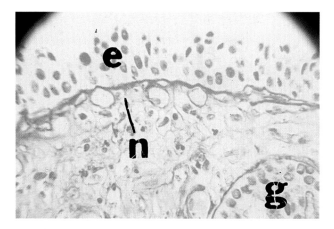

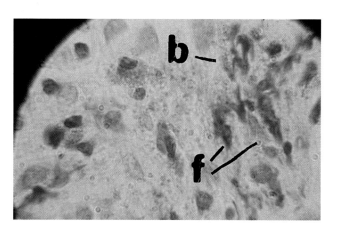

B. **Destroyed basement membrane (n)** shown at 400x magnification reticulum stain. The basement membrane is absent as compared to photograph A. A thin or destroyed basement membrane is seen in symptomatic allergic rhinitis which has been present for at least one to two weeks, in the nasal mucosa of patients who have nasal polyps, and in those with eosinophilic disease of the nose. Epithelium (e), gland (g).

D. Nasal mucosa (Giemsa stain, 1000x magnification) showing broken eosinophils (b) and nuclear fragments (f) from a patient with eosinophilic disease of the nose. Main basic protein released into the tissues from the eosinophil might be responsible for some symptoms and could theoretically cause destruction of the basement membrane. Eosinophils are found in the mucosa of patients with allergic rhinitis in the acute phase, in most patients with nasal polyps, and in patients with eosinophilic disease of the nose even though IgE is normal in the latter group.

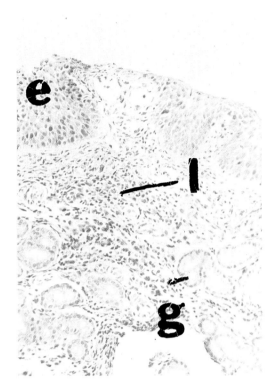

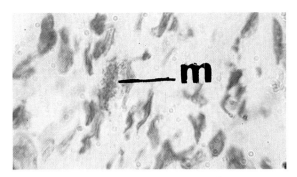

G. Nasal mucosa (Giemsa stain, 1000x magnification). Mucosal mast cell (m), one of many found in this patient with nasal mastocytosis.

E. Nasal mucosa (Giemsa stain, 100x magnification) showing marked lymphocytic infiltrate (l), epithelium (e), gland (g). Patient has normal IgE and severe chronic rhinorrhea. Etiology unknown and classified as "immune disease — unknown etiology." Lymphokins from lymphocytes could cause symptoms.

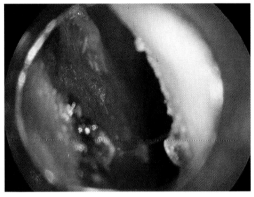

H. Intranasal photograph of patient who is an electrician and works in a cosmetic factory. Mucosa is dry and a dirty brown. Patient's symptom of chronic congestion began six months after he began work. It does not clear on week-ends but does improve after a two week vacation. Patient is believed to have a delayed hypersensitivity to one or more of the many chemicals to which he is exposed in a factory.

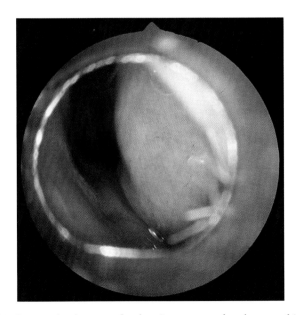

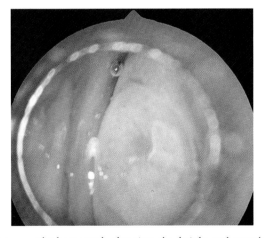

F. Intransal photograph showing very pale almost white mucosa. Patient has severe rhinitis and congestion. IgE is normal. Mucosal biopsy showed marked infiltrate of eosinophils. Pale mucosa is almost always associated with eosinophilic infiltrates; the whiter the mucosa, the greater the number of infiltrating eosinophils.

I. Intranasal photograph showing the bright red membrane associated with longstanding use of neosynephrine nasal spray. There were no infiltrates seen on histological examination of the mucosa. A similarly bright red membrane is seen in many patients with acute coryza. Lymphocytic infiltrates with immune disease of the mucosa are often associated with red membrane.

PSYCHOLOGICAL DISEASE OF THE NOSE

I do not believe that I have ever seen nasal disease caused purely by a psychological abnormality. In a number of cases patients thought to have a psychological nasal condition, psychological treatment was of no avail, and subsequent histological study of the patients' mucosa demonstrated an anatomical lesion. This is not to say that patients with nasal abnormalities cannot be secondarily affected by emotional unheaval. The parasympathetic pathway and its central nervous system connections provide a network for such an occurrence.

On the other hand, I have seen emotionally disturbed patients complain of a nasal problem, yet on examination the nose is usually found to be normal. The probable explanation is use of nasal symptoms as a psychological diversion.

SUMMARY

An overview of nasal disease has been presented based on clinical and histological experiences. Perhaps the greatest lesson to learn is that nasal disease is a heterogeneous mixture of maladies. Except for a few, a significant number of these maladies are unresponsive to our meager pharmacological armamentarium of antihistamines and decongestants, which further emphasizes the multiplicity of mechanisms at work. Steroid therapy is helpful in some of these conditions through its anti-inflammatory action. The clinician will remain frustrated by this multiplicity of diseases comprising chronic rhinitis, since tools currently available may not provide a complete etiological diagnosis.

REFERENCES

1. Goodman LS, Gilman A. The Pharmacological Basis of Therapeutics, 5th Ed. New York: MacMillan Pub. Co., Inc., 1975. pp 425.
2. Connell JT. Nasal mastocytosis (abstract). J Allergy 43:182, 1969.
3. Soter NA, Austen K, Wasserman SL. Oral disodium cromoglycate in the treatment of systemic mastocytosis. N Engl J Med 301:465–469, 1979.
4. Selye H. The Mast Cells. Stoneham, MA: Butterworths, Pubs. Inc. 1965, pp. 6.
5. Knight A, Underdown BJ, Connell JT, Nedzelski J, Elie R. Immunological parameters in perennial rhinitis. Clin Allergy 9:159–66, 1979.
6. Connell JT. Morphological changes in eosinophils in allergic diseases. J Allergy 41:1–9, 1968.
7. Mallory GK, White PD, Salcedo-Salgar J. The speed of healing of myocardial infarction. A study of the pathological anatomy in 72 cases. Am Heart J 18:647, 1939.
8. Connell JT. Allergic rhinitis. In: Weiss EB, Segal MS, eds. Bronchial Asthma: Mechanisms and Therapeutics. Little, Boston: Brown & Co., 1976.
9. Jacobs RL, Freedman PM, Boswell RN. Non-allergic rhinitis with eosinophilia (NARES Syndrome). J Allergy Clin Immunol 67:253–262, 1981.
10. Mullarkey MF, Hill JS, Webb DR. Allergic and non-allergic rhinitis: their characterization with attention to the meaning of nasal eosinophilia. J Allergy Clin Immunol 65:122–126, 1980.
11. Gleich GJ, Loegerings DA, Frigas E, Wassom DL, Solley GO, Mann KG. The major basic protein of the eosinophil granules. Physio-chemical properties, localization and function. In: Mahmoud AA, Austen KF, eds. The Eosinophil in Health and Disease New York: Grune and Stratton, 1980, pp. 79–97.
12. Filley WV, Holley KE, Kephert GM, Gleich GJ. Immunofluorescent and localization of the eosinophil granule major basic protein in lung tissues of patients with bronchial asthma. In press.
13. Connell JT. Unpublished data.
14. Kline BS, Cohen MB, Rudolph JA. Histological changes in allergic and non-allergic wheals. J Allergy 3:531, 1931.
15. Connell JT. Quantitative intranasal pollen challenges: III. The priming effect in allergic rhinitis. J Allergy 43:33–44, 1969.
16. Settipane GA, Chafee FH. Nasal polyps in asthma and rhinitis. A review of 6,037 patients. J Allergy Clin Immunol 59:17–21, 1977.
17. Principato JJ, Ozenberger JM. Cyclical changes in nasal resistance. Arch Otolaryngol 91:71, 1970.
18. Connell JT. Reciprocal nasal congestion-decongestion reflex. Trans Am Acad Ophth Otolaryngol 72:422–426, 1968.

Chapter XIX

Eosinophilic Nonallergic Rhinitis and Vasomotor Rhinitis

Michael F. Mullarkey, M.D.

ABSTRACT

Eosinophilic disease of the upper airways that is not allergic and that responds to therapy with corticosteroids has been described by several workers. Its clinical characteristics are reviewed, as in the possible role of the eosinophil in respiratory diseases in man.

Until recently, nasal eosinophilia had been equated with nasal allergy. Seebohm[1] had expressed a difference of opinion with this tenet, and Knight[2] had reported on seven of 60 patients with nasal eosinophilia and no other findings of nasal allergy in a study of the immunology of perennial rhinitis.

Between October of 1977 and June of 1978, we had the opportunity to prospectively characterize 142 patients with perennial rhinitis.[3] The results of this study indicated that while eosinophilia was present in nasal allergy, it was not unique to or uniformly present in the allergic state. The criteria of classification and evaluation are outlined in detail in our original study. Patients with 3 or more months of congestion and rhinorrhea were evaluated on the basis of history of allergen exacerbation, physical examination with characterization of the nasal mucous membranes, skin tests to common allergens, total serum IgE, and peripheral and nasal eosinophil quantitation. Patients with acute sinusitis and rhinitis medicamentosa were excluded from the study. Forty-

eight patients (34%) had clear-cut allergic rhinitis (Table I). Their histories correlated independently with their skin tests, and their total serum IgEs were elevated. Forty-two percent of these individuals had nasal eosinophilia on initial exam. That left 94 individuals to describe. Twenty-one of these patients had a scattering of findings associated with allergic rhinitis, including positive skin tests and elevated IgEs. However, their histories often did not correlate with their skin tests. This group was considered to have possible or probable allergic rhinitis. Many of these patients, I suspect, had both allergic and nonallergic disease accounting for their symptoms of rhinitis. Fifty-two of the remaining patients (37%) had no historical or laboratory data to suggest allergic disease. For want of a better term, we classified these individuals as having vasomotor rhinitis. Twenty-one of our patients, 15% of the 142 patients evaluated, also had no evidence of nasal disease but demonstrated nasal eosinophilia of at least 25%. These individuals were described as having eosinophilic nonallergic rhinitis (ENR). Their clinical presentations included rhinorrhea, intermittent congestion, and episodes of pruritus which included the nasal and conjunctival mucous membranes. On the basis of their symptoms, these patients were indistinguishable from individuals with allergic rhinitis. One-third of the patients with ENR were noted to have polyps, further fortifying our impression that ENR was a nonallergic condition.[4] There was a significant association between chronic rhinitis and the presence of abnormal sinus x-rays. Twenty-three percent of individuals with allergic rhinitis of 3 months or more duration had 2 mm or more of mucous membrane thickening on a Waters sinus x-ray. For simplicity and convenience we now define ENR as non-

Head, Allergy and Clinical Immunology, Virginia Mason Clinic, Seattle, Washington.

TABLE I

	Allergic Rhinitis	Possible Allergic Rhinitis	Vasomotor Rhinitis	Eosinophilic Non-Allergic Rhinitis
Number (%)	48 (34)	21 (5)	52 (37)	21 (15)
% with nasal eosinophilia ≥25%	42	19	0	100

allergic rhinitis with eosinophilia, lacking historical or laboratory evidence of allergy, nasal polyps, or aspirin sensitivity. As will be discussed later, several groups have confirmed this subset with prospective evaluations in groups of patients with chronic rhinitis.

Our most interesting finding came when response to therapy was evaluated. We arbitrarily accepted a positive response to therapy as the total relief of patient symptoms. Using this strict criteria, we were surprised to note that antihistaminic decongestants, oral corticosteroids, or corticosteroid nose drops gave complete relief of symptoms in only 67% of patients with allergic rhinitis. Individuals with ENR demonstrated an 80% response to antihistaminic decongestants, and a greater than 90% response to therapy with corticosteroids. The presence or absence of nasal eosinophils did not affect the therapeutic response in allergic rhinitis.

We had characterized a subgroup of patients with perennial rhinitis who lacked evidence of allergy in spite of nasal eosinophilia, and who demonstrated a striking response to steroid therapy. Several questions remained about this subgroup of individuals. Was there any evidence that these individuals had "local allergy;" i.e., produced specific IgE in nasal mucous but had circulating levels of specific IgE that were not measured by PRIST or skin tests? Our patients were drawn from an adult population; did pediatric patients present and respond in a similar fashion?

Jacobs[5] and co-workers carefully evaluated 52 individuals presenting to a military facility over many years with recurrent rhinitis, conjunctivitis, nasal eosinophilia, but with no evidence by history, skin test, or serum IgE of allergy, initially confirmed the syndrome of ENR. These patients were also free of nasal polyps.

Dr. Gary Rupp[6] of Cleveland described the syndrome in 12 pediatric patients, aged 6 to 17, and noted excellent response to topical corticosteroid therapy. More recently the syndrome has been described in a prospective series by Settipane and Klein[7] and a retrospective case review by Enberg.[8] Lans and colleagues, in a series of 100 patients have been unable to confirm these observations.[9]

It seems clear that nasal eosinophilia is found in a group of patients with nonallergic rhinitis who may be difficult to distinguish from patients with allergic rhinitis, but who are dramatically responsive to steroid therapy. In retrospect, this observation is not surprising. Eosinophilic disease of the lower respiratory tract is largely idiopathic in Western man. Best estimates indicate that less than 25% of asthma is IgE-mediated.[10] Most of the infiltrative diseases of the chest with peripheral eosinophilia show no evidence of allergic causation, allergic bronchopulmonary aspergillosis being the outstanding exception.[11] Pleural disease with eosinophilia is largely noted with malignancy or infection.[12] Most other diseases accompanied by tissue and peripheral eosinophilia in Western man remain idiopathic with little evidence of Type I mediation.[13] This is not to reduce the importance of IgE-mast cell-mediated eosinophil chemotaxis. Eosinophilia is a hallmark of most Type I diseases, and recent animal data indicate that IgE-mediated eosinophilia is vital in a host defense against parasitism.[14] The observation that most eosinophilic diseases are not IgE-mediated is made to stress the observation that other mechanisms must draw eosinophils into sites of inflammation. Activation of the complement cascade leads to the generation of eosinophilic chemotactic molecules, and recent work from Goetzl's laboratory[15] suggests that metabolites of arachidonic acid in the lipoxygenase pathway are potent stimulators of eosinophil chemotaxis. Aspirin may induce eosinophil chemotaxis in this fashion or may induce eosinophil migration through a nonimmunologic degranulation of mast cells.[16] It is interesting to note that Jacobs challenged 13 of his patients with nonallergic rhinitis and eosinophilia with aspirin and found no responders. We have tested the nasal secretions of some of our ENR patients and have been unable to demonstrate *in vitro* eosinophil chemotaxis.

Clinical studies indicate that a reduction in peripheral eosinophilia[17] leads to better control of asthma, and that the presence of eosinophils in bronchitic sputum indicates a response to steroid therapy.[18] A recent epidemiological study indicates that there is an increased incidence of reversible airway disease in nonsmoking elderly women with blood eosinophilia.[19] Elegant work from Gleich's lab[20] has demonstrated cytotoxicity for tracheal epithelia grown in tissue culture by a protein isolated from eosinophils. This protein constitutes 50% of the cytoplasmic granules found in eosinophils and is known as major basic protein (MBP). Gleigh has gone on to show that the sputum of hospitalized asthmatics is rich in MBP, and that as clinical remission ensues, there is a close and inverse relationship between the concentration of sputum MBP and pulmonary function tests.[21] Are eosinophils then of pathogenic importance in such proliferative changes of the upper airways as nasal polyps? And what is their role in eosinophilic nonallergic rhinitis? It seems probable that the symptoms of congestion, rhinorrhea, and pruritis are due to mediator release and that the accumulation of eosinophils is secondary to such release. Whether the accumulation of eosinophils in the upper airways leads to the proliferative changes of polyps and sinusitis can only be answered by following individuals with ENR for several years.

A final question occurs regarding the efficacy of steroids in clearing eosinophils from secretions. Is this effect and the amelioration of disease coincidental? The mechanism by which corticosteroids act on eosinophils is under study. It is now clear that eosinophils have corticosteroid receptors on their surfaces and that corticosteroids inhibit both eosinophil migration and adherence.[22,23] It remains to be determined if the relief of symptoms noted in ENR after steroid therapy is related to the clearance of eosinophils and their noxious products or is due to another effect of corticosteroids on the primary disease process i.e., on the prevention of nonimmunologic mast cell degranulation.

While the description of patients with ENR has led to more questions than it has answered, its description has led to a simpler classification of nasal disease. Once IgE is defined as participating in the mechanism of nasal disease, we classify according to whether symptoms are perennial or seasonal. Perennial nonallergic rhinitis is classified descriptively, as its etiology is idiopathic. Perennial nasal disease may be due to drugs (rhinitis medicamentosa), metabolic states (the rhinitis of pregnancy), associated with eosinophils and demonstrate steroid responsiveness (ENR), or be unclassifiable; i.e., vasomotor rhinitis. Having these models, we then recognize that most human diseases occur in mixed form. It is not uncommon to see patients with allergic rhinitis plus rhinitis medicamentosa, or patients with positive skin tests, weak histories, and severe symptoms which respond poorly to immunotherapy but well to corticosteroids.

One goal for the further investigation of nasal disease should include the further categorization of subsets of nonallergic nasal disease. After clinical characterization, these subsets should be named descriptively and then defined by serial observations over time. This will allow us to fractionate the remaining category of idiopathic perennial rhinitis into subsets with known therapeutic responses and natural histories.

REFERENCES

1. Seebohm PM. Allergic and nonallergic rhinitis. In: Middleton E, Reed CE, Ellis EF, eds. Allergy: Principles and Practice. St. Louis: CV Mosby Co, 1978, pp 868–876.
2. Knight A et al. Immunologic parameters in perennial rhinitis. Clin Allergy 9:159–166, 1979.
3. Mullarkey MF, Hill JS, Webb DR. Allergic and nonallergic rhinitis: their characterization with attention to the meaning of nasal eosinophilia. J Allergy Clin Immunol 65:22–126, 1980.
4. Settipane GA, Chafee FH. Nasal polyps in asthma and rhinitis: a review 6,037 patients. J Allergy Clin Immunol 59:17–21, 1977.
5. Jacobs RL, Freedman PM, Boswell RN. Nonallergic rhinitis with eosinophilia (Nares Syndrome). J Allergy Clin Immunol 67:253–262, 1981.
6. Rupp GH, Friedman RA. Eosinophilic nonallergic rhinitis in children. Pediatrics (In press).
7. Settipane GA, Klein DE. Nonallergic rhinitis: Demography of eosinophils in nasal smear, blood total eosinophil counts and IgE levels. New Engl Reg Allergy Proc 6:363–366, 1985.
8. Enberg RN. Perennial nonallergic rhinitis: A retrospective review. Ann Allergy 63:513–516, 1989.
9. Lans DM, Alfano N, Rocklin R. Nasal eosinophilia in allergic and nonallergic rhinitis: Usefulness of the nasal smear in the diagnosis of allergic rhinitis. New Engl Reg Allergy Proc 10:275–280, 1989.
10. Stevenson DD, et al. Provoking factors in bronchial asthma. Arch Intern Med 135:777–783, 1975.
11. Schatz M, Wasserman S, Patterson R. Eosinophils and immunologic lung disease. Med Clin North Am 65:1055–1071, 1981.
12. Veress JF, Koss LG, Schreiber K. Eosinophilic pleural effusions. Acta Cytol 23:40–44, 1979.
13. Chusid MJ et al. The hypereosinophilic syndrome: analysis of 14 cases with a review of the literature. Medicine 54:1–27, 1975.
14. Dessein AJ et al. IgE antibody and resistance to infection. I. Selective suppression of the IgE antibody response in rats diminishes the resistance and the eosinophil response to trichinella spiralis infection. J Exp Med 153:423–436, 1981.
15. Goetzl EJ, Weller PF, Sun FF. The regulation of human eosinophil function by endogenous mono-hydroxy-eicosatetraenoic acids (HETEs). J Immunol 24:926–933, 1980.
16. Stevenson DD. Aspirin and rhinosinusitis/asthma: desensitization. NESA Proceedings 2:88–93, 1981.
17. Horn BR et al. Total eosinophil counts in the management of bronchial asthma. N Engl J Med 292:1152–1155, 1975.
18. Shim C, Stover DE, Williams MH Jr. Response to corticosteroids in chronic bronchitis. J Allergy Clin Immunol 62:363–367, 1978.
19. Burrows B et al. Epidemiologic observations on eosinophilia and its relation to respiratory disorders. Am Rev Respir Dis 122:709–719, 1980.
20. Gleich GJ et al. Cytotoxic properties of the eosinophil major basic protein. J Immunol 123:2925–2927, 1979.
21. Frigas E et al. Elevated levels of the eosinophil granule major basic protein in the sputum of patients with bronchial asthma. Mayo Clin Proc 56:345–33, 1981.
22. Altman LC et al. Effect of corticosteroids on eosinophil chemotaxis and adherence. J Clin Invest 67:28–36, 1981.
23. Peterson AP et al. Glucocorticoid receptors in normal human eosinophils: comparison with neutrophils. J Allergy Clin Immunol 68:212–217, 1981.

Chapter XX

Nasal Polyps

Guy A. Settipane, M.D.

ABSTRACT

The pathogenic mechanism of nasal polyps are unknown. They frequently are associated with aspirin intolerance, intrinsic asthma, chronic sinusitis, Young's syndrome, cystic fibrosis, Kartagener's syndrome, and Churg-Strauss syndrome. Children 16 years or younger with nasal polyps should be evaluated for cystic fibrosis. Nasal polyps are frequently bilateral, multiple, freely movable, and pale-gray and arise from the middle meatus of the nose. Histologically, they classically have pseudostratified ciliated columnar epithelium, thickening of the epithelial basement membrane, high stromal eosinophil count, mucin with neutral pH, few glands and essentially no nerve endings. Cells consist of a mixture of lymphocytes, plasma cells, and eosinophils. Polyps from patients with Young's syndrome, Kartagener's syndrome, and cystic fibrosis have predominantly neutrophils with insignificant eosinophils. Chemical mediators found in nasal polyps are as follows: histamine, serotonin, leukotrienes [(SRS-A or LTC_4, LTD_4, LTE_4), LTB_4], ECF-A, norepinephrine, kinins, TAME-esterase, and possibly PGD_2. There is more histamine in nasal polyps than in normal nasal mucosa, and norepinephrine is present in greater concentration in the base of nasal polyps than in normal nasal mucosa. The concentrations of IgA and IgE and, in some cases, IgG and IgM are greater in polyp fluid than in serum. IgE-mediated disease is not the cause of nasal polyps, but when present, may contribute to episodes of exacerbation. Upper respiratory infections also may cause exacerbations. Despite medical or surgical management, a significant number of nasal polyps are recurrent. For treatment, systemic corticosteroids should be tried before surgical polypectomy. Polypectomy does not increase the risk of developing asthma or making asthma worse.

Clinical Professor, Brown University Program in Medicine, and Director, Division of Allergy, Department of Medicine, Rhode Island Hospital, Providence

Nasal polyps are frequently associated with many systemic diseases, the most common of which is nonallergic asthma followed by aspirin intolerance (the bronchospastic type) and chronic sinusitis. The combination of nasal polyps, aspirin intolerance, and asthma is referred to Samter's triad. Other systemic diseases associated with nasal polyps are cystic fibrosis, Kartagener's syndrome (chronic dyskinetic cilia syndrome), Young's syndrome (sinopulmonary disease), azoospermia, and Churg-Strauss syndrome (allergic vasculitis). In some cases, nasal polyps may be visualized only by the use of the rhinoscope. In many situations, the nasal polyp may present as a minor symptom but may represent the "tip of the iceberg" with the major associated syndromes often being severe manifestations of systemic disorders. In this chapter, nasal polyps will be evaluated historically, epidemiologically, anatomically, and histopathologically; in association with systemic diseases and chemical mediators; pathogenesis; relationship to atopy; relationship to aspirin intolerance; and treatment.

HISTORY

Nasal polyps were known as far back as 1000 B.C. Vancil[1] has presented an excellent historical survey of treatment for nasal polyps. In about 400 B.C. Hippocrates developed two surgical methods for nasal polypectomy; extraction by pulling a sponge through the nasal canal and by cauterization. Cato the Censor (234–149 B.C.) developed the first known medical management of nasal polyps using the local application of herbs. Other ancient authors who have written about nasal polyps through the centuries are: Celsus (42 B.C.–37 A.D.), Paulus of Aegina (625–690 A.D.), Avicenna (980–1037 A.D.), Saliceto (1210–1270), Fallopius (1523–1562), Petros Forestus (1522–1597), Fabricius ab Acquapendente (1537–1619), Aranzi (1530–1589),

TABLE I

Frequency of Nasal Polyps in Various Conditions

Diagnosis	Frequency (%)
Aspirin intolerance	36
Adult asthma	7
a. Intrinsic asthma	13
b. Atopic asthma	5
Chronic rhinitis	2
a. Nonallergic rhinitis	5
b. Allergic rhinitis	1.5
Childhood asthma/rhinitis	0.1
Cystic fibrosis	20
Churg-Strauss syndrome	50
Kartagener's syndrome	?
Young's syndrome	?

and Juncker, who in 1721 wrote: "According as the moon fills or wanes, the polypi of the nose increase or decrease in size . . . ," an excellent clinical observation of remissions and exacerbations of polyps but certainly a faulty lunar correlation. Thus, it appears that nasal polyps have been a worrisome medical problem as far back as man can remember.

EPIDEMIOLOGY

Nasal polyps are most commonly found in nonatopic asthmatic patients over 40 years of age, especially in those patients with severe, steroid-dependent asthma. The overall frequency of nasal polyps in asthmatics between the ages of 10 to 50 years is 7% (Tables I and II).[2] In a subgroup of asthmatics, over 40 years old or those with negative skin tests, the frequency ranges from 10–15% (Table III).[2] In patients with aspirin intolerance, the frequency of nasal polyps may be as

high as 36%.[3,4] Slavin's group[5] reported on 33 patients with severe asthma and sinusitis. Fifteen of these patients were receiving corticosteroids: 10 who received continuous corticosteroids and 5 who required intermittent bursts. Of these 33 patients, 30 (or 90%) had a diagnosis of nasal polyps and 17 (52%) had aspirin intolerance. These data demonstrate that the nasal polyps as well as aspirin intolerance found in asthmatic patients usually indicate the presence of a severe asthmatic state. In children, the frequency of nasal polyposis is extremely low, about 0.1%.[2,6] Any child 16 years or younger with nasal polyps should be evaluated for cystic fibrosis.

ANATOMY

Nasal polyps are frequently bilateral and multiple and have a characteristic appearance (Figure 1). They are glistening, pale gray, smooth, soft, semitranslucent, freely movable, attached by a pedicle, and rise from the surfaces of the middle turbinates, the hiatal semilunaries, or ostia of the ethmoid and maxillary sinuses. Most commonly they are found in the middle meatus extending to the nasal cavity filling the nose and finally protruding from the anterior nares. If the polyp projects posteriorly into the nasopharynx, it is called a choanal polyp and may not be seen by routine examination through the anterior nares. Choanal polyps may be single, usually occur during the first two decades of life and are classified in three groups: (1) antrochoanal polyps arising from the antrum; (2) polyps arising from other sinuses; or (3) polyps, which are the posterior part of multiple ethmoidal polyps. Polyps are one of the most common types of mass found in the nasal passage.

HISTOPATHOLOGY

Nasal polyps have pseudostratified columnar epithelium and cellular constituents of normal nasal mucosa (Figure 2). Polyps from patients who do not

TABLE II

Frequency of Nasal Polyps in Asthma and Rhinitis

Diagnosis	Total Patients	Positive Allergy Skin Tests			Negative Allergy Skin Tests			p	Total Polyps		p
		No.	Polyps	%	No.	Polyps	%		No.	%	
Asthma	2,228	1,717	85	5.0	511	64	12.5	<0.01	149	6.7	
Rhinitis only	2,758	2,126	32	1.5	632	30	4.7	<0.01	62	2.2	<0.01*
Total	4,986	3,843	117	3.0	1,143	94	8.2		211	4.2	

* The difference in the frequency of nasal polyps in asthma (6.7%) compared to rhinitis (2.2%) is statistically significant. (Reprinted with permission from Settipane GA, Chafee FH. Nasal polyps in asthma and rhinitis: A review of 6,037 patients. J Allergy Clin Immunol 59:17–21, 1977.)

TABLE III

Frequency of Nasal Polyps in Various Age Groups of Asthmatic Patients

Age when First Seen	No. with Asthma		No. with Nasal Polyps		%		p
10–19	491		9		1.8		
20–29	465	1,374	18	43	3.9	3.1	
30–39	418		16		3.8		<0.01*
40–49	410		41		10.0		
50 and over	444	854	65	106	14.6	12.4	
Total	2,228		149		6.7		

* The difference between the 10–39 year-old group (43/1.374), 3.1% compared to the 40 year-old and over group (106/854), 12.4% is statistically significant.
Reprinted from Settipane GA & Chafee FH. Nasal polyps in asthma and rhinitis: A review of 6,037 patients. J Allergy Clin Immunol 59:17–21, 1977.

have cystic fibrosis have extensive thickening of the epithelial basement membranes with extension into the submucosa as an irregular hyaline membrane, high stromal eosinophil count, and mainly neutral mucin in mucous glands, cysts, and mucous blanket.[8] Glands are few and denervated. Polyp tissue is essentially free of nerve endings, except for nerve terminals in the base of the polyps associated with blood vessels. In most cases, the cells consist of a mixture of lymphocytes, plasma cells, and eosinophils. Occasionally, neutrophils are numerous. Nasal smears from these patients usually reveal "sheets" of eosinophils (Figure 3). In contrast, polyps from patients with cystic fibrosis have a delicate, barely visible basement membrane of surface epithelium without submucosal hyalinization, lack of extensive infiltration of eosinophils, and a preponderance of acid mucin in glands, cysts, and surface mucosa blanket. Polyps from patients with Kartagener's and Young's syndromes usually lack an eosinophilic component and have neutrophils as the predominant cell.

As to non cystic fibrosis polyps, one report[9] demonstrated that all polyps showed evidence of epithelial

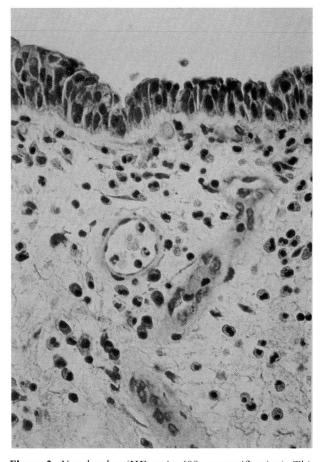

Figure 2. Nasal polyp (HE stain 400× magnification): This high-power view shows orderly pseudostratified columnar epithelium overlying an intact basement membrane. The stroma is edematous, vascular, and contains eosinophils.

Figure 1. Gross photograph of multiple nasal polyps from a 54-year-old male (scale is in centimeters).

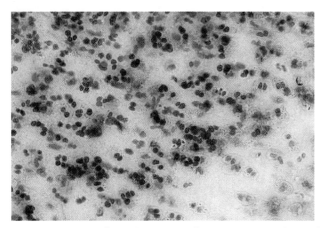

Figure 3. Smear of nasal secretions from a patient with nasal polyps reveals eosinophils.

damage, either ulceration or marked desquamation. In another study,[10] a small proportion of polyps showed a focal dysplastic change of the surface lining of the mucosa with no related changes in the immediately underlying stroma. On follow-up, in none of these patients did an invasive feature supersede, and these changes appear to constitute a local reaction to recurrent irritation.

DIFFERENTIAL DIAGNOSIS

The differential diagnosis of nasal polyps includes chordoma, chemodectoma, neurofibroma, angiofibroma, inverting papilloma, squamous cell carcinoma, sarcoma, and encephaloceles or meningoceles. Most of these present as unilateral lesions. Meningoceles enter the nasal cavity via the cribriform plate. They increase in size with straining, lifting, or crying and may have a pulsating characteristic. The other lesions included in this differential diagnosis are not mobile, bleed easily, and may be sensitive to manipulation.

Nasal polyps are characteristically mobile, rarely bleed, are not sensitive to manipulation, and are frequently bilateral and multiple. Malignant tumors frequently are associated with bony, destructive changes. In rare cases, benign paranasal sinus cysts or polyps also may produce bone destruction (Woakes disease).[11] Diagnostic procedures include angiography, tomographic x-rays, computerized tomography scan, and biopsy.

ASSOCIATION WITH SYSTEMIC DISEASES

The most common systemic disease associated with nasal polyps is nonallergic asthma, followed by aspirin intolerance. The triad of nasal polyps, asthma, and aspirin intolerance will be discussed in a separate category later in this review. Patients with cystic fibrosis have a high frequency of nasal polyps (20%). Children age 16 or younger who have nasal polyps should be evaluated for cystic fibrosis. Similar to cystic fibrosis, the polyps associated with the chronic dyskinetic cilia syndrome and Young's syndrome have the neutrophil as the predominant cell.

Primary ciliary dyskinesia is classically manifested in Kartagener's syndrome, which is an uncommon genetic condition with an estimated incidence of 1 in 20,000 births.[11,12] It appears to be inherited as an autosomal recessive trait and is characterized by bronchiectasis, chronic sinusitis, and situs inversus (complete reversal of internal organs with heart on the right, liver on the left, etc). The ciliary abnormality in these cases usually involves the entire body including the respiratory tract and sperm cells. The disorder is in the cilia itself in which the dynein arms are missing and the cilia remains completely immotile. Situs inversus is found in only 50% of patients with this syndrome. Infection caused by *Pseudomonas aeruginosa* often found in patients with Kartagener's syndrome or cystic fibrosis.[13]

Young's syndrome consists of recurrent respiratory diseases, azoospermia, and nasal polyposis. The respiratory disease consists of severe chronic sinusitis that may be associated with bronchiectasis.[14,15] These patients have normal sweat chloride values and pancreatic function and, therefore, do not have a variant of cystic fibrosis. Cilia structures are normal in sperm tails taken from testicular biopsy specimens and in the cilia from tracheal biopsy specimens and, therefore, these patients do not have a chronic form of immotile cilia syndrome. The azoospermia is due to a block in the epididymis that is distinguishable from the defect in the vas deferens associated with cystic fibrosis. However, spermatogenesis is normal. The prevalence of Young's syndrome is considerably higher than that of cystic fibrosis or Kartagener's syndrome. It is responsible for 7.4% of

---

TABLE IV

Nasal Polyps Associated with Systemic Diseases*

Asthma (nonallergic)

Aspirin intolerance (bronchospastic type)

Samter's triad (asthma, aspirin intolerance, and nasal polyps)

Chronic sinusitis

Churg-Strauss syndrome (vasculitis)

Young's syndrome (sinopulmonary disease, azoospermia, nasal polyps)

Cystic fibrosis

Kartagener's syndrome (bronchiectasis, chronic sinusitis, and situs inversus)

---

* The first four diseases are associated with tissue eosinophilia while in the latter group of diseases the predominant cell is the neutrophil.

ases of male infertility.

Also, 50% of patients with Churg-Strauss disease llergic vasculitis have nasal polyps.

Thus, it is apparent that the presence of nasal polyps nay be a sign that a basic generalized disease may be present and that the nasal polyps may represent just he tip of a deep iceberg. The systemic diseases associted with nasal polyps are listed in Table IV in the rder of frequency found in the general population.

CHEMICAL MEDIATORS

Chemical mediators found in nasal polyps are histamine, serotonin, leukotrienes (slow-reactive subtance of anaphylaxis, LTC^4, LTD^4, LTE^4, LTB^4), eoinophilic chemotactic factor of anaphylaxis (ECF-A), orepinephrine, kinins, TAME-esterase, and possibly rostaglandin PGD^2.

Kaliner et al[18] reported that the release of chemical nediators in nasal polyps is modulated by agents afecting the intracellular concentrations of cyclic nucletides. These authors also stated that the quantity of RS-A released in relation to the amount of histamine eleased from nasal polyps is considerably less than that eleased from the human lung. Bumsted et al.[17] reported nat there is more histamine in nasal polyps than in ormal mucosa and that norepinephrine is present in reater concentration in the base of nasal polyps than n normal mucosa. However, there is no difference in erotonin levels in nasal polyps and normal mucosa. In ddition, there is no difference in levels of histamine, erotonin, and norepinephrine in nasal polyps from roups of patients with or without inhalant allergies or sthma.

An interesting finding is that patients with aspirin ntolerance have levels of histamine in nasal polyps that re much lower than all other types of patients with asal polyps, approximating the histamine levels found n normal mucosa. Chandra and Abrol[19] reported that olyp fluid contains albumin and immunoglobulins IgA, IgE, IgG, IgM, and macroglobulins). The concenrations of IgA and IgE and, in some cases, IgG and gM were greater in the polyp fluid than in the serum. Using the Prausnitz-Kustner procedure, Berdal[20] in 952 reported that skin sensitivity antibody in polyp uid was many times more concentrated than that ound in sera. An explanation for these increased conentrations of serum components found in polyp fluid nay be that the polyp may act as a dialyzing membrane vith water evaporating through the mucosa. This causes n increased concentration of large substances in the olyp sack.

PATHOGENESIS

One theory on the pathogenesis of polyps has been presented by Bumsted et al.[17] Their theory is ased on data that norepinephrine is present in greater concentration in the base of nasal polyps than in normal mucosa. They stated that this norepinephrine at the base of the polyp could produce excessive adrenergic receptor-mediated vasoconstriction that might lead to rebound mucosal congestion and edema, potentiating the effects of histamine and kinins. Norepinephrine through adrenergic receptor activation would lower the effects of cyclic adenosine monophosphate, which would enhance the release of histamine, SRS-A and ECF-A. These mediators would cause an increased vascular permeability, edema, and the leakage of macromolecules out of the vascular system eventually causing the polyp formation. They explain the lower levels of histamine found in polyps of aspirin-intolerant patients, by stating that these patients have an increased sensitivity to histamines.

Mygind[21] believes that polyp formation is related to denervation of blood vessels and to degranulation of mast cells in the nasal mucosa. This process leads to increased vascular permeability, edema, and finally polyp formation. He lists causative factors for denervation to be infection, cystic fibrosis, and aspirin intolerance. He lists contributing factors to be mast cell degeneration and IgE-dependent reactions.

An old theory[22] on polyp formation deals with Bernoulli's theorem that states that gases or fluid passing through a constrictor results in an area of negative pressure in its vicinity. Weakened, denervated tissue such as polyps may theoretically be sucked out by this negative pressure leading to edema and enlargement of the polyp.

Other theories of polyp formation have been established. Tos and Mogensen[23] theory is based on rupture of the epithelium with protrusion of the subepithelial tissue through the epithelial defect and the epithelization of the prolapsed tissue.

A new theory from Bernstein et al.[24] is that a greater rate of transepithelial ion transport occurs in nasal polyps. They suggest that this increased rate may have an effect on movement of water into the cell and interstitial tissue causing edema and formation of nasal polyps. They base their theory on the transepithelial bioelectric potential difference and resistance of nasal polyps and turbinate epithelial cells.

None of these theories may be totally adequate to account for all the known facts involving nasal polyps. The fact that nasal polyps frequently are associated with systemic diseases indicates that the underlying cause of polyposis may be related to a basic generalized biochemical disorder. At present, the pathogenesis of polyp formation is unknown.

RELATIONSHIP TO ATOPY

Nasal polyps are found more frequently in asthmatic/rhinitis patients who have negative skin tests rather than those with positive skin tests (Table

TABLE V

Nasal Polyps (211 Cases): Characteristics

Clinical Categories	No.	%
Males	106	50.2
Females	105	49.8
Asthma	149	70.6
Rhinitis (alone)	62	29.4
Positive allergy skin tests	117	55.5
Total aspirin intolerance	30	14.2
Subtypes of aspirin intolerance		
Bronchospasm	21	70.0
Urticaria	4	13.3
Both bronchospasm and urticaria	2	6.7
Rhinitis	3	10.0

Reprinted from Settipane GA & Charles FH. Nasal polyps and rhinitis: A review of 6,037 patients. J Allergy Clin Immunol 59:17–21, 1977.

II). There is a relationship to asthma in that over 70% of patients with nasal polyps have an associated asthma (Table V). Some patients with nasal polyps not only have no history of asthma but also have negative methacholine challenge tests.[25,26] Therefore, not all patients with nasal polyps have an associated lower-respiratory disease.[27,28] Whiteside et al.[29] reported that in five of six cases of nasal polyps in nonatopic patients, no IgE-bearing lymphocytes were detected in the polyp tissue. However, in atopic patients, IgE-bearing lymphocytes in nasal polyps correlated well with serum IgE levels.

We reviewed[30] 167 patients with nasal polyps, and 143 (86%) of these had one or more polypectomies (Table VI). A number of these patients had a verified history of two, three, four, or even five or more polypectomies. Our preliminary data suggest that patients with positive allergy skin tests (pollen, animal dander, or molds) have a progressively higher rate of repeated

TABLE VI

167 Patients with Verified Polyps and Polypectomies[31]

Total Patients	No. of Polypectomies	No. of Patients	%
167	1 or more	143	86
143	2 or more	57	40
143	3 or more	34	24
143	4 or more	22	15
143	5 or more	17	12
143	6 or more	11	8

TABLE VII

Frequency of Polypectomies in Patients with Positive Allergy Skin Tests

No. of Polypectomies	Total Patients*	No. with Positive Allergy Skin Tests	%
None	24	12	50
One or more	143	81	57
Two or more	57	33	53
Three or more	34	20	59
Four or more	22	15	68
Five or more	17	12	71
Six or more	11	8	73

* Total patients = 167
One patient did not have a skin test

polypectomies, Table VII. However, this trend is not statistically significant possibly because of the small number of patients involved in some categories.

The frequency of one or more positive allergy skin tests (pollens, danders, or molds) in our patient population with nasal polyps is 56%.[2] However, this population was obtained from allergy patients, both in private practice and in the allergy clinic at Rhode Island Hospital where the overall frequency of one or more positive allergy skin tests was 77%.[2] Therefore, the 56% positive allergy skin tests in patients with nasal polyps reflects the positive allergy test frequency in the larger population from which these polyp cases were obtained and is not directly related to polyp formation.

It seems that atopy or IgE-mediated disease is not a

TABLE VIII

Characteristics of the Bronchospastic Type of Aspirin Intolerance

Found in asthmatic patients
Correlated with nasal polyposis
Similar age onset as asthma
Severe rhinorrhea with aspirin reactions
Increased frequency in older age groups
Familial occurrence
Eosinophil in nasal smear
Elevated total (blood) eosinophil count
Nonsteroidal anti-inflammatory drug cross-reaction
No specific IgE (anti-aspiryl)
Normal total IgE
Desensitization possible to aspirin
Pathogenic mechanism: Prostaglandins

TABLE IX

Frequency of Aspirin Intolerance in Various Age Groups of Asthmatic Patients

Age when first seen (years)	No. with asthma	No. with ASA intolerance	%*
10–19	358	5	1.4
29–29	351	13	3.7
30–39	342	12	3.5
40–49	357	24	6.7
50 and over	367	22	6.0
Total	1,775	76	4.3

* The trend of progressive differences by decades is statistically significant ($p < 0.01$).

cause of nasal polyps, but once polyp formation occurs, atopy or IgE-mediated disease may aggravate and increase the risk of nasal polyp formation. Acute upper-respiratory infections are also known to cause an exacerbation or enlargement of nasal polyps.[28]

RELATIONSHIP TO ASPIRIN INTOLERANCE

The full-blown triad of asthma, aspirin intolerance, and nasal polyps usually is associated with a severe type of asthma that is frequently steroid dependent. This type of asthma has the bronchospastic type of aspirin intolerance, not the urticaria/angioedema type (Table VIII). In many cases, only two legs of the triad are present, asthma and aspirin intolerance, which usually occur within one year of each other. Nasal polyps may occur about 10 years later.[30] The mean age of

onset of the asthma and aspirin intolerance part of the triad is about 31 years.[31] However, the cumulative frequency increases with age so that in patients older than 40, the frequency of nasal polyps is 10% and above, table III.

Other characteristics of this triad are listed in Table VIII. It is most commonly associated with nonallergic or negative skin test asthma and with a normal serum IgE level. Specific IgE against aspirin has not been found. During acute bronchospasm produced by aspirin challenge, histamine levels, neutrophil chemotactic activity, and complement activation were not found to be significantly different from baseline levels.[32] Elevated blood eosinophils and a marked eosinophilia in the nasal secretions are also characteristic of this syndrome. There is a hereditary disposition of aspirin intolerance in that clusters of this syndrome are found in certain families.[31] The frequency of aspirin intolerance increases with age, especially over 40. Also, it is the bronchospastic type of aspirin intolerance not the urticaria/angioedema type that increases with age, Tables IX and X.

It is apparent that there are many similarities between aspirin intolerance and nasal polyps. Besides being associated in the triad of asthma, aspirin intolerance (bronchospastic type), nasal polyps are associated with chronic sinusitis and nasal eosinophilia. Both increase in frequency with age, both are associated with negative skin test or nonallergic asthma (Tables II and XI), and both are associated with a high frequency of steroid-dependent asthma. The triad is better described as a tetrad syndrome that includes: aspirin intolerance, nonallergic asthma, nasal polyps, and chronic sinusitis.

Contrary to previous opinion, the surgical removal of nasal polyps does not cause or aggravate asthma

TABLE X

Frequency of Major Types of Aspirin Intolerance in Various Age Groups of Asthmatic Patients

Asthmatic Patients		Major Types of Aspirin Intolerance			
Age when first seen (years)	No. with asthma	No. with bronchospasm	%*	No. with urticaria/ angioedema	%†
10–19	358	3	0.8	2	0.6
20–29	351	6	1.7	6	1.7
30–39	342	11	3.2	3	0.9
40–49	357	18	5.0	7	2.0
50 and over	367	17	4.6	2	0.5
Total	1,775	55	3.1	20	1.1

* The trend of progressive differences by decades is statistically significant ($p < 0.01$).
† The trend of differences is not statistically significant. Included are 3 patients who manifested both bronchospasm and urticaria. Four patients with aspirin intolerance manifested solely by rhinorrhea are not included in this table.

TABLE XI

Frequency of Bronchospasm and Urticaria as Manifestations of Aspirin Intolerance in Asthmatic Patients

	Total No.	No. with Bronchospasm	%	p value	No. with urticaria/ angioedema	%	p value
Extrinsic asthma (positive skin tests)	1,348	30	2.2		17	1.3	
				< 0.01			N.S.
Intrinsic asthma (negative skin tests)	427	25	5.9		3	0.7	
Total asthma	1,775	55	3.1*		20	1.1*	
				< 0.01			< 0.01
Rhinitis alone	2,006	4	0.2†		8	0.4†	

N.S. = not significant.

Three cases who reacted with both bronchospasm and urticaria are included. Four cases of aspirin intolerance manifested solely by rhinorrhea are not included in this table.

* The difference between the number of asthmatics whose symptoms of aspirin intolerance were manifested by bronchospasm (3.1%) as compared to those whose symptoms were manifested by urticaria (1.1%) is statistically significant (p < 0.01).

† Not significantly different.

(Table XII). In our laboratory, 10 patients with nasal polyps and no history of asthma were studied. Results of methacholine challenge tests done before and about five months after polypectomy were similar.[25] In a report by Miles-Lawrence et al.[26] similar data were obtained. They performed methacholine challenge tests one month prior to polypectomy and up to one year following polypectomy. They found essentially no change in methacholine sensitivity, confirming our conclusion that polypectomy does not cause or worsen asthma. However, the occurrence rate for nasal polyps following polypectomy is notoriously high and may be aggravated by many nonspecific factors such as upper respiratory infection and allergies to pollens, danders, and molds (when the chance occurrence of these diseases coexists).[30,33]

To extend these laboratory findings to clinically relevant data, we evaluated pulmonary function tests just prior to polypectomy and up to five months following polypectomy. There was no significant change in pulmonary function tests.[30]

We also evaluated seven steroid-dependent asthmatic patients for steroid requirements before and approximately six months following polypectomy (Table XIII). The steroid requirements were essentially unchanged in five patients and decreased in two, possibly because of less stimulation through the rhinosinobronchial reflex. Thus, our initial data with methacholine sensitivity have been confirmed with subsequent clinical information.

It is important to remember that nonsteroidal anti-inflammatory drugs (NSAID) cross-react with aspirin

TABLE XII

Effect of Polypectomy on Methacholine Sensitivity

Investigators	Total Patients	Diagnosis	Methacholine Sensitivity			Time Interval after Polypectomy
			Same	Increased	Decreased	
Downing, Braman, Settipane (1982)[25]	6	No asthma	6	0	0	Mean 20 wk
	4	Asthma	2	1	1	Mean 20 wk
Miles-Lawrence, Kaplan, Chang (1982)[26]	5	No asthma	2	1	2	1 mo*
	1	Asthma	0	1	0	

* Two patients followed for 6 and 12 months, respectively, had no change in methacholine sensitivity.

TABLE XIII

Effect of Polypectomy on Steroid-Dependent Asthma (6-Month Interval)

| Patient | Age (yr) | Prednisone | | Change in Asthma |
		Preoperative	Postoperative (6 mo)	
M.S.	48	10 mg alt days	10 mg alt days	Same
P.B.	25	10 mg alt days	10 mg alt days*	Same
L.C.	66	10 mg alt days	2.5 mg daily	Better
P.M.	66	5 mg daily	10 mg alt days	Better
F.S.	42	10 mg alt days	10 mg alt days	Same
V.L.	58	10 mg daily	10 mg daily	Same
J.C.	76	10 mg alt days	10 mg alt days	Same

* Data collected at 9 months.

and cause a similar acute bronchospasm in aspirin-intolerant asthmatics. These drugs are cyclooxygenase inhibitors. Some of these NSAID, such as indomethacin and ibuprofen, cross-react with aspirin in intolerant individuals about 100% of the time. Other NSAID cross-react with aspirin in intolerant individuals at a somewhat decreased rate.

The pathological mechanism of aspirin intolerance is unknown. A recent pathogenic hypothesis for aspirin intolerance is based on the association between prostaglandin and SRS-A. It is possible that in certain individuals, inhibition of the cyclooxygenase pathway may cause a preference for the lipoxygenase pathway resulting in increased production of leukotrienes LTC_4, LTD_4, and LTE_4 (SRS-A), which will produce bronchospasm (Figure 4). In addition, products of the lipoxygenase system such as 5-HPETE, 5-HETE, and LTB_4 are chemotactic for eosinophils. Both aspirin intolerance and nasal polyps are associated with eosinophils. A decrease in PGE may allow the bronchospastic effects of PGF and leukotrienes to predominate. A similar mechanism including arachidonic acid and prostaglandins for the formation of nasal polyps has not been developed at this time, but further research is needed in this area.

TREATMENT

Polypectomy is not the treatment of choice for routine nasal polyposis. We reviewed 167 patients with verified nasal polyps (Table VI). Eighty-six percent (143) had polypectomies. Of these 143, 57 (40%) required two or more polypectomies, 34 (24%) required three or more polypectomies, 22 (15%) required four or more polypectomies, 17 (12%) had five or more polypectomies, and 11 (8%) had six or more polypectomies. Three of our patients had a history of 20 or more polypectomies. Therefore, nasal polyposis fre-

quently is a recurrent problem in over 40% of the cases. Other studies[19] have found a recurrence rate of over 31%.

Surgical polypectomy does not permanently eliminate this disease. However in certain selected cases, especially in those in whom corticosteroids are not effective or are contraindicated, surgical polypectomy may be considered. Steroid injection of nasal polyps has been used with some success in the hands of expert otolaryngologists.[34] However, injection of steroids in the nasal turbinates and polyps has resulted in ten instances of visual loss, five of which were permanent as of 1981.[35] Steroid emboli were demonstrated in the retinal vessels in six cases. Certainly, this type of treatment for nasal polyps should be reserved for the very skilled otolaryngologist if it is used at all.

At present, I believe the treatment of choice is a ten-day course of systemic corticosteroid therapy beginning with about 60 mg of prednisone orally and decreasing by 5 mg daily. This short burst of corticosteroids should not cause a clinically significant suppression of the pituitary-adrenal axis. Occasionally, patients may need a second burst of steroids a few weeks later if they don't improve with the first course of corticosteroid treatment.

Afterward patients may be maintained on topical beclomethasone or flunisolide, realizing that long-term use of these topical medications may result in some suppression of the puitary-adrenal axis, which may not be clinically significant. Newer products such as topical fluocortin butyl may help solve these complications since this steroid has not been found to have a significant pituitary-adrenal effect. Fluocortin butyl is still undergoing clinical investigation and has not been released to the practicing physician in the United States.

Even with systemic and topical corticosteroid therapy, nasal polyps frequently still may be a recurrent disease, and periodic bursts of systemic corticosteroids may have to be administered. When treatment with systemic corticosteroids has no effect, or is contraindicated, a surgical procedure may be contemplated.

Patients with nasal polyps deserve an allergic evaluation despite the fact that a large percentage of them are nonatopic. If clinically relevant IgE-mediated disease is found in these patients, a course of hyposensitization may be given, especially in those with recurrent polyposis. IgE-mediated disease is not the cause of nasal polyps, but it may contribute to episodes or exacerbations.[27,36]

SUMMARY

The pathogenic mechanism of nasal polyps are unknown. They frequently are associated with aspirin intolerance, intrinsic asthma, chronic sinusitis, Young's syndrome, cystic fibrosis, Kartagener's syndrome, and Churg-Strauss syndrome. Children 16 years or younger with nasal polyps should be evaluated for cystic fibrosis. Nasal polyps are frequently bilateral, multiple, freely movable, and pale-gray and arise from the middle meatus of the nose. Histologically, they classically have pseudostratified ciliated columnar epithelium, thick-

Arachidonic metabolism: pathogenic mechanism for aspirin intolerance.

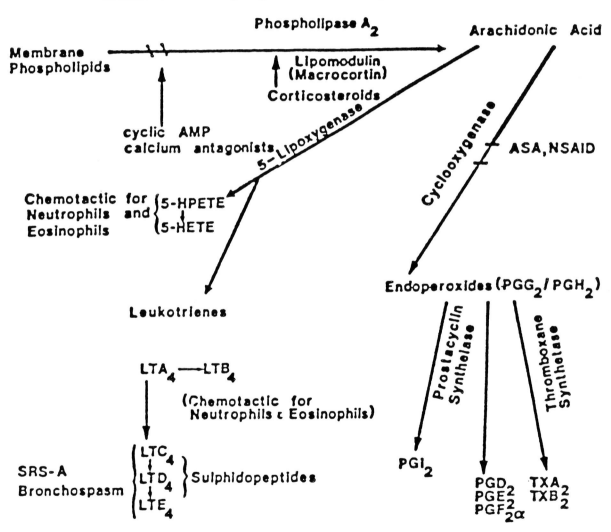

Figure 4. SRS-A induces arachidonic acid metabolism, thus providing a positive feedback mechanism while PGE₁, PGE₂, PGI inhibit SRS-A release, providing a potential negative feedback mechanism. PGE₁, PGE₂ and PGI₂ are bronchodilators. PGF₂, PGD and TXB₂ are bronchoconstrictors. Aspirin and other nonsteroid, anti-inflammatory drugs potentiate 5-lipoxygenase products whil inhibiting cyclooxygenase products. In addition to bronchospasm, LTC₄, LTD₄ and LTE₄ increase cutaneous vasopermeability an elicit a wheal and flare reaction when administered intracutaneously to patients. Elevated cyclic AMP levels, calcium antagonist and glucocorticoids are important inhibitors of arachidonic liberation.

ening of the epithelial basement membrane, high stromal eosinophil count, mucin with neutral pH, few glands and essentially no nerve endings. Cells consist of a mixture of lymphocytes, plasma cells, and eosinophils. Polyps from patients with Young's syndrome, Kartagener's syndrome, and cystic fibrosis have predominantly neutrophils with insignificant eosinophils. Chemical mediators found in nasal polyps are as follows: histamine, serotonin, leukotrienes [(SRS-A or LTC_4, LTD_4, LTE_4), LTB_4], ECF-A, norepinephrine, kinins, TAME-esterase, and possibly PGD_2. There is more histamine in nasal polyps than in normal nasal mucosa, and norepinephrine is present in greater concentration in the base of nasal polyps than in normal nasal mucosa. The concentrations of IgA and IgE and, in some cases, IgG and IgM are greater in polyp fluid than in serum. IgE-mediated disease is not the cause of nasal polyps, but when present, may contribute to episodes of exacerbation. Upper respiratory infections also may cause exacerbations. Despite medical or surgical management, a significant number of nasal polyps are recurrent. For treatment, systemic corticosteroids should be tried before surgical polypectomy. Polypectomy does not increase the risk of developing asthma or making asthma worse.

REFERENCES

1. Vancil ME. A historical survey of treatments for nasal polyposis. Laryngoscope 79:435–445, 1969.
2. Settipane GA, Chafee FH. Nasal polyps in asthma and rhinitis: A review of 6,037 patients. J Allergy Clin Immunol 59:17–21, 1977.
3. Chafee FH, Settipane GA. Aspirin intolerance: I. Frequency in an allergic population. J Allergy Clin Immunol 53:193–199, 1974.
4. Settipane GA, Chafee FH, Klein DE. Aspirin intolerance: II. A prospective study in an atopic and normal population. J Allergy Clin Immunol 53:200–204, 1974.
5. Slavin RG, Linford P, Friedman WH. Sinusitis and bronchial asthma. J Allergy Clin Immunol 69 (Part 2):102, 1982.
6. Lanoff G, Daddono A, Johnson E. Nasal polyps in children: A ten-year study. Ann Allergy 31:551–554, 1973.
7. Ballantyne J. The Nose. In: Grooves, ed. Scott Brown's Diseases of the Ear, Nose and Throat, 3rd ed. Philadelphia: J. B. Lippincott Co, 1971, p. 179.
8. Oppenheimer EH, Rosenstein BJ. Differential pathology of nasal polyps in cystic fibrosis and atopy. Lab Invest 40:445–449, 1979.
9. Wladislavosky-Wasserman P, Kern EB, Holley KE, Gleich GJ. Epithelial damage is commonly seen in nasal polyps. J Allergy Clin Immunol 69 (Part 2):148, 1982.
10. Busuttil A. Dysplastic epithelial changes in nasal polyps. Ann Otol Rhinol Laryngol 87:416–420, 1978.
11. Atzelius BA. Disorders of ciliary motility. Hosp Pract 21:73–80, 1986.
12. Rossman CM, Lee RM, Forrest JB, Newhouse MT. Nasal ciliary ultrastructure and function in patients with primary ciliary dyskinesia compared with that in normal subjects and in subjects with various respiratory diseases. Am Rev Respir Dis 129:161–167, 1984.
13. MacKay DN. Antibiotic treatment of rhinitis and sinusitis. Am J Rhinol 1:83–85, 1987.
14. Schanker HM, Rajfer J, Saxon A. Recurrent respiratory disease, azoospermia, and nasal polyposis. Arch Intern Med 145:2201–2203, 1985.
15. Handelsman DJ, Conway AJ, Boylan LM, Turtle JR. Young's syndrome. Obstructive azoospermia and chronic sinopulmonary infections. N Engl J Med 310:3–9, 1984.
16. Pelletier G, Hebert J, Bedard PM, Salari H, Borgeat P. Profile of leukotrienes and histamine from human nasal polyps (abst). J Allergy Clin Immunol 77 (Part 2):177, 1986.
17. Bumsted RM, El-Ackad T, Smith JM, Brody MJ. Histamine, norepinephrine and serotonin content of nasal polyps. Laryngoscope 89:832–843, 1979.
18. Kaliner M, Wasserman SI, Austen KF. Immunologic release of chemical mediators from human nasal polyps. N Eng J Med 289:277–281, 1973.
19. Chandra RK, Abrol BM. Immunopathology of nasal polypi. J Laryngol Otol 88:1019–1024, 1974.
20. Berdal P. Serologic investigations on the edema fluid from nasal polyps. J Allergy 23:11–14, 1952.
21. Mygind N. Nasal polyps. In: Mygind W, ed. Nasal Allergy, 2nd ed. Oxford, London: Blackwell Scientific Publications, 1979, pp. 233–238.
22. Gray L. Deviated nasal septum. III. Its influence on the physiology and disease of the nose and ear. J Laryngol 81:953–986, 1967.
23. Tos M, Mogensen C. Density of mucous glands in normal adult nasal septum. Arch Otorhinolaryngol 215:101, 1977.
24. Bernstein JM, Cropp JA, Nathanson I, Yankaskas JR. Bioelectric properties of cultured human nasal polypi and turbinate epithelial cells. Am J Rhinol (in press).
25. Downing ET, Braman S, Settipane GA. Bronchial reactivity in patients with nasal polyps before and after polypectomy. J Allergy Clin Immunol 69 (Part 2):102, 1982.
26. Miles-Lawrence R, Kaplan M, Chang K. Methacholine sensitivity in nasal polyposis and the effects of polypectomy. J Allergy Clin Immunol 69 (Part 2):102, 1982.
27. Connell JT. Nasal disease. N Engl Soc Allergy Proc 3:389–396, 1982.
28. Settipane GA. Aspirin intolerance presenting as chronic rhinitis. R I Med J 63:63–65, 1980.
29. Whiteside TL, Rabin BS, Zetterberg J, Criep L. The presence of IgE on the surface of lymphocytes in nasal polyps. J Allergy Clin Immunol 55:186–194, 1975.
30. Settipane GA, Klein DE, Lekas MD. Asthma and nasal polyps. In: Myers E, ed. New Dimensions in Otorhinolaryngology, Head and Neck Surgery. Amsterdam: Excerpta Medica, 1987, pp. 499–500.
31. Settipane GA, Pudupakkam RK. Aspirin intolerance. III. Subtypes, familial occurrence and cross-reactivity with tartrazine. J Allergy Clin Immunol 56:215–221, 1975.
32. Simon R, Pleskow W, Kaliner M, Wasserman S. Plasma mediator studies in aspirin sensitive asthma. J Allergy Clin Immunol 71 (Part 2):146, 1983.
33. Settipane GA. Nasal polyposis. N Engl Soc Allergy Proc 3:497–504, 1982.
34. McCleve D, Gatos L, Goldstein J, Silvers S. Corticosteroid injections of the nasal turbinates: Past experience and precautions. ORL J Otorhinolaryngol Relat Spec 86:851–857, 1978.
35. Mabry RL. Visual loss after intranasal corticosteroid injection. Arch Otolaryngol 107:484–486, 1981.
36. Settipane GA. Nasal polyps: Epidemiology, pathology, immunology and treatment. Am J Rhinol 1:119–126, 1987.

Chapter XXI

Chronic Sinusitis and Nonallergic Rhinitis

Howard M. Druce, M.D.

ABSTRACT

Syndromes of chronic sinusitis (CS) and nonallergic rhinitis (NAR) are poorly defined. There is a paucity of epidemiologic studies, and long-term treatment outcome remains based mainly on anecdotal evidence. Clinical diagnoses must be differentiated from those made solely on radiographic criteria. The role of allergic disease in CS is undetermined. Many factors such as vascular reactivity, cellular infiltration, modifications of nasal secretions, anatomic abnormalities, deficiency of mucociliary clearance, immunodeficiency, and nasal reflexes contribute to symptom pathogenesis. The question whether NAR is a disease or an exaggerated physiologic response is controversial and is addressed in this contribution. Ultimately, enhanced knowledge of the pathophysiology of CS and NAR may lead to novel therapeutic approaches. Patients readily attribute a variety of symptoms such as postnatal drainage, facial fullness or swelling, head pressure, and nasal congestion to the paranasal sinuses. Unfortunately, many practitioners do not adopt a critical attitude to diagnosing sinus pathology and differentiating it from exaggerated physiologic responses to environmental factors. In this paper I will try to highlight some of the difficulties in this area.

CHRONIC SINUSITIS

Chronic sinusitis (CS) is one of the most common chronic diseases and has significant morbidity to warrant study.[1,2] Clinically, patients who complain of purulent postnasal drainage, facial pain, frontal head-

Assistant Professor of Internal Medicine and Otolaryngology, and Director, Nasal and Paranasal Sinus Physiology Laboratory, St. Louis University School of Medicine, St. Louis, MO.

aches, nasal congestion, and halitosis are considered to have CS.[3] A sinus radiograph (SXR) in this condition is usually abnormal and they may be considered the hallmark of the disease.[4] Radiographic abnormalities generally accepted for diagnosis include opacification, air-fluid levels, or mucoperiosteal thickening in at least one sinus. The degree of thickening considered significant is debatable.[5,6] Air-fluid levels are less commonly seen in CS compared to acute sinusitis.

Symptoms overlap between CS and nonallergic rhinitis (NAR). It is not possible to make a differential diagnosis on the basis of symptoms, taken either individually or in combination,[7] and predict the presence of an abnormal SXR. Even with the classical symptoms as mentioned above, it has been estimated that at least 10% of sinusitis patients have a normal SXR, according to Melén et al.[8] There is also a marked disparity between radiologists' interpretations of SXRs, even when standardized study conditions are adopted.[9] In sinusitis in general, it has been considered that an abnormal SXR predicts the finding of fluid or organisms in the affected sinus,[6] however, antral puncture is generally not performed in CS and is only feasible for the maxillary sinuses.

Our clinical strategy is to categorize patients depending on five clinical syndromes they may exhibit (Table I). To make a definitive diagnosis, a SXR is generally required, although in cases with a first episode it is rational to treat symptomatically.

Acute sinusitis may be described as a constellation of symptoms, including purulent postnatal drainage and/ or rhinorrhea, nasal congestion, facial pain, tenderness and/or swelling, and halitosis. These usually occur as the prolongation of a febrile upper respiratory infection but may also be the consequence of barotrauma or facial injury.[10] A first episode may be treated initially by an antibiotic course of sufficient duration and dosage,[11] decongestants, and nasal toilet measures, including steam inhalations and saline irrigation.

Recurrent acute sinusitis may be defined as a condition with recurrent episodes, with an abnormal SXR during exacerbations, but normal films during the symptom-free intervals. Depending on the frequency of attacks, a course of treatment may be given for each episode and medical prophylaxis to maintain ostial patency is not always recommended.

Patients with clinical chronic sinusitis are considered to have exhibited continuous symptoms for more than 3 months. The SXR is generally abnormal and patients often make a good short-term response to adequate medical treatment.[3] However, it is important to detect underlying conditions, such as anatomic defects, polyps, or coexisting chronic rhinitis, either allergic or nonallergic. Failure of medical therapy with continued symptoms is an indication for sinus surgery.[12] Acute exacerbations frequently occur in addition to CS and for this reason we usually maintain CS patients on prophylactic therapy designed to maintain ostial patency,[13,14] such as oral decongestants and/or topical nasal steroids.

Diagnostic difficulty arises when symptoms are presented and the SXR is normal. Frequently, isolated frontal headaches, facial pain, or nasal congestion is ascribed to sinus pathology. In such patients we try carefully to look for a pathologic condition not directly related to the sinuses. Chronic dental infection may produce symptoms in a significant number of patients.[15] Intermittent occlusion of the sinus ostia by nasal mucosal swelling may produce vacuum headaches. This is especially marked when the middle turbinate occludes the nares, often with the coexistence of a deviated nasal septum. Eustachian tube dysfunction, temporomandibular joint syndromes, nonerupted wisdom teeth, and visual acuity changes may also be involved.[3] To reassure such patients that no underlying sinus pathology is present, we obtain a SXR and perform skin-prick tests to environmental allergens. When symptoms are isolated, such as copious clear rhinorrhea

---

TABLE I

Sinusitis Syndromes

1. Acute sinusitis
2. Recurrent acute sinusitis
3. Chronic sinusitis
4. Acute-on-chronic sinusitis
5. Sinus-related symptoms (includes chronic rhinitis, eustachian tube dysfunction, middle turbinate squeeze, etc.)

---

or shifting nasal congestion, an exaggerated physiologic response that does not imply a pathologic condition must be considered.

Population studies have determined that groups of patients with nonrespiratory complaints may still have an abnormal SXR.[5] Such a finding has also been demonstrated for other imaging tests such as magnetic resonance imaging,[16] and this has led to some controversy in interpretation of the role of asymptomatic sinus disease in exacerbations of asthma.[17] Can chronic sinusitis be asymptomatic, and do abnormal SXRs always denote disease? Only ready availability of a pathologic test (abnormal microbial culture or biopsy) can provide a definitive diagnosis. In the absence of such a finding, diagnoses are inferential, at best.

There are no good prospective studies of CS to assess treatment outcome on medical therapy. It is clear that treatment for sinusitis ameliorates asthmatic symptoms[18] and reduces prednisone requirements in such subjects.[19,20] Our data to date indicate a 60–70% rate of significant improvement in symptoms using medical therapy for one month, followed by long-term prophylaxis as detailed above.[21]

Another confounding issue is that of superimposed allergic disease. Clearly, if the classical symptoms of allergic rhinitis are present (clear rhinorrhea, episodic sneezing paroxysms, and nasal itching), the diagnosis is easy. However, patients with only classical symptoms of CS have an appreciable incidence of positive epicutaneous skin tests to environmental allergens.[22] Do these skin tests denote participation of the sinus mucosa in the allergic process? One suggestion that this may be the case has been advanced in a preliminary study by Slavin et al.[23] In this study a hyperemic response of the sinus mucosa was demonstrated during the ragweed season which returned to normal once the season was over, implying a direct participation of the sinus mucosa in an allergic reaction. The finding of major basic protein in biopsies of sinus mucosa, in both allergic and nonallergic patients, also suggests a hypersensitivity-type reaction.[24]

Whereas many symptoms of CS (nasal obstruction, headache, and postnasal drainage) may be accounted for by sinus ostial occlusion, it has been postulated that the key to the pathogenesis can be found in this anatomic location.[25] It is unclear to what extent abnormal anatomy, mucosal inflammation, and hyperreactivity processes contribute to genesis of the symptoms. Since nasal steroids can relieve nasal congestion in many cases, it is tempting to assume that significant ostial inflammation is present.

NONALLERGIC RHINITIS (NAR)

Classically, such patients have been divided into those with predominant nasal obstruction (blockers) and those with rhinorrhea (drippers).[26] However, symptoms may include vacuum or sinus-type headaches and post-nasal drainage. In patients with symptoms exacerbated by temperature changes, hot or spicy foods, alcohol, bright lights, or odors, a diagnosis of vasomotor rhinitis, which is considered to be a subset of NAR, is made. There is no good evidence that these patients have increased sympathetic afferent neural impulses to produce "vasomotor" effects. Indeed, the lack of response to oral decongestants may suggest that factors other than vascular reactivity are involved in its pathogenesis.[27] NAR symptoms in patients are often diagnosed as "sinusitis" and limited or temporary relief is obtained from antibiotics. Is NAR a true disease or an exaggerated physiological response to an as-yet-undefined stimulus?

There are other specific subsets of NAR. Jacobs et al.[28] have described patients with a characteristic pattern of nasal obstruction, sneezing, and rhinorrhea, who, despite negative skin tests, display nasal eosinophilia. It is not clear how prevalent this syndrome (nonallergic rhinitis with eosinophilia) is in the general population.[29] Occasionally, patients with pure rhinorrhea are seen with pronounced nasal eosinophilia, but with negative skin tests and normal range serum IgE.

How can we determine whether NAR is an exaggerated physiologic response or a pathologic one? Three areas may be addressed:

1. Vascular response. Microvascular parameters (blood flow, blood volume, and speed of red blood cells) can be measured directly in human nasal mucosa.[30] In this way, it may be determined if autonomic responses are similar to those in subjects with hyperreactive or normal airways. Plasma proteins or chemical mediators produced by local cells may be measured in nasal lavage.[31] So far, data obtained from an α-adrenergic topical nasal provocation challenge are not different in NAR patients from those seen in normal subjects, whereas cholinergic challenge with methacholine yields an intermediate response between normal and allergic subjects.[22,32]

2. Cellular response. Prolonged nasal and/or sinus ostial occlusion may be accounted for by an abnormal cellular infiltration. This process may constitute an inflammatory response, either triggered by an as yet undefined stimulus or may be part of a mast cell-mediated process. It has been hypothesized that chronic allergic rhinitis is a continuously triggered "late-phase" mast cell-mediated reaction.[33] Nonimmunologic degranulation of mast cells by physical stimuli such as cold dry air and hyperosmolarity have been well demonstrated.[34] A link between the latter reaction and a late phase has yet to be clearly demonstrated.

The role of the eosinophil has to be further clarified. Its role in acute allergic reactions is not totally certain. The major toxic product of the eosinophil granules, major basic protein, has been found in biopsy specimens of sinus mucosa of allergic and nonallergic subjects.[34] Eosinophils are found in both allergic rhinitis and nonallergic forms of rhinitis.[29] Cellular recovery from nasal lavage is scant, but further cytologic studies may be expected to add to our knowledge.

3. Nasal secretions. Are these normal or abnormal in these clinical syndromes? Since the normal composition of upper airway secretions is complex and variable,[36,37] the advent of controlled experiments designed to recover nasal lavage after topical nasal provocation challenge has yielded useful information.[31] Techniques are now available to assay the minute quantities of products secreted by mast cells, neutrophils, and eosinophils, such as leukotrienes and prostaglandins. The difficulty of quantitating the volume of nasal secretions accurately[31] has hampered studies. The concentrations of mediators recovered from nasal lavage indirectly reflect cellular processes occurring deep in the nasal mucosa. Analyses of mediators such as neuropeptides and metabolic nucleotides have been undertaken.

ANATOMIC CONSIDERATIONS

The role of physiologic aberrations is as uncertain in these diseases as is the role of anatomic abnormalities. Most practitioners have seen patients unsuccessfully treated for sinusitis by correction of a nasal septal deflection. Clearly, a marked deflection may occlude a sinus ostium directly or may cause synechiae with the lateral nasal wall or the middle turbinate. It is often not appreciated that most septal deflections are S-shaped, with the main resistance to airflow occurring at the narrowest bony portion of the nose by the bridge.[38] This area is not visualized by simple anterior rhinoscopic examination. For complete evaluation of the nasal airway fiberoptic rhinoscopy with topical decongestion is useful.[39] Although there is often a lack of correlation between subjective symptoms of nasal obstruction and objective measurements of airflow resistance,[40] measurement of nasal airflow resistance is often useful.[41] We utilize the technique of active anterior rhinomanometry in our laboratory, pre- and post-topical decongestion, to assess not only the severity of obstruction, but also to what degree it is reversible by vascular constriction. In this way, many patients who benefit from extended efforts to promote decongestion are discovered.[42]

The recent interest in functional endoscopic sinus surgery has demonstrated the importance of sinus ostial occlusion[25] not only in maxillary disease but also in ethmoid sinusitis. Mere correction of abnormal anatomy may lead to resolution of chronic sinusitis.

In addition to surgical intervention, α-adrenergic agonists have been shown to improve sinus ostial patency.[14] It is also likely that topical intranasal corticosteroids affect ostial patency, as well as cellular recruitment.

TABLE II

Pathophysiology of Nasal Symptoms in CS and NAR

Syndrome	Pathophysiology	Response	Exaggerated
Nasal obstruction	Vascular dilatation, 2° sympathetic stimulation	Nasal cycle (insensible)	Shifting congestion
Rhinorrhea	a. Glandular secretion, 2° parasympathetic stimulation	Insensible secretions	Clear rhinorrhea
	b. Transudation from vascular compartment	Insensible	Clear rhinorrhea
Postnasal drip	Normal glandular secretions	Normal glandular secretions insensibly cleared (evaporation; ciliary transport)	Nasal obstruction forces postnasal drip

The detailed microanatomy around the sinus ostia is unknown. It would be of interest to know more about the configuration of the blood vessels in this region. For instance, precise ascertainment of the ratio of arteriovenous shunt vessels to capacitance vessels and their spatial disposition should lead to a more detailed interpretation of microvascular physiologic measurements.

In addition, this work can be combined with an enhanced analysis of vessel receptors. The use of competitive receptor antagonism with dose-response assessment and receptor-specific agents would be of value. α_1 and α_2 specific adrenergic sympathomimetics and antagonists, and histamine H_1 and H_2 agents may be useful agents to study in vitro. Ligand-binding studies of nasal tissue are another promising method for receptor analysis.[43]

OTHER ETIOLOGIC FACTORS

The role of mucociliary clearance has not been fully considered in the genesis of these syndromes. When there is a profound defect such as Kartagener's syndrome,[44] sinusitis is common. More subtle changes are difficult to detect because tests of mucociliary function are either not quantitative (electron microscopy)[45] or not sufficiently precise (saccharin taste test). α-Adrenergic agonist medications have been withheld by some practitioners, because they have the potential to promote ciliary stasis. The clinical evidence is unclear[46]; however, in our experience, this has not proved to be a problem.

The persistence of symptoms, especially purulent drainage, should suggest the presence of an organism resistant to the antibiotic therapy previously employed.[47,48] There is certainly an increase in the incidence of β-lactam resistant Branhamella catarrhalis especially in children.[49] In adult patients, there has been an increased appearance of fungal sinusitis, possibly on the basis of a true infection or as a sign of a hypersensitivity reaction.[50,51]

Immunodeficiency may also lead to sinusitis in certain cases. Generalized immunodeficiency states lead to chronic infections with specific organisms[52] and the sinuses may be frequently infected.[53] Selective immunodeficiency, such as IgG2 or IgG4 deficiencies, may be found in CS, but it is unclear if this is a sole causative factor in these patients.[54] Localized immunodeficiency may occur in the nose, either by reduced production of IgE or secretory IgA. It has not been determined if this defect is an important factor in the development of CR and CS.

Nasobronchial reflexes and local nasal reflexes may underlie some of the symptoms seen in these patients.[55] Connell[56] described a congestion-decongestion reflex affter unilateral antigen challenge. The well-described nasal cycle, when exaggerated, may be perceived as the shifting congestion in NAR[57] (Table II). Other reflexes need further elucidation.

In summary, our knowledge of CS and NAR is still in an embryonic state. Until our terms are well defined and prospective studies are carried out, it will prove difficult to analyze data in these heterogeneous groups. However, novel methods and technology are providing new insights that may ultimately lead to therapeutic developments.

ACKNOWLEDGMENTS

The author thanks Vernon W. Fischer Ph.D. for his valuable editorial suggestions and counsel, and Margaret Smith for typing the manuscript.

REFERENCES

1. Department of Health and Social Security. Digest of Health Statistics, London: HMSO, 1971.
2. NIH Data Book. U.S. Department of Health and Human Services. 1984, Table 35, p. 57.
3. Druce HM. Diagnosis and management of chronic sinusitis

and its complications. Immunol Allergy Clin North Am 7:117–132, 1987.

4. Axelsson A, Jensen C. The roentgenologic demonstration of sinusitis. AJR 122:621–627, 1974.

5. Kovatch AL, Wald ER, Ledesma-Medina J, Chiponis DM, Bedingfield B. Maxillary sinus radiographs in children with nonrespiratory complaints. Pediatrics 73:306–308, 1984.

6. Evans FO, Sydnor JB, Moore WEC, et al. Sinusitis of the maxillary antrum. N Engl J Med 293:735–739, 1975.

7. Rutledge J, Druce HM. Epidemiology of chronic rhinitis and sinusitis. J Allergy Clin Immunol 81:172, 1988.

8. Melén I, Lindahl L, Andréasson L. Short and long-term treatment results in chronic maxillary sinusitis. Acta Otolaryngol 102:282–290, 1986.

9. Druce HM, Heiberg E, Rutledge J. Disparity between radiographic and ultrasound interpretation in chronic sinusitis. J Allergy Clin Immunol 81:284, 1988.

10. Slavin RG. Nasal polyps and sinusitis. In: Middleton E Jr, Reed CE, Ellis EF, Atkinson NF Jr, Yuninger JW 3rd, eds. Allergy, Principles and Practice. St. Louis, C. V. Mosby, 1988, Chap. 54, pp. 1291–1303.

11. Siegel JD. Diagnosis and management of acute sinusitis in children. Pediatr Infect Dis 6:95–99, 1987.

12. Friedman WH, Slavin RG. Diagnosis and medical and surgical treatment of sinusitis in adults. Clin Rev Allergy 2:409–428, 1984.

13. Melén I, Friberg B, Andréasson L, Ivarsson A, Jannert M, Lindahl L. Ostial and nasal patency in chronic maxillary sinusitis. A long-term post-treatment study. Acta Otolaryngol 102:500–508, 1986.

14. Melén I, Friberg B, Andréasson L, Ivarsson A, Jannert M, Johansson C-J. Effects of phenylpropanolamine on ostial and nasal patency in patients treated for chronic maxillary sinusitis. Acta Otolaryngol 101:494–500, 1986.

15. Melén I, Lendahl L, Andréasson L, Rundcrantz H. Chronic maxillary sinusitis: definition, diagnosis and relation to dental infections and nasal polyposis. Acta Otolaryngol 101:320–327, 1986.

16. Conner BL, Phillips K, Roach ES, Georgitis JW. Nuclear magnetic resonance (NMR) imaging of paranasal sinuses: frequency of abnormalities. J Allergy Clin Immunol 77:139, 1986.

17. McFadden ER Jr. Nasal-sinus-pulmonary reflexes and bronchial asthma. J Allergy Clin Immunol 78:1–3, 1986.

18. Phipatanakul CS, Slavin RG. Bronchial asthma produced by paranasal sinusitis. Arch Otolaryngol 100:109–112, 1974.

19. Rachelefsky GS, Katz RM, Siegel SC. Chronic sinus disease with associated reactive airway disease in children. Pediatrics 73:526–529, 1984.

20. Friedman R, Ackerman M, Wald E, Casselbrant M, Friday G, Fireman P. Asthma and bacterial sinusitis in children. J Allergy Clin Immunol 74:185–9, 1984.

21. Druce HM, Rutledge JL. Unpublished data.

22. Druce HM, Ellington-Harris L, Cressman W, Glenn J. Perennial rhinitis and chronic sinusitis: overlapping syndromes. J Allergy Clin Immunol 79:243, 1987.

23. Salvin RG, Zilliox AP, Samuels LD. Is there such an entity as allergic sinusitis? J Allergy Clin Immunol 81:284, 1988.

24. Harlin SL, Ansel DG, Lane SR, Myers J, Kephart GM, Gleich GJ. A clinical and pathological study of chronic sinusitis: the role of the eosinophil. J Allergy Clin Immunol 79:128, 1987.

25. Kennedy DW, Zinreich SJ, Rosenbaum AE, Johns ME. Functional endoscopic sinus surgery: theory and diagnostic evaluation. Arch Otolaryngol 111:576–582, 1985.

26. Mygind N. Perennial rhinitis. In: Nasal Allergy, 2nd ed. Oxford: Blackwell, 1979, Chap. 15, pp. 224–232.

27. Druce HM. Measurement of nasal mucosal blood flow. J Allergy Clin Immunol 81:505–508, 1988.

28. Jacobs RL, Freedman PM, Boswell RN. Nonallergic rhinitis with eosinophilia (NARES syndrome). Clinical and immunologic presentation. J Allergy Clin Immunol 67:253–262, 1981.

29. Mullarkey MF. The classification of nasal disease: an opinion. J Allergy Clin Immunol 67:251–252, 1981.

30. Druce HM, Bonner RF, Patow C, Choo P, Summers RJ, Kaliner MA. Response of nasal blood flow to neurohormones as measured by laser-Doppler velocimetry. J Appl Physiol 57:1276–1283, 1983.

31. Druce HM. Nasal provocation challenge—strategies for experimental design. Ann Allergy 60:191–196, 1988.

32. Druce HM, Wright RH, Kossoff D, Kaliner MA. Cholinergic nasal hyperreactivity in atopic subjects. J Allergy Clin Immunol 76:445–452, 1985.

33. Kaliner M. Hypotheses on the contribution of late-phase allergic responses to the understanding and treatment of allergic diseases. J Allergy Clin Immunol 73:311–315, 1984.

34. Togias AG, Proud D, Lichtenstein LM, Adams GK III, Norman PS, Kagey-Sobotka A, Naclerio RM. The osmolality of nasal secretions increases when inflammatory mediators are released in response to inhalation of cold, dry air. Am Rev Respir Dis 137:625–629, 1988.

35. Gleich GJ. Current understanding of eosinophil function. Hosp. Pract. 23:137–160, 1988.

36. Kaliner M, Marom Z, Patow C, Shelhamer J. Human respiratory mucus. J Allergy Clin Immunol 73:318–323, 1984.

37. Shelhamer J, Marom Z, Kaliner M. The constituents of nasal secretion. Ear Nose Throat J 63:82–84, 1984.

38. Gray L. Dedicated nasal septum. III. Its influence on the physiologic and disease of the nose and ear. J Laryngol Otol 20:953–986, 1967.

39. Selner JC, Koepke JW. Rhinolaryngoscopy in the allergy office. Ann Allergy 54:479–482, 1985.

40. Eccles R, Lancashire B, Tolley NS. Experimental studies on nasal secretion of airflow. Acta Otolaryngol 103:303–306, 1987.

41. McLean JA. Nasal rhinomanometry and experimental nasal challenges. In: Settipane GA, ed. Rhinitis. Providence, RI: The New England Regional Allergy Proceedings 1984, pp. 62–69.

42. Solomon WR, McLean JA. Nasal provocative testing. In: SL Spector, ed. Provocative Challenge Procedures: Bronchial, Oral, Nasal and Exercise. Boca Raton, FL: CRC Press, 1983, Vol. 2, pp. 133–167.

43. Ishibe T, Yamashita T, Kumazawa T, Tanaka C. Adreneric and cholinergic receptors in human nasal mucosa in cases of nasal allergy. Arch Otorhinolaryngol 238:167–173, 1983.

44. Wasserman SJ. Ciliary function and disease. J Allergy Clin Immunol 73:17–19, 1984.

45. Rossman CM, Lee RMKW, Forrest JB, Newhouse MT. Nasal ciliary ultrastructure and function in patients with primary ciliary dyskinesia compared with that in normal subjects and in subjects with various respiratory diseases. Ann Rev Respir Dis 129:161–167, 1984.

46. Paula D, Sutton PP, Lopez-Vidriero MT, Agnew JE, Clarke SW. Drug effects on mucociliary function. Eur J Respir Dis 64(Suppl 128):304–317, 1983.

47. Karma P, Jokipii L, Sipilä P, Luotonen J, Jokipii AMM. Bacteria in chronic maxillary sinusitis. Arch Otolaryngol 105:386–390, 1979.

48. Frederick J, Braude AI. Anaerobic infection of the paranasal sinuses. N Engl J Med 290:135–137, 1974.

49. Nelson JD. Changing trends in the microbiology and management of acute otitis media and sinusitis. Pediatr Infect Dis 5:749–753, 1986.

50. Katzenstein A-LA, Sale SR, Greenberger PA. Allergic aspergillus sinusitis: a readily recognized form of sinusitis. J Allergy Clin Immunol 72:89–93, 1983.

51. Nishioka G, Schwartz JG, Rinaldi MG, Aufdemorte TB, Mackie E. Fungal maxillary sinusitis caused by Curvularia lunata. Arch Otolaryngol Head Neck Surg 113:665–666, 1987.

52. Schlanger G, Lutwick LI, Kurzman M, Hoch B, Chandler FW. Sinusitis caused by Legionella pneumophilia in a patient with the acquired immune deficiency syndrome. Am J Med 77:957–960, 1984.

53. van de Plassche-Boers EM, Drexhage HA, Kokjé-Kleingeld M, Leezenberg HA. Parameters of T cell mediated immunity to commensal micro-organisms in patients with chronic purulent rhinosinusitis: a comparison between delayed type hypersensitivity skin tests, lymphocyte transformation test and macrophage migration inhibition factor assay. Clin Exp Immunol 66:516–524, 1986.

54. Umetsu DT, Ambrosino DM, Quinti I, Siber GR, Geha RS. Recurrent sinopulmonary infection and impaired antibody response to bacterial capsular polysaccharide antigen in children with selective IgG-subclass deficiency. N Engl J Med 313:1247–1251, 1985.

55. Patow CA, Kaliner M. Nasal and cardiopulmonary reflexes. Ear Nose Throat J 63:78–81, 1984.

56. Connell JT. Reciprocal nasal congestion-decongestion reflex. Trans Am Acad Ophthalmol Otolaryngol 72:422–426, 1968.

57. Stoksted P. Rhinometric measurements for determination of the nasal cycle. Acta Otolaryngol [Suppl] 109:159–175, 1953.

Chapter XXII

Gustatory Rhinitis

Gordon D. Raphael, M.D., Mindy Hauptschein-Raphael, M.S., R.D., and Michael A. Kaliner, M.D.

ABSTRACT

Gustatory rhinitis is a syndrome characterized by the profuse watery rhinorrhea produced by consumption of certain spicy, hot foods. In order to investigate the pathogenesis of this common disorder, 18 subjects underwent food challenges with control (bland) foods and positive (spicy) foods. Positive foods, but not control foods, produced rhinorrhea and increased the secretion of albumin and total protein into nasal lavage fluid. Nasal pretreatment with atropine clinically blocked the positive food-induced rhinorrhea and significantly reduced albumin and total protein secretion. Thus, gustatory rhinitis is produced by spicy foods which stimulate atropine-sensitive muscarinic receptors, and this syndrome can be prevented by pretreatment with topical atropine.

There are several well-recognized stimuli or situations which reliably cause rhinitis in many individuals. These include allergic rhinitis, exposure to cold air,[1] assuming the recumbent position,[2] recovering from performing vigorous exercise,[3,4] and inhaling irritating or noxious gases, dust, or fumes.[5] In addition, another syndrome commonly produces rhinorrhea but has received little attention. This syndrome involves the profuse watery rhinorrhea which is produced after eating certain foods and is generally unaccompanied by sneezing, congestion, or pruritus. A study was performed at the National Institutes of Health in order to investigate the pathogenesis of this food-induced rhinorrhea, referred to as gustatory rhinitis.[6]

Eighty-five adult subjects completed a questionnaire about food-related rhinitis symptoms. Out of this group, 18 subjects underwent food and nasal provocations. Atopic subjects had seasonal symptoms of rhinitis and/or asthma, were skin prick test positive to relevant aeroallergens, and were studied outside of their allergy season, when they were asymptomatic. Nonatopic subjects had no allergy symptoms (other than gustatory rhinitis) and were skin test negative. Subjects were skin tested to the foods which were implicated by history as provoking gustatory rhinitis.

A questionnaire was developed in order to determine the prevalence of rhinorrhea produced by the consumption of foods and/or beverages. The questionnaire consisted of 127 items, which were divided into several broad categories: meats, milk and milk products, fruits and juices, breads and grains, vegetables, fats, nuts and seeds, desserts, spices, and miscellaneous. Responders indicated the frequency with which each item produced rhinorrhea.

Nasal challenge solutions consisted of normal saline and atropine sulfate. Foods were commercially obtained or provided by subjects. Control foods were those which historically produced no symptoms upon ingestion, whereas positive foods were those which by history reliably caused rhinorrhea.

CHALLENGE METHODS

Subjects were seated comfortably in an upright position. A soft 8-Fr rubber catheter was atraumatically inserted along the floor of one or both nasal cavities and was connected to suction in order to collect nasal secretions and lavage fluid. In each experiment, four prewashes with normal saline (4 ml each) were performed at 1-minute intervals in order to remove preexisting nasal secretions. A hand-held nebulizer was used to deliver nasal prewashes, saline challenges, atropine treatments, and nasal lavages, and these were sprayed into one nasal cavity at a time. Nasal lavage samples were kept on ice until the end of the experiment at which point they were stored at −70°C for subsequent analysis.

Three protocols were used in this study. In the first protocol, subjects initially received a control nasal challenge with normal saline (0.3 ml). Then they ate a

From the Allergic Diseases Section, Laboratory of Clinical Investigation, and the Clinical Nutrition Service, National Institutes of Health, Bethesda, MD

control food followed by a positive food. In the second protocol, subjects underwent the same control food and positive food challenges, the nasal mucosa was treated unilaterally with 100 μg of atropine (0.3 ml), and then the positive food challenge was again repeated. The third protocol was similar to the second protocol except that catheters were inserted into both nasal cavities and lavages were therefore collected bilaterally. After the first positive food challenge, atropine was sprayed into the right nasal cavity only prior to repeating the positive food challenge.

In each of these protocols, the nasal challenges, atropine treatments, and food challenges were performed at 10-minute intervals, each challenge being followed by a 4-ml nasal lavage prior to the next challenge.

ASSAYS

Total protein in each sample was measured by the method of Lowry et al.[7] using bovine serum albumin as the protein standard.

Human albumin was measured by a specific, competitive enzyme-linked immunosorbent assay.[8] The assay range is between 1 and 100 μg/ml.

Histamine was measured by a single isotope radioenzyme assay as described by Shaff and Beaven[9] and modified by Dyer et al.[10] The sensitivity of this assay is <1.0 ng/ml.

All assay results are recorded as the mean ± SEM. Student's t test was used for statistical comparison.

RESULTS

The food questionnaire was distributed to 85 adults (45 women, 40 men) between the ages of 21 and 68 years (median age 34). According to the questionnaire, the majority of food items did not produce rhinorrhea. Some foods, however, stimulated rhinorrhea in some people some of the time, while a smaller, select group of foods produced rhinorrhea in many subjects virtually all of the time (Table I). Hot chili peppers were the most frequent offenders and produced rhinorrhea in greater that 60% of all responders, followed closely by several other spicy "hot" foods.

Eighteen subjects (10 women and 8 men) between the ages of 21 and 45 participated in nasal and food challenges. The group included nine atopic subjects, eight nonatopic subjects, and one subject with vasomotor rhinitis. Each subject indicated that the consumption of at least one food item reliably produced rhinorrhea without any other symptoms suggestive of food allergy (such as nasal pruritus or sneezing; anosmia; swelling or pruritus of the lips, tongue, or oropharynx; gastrointestinal symptoms including nausea, vomiting, or diarrhea; urticaria; or respiratory symptoms). All subjects were skin test negative to the foods used in the food challenge.

Each subject first consumed a control food consisting of wheat crackers, potato chips, pretzels, hot tea, or gefilte fish balls, followed by a positive food challenge which consisted of hot chili peppers, horseradish, or hot and sour soup. Subjects were instructed to maximize exposure of the food within the mouth rather than quickly swallow it.

Control food challenge did not produce any subjective symptoms or clinical signs. Positive food challenge, on the other hand, produced bilateral rhinorrhea in all subjects (Table II). There were no complaints of nasal or oropharyngeal pruritus, the urge to sneeze, lip swelling, gastrointestinal symptoms, or pulmonary symptoms throughout the study. Facial flushing developed in about half of the subjects, but was unassociated with any cardiovascular changes. Postchallenge nasal examinations revealed, in all subjects, watery secretions with variable amounts of mucus. Minimal mucosal edema was noted in a few subjects (on the side of the nose containing the nasal catheter).

Saline challenge in eight subjects resulted in 72 ± 14 μg/ml of protein while control food challenge failed to affect the measurement significantly (61 ± 9 μg/ml). The effect of control food challenge and positive food challenge (in 18 subjects) on nasal lavage protein, albumin, and albumin percent are shown in Figure 1. Positive food challenge significantly increased the total protein in every subject, increasing from an mean or 78 ± 9 to 255 ± 34 μg/ml ($p < 0.005$). The albumin concentration likewise increased from 7.0 ± 1.6 to 21.0 ± 6.4 μg/ml ($p < 0.025$). On the other hand, the albumin percent, which represents the ratio of albumin to total protein, went from 10.0 ± 2.4 to 8.8 ± 2.0 and

TABLE I

Foods Which Produce Gustatory Rhinitis

Food	Nose Runs Sometimes (%)*	Nose Runs Always (%)*
1. Hot chili peppers	36	27
2. Spicy foods	63	10
3. Horseradish	41	20
4. Hot and sour soup	29	18
5. Red cayenne pepper	38	11
6. Tabasco sauce	36	9
7. Black pepper	38	4
8. Onion	12	8
9. Vinegar	29	0
10. Mustard	13	4

Percentage of total population who scored this result.

TABLE II

Symptoms after Food Challenge

Symptoms	No. Positive/Total (%)		
	Control Food Challenge	Positive Food Challenge	Positive Food Challenge after Atropine
Rhinorrhea on right	0/18 (0)	18/18 (100)	0/10 (0)*
Rhinorrhea on left	0/18 (0)	18/18 (100)	7/10 (70)
Facial flush	0/18 (0)	13/18 (72)	5/10 (50)
Nasal congestion	0/18 (0)	5/18 (28)	3/10 (30)
Tearing	0/18 (0)	5/18 (28)	2/10 (20)
Perspiration	0/18 (0)	2/18 (11)	1/10 (10)

Decrease significant at $p < 0.002$.

was virtually unchanged from control food challenge values.

As noted in a previous study,[8] this secretory pattern (i.e., proportional increases in both albumin and total protein) is most consistent with cholinergically induced secretions. Therefore, the effect of topical atropine on gustatory rhinitis was next examined. Ten subjects received control food challenges, positive food challenges, and then repeat positive food challenges after topical nasal atropine treatment (Fig. 2). Nasal lavages after control food challenges contained 96 ± 10 μg/ml of protein while positive food challenge dramatically increased the protein to 295 ± 43 μg/ml ($p < 0.001$). Atropine treatment reduced this response to 141 ± 21 μg/ml ($p < 0.025$) as compared to no atropine treatment. Atropine also significantly reduced food-induced albumin secretion from 15.3 ± 4.5 μg/ml before treatment to 5.4 ± 2.1 μg/ml after treatment ($p < 0.05$). The albumin percent, however, was unchanged by atropine treatment and remained at control levels.

Four subjects underwent the same second food challenge protocol with nasal catheters inserted into both sides of the nose. In this manner the specific effect of unilaterally applied atropine on gustatory rhinitis was examined, and each subject served as his or her own control. After the first positive food challenge, atropine sulfate (0.1 mg) was applied to the right side of the nose while saline (placebo) was applied to the left side. Then the positive food challenge was repeated. Total protein results from this experiment are shown in Figure 3. On both sides of the nose, positive food challenge significantly increased total protein secretion as compared to control food challenge ($p < 0.05$). Atropine treatment significantly reduced this positive food-induced protein secretion, while the placebo-treated side showed virtually no change.

Histamine was measured in nasal lavages in order to explore the possibility that mast cell degranulation may cause or be associated with gustatory rhinitis. Baseline histamine levels were 1.4 ± 0.6 ng/ml (within normal range) in 15 challenges. Control food challenge, positive food challenge, and positive food challenge after atropine all failed to alter the histamine level significantly, suggesting that gustatory rhinitis does not cause mast cell degranulation.

DISCUSSION

Ingestion of hot, spicy foods elicits rhinorrhea due to stimulation of atropine-inhibitable muscarinic receptors. This phenomenon has been termed "gustatory rhinitis." Gustatory rhinitis is a common phenomenon characterized by the acute onset of watery (and sometimes mucoid) rhinorrhea precipitated by the ingestion of certain foods. Although most foods do not cause gustatory rhinitis, it is clear that certain foods produce this condition in a large portion of the population.

Gustatory rhinitis differs from allergic rhinitis in several important respects. Symptoms invariably begin within a very few minutes of eating the particular food, and last only as long as the food is eaten. Subjects with gustatory rhinitis do not complain about nasal or oropharyngeal pruritus even though the food may actually cause a burning sensation in the mouth. In addition, they do not complain about nasal congestion, the urge to sneeze, or conjunctival itching, all of which are characteristic of allergic rhinitis. And finally, skin tests with extracts of implicated foods are consistently negative in subjects with gustatory rhinitis.

Positive food challenge consistently produced symptoms and nasal secretions containing increased levels of albumin and protein, without changing the albumin

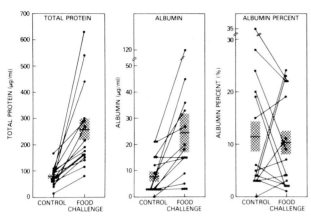

Figure 1. *The effect of food challenge on total protein, albumin, and albumin percent. Open circles represent values of total protein, albumin, and albumin percent from lavage fluids from 18 subjects. Solid lines connect values from each subject after control food challenge followed by positive food challenge. The bars represent mean values.*

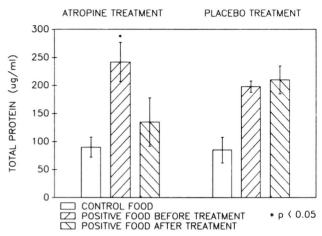

Figure 3. *The effect of atropine versus placebo on food-induced protein secretion. Four subjects were challenged with a control food, a positive food, and then again with a positive food after treatment of one side of the nose with atropine and the other side with saline. Bars represent mean values ± SEM.*

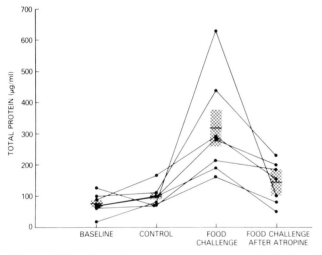

Figure 2. *The effect of atropine pretreatment on food-induced protein secretion. Ten subjects were challenged with a control food, a positive food, and then the same positive food after nasal pretreatment with atropine (0.1 mg). Protein values for each subject are represented by open circles connected by solid lines.*

percent. In contrast, control food challenge produced neither clinical symptoms nor changes in baseline nasal secretions. Prior treatment with atropine blocked food-induced albumin and protein secretion without altering the albumin percent, a pattern which was seen previously with methacholine-induced secretions.[8] These results suggest that gustatory rhinitis provokes a muscarinically mediated secretion of glandular proteins which can be inhibited by atropine. The following sequence of events may explain the syndrome of gustatory rhinitis. Certain food, particularly spicy "hot" foods, contain chemicals (such as capsaicin) which stimulate af-

ferent sensory nerves in the mucosa of the mouth and oropharynx by interacting with chemical or irritant receptors or by eliciting the release of neuropeptides from sensory nerves.[11] A neural reflex arc is initiated which stimulates atropine-inhibitable parasympathetic efferent nerves supplying: the nasal mucosa and glands, producing nasal secretions and congestion; the lacrimal glands in the eyes, producing tears; the sweat glands on the head and forehead, producing perspiration; and the vasculature of the head and neck, causing a facial flush.

In subjects who are particularly sensitive to gustatory rhinitis, there are now two options. They can either avoid the provocative foods, or they can apply topical nasal atropine prophylactically (once it becomes available). Thus, for people with a passion for spicy foods, there may soon be an effective therapy which will allow them to eat to their heart's (and nose's) content.

REFERENCES

1. Togias AG, Naclerio RM, Proud D, Fish JE, Adkinson NF, Kagey-Sobotka A, Norman PS, Lichtenstein LM. Nasal challenge with cold, dry air results in the release of inflammatory mediators. Possible mast cell involvement. J Clin Invest 76:1375–1381, 1985.
2. Cole P, Haight SJ. Posture and nasal patency. Am Rev Respir Dis 129:351–354, 1984.
3. Olson LG, Strohl KP. The response of the nasal airway to exercise. Am Rev Respir Dis 135:356–359, 1987.
4. Syabbalo AK, Bundegaard A, Widdicombe JG. Effects of exercise on nasal airflow resistance in healthy subjects and in patients with asthma and rhinitis. Bull Eur Physiopath Respir 21:507–513, 1985.
5. Patow CA, Kaliner M. Nasal and cardiopulmonary reflexes ENT J 63:78–81, 1984.
6. Raphael GD, Hauptschein-Raphael ML, Kaliner MA. Gus-

tatory rhinitis: A syndrome of food-induced rhinorrhea. J Allergy Clin Immunol 83:110–115, 1989.

7. Lowry OH, Rosebrough NJ, Farr AL, Randall RJ. Protein measurement with the Folin phenol reagent. J Biol Chem 193:265–275, 1951.

8. Raphael GD, Druce HM, Baraniuk JN, and Kaliner MA. Pathophysiology of rhinitis. I. Assessment of the sources of protein in methacholine-induced nasal secretions. Am Rev Respir Dis 138:413–420, 1988.

9. Shaff RE, Beaven MA. Increased sensitivity of the enzymatic isotopic assay of histamine: measurement of histamine in plasma and serum. Anal Biochem 94:425–430, 1979.

10. Dyer J, Warren K, Merlin S, Metcalfe DD, Kaliner M. Measurement of plasma histamine: description of an improved method and normal values. J Allergy Clin Immunol 70:82–87, 1982.

11. Lundblad L, Saria A, Lundberg JM, Anggard A. Increased vascular permeability in rat nasal mucosa induced by substance P and stimulation of capsaicin-sensitive trigeminal neurons. Acta Otolaryngol 96:479–484, 1983.

Chapter XXIII

Nasal Manifestations of Systemic Diseases

Guy A. Settipane, M.D.

ABSTRACT

Many systemic diseases are associated with nasal symptoms. Rhinitis associated with asthma is probably the most common with leprosy and fungal infections being the rarest.

A careful history and nasal examination in a patient with rhinitis may lead to the discovery of more significant systemic diseases. Proper treatment of systemic disease will often cure or improve the associated rhinitis. Similarly, appropriate treatment of the rhinitis/sinusitis may reduce systemic complaints such as asthma. At times, identification of the cause of rhinitis as in CSF rhinorrhea, Wegeners' syndrome, etc., alerts one to a life-threatening entity.

Thus, it is apparent that the nose is an excellent mirror of some systemic diseases and identifying and understanding the differential diagnosis of nasal symptoms may be a tremendous help in diagnosing the disease and treating the whole patient.

Nasal symptoms may be an excellent mirror and diagnostic aid for suspecting the presence of certain generalized or systemic diseases. By examining and evaluating the nose, one may suspect the presence of asthma, aspirin intolerance, endocrine disorders, neoplasms, chest tumors, lung cavities, widespread granulomatous disease, certain chronic infections, dyskinetic cilia syndrome, recurrent meningitis, frequent respiratory infections, and even risk factors for developing asthma. Indeed, the nose, the most anterior part of the body, should be in the forefront for suspicion of systemic diseases.

Clinical Professor, Brown University and Director, Division of Allergy, Department of Medicine, Rhode Island Hospital, Providence, RI 02906

ASTHMA

When a patient is seen with signs of perennial or seasonal rhinitis, it is important to examine the lungs and question the patient for any symptoms of asthma. Pulmonary function tests should be performed in suspected cases, and pulmonary metacholine challenge tests may be done in those patients in whom a diagnosis of asthma is still in question. Perennial or seasonal rhinitis has been associated with asthma in as many as 74% of epidemic studies (Table I). Davies et al.[1] reported that 66% of patients with extrinsic asthma and 40% of patients with nonallergic (cryptogenic) asthma had symptoms of perennial/seasonal rhinitis. Pederson and Weeke[2] in an epidemiology study involving over 7,000 patients in Denmark found that 28% of patients with asthma consulted a general practitioner because they also had allergic rhinitis. This incidence appears low and may be explained by a number of patients who had mild rhinitis and self-medicated rather than consulted a physician.

Another reason to evaluate the lungs and rule out asthma in rhinitis patients is that patients with hay fever have four times the risk of developing asthma than nonallergic individuals. In a 7-year follow-up study[3] of Brown University freshmen, 6.0% of those with allergic rhinitis developed asthma compared to 1.3% of asymptomatic freshmen. In addition, Townley[4] feels that 5% of patients with allergic rhinitis will develop asthma at a later date. He bases this prediction on his methacholine challenge studies in which he found that although 50% of patients with allergic rhinitis showed a greater than 20% decrease in FEV_1, many of these patients reached a "plateau" and further increases in methacholine did not result in a further decrease in FEV_1. Only 5% showed a positive response

TABLE I

Asthma in College Students

Investigators and Population Source	Year of Study	Total No. Students	Asthma %	Asthma % with Allergic Rhinitis
Van Arsdel and Motulsky, University of Washington	1959	5,818	4.7	57
Maternowski and Mathews, University of Michigan	1962	434	5.7	56
Hagy and Settipane, Brown University	1969	1,836	5.3	74

Reprinted with permission from Settipane GA. Current Treatment of Ambulatory Asthma. Providence, New Engl Reg Allergy Proceedings, 1986.

without a plateau phenomenon and these 5% may be the ones that would develop overt asthma at a later time. Townley feels that a partial β-adrenergic blockage exists in patients with allergic rhinitis but not to the degree found in asthmatic patients. Braman et al.[5] reported that 7.5% of patients with allergic rhinitis developed asthma within 5 years. The mean age of these patients was 27 years. Initially, these patients had a positive methacholine test as judged by the PD_{20}. With this background information, all rhinitis patients should be evaluated for early, latent, or silent asthma.

NASAL POLYPS

Nasal polyps may be associated with aspirin intolerance, nonallergic asthma,[6] sinusitis, cystic fibrosis, Kartagener's syndrome, Churg-Strauss syndrome, and Young's syndrome. Detailed information on epidemiology, pathology, pathogenesis and treatment are described in Chapter XX, *Nasal Polyps*. About 23% of patients with nasal polyps have aspirin intolerance as described by acute bronchospasm, severe rhinorrhea, or urticarial/angioedema occurring within 3 hours of ingestion. Nasal polyps are usually the last leg of the triad of asthma, aspirin intolerance, and nasal polyps, but occasionally they can be the first manifestation of this triad.[6] Chronic sinusitis also is associated with this triad. About 71% of patients with nasal polyps have an associated history of asthma. Nasal polyps are frequently found in nonallergic asthma and are associated with "sheets" of eosinophils in nasal secretions. The pathogenesis of nasal polyps is unknown, but since this condition is so intimately involved with aspirin intolerance, it may be associated with an abnormal arachidonic metabolism. Metabolism of arachidonic acid is through two major pathways: 5-lipoxygenase and cyclooxygenase. In aspirin intolerance, the cyclooxygenase pathway is inhibited, resulting in the reduced production of prostaglandin E and increased production of products of the lipoxygenase pathway including leu-

kotrienes B_4 whose actions are chemotactic for neutrophils and eosinophils. This may explain the mechanism that produces the marked eosinophilia in nasal secretions. It is important to know that patients with nasal polyps who have aspirin intolerance also may have adverse reactions to other nonsteroidal anti-inflammatory drugs. In addition, recent investigators have shown that polypectomy does not appear to precipitate asthma.[6]

Nasal polyps are most frequently found in patients over 40 years of age. Children aged 16 years or younger who have nasal polyps should be evaluated for cystic fibrosis. About 20% of patients with cystic fibrosis have nasal polyps. Polyps found in cystic fibrosis are usually characterized by nasal neutrophilia, purulent secretions, lack of response to corticosteroids, a delicate barely visible basement membrane without submucosal hyalinization, lack of extensive infiltration of eosinophils, and a preponderance of acid mucin in glands, cysts, and surface mucosa blanket. Polyps from noncystic fibrosis patients show extensive thickening of the basement membrane with extension into the submucosa as an irregular hyaline membrane, high stromal eosinophil count, and mainly neutral mucin in mucous glands, cysts, and mucous blanket. A sweat chloride test or iontophoresis will help rule out cystic fibrosis.

The occasional association of Kartagener's syndrome with nasal polyps has been reported; detailed information about this syndrome will be given under the heading "Dyskinetic Cilia Syndrome." Polyps found in Kartagener's syndrome also are associated predominantly with neutrophils.

The differential diagnosis of nasal polyps includes chordoma, chemodectoma, neurofibroma, angiofibroma, inverting papilloma, squamous cell carcinoma, sarcoma, and encephaloceles or meningoceles. Most of these lesions present as unilateral lesions. Meningoceles enter the nasal cavity via the cribriform plate. They increase in size with straining, lifting, or crying and may have a pulsating characteristic. The other lesions included in this differential diagnosis are not mobile, bleed easily, and may be sensitive to manipulation. Nasal polyps are characteristically mobile, rarely bleed, and are not sensitive to manipulation, and are frequently bilateral and multiple. Malignant tumors frequently are associated with bony, destructive changes. In rare cases, benign paranasal sinus cysts or polyps may also produce bone destruction. Diagnostic procedures include angiography, tomographic x-rays (CT scan), and biopsy.

The treatment of nasal polyps initially should be medical and include a tapering dose of oral corticosteroids with maintenance of remission by topical nasal steroids. Oral decongestants are supportive treatment but are ineffective when used alone. Nasal cromolyn and anticholinergic drugs appear to be ineffective. Surgical polypectomy is indicated when corticosteroid treatment fails. Evaluation of paranasal sinuses is mandatory to rule out polyps in the sinuses and an associated purulent sinusitis.

Despite medical and surgical treatment, nasal polyps have a high recurrence rate. Approximately 40% of patients who have had one polypectomy eventually require additional surgery because of recurrences.

ENDOCRINE DISORDERS

Endocrine disorders are often reflected by abnormalities in nasal function. These endocrine disorders are pregnancy, high levels of estrogen from oral contraceptives, and hypothyroidism. Proctor[7] states that nasal obstruction and hypersecretion are often associated with puberty, sexual excitement, menstruation, and pregnancy. In some women, the nasal mucosa becomes hyperemic and swollen during menstruation, pregnancy, and use of estrogen contraceptives. Epistaxis may occur with menstruation. Other symptoms during pregnancy are similar to those of vasomotor rhinitis and may or may not disappear after delivery. This type of nasal congestion can be refractory to treatment and may occur early in pregnancy, and at times, even before the diagnosis of pregnancy has been confirmed.

Hypothyroidism can produce extremely boggy nasal mucosa with large whitish turbinates. Nasal symptoms are similar to those of vasomotor rhinitis. In these patients, serum total IgE, allergy skin tests, and blood eosinophil counts are normal. There are no eosinophils in the nasal smear. Thyroxine and thyroxine-specific activity thyroid tests are diagnostic. In a consecutive series of 68 patients with nonallergic rhinitis one patient was found to have hypothyroidism as the cause.[8] The authors excluded a second patient with hypothyroidism manifesting as rhinitis, because of associated bronchitis. The diagnosis becomes clinically apparent when hypothyroidism is considered because these patients exhibit the other classical symptoms: periorbital edema, dry skin, constipation, lethargy, and preference for warm weather as well as other symptoms associated with this disease. Thus, in about 2–3% of patients with nonallergic rhinitis the diagnosis is hypothyroidism. Treatment consists of thyroid replacement therapy.

TUMORS

Tumors of the nasal pharyngeal and sinus areas may start with symptoms of simple progressive nasal blockage or those resembling vasomotor rhinitis. Frequently these lesions are unilateral, painful, and manifest hemorrhagic secretions. Paranasal sinus x-rays, rhinoscopy, and computed tomography may be extremely helpful in making the diagnosis. A particularly disturbing tumor is the juvenile nasopharyngeal angiofibroma, which is a highly vascular, noninfiltrating benign neoplasm occurring in the nasopharynx or posterior nasal cavity. This tumor usually occurs at about the time of puberty and is present almost exclusively in males. It can be a very aggressive tumor, invading the orbit, sinus, sphenoid, and intracranial cavity. It does not infiltrate bone but rather erodes it by direct pressure. Microscopically, this tumor has two major components: a fibrous stroma and a rich vascular network. It has a great tendency to bleed, sometimes massively, especially when biopsied or surgically excised. The initial symptoms of juvenile nasopharyngeal angiofibroma have been mistaken for allergic rhinitis in the past.[9]

SUPERIOR VENA CAVA SYNDROME

Another important syndrome that may be mistaken for allergic conjunctivitis, allergic rhinitis, or angioedema is the superior vena cava syndrome. Initially, this syndrome may be manifested by periorbital erythema and edema, nasal stuffiness, headache, and progressive facial swelling. This syndrome may so mimic allergic symptoms that frequently these patients are referred for an allergic workup by emergency rooms and primary care physicians.[10] Pathognomonic signs are progressive telangiectasia of the chest wall ("venous stars"), plethora and facial edema, and distended, prominant jugular veins. Frequently, these patients are unable to sleep or lie down because of excruciating headaches that are aggravated by nose blowing. Usually a routine chest x-ray will reveal the presence of a mass encroaching on the superior mediasternum. However, in some cases the initial chest x-ray has been reported as normal but pathognomonic signs should be sufficient to make the diagonsis.[10] The cause of superior vena cava obstruction is a malignancy in 97% of cases. External pressure on the superior vena cava may cause thrombosis, resulting in the full blown manifestation of this syndrome.

SYSTEMIC IMMUNOLOGIC DISEASES

Systemic immunologic diseases that have a nasal manifestation include general granulomatosis, midline granuloma, sarcoidosis, relapsing polychondritis, Sjogren's syndrome, and systemic lupus erythematosis.

Wegener's granulomatosis is a necrotizing granulomatous lesion with classical symptoms of vasculitis involving the upper and lower respiratory tract and glomerulonephritis. In most patients the upper airway and less frequently the pulmonary symptoms dominate the presenting clinical features. These symptoms include paranasal sinus pain, purulent or bloody nasal discharge, serous otitis media, and in the later stages nasal mucosal ulceration. Septal perforation may occur, resulting in the saddle nose deformity. The nasal mucosa has a red raised granular appearance, is friable, and bleeds easily. Pulmonary symptoms are cough, hemoptysis, pleuritis, and shortness of breath. Chest x-ray may reveal pulmonary infiltrates with cavitation. Other signs include fever, malaise, anorexia, weight loss, arthritis, skin lesions, and eye disorders including proptosis. Eosinophilia is not characteristic of this disease. The diagnosis is established by biopsy especially of the renal tissue. The treatment consists of cytotoxic agents such as cyclophosphamide and an initial treatment with corticosteroids. This disease that formerly was universally fatal now has a good prognosis. Long-term remissions may occur with proper therapy.

Another disease that sometimes is confused with Wegener's granulomatosis is midline granuloma, a rare disease manifested by a progressive localized destructive process that predominantly involves the nose, paranasal sinuses, and palate with erosion of contiguous structures such as soft tissue, cartilage, and bone. The cause is unknown. It is characterized by nonspecific acute and chronic inflammation and necrosis with or without granuloma formation. It usually occurs in patients in the fifth and sixth decades of life and is slightly more common in women. Early symptoms are rhinorrhea and nasal stuffiness followed by purulent discharges, nonhealing ulcerations of the nasal mucosa, and perforation of the nasal septum. The necrotic tissue is malodorous and may result in dramatic mutilation of facial structures. Laboratory findings are nonspecific, such as leukocytosis, elevated erythrocyte sedimentation rate, anemia, and hyperglobulinemia. X-rays reveal pansinusitis with destruction of cartilaginous and bony structures of the upper airways. It differs from Wegener's granulomatosis in that midline granuloma is a localized disease without pulmonary and renal involvement. If untreated, this disease is uniformly fatal. With high-dose local radiation, the prognosis for survival is excellent with a greater than 70% remission rate and cures lasting more than 10 years.

Nasal manifestations of sarcoidosis include mucosal hypertrophy, mucosal yellowish and bluish plaques, solitary nasopharyngeal mass, saddle nose deformity, and nasal septal perforation. The nasal mucosa reportedly has pinhead size nodules forming diffuse infiltrates.

Nasal signs of relapsing polychondritis (recurrent episodes of inflammation of all cartilages) include saddle-nose deformity and retraction of the columella with flattening of the nasal tip. The mechanism of these signs is due to the fibrous connective tissue replacement of cartilage leading to painless collapse of the nasal septum.

Sjögren's syndrome is a general dryness of mucosa associated with rheumatoid arthritis or other connective tissue disease. The diagnosis frequently is established by a positive Schirmer's test in tears. Nasal signs are dryness, crusting, and atrophy of the nasal mucosa. Nasal septal perforation is usually not found.

The nasal manifestations of systemic lupus erythematosis (SLE) are mucosal petechiae, purpura, and ulcerations. SLE affects many other tissues such as skin, joints, kidney, neurological system, and hematology. Exacerbation of the mucosal membrane lesions are associated with exacerbation of other systemic manifestations.

CHRONIC INFECTIONS

The chronic infections of the nose that may masquerade as allergic rhinitis are mucormycosis, blastomycosis, aspergillosis, histoplasmosis, coccidiodomycosis, late stage syphilis, tuberculosis, and leprosy. Fungus infections of the paranasal sinus and nose are usually found in the uncontrolled diabetic and in patients with a compromised immune system.[11] Fungus infections should be considered in the differential diagnosis of patients presenting with nasal stuffiness, blood-tinged nasal discharges, unilateral orbital painful swelling, cellulitis, and sinusitis. The nasal mucosa may by "dirty red" with black necrotic turbinates. This appearance may be a major clue to the diagnosis. Fungus infections may be rapidly progressive. Rhinocerebral mucormycosis accounts for about half of all cases of mucormycosis. Over 75% of cases of rhinocerebral mucormycosis occur in patients with acidosis, especially diabetic ketoacidosis. Mycormycosis (Rhizopus) contains a ketone reductase system and grows well in a media of elevated glucose levels and acid pH. For this reason, it has a predilection for patients with poorly controlled diabetes mellitus and metabolic acidosis. Treatment consists of amphotericin B, control of metabolic acidosis, and surgical debridement when necessary. For treatment details, the reader is referred to standard infectious disease textbooks. If untreated, these fungal infections can be fatal within 2-10 days.

Coccidiodomyocosis and histoplasmosis can produce

nasal mucosa ulcerations and should be considered in the differential diagnosis of rhinitis. Both of these mycotic infections have pulmonary and other organ involvement. Coccidiodomycosis occurs in the southwestern United States and neighboring Mexico and parts of Central and South America. In parts of California and Arizona about 80-95% of the population have positive skin tests. The diagnosis is made by demonstrating endosporulating spheres in 10% KOH wet mounts of sputum or inflammatory exudates. Biopsy specimens with the appropriate stain may demonstrate the fungi. Treatment consists of amphotericin B, miconazole, or ketoconazole.

The suggestive features of histoplasmosis include mucous membrane ulceration, leukopenia, adrenal insufficiency, buckshot pulmonary calcifications, and splenic calcifications. About 80-95% of the population in the Mississippi, Missouri, and Ohio River Valley areas have positive skin tests to histoplasmin. The diagnosis can be made by positive sputum smears or cultures. This disease is usually self-limiting and may not require treatment.

Cutaneous gummas may involve the nose and are associated with a plethora of systemic diseases, such as late syphilis, tuberculosis, sarcoidosis, leprosy, and deep fungal infections. Most of these disorders have systemic manifestations that also act as an aid in diagnosis of the nasal lesion. They appear as chronic granulomatous ulcerative lesions that may destroy surrounding tissue. Gummas of the nose and palate may result in septal perforations and disfiguring facial lesions. Histologically, the gummas may be nonspecific and associated with central necrosis surrounded by epithelioid and fibroblastic cells and occasional giant cells. Microorganisms may not be detectable. The syphilitic gumma is the only such lesion to heal dramatically with penicillin therapy. Tuberculosis orificialis responds well to isoniazid. It is associated with an underlying tuberculous node.

Early in lepromatous leprosy, the patient complains of nasal stuffiness and rhinorrhea that may be bloody and may have a fetid odor. The nasal secretions may contain up to 2×10^8 Mycobacterium leprae in a single nose blow. Transmission of this disease most often is via the infected nasal discharge. Classically, anesthetic or hypoesthesia skin lesions together with other skin lesions should suggest the diagnosis of leprosy.

An unusual nasal disorder is mucocutaneous leishmaniasis. It begins as a progressive destructive ulcer of the nose by a protozoan parasite. Polypoid lesions may occur. The infection usually progresses to the lower respiratory tract. It is found in Central and South America. The diagonsis is made by biopsy. The infection is difficult to treat.

Rhinoscleroma, rhinosporidiosis, and localized mucocutaneous herpes are limited to the nose. Rhinoscle-roma is a chronic granulomatous disease found in Central and Southern Europe, Egypt, Central and South America, and the East Indies. It is caused by Klebsiella rhinoscleromatis, a Gram-negative rod of the coliform group. The characteristic cell is the Mikulicz cell, a foamy lacy cell containing the Gram-negative organism. Early signs are nasal obstruction or deformity, which may be associated with hoarseness. The mucosa is hypercmic and has a raw granular appearance with a crusty, yellow purulent exudate. Hypertrophy of tissue may be present leading to formation of polypoid lesions. Treatment consists of gentamicin and kanamycin with cephalothin. Surgical removal of polypoid tissue may be necessary.

Rhinosporidiosis is caused by an endosporulating fungus. It is associated with a pedunculated, red, polypoid, sessile mass involving predominantly the nose and nasopharynx. It is endemic in India and is acquired by swimming in contaminated water. The diagnosis is made by biopsy identifying the fungus. Early cauterization of the lesion is curative.

DRUGS

Anti-hypertensive drugs have been known to have an adverse effect on the nose, either causing nasal stuffiness or producing a significant drying effect (Tables II and III). These drugs can be divided into three major categories. The first category is centrally acting drugs that interfere with adrenergic neuronal function. Examples of these are methyldopa, clonidine, guanabenz, and guanfacine. The second category is adrenergic neuron blocking agents such as reserpine, guanethidine, guanadrel, bretylium, bethanidine, and debrisoquine. The third category is inhibitors of catecholamine synthesis such as metyrosine.

Drugs in the first category act on neurons in the brainstem that are adrenergic and are involved in regulation of peripheral sympathetic activity. These drugs have a direct postsynaptic α_2-agonist effect on the central nervous system. As a consequence, neural release of norepinephrine is inhibited, which leads to a reduction of central and peripheral sympathetic activity.

Drugs in the second category, adrenergic neuron blocking agents, function either by depletion of the stores of mediator or direct prevention of its release. Many drugs in this category may act by more than one mechanism. However, the end result appears to be reduced norepinephrine content causing less stimulation of the α_2-adrenoceptors with decreased vasoconstriction of blood vessels in the nose resulting in nasal congestion. Reserpine is the classical drug in this category. Depletion of norepinephrine by reserpine is well known. Nasal vasoconstrictor response to nerve stimulation is completely abolished after administration of reserpine. In addition, it is important to note that drugs such as cocaine and desmethylimipramine act in a

TABLE II

Antihypertensive Drugs Causing Rhinitis

Trade Name	Generic Name	Symptoms
1. Aldomet Ester HCl Injection	Methyldopate hydrochloride	Nasal stuffiness
2. Aldomet Oral Suspension	Methyldopa, MSD	Nasal stuffiness
3. Aldomet Tablets	Methyldopa, MSD	Nasal stuffiness
4. Apresoline Hydrochloride	Hydralazine hydrochloride USP	Nasal congestion, dyspnea
5. Apresoline Hydrochloride Parenteral	Hydralazine hydrochloride parenteral	Nasal congestion, dyspnea
6. Catapres	Clonidine hydrochloride USP	Dryness of nasal mucosa
7. Corgard	Nadolol, β-blocker	Nasal stuffiness, bronchospasm, cough
8. Demi-Regroton	Chlorthalidone and reserpine	Nasal congestion, dyspnea
9. Harmonyl	Deserpidene	Bronchospasm in asthmatic patients, nasal congestion, dyspnea
10. Ismelin	Guanethidine monosulfate	Dyspnea, asthma in susceptible individuals, nasal congestion
11. Minipress	Prazosin hydrochloride	Nasal congestion, dyspnea
12. Minizide	Prazosin hydrochloride, polythiazide	Nasal congestion, dyspnea
13. Moderil	Riscinnamine, ester of methyl reserpate	Nasal congestion (frequently), dyspnea
14. Moduretic	Amiloride HCl-hydrochlorothiazide	1% nasal congestion, 1% dryness
15. Normodyne injection	Brand of labetalol hydrochloride	Nasal stuffiness, wheezing in 1
16. Normadyne Tablets	Brand of labetalol hydrochloride	Nasal stuffiness, dyspnea
17. Raudixin	Rauwolfia serpentina tablets USP	Nasal congestion, dyspnea
18. Regroton Tablets	Chlorthalidone and reserpine	Nasal congestion, dyspnea
19. Serpasil Tablets	Reserpine USP	Nasal congestion (frequently), dyspnea
20. Serpasil, Parenteral Solution	Reserpine	Nasal congestion, dyspnea
21. Serpasil-Apresoline	Reserpine and hydrolazine hydrochloride	Nasal congestion, dyspnea
22. Trandate	Labetalol hydrochloride, α- and β-blocker	Nasal stuffiness, dyspnea, bronchospasm
23. Wytensin	Guanabenz acetate	Nasal stuffiness, dyspnea

manner opposite to reserpine-type drugs in that they interfere with the uptake of noradrenaline into nerve endings, thus greatly potentiating the nasal vasoconstriction induced by sympathetic nerve stimulation.

Drugs that cause nasal stuffiness also may act directly through neurochemical receptors in the nose. These receptors are found in the smooth muscle around blood vessels. They cause either vasodilation or vasoconstriction resulting in nasal congestion or clearing of the nasal canals. There are five functional neurochemical receptors in the nose: the α-adrenoceptor, the β_2-adrenoceptor, the cholinoreceptor, the H_1-histamine receptor, and the irritant receptor.[12] The H_2-histamine receptor is essentially nonfunctional. Stimulation of the α-adrenoceptor causes nasal airway clearing and inhibition of the α-adrenoceptor causes nasal congestion.

Norepinephrine and phenylephrine stimulates this receptor, causing decreased nasal airway resistance. Inhibition of this receptor (interfering with the neurotransmitter norepinephrine) causes nasal congestion. Also, drugs containing iodides, which may be used for expectoration, can cause nasal stuffiness by stimulating nasal secretions.

DYSKINETIC CILIA SYNDROME

Dyskinetic cilia syndrome can be divided into transient and chronic types.[13,14] The acute transient variety is caused by a virus associated with the common cold that causes an inhibition of ciliary movement. Restoration of normal mucociliary clearance occurs between 2-6 weeks after a viral infection. The chronic variety, primary ciliary dyskinesia, is classically mani

TABLE III

Antihypertensive Drugs with Diuretics Causing Rhinitis

Trade Name	Generic Name	Symptoms
1. Aldoclor	Combination of methyldopa and chlorothiazine	Nasal stuffiness
2. Aldoril	Methyldopa-hydrochlorothiazide, MSD	Nasal stuffiness
3. Apresazide	Hydralazine hydrochloride and hydrochlorothiazide	Conjunctivitis, eosinophilia, dyspnea, nasal congestion
4. Apresoline-Esidrix	Hydralazine hydrochloride and hydrochlorothiazide	Eosinophilia, dyspnea, nasal congestion, conjunctivitis
5. Combipres	Clonidine hydrochloride and chlorthalidone	Dryness of nasal mucosa
6. Corzide	Nadolol bendroflumethiazide	Bronchospasm, cough, nasal stuffiness
7. Diupres	Chlorothiazide, MSD and reserpine	Nasal congestion, dyspnea
8. Diutensen-R	Methyclothiazine and reserpine	Frequent nasal congestion, dyspnea
9. Enduronyl Forte	Methylclothiazide and deserpidine	Asthma in asthmatic patients, nasal congestion, dyspnea
10. Enduronyl Tablets	Methylchothiazide and deserpidine	Asthma in asthmatic patients, nasal congestion, dyspnea
11. Esimil	Guanethidine monosulfate hydrochlorothiazide	Dyspnea, nasal congestion, asthma in susceptible individuals
12. Hydromox-R	Quinethazone with reserpine	Nasal congestion
13. Hydropres	Reserpine-hydrochlorothiazide, MSD	Nasal congestion, dyspnea
14. Metatensin	Trichlormethiazide USP and reserpine	Nasal stuffiness
15. Naquival	Trichlormethazide USP and reserpine	Nasal stuffiness
16. Oreticyl	Hydrochlorothiazide and deserpidine tabs	Asthma in asthmatic patients, nasal congestion, dyspnea
17. Rauzide	Powdered rauwolfia serpentina with bendroflumethiazide	Nasal congestion, dyspnea
18. Renese-R	Polythiazide and reserpine	Frequent nasal congestion
19. Salutensin	Hydroflumethiazide reserpine	Dyspnea, nasal congestion
20. Salutensin-Demi	Hydroflumethiazide reserpine	Dyspnea, nasal congestion
21. Ser-Ap-Es	Reserpine, hydralazine hydrochloride, hydrochlorothiazide	Dyspnea, nasal congestion
22. Serpasil-Esidrix	Reserpine, hydrochlorothiazide	Dyspnea, nasal congestion

fested in Kartagener's syndrome, which is an uncommon genetic condition with an estimated incidence of 1 in 20,000 births. It appears to be inherited as an autosomal recessive and is characterized by bronchiectasis, chronic sinusitis, and situs inversus (complete reversal of internal organs with heart on the right, liver on the left, etc.). The ciliary abnormality in these cases usually involves the entire body including the respiratory tract and sperm cells. The disorder is in the cilia itself in which the dynein arms are missing and the cilia remain completely immotile. Situs inversus is found in only 50% of patients with this syndrome. Also there appears to be an increased frequency of nasal polyps in Kartagener's syndrome and Young's syndrome, as described in chapter XX of this book.

CEREBROSPINAL FLUID (CSF) RHINORRHEA

Leakage of CSF into the nose presents a condition that can be confused with rhinorrhea or rhinitis. CSF rhinorrhea may be due to spontaneous, traumatic, or postoperative events or may be a result of tumors.

TABLE IV

Nasal Reflexes

Type	Action
1. Rhinobronchial	Bronchospasm
2. Sneezing (5th nerve)	Clears nasal passages
3. Rhinosalivary	↑ Salivation
4. Rhinogastric	↑ Gastric secretion
5. Exercise (hypothalamus)	↓ Nasal resistance (↑ sympathetic tone)
6. ↑ CO_2 (arterial chemoreceptors)	↓ Nasal resistance
7. ↓ CO_2 (arterial chemoreceptors)	↑ Nasal resistance
8. Vasomotor rhinitis (parasympathetic overactivity)	↑ Nasal resistance
9. Nasal ocular	↑ Tearing, sneezing
10. Pain/fear (adrenalin)	↓ Nasal resistance
11. Recumbent position	↑ Nasal resistance
12. Lateral recumbent position	↑ Nasal resistance (on down side)
13. Submersion reflex	Apnea, bradycardia, and ↑ blood pressure (CNS)

Reprinted with permission from Settipane GA. Nasal neural-chemical receptors. New Engl Reg Allergy Proc 5:329, 1984.

Most CSF fistulas (80%) are caused by head injuries, and 16% occur as complications of operations in nasal and paranasal cavities or in the skull base. Spontaneous CSF fistulas occur only 3-4% of the time.[15] Post-traumatic CSF rhinorrhea has been reported to occur up to 41 years after the trauma.[16] Classically, marked CSF rhinorrhea occurs when the patient is leaning forward or bending down. Analysis of nasal fluid reveals glucose and protein levels similar to that found in CSF. Free air may occur within the cranial cavity and cisternal and ventricular system. There may be a history of repeated episodes of meningitis. CSF rhinorrhea is present in about 5% of patients with pneumococcal meningitis.

CT scan with contrast media is needed for definitive diagnosis.

IgA DEFICIENCY

Secretory IgA is a major component of mucous secretion of the nose. Absence of IgA is one of the most common immunodeficiency disorders with a frequency of 1 in 886 individuals. Deficiency in secretory IgA can be related to nasal and sinus problems. Patients with a low IgA level have an increased risk of upper respiratory infection and possibly allergy. Several reports[17–20] from different parts of the world indicate that the normal transient IgA deficiency in the first few months of life may have long-term implications as far as allergic rhinitis is concerned. These reports suggest that newborns delivered in months of heavy atmospheric pollen exposure have an increased risk of developing hay fever in later life. The hypothesis is that IgA in secretions of the upper respiratory tract provides a protective barrier that prevents pollen proteins from interacting with macrophages, lymphocytes, and other cells. Absence of IgA increases the risk of IgE sensitization in later years. This theory is still speculative but affirmative reports have appeared in Great Britain, Australia, Scandinavia, and the United States.[17–20]

VIRAL INFECTIONS

Lastly, many acute viral infections began as coryza, and these result in rhinorrhea, nasal congestion, sinusitis, fever, and generalized malaise. Most of these viruses are relatively small, RNA type, heat stable, and acid labile. These viruses include rhinovirus, influenza, parainfluenza, respiratory syncytial, *Coronavirus, Reovirus*, coxsackievirus, echovirus, and adenovirus. Infections of the nose and sinuses with these viruses can trigger the rhinosinobronchial reflex in some asthmatics causing acute bronchospasm. Also, viral upper respiratory infections can cause cough and bronchospasm directly because of the physical irritation from the postnasal drip and excessive nasal secretion associated with these infections. The reflex mechanism is through the irritant and H_1-histamine receptors found in the nose and upper respiratory tract. These receptors transmit afferent neural impulses through the trigeminal, facial, and glossopharyngeal nerves to the medulla oblongata where the vagal nucleus is stimulated. The efferent arm of this reflex is the vagal nerve with its ramifications sending neural impulses to the bronchial tree causing bronchospasm (Fig. 1). It is not uncommon to have generalized reflexes beginning in or associated with the nose. Other reflexes associated with the nose are listed in Table IV.

SUMMARY

In summary, many systemic diseases are associated with nasal symptoms (Table V). Rhinitis associated with asthma is probably the most common with leprosy and fungal infections being the rarest.

A careful history and nasal examination in a patient with rhinitis may lead to the discovery of more significant systemic disease. Proper treatment of systemic disease will often cure or improve the associated rhinitis. Similarly, appropriate treatment of the rhinitis/sinusitis may reduce systemic complaints such as asthma. At times, identification of the cause of rhinitis

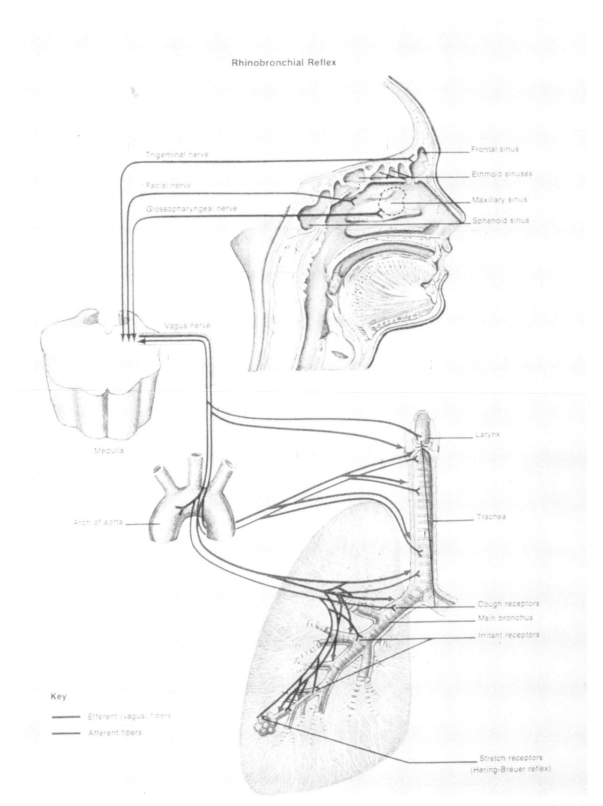

Figure 1. Stimulation of receptors found in the nose, pharyngeal, and sinus areas can produce bronchospasm through neural reflexes. The receptors involved are the histamine (H_1) and irritant receptors which send afferent neural impulses through the trigeminal, facial, and glossopharyngeal nerves to the medulla oblongata where the vagal nucleus is stimulated. The efferent arm of this reflex is the vagal nerve with its ramifications sending neural impulses to the bronchial tree causing bronchospasm.

TABLE V

Rhinitis as a Manifestation of Systemic Diseases

Nasal Signs/Symptoms	Systemic Disorders
Nasal polyps	Samter's triad (asthma, aspirin intolerance & nasal polyps) Churg-Strauss syndrome (vasculitis) Young's syndrome (sino-pulmonary disease, azoospermia, nasal polyps) Cystic fibrosis Kartagener's syndrome (bronchiectasis, sinusitis, & situ inversus)
Allergic rhinitis	↑ Risk for asthma

Nonallergic rhinitis	Endocrine disorders
	   Pregnancy
	   Estrogen contraceptives
	   Hypothyroidism
	Rhinitis medicamentosa
	   Antihypertensive drugs
	   Decongestant nose drops/spray
	Systemic Immunologic Diseases
	   Wegener's Granulomatosis (sinus, lung, & kidney involvement)
	   Midline granuloma
	   Sarcoidosis
	   Relapsing polychrondritis
	   Sjögren's syndrome
	   Systemic lupus erythematosis
	Tumors (e.g., juvenile angiofibroma)

Purulent rhinitis/sinusitis (Mucormycosis)	Uncontrolled diabetes
Infectious gummas of the nose	Late syphilis Tuberculosis Fungal infection Leprosy
Cerebral spinal fluid (CSF) rhinorrhea	CSF fistula, old skull fractures
Recurrent infections of the nasal/sinus area	IgA deficiency (most frequent immunologic defect)
Acute infections	Viruses (common cold)

as in CSF rhinorrhea. Wegener's syndrome, etc., alerts one to a life threatening entity.

Thus, it is apparent that the nose is an excellent mirror of some systemic diseases and identifying and understanding the differential diagonsis of nasal symptoms may be a tremendous help in diagnosing the disease and treating the whole patient.

REFERENCES

1. Davies RJ, et al. Rhinitis and asthma. In Mygind N, ed. Allergic and Vasomotor Rhinitis: Clinical Aspects. Copenhagen: Munksgaard, 1985, p. 65.
2. Pederson PA, Weeke ER. Asthma and allergic rhinitis in the same patients. Allergy 38:25–29, 1983.
3. Hagy GW, Settipane GA. Risk factors for developing asthma and allergic rhinitis: a 7-year follow-up study of college students. J Allergy Clin Immunol 58:330–336, 1976.
4. Townley RG. Allergic rhinitis and airway reactivity to mediators. New Engl Soc Allergy Proc 3:459–467, 1982.
5. Braman SS, Barrows AA, DeCotiis BA, Settipane GA, Corrao WM. Airway hyperresponsiveness in allergic rhinitis—A risk factor for asthma. Chest 91:671–674, 1987.
6. Settipane GA, Klein DE, Lekas MD. Asthma and nasal polyps. In Myers EN ed. New Dimensions in Otorhinolaryngology—Head and Neck Surgery. International Congress Series. Amsterdam: Elsevier Biomedical Press, 1985, p. 499.
7. Proctor DF. The Nose: Upper Airway Physiology and the Atmospheric Environment. Amsterdam: Elsevier Biomedical Press, 1982, p. 207.
8. Settipane GA, Klein DE. Nonallergic rhinitis: demography of

eosinophils in nasal smears, blood total eosinophil counts and IgE levels. New Engl Reg Allergy Proc 6:363–366, 1985.

9. Pitel PA, Smith PA, Bhat D. An unusual case of nasal obstruction. New Engl Reg Allergy Proc 3:410–414, 1982.

10. Settipane GA. "Venous stars," an important diagnostic sign: case report. New Engl Soc Allergy Proc 3:260–266, 1982.

11. Lekas MD, Tsiaras WG, Barone AJ. Rhinocerebral mucormycosis presenting as an orbital apex syndrome: a case report. New Engl Soc Allergy Proc 3:505–508, 1982.

12. Settipane GA. Allergic rhinitis—update. Otolaryngol-Head Neck Surg 94:470–475, 1986.

13. Atzelius BA. Disorders of ciliary motility. Hosp Practice 21:73–80, 1986.

14. Rossman CM, Lee RMKW, Forrest JB, Newhouse MT. Nasal ciliary ultrastructure and function in patients with primary ciliary dyskinesia compared with that in normal subjects and in subjects with various respiratory diseases. Am Rev Respir Dis 129:161–167, 1984.

15. Loew F, Pertuiset B, Chaumier EE, Jaksche H. Traumatic, spontaneous and postoperative CSF rhinorrhea. Adv Tech Stand Neurosurg 11:169–207, 1984.

16. Calhoun KH, Weiner R, Theilen F, Quinn FB, Stiernberg CM. CSF rhinorrhea 41 years after injury (abstract). Otolaryngol-Head Neck Surg Special Issue, 1986 Annual Program, 1986, p. 86.

17. Bjorksten F, Suoniemi I. Dependence of immediate hypersensitivity on the month of birth. Clin Allergy 6:165–171, 1976.

18. Pearson DJ, Freed DL, Taylor G. Respiratory allergy and month of birth. Clin Allergy 7:29–33, 1977.

19. Smith JM, Springett VH. Atopic disease and month of birth. Clin Allergy 9:153–157, 1979.

20. Settipane RJ, Hagy GW. Effect of atmospheric pollen on the newborn. RI Med J 62:477–482, 1979.

Chapter XXIV

Rhinologic Manifestations of Acquired Immunodeficiency Syndrome

Frank E. Lucente, M.D., F.A.C.S., Lawrence Z. Meiteles, M.D., and Philip S. Schoenfeld, B.S.

ABSTRACT

Among the more common manifestations of acquired immunodeficiency syndrome (AIDS) are infections and tumors that occur in regions treated by the otorhinolaryngologist. In this article we discuss the various infections and tumors of the nose and paranasal sinuses that have been reported among AIDS patients. Many of these disease entities may be the presenting signs of human immunodeficiency virus seropositivity and AIDS. The rhinologist should be able to recognize and diagnose these diseases so that proper testing and treatment may ensue. We also review the universal precautions and specific guidelines recommended for safeguarding the rhinologist and other health care workers who treat these patients.

One of the most significant diseases to affect the world in the last 100 years is AIDS (acquired immune deficiency syndrome). This disease is important to the otorhinolaryngologist both because of the frequency with which presenting symptoms and signs affect the head and neck region and because of the devastating impact the disease will have on the health care system in general.

Although this disorder has only been recognized since 1981, it is already widespread and it is estimated that by 1991, at the end of the "AIDS decade," there will be 50–100 million persons infected with the AIDS virus throughout the world.

Department of Otolaryngology, SUNY–Health Science Center at Brooklyn, Brooklyn, New York

Some of the statistics currently available about AIDS demonstrate the significant impact it will have on the United States and the world. In 1988 there were estimated to be about 10 million infected persons in the world and up to 1,500,000 in the United States. To date the disease has occurred principally among homosexual or bisexual males and intravenous drug abusers, but other groups are also involved, including sexual partners of these groups, children born to mothers who are infected, and recipients of blood and blood products such as hemophiliacs.

AIDS has generally come to be recognized as a syndrome characterized by the presence of one or more opportunistic diseases indicative of an underlying cellular immunodeficiency without any other known underlying cause of immunodeficiency. The condition strongly correlates with the presence of human immunodeficiency virus (HIV) antibody.

Currently (1988) 93% of affected persons are male and 7% female. With regard to age, 68% have been between 20 and 39 and 31% 40 or over. About 1% have been under the age of 20, principally infants born to infected mothers. With regard to race, 61% have been white, 25% black, and 14% Hispanic. Presently, approximately 74% of cases have been reported in homosexuals or bisexuals, 16% in drug abusers, and 10% in heterosexuals including infants.[1]

On the basis of information available at that time there appeared to be three modes of transmission: (1) sexual, (2) contaminated blood or blood products, and (3) perinatal.

The inapparent-to-apparent disease ratio with the AIDS virus is not completely known. It is estimated that there may be as many as 50 times more HIV infections as there are actual cases of AIDS. Estimates are complicated by the long incubation period of AIDS, which may be 4 years or more until opportunistic infections and other clinical manifestations of the disease occur. Currently it appears that AIDS will develop in approximately 35% of HIV-infected persons. This percentage may increase as more experience is gained and a lengthening of the incubation period may be noted. In addition to the 35% who develop AIDS, approximately 25% develop other signs of HIV infection, such as AIDS-related complex (ARC) with lymphadenopathy, fever, night sweats, or diseases directly related to HIV infection such as encephalopathy or myocardiopathy. It appears that some ARC patients eventually develop full-blown AIDS, but not necessarily all will do so. The outcome for the 40% of HIV-positive patients who do not currently have AIDS or ARC remains to be seen.[1]

Most reports indicate that more than 40% of AIDS patients present with lesions in the head and neck region. In view of the frequency of these otorhinolaryngologic complaints, it is important for the otorhinolaryngologist to be conversant with the various manifestation of AIDS, to understand the primary and supportive therapies currently in use for the treatment of the AIDS patient, and to understand the optimal methods of protecting health care personnel from infection with HIV.

RHINOLOGIC MANIFESTATIONS

Rhinosinusitis

The mucosa of the nose, paranasal sinuses, and nasopharynx are possible portals of entry for systemic disease and as such diseases of these regions should be diagnosed and treated promptly in the immunocompromised host. One would expect a multitude of opportunistic infections of the nose and paranasal sinuses in hosts whose main defense against such infection is cell-mediated immunity. Yet, there has been a paucity of information regarding sinusitis in the AIDS patient. Table I lists the encountered organisms reported in the medical literature.

A case of cytomegalovirus (CMV) rhinitis was reported by Kotler and co-workers[2] in a patient with a concomitant *Pneumocystis carinii* pneumonia. The patient had purulent rhinitis and sinus x-rays were normal. Nasal mucosa was erythematous and granular. Mucosal biopsy revealed multiple CMV inclusions in endothelial cells and squamous metaplasia of the mucosa plus patchy acute and chronic inflammation. Viral inclusions were not found in rectal biopsy specimens. Cytomegalovirus infection can be identified histologically by intranuclear inclusion bodies in vascular endothelial cells.

Legionella pneumophila rhinosinusitis was reported by Schlanger and co-workers[3] in a patient with disseminated CMV. Open lung biopsy and liver biopsy revealed intranuclear inclusion bodies of CMV. The patient had purulent nasal discharge and air fluid levels were seen in the antrum on sinus radiography. Caldwell-Luc surgical biopsy and drainage were performed. Culture revealed a few colonies of *Staphylococcus epidermidis*. Direct immunofluorescence staining using group 1 *L. pneumophila* antiserum revealed brightly fluorescent bacilli. Direct immunofluorescence of lung and hepatic biopsy specimens were negative. Treatment with oral erythromycin for 10 days resulted in resolution of the drainage. *L. pneumophila* is a facultative intracellular pathogen and a probable etiologic factor in a deficient host cell-mediated immunity.

Rhinosinusitis due to *Acanthamoeba castellanii* was reported by Gonzalez and co-workers[4] in a patient with concomitant *Pneumocystis carinii* pneumonia. The patient presented with a complaint of progressive nasal obstruction, epistaxis, nasal tenderness, and frontal headaches. Physical examination revealed nasal obstruction with crusted mucosa over the turbinates. Biopsy of the left inferior turbinate revealed granulomatous inflammation containing *A. castellanii*. Computed tomographic (CT) scan revealed mucosal swelling of the turbinates, soft tissue swelling in the maxillary sinuses, and partial opacification of the ethmoid sinuses. The patient was treated with rifampin and ketaconazole and succumbed 3 months later to *Salmonella* sepsis. Autopsy revealed abundant edematous pale yellow mucosa with focal areas of hemorrhage in all sinus cavities. The patient also had a right calf lump which proved to be an abscess cavity containing *Acanthamoeba*, most likely due to hematogenous spread of the infection. *Acanthamoeba* has been isolated from the nasopharynx of healthy individuals and the transition from colonization to infection probably occurs only in the immunocompromised host.

Poole and co-workers[5] reported a case of sinusitis in a patient with central nervous system toxoplasmosis and mucosal candidiasis. The patient had purulent nasal discharge and opacified paranasal sinuses on radiologic examination. Antral aspiration cultures revealed *Pseudomonas aeruginosa*, *Staphylococcus aureus*, and *Streptococcus pneumoniae*. Surgical drainage resulted in cessation of symptoms. The authors noted that AIDS patients with fungal and parasitic infections respond poorly to antimicrobial therapy and recommend early surgical intervention.

Sooy[6] reported that *Haemophilus influenzae* and *S. pneumoniae* were the most common bacterial organisms encountered in AIDS patients with sinusitis and *Pseudallescheria boydii* was the most common fungal pathogen in a series of 12 case studies. He recommended that sinus irrigation was both diagnostic and therapeutic and should be done early, particularly in

TABLE I

Reported Infectious Agents

Agent	No. of Cases	
Cytomegalovirus	1	Kotler et al.[2]
Legionella pneumophila	1	Schlanger et al.[3]
Acanthamoeba castellanii	1	Gonzalez et al.[4]
Pseudomonas aeruginosa		
Staphylococcus aureus	1	Poole et al.[5]
Streptococcus pneumoniae		
Haemophilus influenzae	12 patients	Sooy[6]
Streptococcus pneumoniae	most common	
Pseudallescheria boydii	organisms	
Alternaria alternata	1	Wiest et al.[7]
Cryptococcus neoformans	1	Choi et al.[8]
Staphylococcus aureus (nasal abscess)	1	Henry et al.[9]

the patient who is in a toxic condition. He also noted that tumor should be included in the differential diagnosis of sinus opacification and listed Kaposi's sarcoma and lymphoma as possible causes.

Rhinosinusitis secondary to infection with *Alternaria*, a ubiquitous filamentous fungus primarily recognized as a plant pathogen and soil saprophyte, was described in a patient with AIDS by Wiest and co-workers.[7] Two months prior to diagnosis the patient was treated for *P. carinii* pneumonia and esophageal candidiasis. Two months after discharge, while the patient was being treated for recurrent symptoms with ketaconazole and oral acyclovir for herpes zoster of the right second branch of the trigeminal nerve, he complained of tenderness over the right side of his nose. The patient also noted a persistent clear nasal discharge and a sinus radiograph showed a thickened lining of the right antrum. Physical examination revealed a sharply circumscribed 0.5-cm black necrotic lesion on the right nasal septum. Culture and biopsy revealed *Alternaria alternata*. CT scan revealed a right antral soft tissue density. The nasal lesion was completely excised and a right Caldwell-Luc procedure was performed. Biopsy of the maxillary sinus showed only chronic inflammation. The patient was treated with amphotericin B. Because of persistent pain the patient underwent repeat biopsies of the right antrum and again no evidence of fungal infection was found. The patient did not experience a recurrence for 8 months after receiving amphotericin B at which point he died, and autopsy revealed no fungal infection. This patient developed *Alternaria* rhinitis while receiving ketaconazole for mucosal candidiasis. The average reported serum concentration of ketaconazole for patients receiving 400 mg/day is 3.32 mg/ml, a level well below the

minimal inhibitory concentration for *Alternaria.*[7] There are two distinct histologic appearances of *Alternaria.*[7] In the first, broad hyphae with occasional branching and chains of conidia are seen in the presence of a granulomatous or suppurative tissue reaction. In the second, granulomatous inflammation with numerous giant cells are seen. The giant cells contain periodic acid-Schiff positive rounded fungal forms, hyphae, or chains of conidia. Treatment of *Alternaria* rhinosinusitis should include surgical excision and intravenous administration of amphotericin B.

Choi and co-workers[8] reported a case of cryptococcosis secondary to cryptococcal sinusitis. The patient, who had been healthy previously, presented with a complaint of frontal headaches, intermittent fever, nausea, and vomiting of 2 weeks' duration. He also noted the onset of malaise, anorexia, and a 14-pound weight loss 3 months prior to admission. Significant findings on physical examination were oral thrush and diffuse spotty cervical lymphadenopathy. A CT scan performed prior to lumbar puncture revealed an air-fluid level in the right frontal and maxillary sinus, as well as opacification of bilateral sphenoids and left maxillary sinus. India ink preparation of cerebrospinal fluid was positive. Cerebrospinal fluid cultures grew *Cryptococcus neoformans*. Despite therapy with amphotericin B and 5-flucytosine the patient did not improve and underwent bilateral intranasal sphenoethmoidectomies, bilateral antrostomies, and a right frontal sinus trephination. Biopsies from all sinuses were positive for *C. neoformans*. After 8 weeks of amphotericin B and 5-flucytosine therapy the patient was discharged on a regimen of intermittent amphotericin B and 5-flucytosine treatment for 6 months. The patient was followed for 14 months without relapse.

The diagnosis of cryptococcosis is made by India ink preparation and culture of appropriate body fluids.[8] Another useful test is a latex agglutination procedure for detection of the cryptococcal antigen. The treatment of disseminated cryptococcosis consists of intravenous amphotericin B with or without oral 5-flucytosine.[8]

Nasal septal abscess due to *S. aureus* in a patient with concomitant *P. carinii* pneumonia was reported by Henry and associates.[9] The patient presented with nasal obstruction, marked maxillary tenderness, and purulent posterior nasal drainage. CT scan revealed a large mass in the nasal septum and 10 ml of purulent material was drained. Cultures revealed *S. aureus*. The patient recovered with pentamidine and cephalexin antibiotic treatment.

Of interest, the AIDS patients with rhinosinusitis reviewed above had multiple concurrent infections. In such patients special stains and ultrastructural examination should be considered before surgical excision and biopsy. Perhaps isolated rhinosinusitis in AIDS patients may be due to conventional organisms and is amenable to conventional medical treatment. When conventional medical treatment fails or when the rhinosinusitis is associated with concurrent multiple systemic infections aggressive combined surgical-medical treatment is necessary.

Kaposi's Sarcoma

Prior to the onset of the AIDS epidemic, Kaposi's sarcoma was a rare neoplasm that affected elder men of Italian ancestry and Eastern European Jews. Those patients typically had cutaneous involvement of the lower extremities. A more fulminant form of Kaposi's sarcoma now occurs in up to 40% of patients with AIDS.[10] Rarely had Kaposi's sarcoma been known to affect the respiratory tract. Pulmonary involvement with Kaposi's sarcoma has been reported as high as 47% at autopsy.[10] Isolated cases of Kaposi's sarcoma involving the upper respiratory tract have been reported. Sooy[6] reported a case of paranasal sinus involvement with Kaposi's sarcoma. This tumor has been noted to occur in the nasal cavity, nasal vestibule, on the nasal septum, and in the nasopharynx.[6,11] In a report by Patow and co-workers[12] on 13 AIDS patients with Kaposi's sarcoma 11 of the 13 patients had facial cutaneous lesions and at least two of these patients had nasal skin involvement. Patients with nasal Kaposi's sarcoma generally complain of nasal obstruction, drainage, and epistaxis. On direct visualization one notes discrete nodular violaceous tumors. Diagnosis can be made by excisional biopsy of a cutaneous lesion. Histologic examination reveals fascicles of spindle cells surrounding cleft-like spaces containing extravasated erythrocytes. Other areas show hemosiderin deposition, plasma cell and polymorphonuclear cell clusters, and dilated lymphatic and capillary channels. Identical histologic findings are present regardless of where the lesion is located.[13] Chemotherapy and radiation therapy are recommended as the treatment of choice. In a recent report,[14] virus particles ultrastructurally identical to HIV were seen in electron microscopic examination of Kaposi's sarcoma of the oral mucosa.

Candidiasis

Oral candidiasis is often the presenting symptom in ARC and can forebode the development of AIDS. Candidiasis can be diagnosed in its most typical pseudomembranous form, by its cheesy white plaques that can be scraped off, leaving an erythematous base. Less characteristic variants have been recognized, including a hyperplastic form that does not scrape off, an erythematous or atrophic form, and a form that presents as angular cheilitis.[15] Oral candidiasis has been reported as a marker for esophageal candidiasis in AIDS patients.[16] Oral candidiasis can spread caudally toward the hypopharynx and esophagus and cephalad into the nasopharynx. Nasopharyngeal candidiasis can be confirmed by smear and culture. Oral and oropharyngeal candidiasis can often be successfully managed with oral cystatin rinse. However, this preparation will not enter the nasopharynx and therefore candidiasis in this region is generally best managed with oral ketaconazole.

Seborrheic Dermatitis

The prevalence of seborrheic dermatitis in AIDS patients has been reported to range from 22 to 83%.[17] The most common site of involvement is the head and neck and a malar rash is often seen involving the nose and cheeks.[18,19] Other sites of involvement include the chest, back, groin, and extremities. The skin eruption is characterized by indurated erythematous scaly plaques. Soeprono and co-workers[19] showed that the seborrheic dermatitis of AIDS is a entity histologically distinct from ordinary seborrheic dermatitis. Histologic examination reveals spotty keratinacytic necrosis, leukoexocytosis, superficial perivascular infiltrate of plasma cells, and neutrophils that show occasional leukoexocytosis.[19] These histologic features are not encountered in ordinary seborrheic dermatitis, yet, clinically, seborrheic dermatitis of AIDS is indistinguishable from ordinary seborrheic dermatitis. Additional differences include its occurrence in a younger population, greater severity, and involvement of sites such as the extremities and chest not usually affected by seborrheic dermatitis. Seborrheic dermatitis may be a marker for AIDS or ARC, and it may be somewhat refractory to treatment with topical corticosteroids.[18]

Nasopharyngeal Lymphoid Proliferation

In a recent report from our institution by Stern and co-workers,[20] nasopharyngeal lymphoid proliferation was found to be a presenting sign of HIV infection. Patients presented with a complaint of nasal obstruction and some also had hearing loss due to otitis media with effusion. Flexible fiberoptic nasopharyngoscopy revealed large mucosal covered nasopharyngeal masses occluding the choana and torus tubaris. Nasopharyngeal biopsy revealed benign lymphoid hypertrophy. All patients tested positive for HIV, and all were asymptomatic for AIDS or ARC. Adenoidectomy was found to relieve symptoms. The authors recommend adenoidectomy and HIV testing of high-risk patients with nasal obstruction secondary to benign lymphoid hypertrophy.

Lymphoma

Leess and co-workers[21] reported a case of high-grade undifferentiated, large cell lymphoma involving the nasal cavity and maxillary antrum in an AIDS patient. The patient presented with nasal obstruction and a persistent foul smelling discharge from the left nostril and a 20-pound weight loss. On physical examination he was noted to have a large necrotic mass that filled the left nostril and caused flaring of the ala. CT scan revealed a soft tissue density in the left nasal cavity and maxillary antrum and no bony destruction. Follow-up CT scan showed enlargement of the sinus mass and a right-sided temporo-occipital lesion. The patient responded poorly to chemotherapy and was subsequently lost to follow-up. Leess and co-workers[21] also reported a case of high-grade, small, noncleaved B-cell lymphoma involving the palate and antrum. The patient presented with a complaint of an enlarging lesion of the left maxillary molar region. CT scan demonstrated that the mass extended into the maxillary antrum with bony destruction. The patient responded well to chemotherapy with resolution of the mass. The authors note a high incidence of central nervous system involvement in association with non-Hodgkin's lymphomas of the head and neck and recommended lumbar puncture and brain CT scan to aid diagnosis. They also recommend aggressive radiation and chemotherapy as the mode of treatment.

Herpes Zoster and Herpes Simplex

Herpes zoster infection is due to reactivation of latent varicella zoster virus in dorsal root ganglia in patients with previous infection. Localized herpes zoster is usually a disorder of elderly and immunocompromised patients and is thought to be secondary to deficient cell-mediated immunity.[22,23] It has been documented that herpes zoster infection in asymptomatic individuals at high risk for AIDS may be a presenting sign of HIV infection.[22,23] Friedman-Kien and associates[23] found that among 48 patients in high-risk groups for AIDS, who presented with herpes zoster, 35 or 73% were found to be seropositive for HIV. Seven patients subsequently became HIV positive during follow-up of 1 to 28 months after their zoster infection was diagnosed. Herpes zoster infection in HIV-positive patients and AIDS patients tend to be of greater severity and tend to become generalized.[18] At our institution we have noted the presentation of herpes zoster ophthalmicus in high risk individuals who subsequently were found to be HIV positive.[24] Treatment is with acyclovir. The postherpetic neuralgia is found to be no greater than that in the general population.

AIDS patients have also been seen to have a new entity of giant herpetic nasal ulcers.[6] The ulcers begin in the vestibule and may extend onto the face or septum reaching a size of up to 3 cm. Treatment of choice is acyclovir.

We have also encountered an AIDS patient with molluscum contagiosum extensively involving the skin of the nose and midface. The lesions were typically well-circumscribed and elevated with central umbilication.

PRECAUTIONS FOR HEALTH CARE WORKERS

The risk to the health care worker comes more from the unknown carrier of HIV than from the known AIDS sufferer during the care of whom one may observe optimal precautions. To be sure, the risks to the prudent health care worker appear to be minimal. To date only 33 cases through occupational exposure have been reported and the majority have been in housekeeping and other support personnel.[1] Since the time for seroconversion after inoculation may be up to 6 months, we should consider all patients as potentially infected. Therefore, we too must learn and practice those measures which will reduce the hazards for any virus infection by percutaneous or mucous membrane inoculations whether the virus be infectious hepatitis virus, human immunodeficiency virus, or some other lethal virus not yet identified. The following precautions are recommended:

1. In the office when treating *any* patient, frequent handwashing before and after examining patients remains the most important precaution, but remember that viruses do not traverse intact skin. There is no reason to avoid shaking hands with a patient or touching the ear, nose, face, or neck of *any* patient.
2. Wear gloves when touching mucous membrane surfaces, blood and body fluids, and non-intact skin of all patients.

3. Change gloves after contact with each patient or if they are torn.
4. Avoid unprotected patient contact if you have broken skin.
5. Wear masks and protective eyewear or face shields when aerosolization is a risk.
6. Wear gloves when performing venipuncture.
7. Do not recap needles—throw them away.
8. Lay out instruments before beginning examination, rather than reaching into the instrument drawer with contaminated hands.
9. Reduce the number of sharp objects in any operative field and allow only one person to handle a scalpel at any time.
10. Clean all instruments thoroughly and disinfect in a dilute solution of sodium hypochlorite or glutaraldehyde.
11. Communicate infection control facts to staff members *and* patients even if they seem unnecessary or frightening. They will respect us for this if we serve as models for careful practice.
12. Try to convey to all patients that these are the precautions that you as a prudent physician need to observe and the precautions that they should extrapolate to their own lifestyle so that hematogenous or transmucosal inoculation by infectious agents does not occur.

CONCLUSION

In conclusion, we have reviewed some of the nasal, sinus, and nasopharyngeal manifestations of AIDS. We have also presented a summary of the precautions to be observed in the office and operating room in order to treat patients carefully while simultaneously avoiding unnecessary hazards to the health care worker. The AIDS epidemic poses a serious challenge to the rhinologist who will need to remember three important watchwords if he is to continue to be a careful and productive practitioner: vigilance (to recognize manifestations of AIDS as early as possible), prudence (to protect all health care workers), and compassion (to continue to render the highest standards of care to all patients).

REFERENCES

1. Lucente FE, Dull HB, Pincus RL. Acquired immunodeficiency syndrome in otolaryngology. In: Cummings CW, et al., eds. Otolaryngology—Head and Neck Surgery. St. Louis: Mosby, 1988.
2. Kotler DP, Scholes JV, Jacob AL, Edelheit W. Disseminated CMV infection. JAMA 253:3093–3094, 1985.
3. Schlanger G, Lutwick LI, Kurzman M, Hoch B, Chandler FW. Sinusitis caused by *Legionella pneumophila* in a patient with the acquired immune deficiency syndrome. Am J Med 77:957–960, 1984.
4. Gonzalez MM, Gould E, Dickinson G, Martinez AJ, Visvesvara G, Cleary TJ, Hensely GT. Acquired immunodeficiency syndrome associated with *Acanthamoeba* infection and other opportunistic organisms. Arch Pathol Lab Med 110:749–751 1986.
5. Poole MD, Postma D, Cohen MS. Pyogenic otorhinologic infections in acquired immune deficiency syndrome. Arch Otolaryngol 110:130–131, 1984.
6. Sooy CD: The impact of AIDS in otolaryngology–head and neck surgery. Adv Otolaryngol Head Neck Surg 1:1–27, 1987.
7. Wiest PM, Wiese K, Jacobs MR, Morrissey AB, Abelson TI Witt W, Lederman MM: *Alternaria* infection in a patient with acquired immunodeficiency syndrome: case report and review of invasive *Alternaria* infections. Rev Infect Dis 9:799–803, 1987.
8. Choi SS, Lawson W, Bottone EJ, Biller HF: Cryptococcal sinusitis: a case report and review of literature. Otolaryngol Head Neck Surg 99:414–418, 1988.
9. Henry K, Sullivan C, Crossley K: Nasal septal abscess due to *Staphylococcus aureus* in a patient with AIDS. Rev Infect Dis 10:428–430, 1988.
10. Zibrak JD, Silvestri RC, Costello P, Marlink R, Jensen WA Robins A, Rosc RM: Bronchoscopic and radiologic features of Kaposi's sarcoma involving the respiratory system. Chest 90:476–479, 1986.
11. Marcusen DC, Sooy CD: Otolaryngologic and head and neck manifestations of acquired immunodeficiency syndrome (AIDS). Laryngoscope 95:401–405, 1985.
12. Patow CA, Steis R, Longo DL, Reichert CM, Findlay PA Petter D, Masur H, Lane HC, Fauci AS, Macher AM: Kaposi's sarcoma of the head and neck in the acquired immune deficiency syndrome. Otolaryngol Head Neck Surg 92:255–260, 1984.
13. Hymes K: Kaposi's sarcoma in AIDS: In: Wormser GP, Stahl RE, Bottone EJ, eds. Acquired Immune Deficiency Syndrome and Other Manifestations of HIV Infection. Park Ridge, NJ Noyes Publications, 1987, pp 747–766.
14. Schenk P: Retroviruses in Kaposi's sarcoma in acquired immune deficiency syndrome (AIDS). Acta Otolaryngol (Stockh) 101:295–298, 1986.
15. Lucente FE, Meiteles LZ, Pincus RL: Bronchoesophageal manifestations of acquired immunodeficiency syndrome Ann Otol Rhinol Laryngol 97:530–533, 1988.
16. Tavitan A, Raufman JP, Rosenthal LE: Oral candidiasis as a marker for esophageal candidiasis in the acquired immunodeficiency syndrome. Ann Intern Med 104:54–55, 1986.
17. Matis WL, Triana A, Shapiro R, Eldred L, Polk BF, Hood AF: Dermatologic findings associated with human immunodeficiency virus infection. J Am Acad Dermatol 17:746–751 1987.
18. Cockarell CJ: Cutaneous manifestations of AIDS other than Kaposi's sarcoma. In: Wormser GP, Stahl RE, Bottone EJ eds. Acquired Immune Deficiency Syndrome and Other Manifestations of HIV Infection. Park Ridge, NJ: Noyes Publications, 1987, pp 808–811.
19. Soeprono FF, Schinella RA, Cockarell CJ, Comite SL: Seborrheic-like dermatitis of acquired immunodeficiency syndrome. J Am Acad Dermatol 14:242–248, 1986.
20. Stern J, Lin PT, Lucente FE: Symptomatic benign nasopharyngeal lymphoid proliferation and human immunodeficiency virus (HIV) infection. Presented at the Second International Conference on Head and Neck Cancer, Boston, Aug 1, 1988.
21. Leess FR, Kessler OJ, Mickel RA: Non-Hodgkin's lymphoma of the head and neck in patients with AIDS. Arch Otolaryngol Head Neck Surg 113:1104–1106, 1987.

22. Cone LA, Schiffman MA: Herpes zoster and the acquired immunodeficiency syndrome. Ann Intern Med 100:462, 1984.

23. Friedman-Kien AE, Lafleur FL, Gendler E, Hennessey NP, Montagna R, Halbert S, Rubinstein P, Krasinski K, Zang E, Polesz B: Herpes zoster: a possible early clinical sign for development of acquired immunodeficiency syndrome in high-risk individuals. J Am Acad Dermatol 14:1023–1028, 1986.

24. Unpublished data. ☐

TREATMENT

Chapter XXV

Classical Antihistamines and Decongestants in the Treatment of Chronic Rhinitis

James W. Cooper, Jr., Ph.D., F.C.P., F.A.S.C.P.

ABSTRACT

Antihistamines and decongestants are most effective in chronic non-infectious rhinitides. Chronic rhinitic symptomology includes nasal congestion and pruritus, sneezing, rhinorrhea and "post-nasal" drip. Decongestants are typically thought to decrease congestion by stimulation of alpha adrenergic receptors of the nasal mucosa, while antihistamines decrease the latter symptoms by preventing the mediator effects of released histamine.

Misuse of decongestants and detoxification are perplexing problems facing the clinician, as well as tolerance to antihistamine effect. Anticipation and avoidance of decongestant toxicity in patients with high blood pressure, cardiovascular disease, diabetes, thyroid disease as well as neurological and psychologic drug effects are discussed. Tabulation of currently used single antihistamine and decongestants as well as most commonly used combinations of both are also presented.

INTRODUCTION

Chronic rhinitis may be associated with the interplay of a variety of factors (Figure 1) to include infectious processes (not infrequently sinusitis), inflammatory response to chemical vapors or physical changes in temperature and humidity, allergic responses (e.g. identifiable antigens), and/or emotional response to life situations.

Professor and Head of Department of Pharmacy Practice, The University of Georgia College of Pharmacy, and Assistant Clinical Professor, Department of Family Medicine, Medical College of Georgia, Athens, GA 30602.

Figure 1

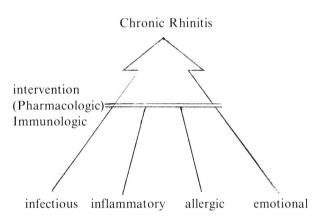

Pharmacotherapeutic intervention in chronic noninfectious rhinitis takes two forms: pharmacologic with antihistamines and decongestants, and immunologic with corticosteroids.

Pharmacologic intervention in chronic rhinitis is directed at either autonomic imbalance of parasympathetic predominance (decongestants) or prevention of release (cromolyn) or the physiologic mediator effects of histamines (antihistamines) or other autacoids released (e.g. ECF-A and SRS-A).

Chronic rhinitis symptomology includes nasal congestion and pruritus, sneezing, rhinorrhea, and "post-nasal drip". Decongestants are typically thought to decrease congestion while antihistamines decrease the frequency of the latter symptoms.

Nasal Decongestants (Sympathomimetics) Table I.

Sympathomimetics cause decongestion by stimulation of alpha adrenergic receptors in blood vessels of the nasal mucosa. They also cause elevation of blood pressure, increased heart rate and CNS stimulation.

Decongestants may be used in topical or oral (systemic) form. While topical forms may be useful for three to five days at the most, longer use of topical decongestants for chronic rhinitis is generally discouraged due to the development of overuse and abuse associated with "rebound" phenomena (rhinitis medicamentosa).

Misuse of Decongestants

A further problem facing the physician is how to deal with the individual who presents with chronic rhinitis *and* rhinitis medicamentosa. While a "detoxification" plan of weekly to biweekly changes from the longest acting [6-12 hrs. — Afrin, Otrivin, Neo-Synephrine II] to shorter acting, [4-6 hrs. — Privine] then Neo-Synephrine, [2-4 hrs. 1%, 0.5%, .25% and .125%] to normal saline spray may be "clinically" recommended, with or without intercurrent use of newer nasal corticosteroids (Vancenase, Beconase), there is no current objective documentation of the benefit of this treatment. Chronic topical decongestants should be especially avoided in the very young

(less than six years) or elderly (over 60 years), due to the high incidence of adverse reactions.

Efficacy

Oral decongestant agents (phenylpropanolamine and pseudoephedrine) may constrict nasal mucosa on a short-term basis with less likelihood of rebound than topical treatment but have not been extensively studied for chronic therapy. They are, nevertheless, extensively used as single agents or in combination with antihistamines for chronic "cyclic" therapy. Oral phenylephrine is unreliably absorbed due to gut degradation and has no use in single or combination oral antihistamines/decongestants.[1]

Anticipation and Avoidance of Toxicity

Topical and systemic decongestants can cause stinging, burning and dryness of the nasal mucosa. Normal saline spray (ten to twenty minutes after topical administration) may help lessen this problem, which tends to be transitory and decreases after several days of use. Again, however, topical sympathomimetic forms should not be used for more than three to five days. Topical forms can be particularly hazardous in infants and children as well as

Table I

Nasal Decongestants*

Generic Name	Trade Name	Onset (hr.)	Duration (hr.)	Comments
Topical**				
Phenylephrine HCl	Neo-synephrine	0.1	1-4	Effective topically. Ineffective orally.
Naphazoline	Privine	0.1	2-6	Rebound congestion, more common in 4 to 6 hr. Not recommended for more than 3 days or in children.
Oxymetazoline	Otrivin	0.1	5-12	Negligible rebound on short-term use.
Xylometazoline	Afrin	0.1	6-12	Less rebound over 6 hours than Naphazoline.
Oral*				
Phenylpropanolamine	Propadrine	0.25-0.5	3-4	Available in sustained-released form (8-12 hr.) (Watch for weight reduction use).
Pseudoephedrine	Sudafed	0.25-0.5	4-8	Available in sustained-released form (8-12 hr.)

For complete prescribing information, please consult standard sources.
**Not recommended for more than 3 to 5 days for regular usage.*
***Commonly used in combination with antihistamine.*

the elderly due to excessive nasal mucosal absorption and/or swallowing of the solution. Severe reactions that include diaphoresis, drowsiness, and coma and "shocky" states with bradycardia have been seen with overdosage of naphazoline and tetrahydrozoline.[2]

Blood Pressure

Pressor amines or sympathomimetics such as phenyl-propanolamine and pseudoephedrine do not commonly increase blood pressure in normotensive persons. In persons with labile or overt high blood pressure, vasoconstrictor activity through alpha receptor stimulation may increase diastolic pressure.[1,2] Severe blood pressure increases may be seen in persons taking monoamine oxidase inhibitor (MAOI) within two weeks. Examples include isocarboxazid (Marplan), Pargyline (Eutonyl), phenelezine (Nardil) and tranylcypromine (Parnate).[3,5]

In addition, sympathomimetics can reduce the effect of antihypertensives such as guanethidine (Ismelin), beta-blockers and reserpine.[5]

Heart Disease

Persons with cardiovascular disease may suffer worsening angina due to sympathomimetic vasoconstriction. Prior myocardial infarctions should be a contraindication to pressor amine usage. Atrial fibrillation will also show an exaggerated heart response. "Palpitations" are a common complaint in persons taking oral sympathomimetics and should be taken seriously if a history of heart disease, "light-headedness" or dizziness is present.[2,3,4]

Endocrine Problems

The diabetic patient may experience difficulty in blood sugar control due to sympathomimetic increase in glycogenolytic sugar release. The hyperthyroid patient may be more difficult to control with thyroid inhibitors when exogenous sympathetic amines are given and may show heart rate increase, sweating and palpitations suggesting the need for an increase in antithyroid therapy. On the other hand, in the hypothyroid patient, levothyroxine may increase sympathomimetic effects on the heart when sympathomimetics are used concurrently.[2,3,4]

Neurologic/Psychologic Problems

Anxiety, nervousness, restlessness, dizziness as well as headache and nausea are common with higher doses of the oral agents. The drug history of persons on long-term decongestants may also show antianxiety agents such as the benzodiazepines used for sedation and sleep (e.g. Valium and/or Dalmane).

An often under-recognized problem is the patient on acute or long-term decongestants who complains of altered sleep patterns to include more frequent or earlier awakenings, "lighter" sleep, and bizarre dreams or nightmares. In the child, night-time crying or "fitful" restless sleep is a clinical clue to this problem. Decrease in dosage, a change to another sympathomimetic, or avoidance of doses after 6 P.M. may decrease this problem.

In addition, tricyclic antidepressants may also exaggerate sympathomimetic effects.

Elderly Considerations

Those over 60 years of age are more prone to sympathomimetic adverse effects to include blood pressure increase, tachycardia, seizures, paradoxical CNS excitation or depression, and death. Safe use of shorter-acting drugs or dosage forms in lower dose (e.g. 30mg pseudoephedrine, two to three times a day) should be established before longer-acting dosage forms are used in the older patient.

In addition, prostatic hypertrophy may become worse by sympathomimetic usage.

Other CNS Stimulants

Combined use of two sympathomimetics should usually be avoided. This includes combined oral forms such as phenylpropanolamine plus phenylephrine (which is fortunately ineffective and has no significant absorption, e.g. Dimetapp), combined, long acting oral use (e.g., Afrinol plus Drixoral), or combined oral and topical, (Ornade plus Afrin) which is a commonly used combination in acute rhinitic conditions.

A currently popular over-the-counter use of phenylpropanolamine is for short-term weight reduction. Brandnames include Control, Prolamine, Dietac, Dexatrim, etc. Patients should be cautioned against both prescription and OTC (over-the-counter) use of these anorexiant products if they are on chronic decongestant therapy. Prescription anorexiants include amphetamines, and their congeners, such as Preludin, Pre-Sate, Tepanil, Tenuate, Sanorex and Fastin. The chief danger is severe high blood pressure, and tachycardia, and their consequent damage to the heart and brain.

Antihistamines

Antihistamines are H_1 receptor inhibitors which have demonstrated utility in nonseasonal (perennial) allergic rhinitis. They are less effective in vasomotor (nonallergic rhinitis) and essentially ineffective in infectious rhinitis. Varying anticholinergic and antiemetic properties are also characteristic of antihistamine overall effect. In addition, all commonly produce some degree of sedation, dry mouth, irritability, mood changes, and dizziness on acute and chronic use. The main drug interaction is to increase the sedative effects of the CNS depressants, which includes alcohol (Table II).

Anticipation of excessive sedation is best accomplished by forewarning the patient and encouraging increased caffeine intake until tolerance to sedative effects takes place (over several days).

The therapeutic effect of antihistamines in rhinitis has been reviewed[1] and found to be unrelated to drug half-life and dosing schedule. Hydroxyzine (Atarax, Vistaril) suppress wheal size to the greatest extent and for the longest period of time (four days) compared with other com-

Table II

Antihistamine Classes

Chemical Class	Generic Name	Trade Name	Comments
Ethanolamine	bromodiphenhydramine HCl	Ambodryl	Frequent sedation and anticholinergic effect
	carbinoxamine maleate	Clistin	Lowest sedation effect of class
	clemastine fumarate	Tavist	Frequent drowsiness
	diphenhydramine HCl	Benadryl	Frequent drowsiness and anticholinergic effect
	doxylamine succinate	Decapryn	Frequent drowsiness
Alkylamine	brompheniramine maleate	Dimetane	This class has less sedation than with other classes.
	chlorpheniramine maleate	Chlor-Trimeton	
	dexchlorpheniramine maleate	Polaramine	
	dimethindene maleate	Forhistal	
	triprolidine HCl	Actidil	
Ethylenediamine	tripelennamine citrate	PBZ	Moderate sedation, dizziness, and other GI effects common.
	pyrilamine	usually in combination products	
	methapyriline	Histadryl	
Phenothiazine	methdilazine	Tacaryl	Primarily used as antipruritic, least sedating phenothiazine.
	promethazine HCl	Phenergan	Most sedating phenothiazine, also extrapyramidal effects plus photosensitization
	trimeprazine tartrate	Temaril	Used primarily as antipruritic
Piprazine	hydroxyzine HCl pamoate	Atarax	May be preferred in chronic therapy.
		Vistaril	Anticholinergic effects and drowsiness common.
Miscellaneous	azatadine maleate	Optimine	Less sedation than many other drugs.
	cyproheptadine	Periactin	Weight gain common, pronounced sedation (especially useful in cold urticaria).
	Terfenadine	Seldane	Both take 2–3 weeks of regular use for full effectiveness to be evident
	Astemizole	Hismanal	

monly used antihistamines (diphenhydramine, cyproheptadine, and chlorpheniramine). This should be borne in mind when skin testing for skin sensitivity (reaginic or IgE) antibodies. Antihistamines do not appear to interfere with serologic IgE or RAST.

THERAPEUTIC CONSIDERATIONS

Several therapeutic points should be emphasized in the use of decongestants and antihistamines in chronic rhinitis:

Table III

Selected Combination Antihistamine/Decongestants

Product Brand Name	Antihistamine(s)	Decongestants		
		Phenylephrine	Phenylpropanolamine	Pseudoephedrine
Actifed	triprolidine	—	—	yes
Deconamine	chlorpheniramine	—	—	yes
Demazin	chlorpheniramine	yes	—	—
Dimetapp	brompheniramine	yes	yes	—
Disophrol	dexbrompheniramine	—	—	yes
Drixoral	brompheniramine	—	—	yes
Naldecon	chlorpheniramine phenyltoloxamine	yes	yes	—
Ornade	chlorpheniramine	—	yes	—
Rondec	carbinoxamine	—	—	yes
Triaminic	pyrilamine pheniramine	—	yes	—

1. While hydroxyzine may be the preferred antihistamine for long term use, tolerance to sedation and therapeutic effect may develop over days to two weeks. The latter effect may be avoided by periodically (every one to two weeks) changing the chemical class of antihistamine used (Table II). (Seldane and Hisminal should be included)

2. Using more than one antihistamine at a time has no basis in therapeutics.

3. If events that would *worsen* rhinitis are anticipated, a dose of antihistamine should be taken one to three hours before the event.

4. Patient compliance and medication errors should be assessed by calling the pharmacist and checking refill dates by prescription number to ensure timely refills as well as appropriate use. Encourage the pharmacist to reinforce your counseling on appropriate use of the drugs, and recognize and report to you drug-related adverse effects as well as misuse.

5. Chronic problems may require *chronic, regular not prn* usage of antihistamine and/or decongestant.

6. Treat specific symptoms with single drugs when possible or use effective combinations of single ingredients when indicated (Table III).

7. Use precautions as previously discussed especially when chronic decongestants are used.

8. Recognize and check for adverse effects of your prescribed medication, and caution patient to keep and present a complete record of all prescription and OTC drugs to each potential prescriber or pharmacist they see with problems or prescriptions.

9. Especially caution patients to check with you or their pharmacist before using any new medication whether prescription or OTC.

10. Caution patients who are on other psychoactive medication (e.g., sympatholytics, psychotropics, and narcotic analgesics) to carefully limit their concurrent use with antihistamines.

REFERENCES

1. Hendeles L, Weinberger M, Wong L. Medical management of noninfectious rhinitis. Am J Hosp Pharm 37:1496-1504, 1980.
2. Nasal Decongestants. Ch. 29. In: AMA Drug Evaluations, 4th ed. Prepared by AMA Dept. of Drugs. John Wiley & Sons Inc. N.Y., 1980, p. 453.
3. United States Pharmacopeia Dispensing Information. About Your Medicines. Easton Mack, Penn., 1980.
4. Facts and Comparisons, 1981 Edition, Facts and Comparisons Inc., St. Louis, Mo.
5. Hansten PD. Drug Interactions. 4th ed. Lea & Febiger, Philadelphia, Penn., 1979.
6. Karmody CS. Nasal decongestants. In: Handbook of Drug Therapy. Miller RR, Greenblatt DJ. (Eds.) Elsevier Pub. Co., N.Y., 1979.
7. Pearlman DS. Antihistamines useful in allergic disorders. In: Handbook of Drug Therapy. Miller RR, Greenblatt DJ. (Eds.) Elsevier Pub. Co., N.Y., 1979.
8. Antihistamines. Ch. 28. In: AMA Drug Evaluations, 4th ed. Prepared by AMA Dept. of Drugs. John Wiley & Sons Inc., N.Y., 1980, p. 440-448.

Chapter XXVI

New Nonsedating Antihistamines

F. Estelle R. Simons, M.D., FRCPC* and **Keith J. Simons, Ph.D.

ABSTRACT

The new H₁-receptor antagonists such as terfenadine, astemizole, cetirizine, loratadine, levocabastine, ketotifen, and azelastine have diverse pharmacokinetics, pharmacodynamics, and potency. Astemizole, for example, is the most long-acting of the new drugs and is not suitable for sporadic use. Cetirizine, the carboxylic acid metabolite of hydroxyzine, unlike other H₁-receptor antagonists, is minimally metabolized in the body and is primarily excreted in unchanged form in the urine. Levocabastine is the most potent of the new drugs and can be applied topically to the conjunctivae or to the nasal mucosa for relief of allergic rhinoconjunctivitis. Cetirizine, terfenadine, loratadine, ketotifen, and azelastine have antiallergic effects in addition to their antihistaminic effects. Cetirizine also has potent anti-inflammatory effects. The new H₁-receptor antagonists are no more effective in relieving nasal congestion than are the first-generation H₁-receptor antagonists. Most, but not all, of the new H₁-receptor antagonists lack anticholinergic effects and are relatively nonsedating.

The perfect H₁-receptor antagonist would be highly potent and would produce clinical benefits within an hour after ingestion. It would have a duration of action of at least 24 hours. It would be completely devoid of undesirable anticholinergic or central nervous system adverse effects. No first-generation H₁-receptor antagonist fulfills all these criteria, but some of the newer, second-generation H₁-receptors antagonists may meet these expectations.[1]

In addition to being pharmacologic antagonists of histamine, many H₁-receptor antagonists such as cetirizine, terfenadine, loratadine, ketotifen, and azelastine prevent release of inflammatory mediators from IgE sensitized mast cells and basophils. In therapeutic concentrations readily achieved *in vivo*, cetirizine also has anti-inflammatory effects, including the ability to inhibit eosinophil recruitment. Ketotifen inhibits calcium transport across cell membranes, has a weak antiserotonin effect and reduces human neutrophil activation induced by PAF-acether. Azelastine antagonizes the action of leukotrienes, serotonin, acetylcholine, and bradykinin, at least in animals.[2-5]

PHARMACOKINETICS AND PHARMACODYNAMICS

There are considerable differences in the pharmacokinetics and pharmacodynamics of the newer, relatively nonsedating, H₁-receptor antagonists. Our understanding of these differences facilitates optimal use of these medications.

Terfenadine[6-8] is well-absorbed when administered by mouth. Peak serum concentrations are low, usually around 1–2 ng/mL following a 60 mg dose. For this reason, the active human carboxylic acid metabolite of terfenadine, terfenadine metabolite I, is usually quantitated instead of the parent compound. Due to difficulties in measuring low levels of terfenadine metabolite I, different half-life values have been reported; it is less than 24 hours in young adults. A single 60 mg dose of terfenadine has not suppressed the histamine-induced wheal and flare significantly for 24 hours in all studies, but a single 120 mg dose does suppress the wheal and flare significantly for 24 hours. A dose of 120 mg daily therefore is being recommended in many countries; once-daily dosing probably facilitates patient compliance with the treatment regimen.

Astemizole.[9-11] Initially, it was reported that absorption of astemizole from the gastrointestinal tract was

*Professor and Head, Section of Allergy and Clinical Immunology, Department of Pediatrics and Child Health, University of Manitoba. **Professor, Faculties of Pharmacy, Medicine, and Science, University of Manitoba, Winnipeg, Manitoba, Canada R3A 1S1.*

decreased in the presence of food, but this is no longer believed to be true. Astemizole seems to undergo extensive first-pass metabolism, and practically none of an oral dose is excreted in unchanged form in urine or feces. Desmethylastemizole is the main active human metabolite; norastemizole and 6-hydroxydesmethyl-astemizole also are produced. Peak serum concentrations of astemizole after a conventional 10 mg dose are extremely low, approximately 1–3 ng/mL. The mean serum elimination half-life value of astemizole plus desmethylastemizole is 9.5 days. Steady-state serum concentrations of 5–6 ng/mL of astemizole plus hydroxylated metabolites are achieved after 4–6 weeks of daily dosing, and apparently further accumulation does not occur after this time. Astemizole binds to peripheral H_1-receptor sites with far greater affinity than do any other existing H_1-receptor antagonists. A short course of astemizole, 10 mg daily, suppresses the histamine-induced wheal and flare significantly for weeks after the astemizole has been discontinued.

Loratadine,[12–14] like terfenadine and astemizole, results in extremely low maximum serum concentrations after a single 10 mg dose. It, too, is rapidly transformed into various metabolites, including descarboethoxyloratadine, which is active in humans and is itself further metabolized. The serum elimination half-life value of loratadine in normal adults has been reported as 7.8 to 11 hours; the serum elimination half-life of the active metabolite is 17–24 hours. A single 10 mg dose of loratadine suppresses the histamine-induced wheal and flare for 12–24 hours; a 20 mg dose suppresses the wheal and flare for 24 hours or more. The serum elimination half-life value of loratadine and of its active metabolites may be prolonged in some elderly patients.

Cetirizine[15–17] is a carboxylic acid metabolite of the first-generation H_1-receptor antagonist, hydroxyzine, and is only minimally further metabolized in humans. A single 10 mg dose of cetirizine in adults results in maximum serum concentrations of approximately 300 ng/mL. Within 72 hours of a single cetirizine dose, 70% of the medication appears unchanged in the urine. The serum elimination half-life of cetirizine is approximately 7.4 hours in adults, being slightly shorter in children and slightly longer in normal elderly adults. In adults with renal failure, it is approximately 19 hours. Cetirizine 10 mg has prompt onset of action and effectively suppresses the wheal and flare for 24 hours.

Levocabastine,[18–19] in animal studies, is 15,000 times as potent as chlorpheniramine, 1,500 times as potent as terfenadine, and 65 times as potent as astemizole. It is water-soluble and effective when applied topically to the nasal mucous membrane and the conjunctivae. A single topical application of levocabastine blocks the nasal and conjunctival response to histamine or antigen challenge for 24–72 hours. Some systemic absorption occurs from the mucosa, the serum concentrations

being about 1/30 of the steady-state level achieved after giving 0.5 mg of levocabastine by mouth.

Ketotifen[20] has a serum elimination phase half-life value of 20.4 hours and a duration of action of at least 12 hours. In asthma treatment, it is maximally effective after 6 to 12 weeks.

Azelastine[21,22] has a serum elimination half-life of approximately 12 hours and twice daily dosage is required.

ADVERSE EFFECTS

Terfenadine, 60 mg or 120 mg, causes no higher incidence of dry mouth, other anticholinergic effects, or central nervous system effects than does placebo.[6–8] Even in patients taking massive terfenadine overdoses, adverse reactions have been extremely rare. In the manufacturer's recommended doses, terfenadine does not interact with, or potentiate, the effects of alcohol, diazepam, or other central nervous system-active medications. For use in pregnancy, it is classified as a Schedule C drug, and therefore should be used only if the potential benefit justifies the potential risk to the fetus.

Astemizole, 10 mg does not produce any more sedation or anticholinergic effects than does placebo.[9–11] In some studies, it has been reported to cause increased appetite and excess weight gain. A few patients on astemizole, most of whom have admitted to taking overdoses of approximately 200 mg, have had torsade de pointes, syncope, and cardiac arrest. Astemizole does not interact with, or enhance, central nervous system suppression effects of alcohol, diazepam, or other central nervous system-active medications. No teratogenic effects have been observed in animal studies with astemizole, however, some physicians, concerned about its long serum elimination half-life value, believe that this medication should not be used by pregnant or lactating women.

TABLE I

Serum Elimination Half-life Values for Second-Generation H_1-Receptor Antagonists and Metabolites

Agent	Dose	Half-Life Adults
Terfenadine	60 mg	
Metabolite I		17.0 hrs
Astemizole*	30 mg	9.5 days
Loratadine	10 mg	7.8 to 11.0 hrs
Metabolite**		17 to 24 hrs
Cetirizine	10 mg	7.4 hrs***

* *Plus desmethylastemizole*
** *Descarboethoxyloratadine*
*** *In adults with renal insufficiency, half-life is 19 hrs*

Loratadine 10 mg does not cause a higher incidence of sedation or anticholinergic effects than does placebo.[12-14] Some sedation may occur with higher loratadine doses. Loratadine does not appear to interact with or potentiate the effects of central nervous system-active substances, although it has not been as extensively studied in this regard as have terfenadine and astemizole. Loratadine concentrations in breast milk parallel loratadine concentrations in serum. Loratadine has not caused teratogenic effects in animals.

Cetirizine 10 mg produces an incidence of anticholinergic effects similar to that produced by placebo and an incidence of central nervous system adverse effects slightly greater than that produced by placebo. Serious adverse effects have not been attributed to cetirizine. Although this medication has been introduced fairly recently into therapeutic usage, in fact, in the past 40 years there has been considerable worldwide experience with cetirizine arising *in vivo* as a metabolite of hydroxyzine.[15-17]

Levocabastine causes sedation when administered by mouth but not when applied topically.[18,19]

Ketotifen causes sedation in about 15% of adults, when given in the usual dose of 1 mg twice daily; this tends to be worse in the first week of treatment and ameliorates over time. It may cause excessive weight gain, possibly due to its anti-serotonin effects.[20]

Azelastine occasionally causes drowsiness, and it may cause a dose-related, dry, metallic taste in the mouth.[22]

EFFICACY

The new second-generation H_1-receptor antagonists are effective in the management of seasonal and perennial allergic rhinitis symptoms such as rhinorrhea, nasal itching, and sneezing but are much less effective in prevention or relief of nasal congestion. In most prospective, double-blind studies of the efficacy of the new H_1-receptor antagonists, effectiveness has been determined with patient- and physician-recorded symptom scores, either in a closely monitored field trial of short duration or, more commonly, recorded at home over one or more weeks.

In adults, terfenadine, 60 mg twice daily, has been found in most (but not all) studies to be equal in efficacy to chlorpheniramine, 8 mg twice daily (Figure 1), or loratadine, 10 or 40 mg daily. Terfenadine generally is administered in a dose of 60 mg every 12 hours, but 120 mg every 24 hours is just as effective.

Astemizole, 10 mg daily, is more potent than placebo, pheniramine, chlorpheniramine, or terfenadine, 60 mg twice daily. Astemizole has a longer lag time to peak onset of action than any other H_1-receptor antagonist and is not suited for sporadic use. For optimal effectiveness of astemizole, either a loading dose of 30 mg daily should be administered in the first week of treatment or astemizole treatment should be started well in

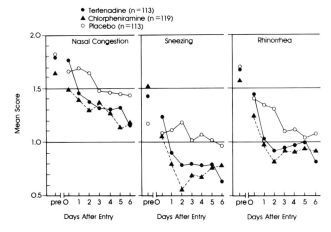

Figure 1. *Efficacy of terfenadine and chlorpheniramine versus placebo in patients with allergic rhinoconjunctivitis. Both H_1-receptor antagonists were effective in reducing sneezing and rhinorrhea but were not significantly more effective than placebo in relieving nasal congestion. The incidence of sedation in the terfenadine-treated group (7.6%) and in the placebo-treated group (2.4%) did not differ significantly. The incidence of sedation in the chloropheniramine-treated group was 19%, significantly higher than in either the terfenadine- or the placebo-treated group. The physicians' pretreatment severity scores are presented in the upper left corners of each plot since no pretreatment severity of symptoms was obtained from the patients' diaries. Kemp JP, Buckley CE, Gershwin ME et al. Multicenter, double-blind, placebo-controlled trial of terfenadine in seasonal allergic rhinitis and conjunctivitis. Ann Allergy 54:502–509, 1985.*

advance of the peak pollen season in patients with chronic allergic rhinitis.

Loratadine, 10 mg once daily, is superior to placebo and equal in efficacy to chlorpheniramine twice daily; terfenadine, 60 mg twice daily; clemastine, 1 mg twice daily; or mequitazine, 5 mg twice daily.

Cetirizine, 5 to 20 mg daily, is superior to placebo, and in a 10 mg daily dose, it is as effective as terfenadine, 60 mg twice daily, in controlling the symptoms of seasonal and perennial allergic rhinitis.

In prospective, controlled, double-blind studies in patients with allergic rhinoconjunctivitis, H_1-receptor antagonists administered by mouth generally are found to be less potent than intranasal corticosteroids in the treatment of rhinitis symptoms but more potent than intranasal corticosteroids in relief of ocular symptoms such as itching, tearing, and erythema (Figure 2). No satisfactory comparison exists of new H_1-receptor antagonists with topical cromolyn sodium treatment in allergic rhinoconjunctivitis.

While some of the new H_1-receptor antagonists will no doubt be used in a traditional role for control of itching, sneezing, and rhinorrhea in patients with allergic rhinitis, one can envision expanded and different

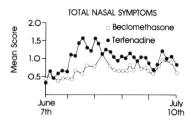

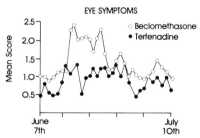

Figure 2. Total nasal symptom and eye symptom diary scores in a double-blind, parallel group comparison of beclomethasone dipropionate aqueous nasal spray and terfenadine tablets, 60 mg twice daily. The terfenadine-treated group had lower eye symptom scores than did the beclomethasone-treated group, and these differences were statistically significant during the first half of the study. The beclomethasone-treated group had lower nasal symptom scores than the terfenadine-treated group, and these differences reached statistical significance on high pollen-count days. Beswick KBJ, Kenyon GS, Cherry JR. A comparative study of beclomethasone dipropionate aqueous nasal spray with terfenadine tablets in seasonal allergic rhinitis. Curr Med Res Opin 9:560–567, 1985.

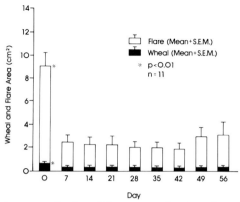

Figure 3. Mean wheal-and-flare areas after intradermal injection of 0.01 mL of histamine, 0.1 mg/mL at study entry (day 0), and 12 hrs after a dose of terfenadine, 60 mg, on days 7, 14, 21, 28, 35, 42, 49, and 56. The subjects were taking terfenadine, 60 mg twice daily, regularly, throughout the 56-day study. The wheal-and-flare areas did not differ significantly on days 7, 14, 21, 28, 35, 42, 49, and 56, and remained significantly suppressed compared to pretreatment wheal-and-flare size. No evidence of subsensitivity to terfenadine was found during long-term treatment. Simons FER, Watson WTA, Simons KJ. Lack of subsensitivity to terfenadine during long-term terfenadine treatment. J Allergy Clin Immunol 82:1068–1075, 1988.

roles for others. For example, levocabastine as a topical agent will be extremely useful in the management of allergic conjunctivitis, as well as in the management of allergic rhinitis. Ketotifen and azelastine probably will find their chief applications in the treatment of patients with mild asthma who also have allergic rhinoconjunctivitis.

CLINICAL INVESTIGATION FACILITATED BY THE NEW, NONSEDATING H_1-RECEPTOR ANTAGONISTS

The nonsedating H_1-receptor antagonists provide useful insights into the class of medications as a whole, for example, by facilitating studies of subsensitivity to H_1-receptor antagonists and studies of H_1-receptor antagonists in asthma.

Long-term administration of first-generation H_1-receptor antagonists has been associated with apparent decreased efficacy after weeks or months, attributed to autoinduction of hepatic metabolism and increased hepatic clearance of the H_1-receptor antagonist. Autoinduction and subsensitivity have not been reported with the second-generation H_1-receptor antagonists; recent

studies have shown that patients do not eliminate terfenadine or cetirizine more rapidly after weeks of treatment than at the onset of treatment. After long-term treatment with terfenadine, cetirizine, and loratadine during which compliance is monitored regularly, the efficacy of the H_1-receptor antagonists in suppression of the wheal and flare (Figure 3) and in suppression of allergic rhinoconjunctivitis symptoms is not diminished. The apparent subsensitivity noted with the first-generation H_1-receptor antagonists may have been due to lack of compliance with medication regimens that caused sedation yet did not completely relieve symptoms.[1]

The new, nonsedating H_1-receptor antagonists terfenadine, astemizole, loratadine, cetirizine, ketotifen, and azelastine have been tested in a truly double-blind fashion in patients with asthma. They have a modest, dose-related beneficial effect. H_1-receptor antagonists are no longer considered to be harmful to patients with asthma who happen to require these medications for a disorder such as chronic allergic rhinitis.[20,22,23]

SUMMARY

H_1-receptor antagonist research has entered a phase of unprecedented activity. Information about individual new H_1-receptor antagonists is exciting, but, best of all, this information is contributing to our increased understanding of these medications as a class and is helping investigators to shed light on many of the old, intriguing questions about these most useful pharmacologic compounds.

REFERENCES

1. Simons FER. H$_1$-receptor antagonists: Clinical pharmacology and therapeutics. J Allergy Clin Immunol 84:845–861, 1989.
2. Michel L, De Vos C, Rihoux J-P, Burtin C, Benveniste J, Dubertret L. Inhibitory effect of oral cetirizine on in vivo antigen-induced histamine and PAF-acether release and eosinophil recruitment in human skin. J Allergy Clin Immunol 82:101–109, 1988.
3. Bousquet J, Lebel B, Chanal I, Morel A, Michel F-B. Antiallergic activity of H$_1$-receptor antagonists assessed by nasal challenge. J Allergy Clin Immunol 82:881–887, 1988.
4. Martin U, Römer D. The pharmacological properties of a new orally active antianaphylactic compound: Ketotifen, a benzocycloheptathiophene. Arzneimittel-Forschung Drug Res 28:770–782, 1978.
5. Little MM, Casale TB. Azelastine inhibits IgE-mediated human basophil histamine release. J Allergy Clin Immunol 83:862–865, 1989.
6. Sorkin EM, Heel RC. Terfenadine: a review of its pharmacodynamic properties and therapeutic efficacy. Drugs 29:34–56, 1985.
7. Simons FER, Watson WTA, Simons KJ. Lack of subsensitivity to terfenadine during long-term terfenadine treatment. J Allergy Clin Immunol 82:1068–1075, 1988.
8. Shall L, Newcombe RG, Marks R. Assessment of the duration of action of terfenadine on histamine-induced wheals. Br J Dermatol 119:525–531, 1988.
9. Richards DM, Brogden RN, Heel RC, Speight TM, Avery GS. Astemizole: A review of its pharmacodynamic properties and therapeutic efficacy. Drugs 28:38–61, 1984.
10. Heykants J, Van Peer A, Woestenborghs R, Jageneau A, Vanden Bussche G. Dose-proportionality, bioavailability, and steady-state kinetics of astemizole in man. Drug Develop Res 8:71–78, 1986.
11. Malo J-L, Fu CL, L'Archeveque J, Ghezzo H, Cartier A. Duration of the effect of astemizole on histamine-inhalation tests. J Allergy Clin Immunol 85:729–736, 1990.
12. Clissold SP, Sorkin EM, Goa KL. Loratadine: A preliminary review of its pharmacodynamic properties and therapeutic efficacy. Drugs 37:42–57, 1989.
13. Kassem N, Roman I, Gural R, Dyer JG, Robillard N. Effects of loratadine (SCH 29851) in suppression of histamine-induced skin wheals. Ann Allergy 60:505–507, 1988.
14. Simons FER. Loratadine, a non-sedating H$_1$-receptor antagonist (antihistamine). Ann Allergy 63:266–268, 1989.
15. Rihoux JP, De Vos C, Baltes E, de Lannoy J. Pharmacoclinical investigation of cetirizine, a new potent and well-tolerated anti-H$_1$. Ann Allergy 55:392, 1985.
16. Watson WTA, Simons KJ, Chen XY, Simons FER. Cetirizine: A pharmacokinetic and pharmacodynamic evaluation in children with seasonal allergic rhinitis. J Allergy Clin Immunol 84:457–464, 1989.
17. Matzke GR, Yeh J, Awni WM, Halstenson CE, Chung M. Pharmacokinetics of cetirizine in the elderly and patients with renal insufficiency. Ann Allergy 59:II:25–30, 1987.
18. Bende M, Pipkorn U. Topical levocabastine, a selective H$_1$ antagonist, in seasonal allergic rhinoconjunctivitis. Allergy 42:512–5, 1987.
19. Pécoud A, Zuber P, Kolly M. Effect of a new selective H$_1$-receptor antagonist (levocabastine) in a nasal and conjunctival provocation test. Int Arch Allergy Appl Immunol 82:541–543, 1987.
20. Simons FER, Luciuk GH, Becker AB, Gillespie CA. Ketotifen: a new drug for prophylaxis of asthma in children. Ann Allergy 48:145–50, 1982.
21. Meltzer EO, Storms WW, Pierson WE et al. Efficacy of azelastine in perennial allergic rhinitis: Clinical and rhinomanometric evaluation. J Allergy Clin Immunol 82:447–455, 1988.
22. Kemp JP, Meltzer EO, Orgel HA, et al. A dose-response study of the bronchodilator action of azelastine in asthma. J Allergy Clin Immunol 79:893–899, 1987.
23. Rafferty P, Holgate ST. Histamine and its antagonists in asthma. J Allergy Clin Immunol 84:144–151, 1989.

Chapter XXVII

Topical Corticosteroids in the Management of Rhinitis

Sheldon C. Siegel, M.D.

ABSTRACT

The newer topical corticosteroids have proved extremely valuable in the management of several types of rhinitis. Patients who show a clear indication for their use appear to be relatively few of major side effects with the recommended dosages; nevertheless, long-term effects remain unknown. Thus their use should be limited to properly selected patients, using the lowest possible dose, and for the shortest period of time for the control of symptoms.

It has been known since 1949 that corticosteroids are highly effective in treating both asthma and allergic rhinitis. However, because of serious adverse effects associated with prolonged systemic administration of corticosteroids, they have been used primarily for the treatment of severe asthma. Early on after their discovery, attempts were made to circumvent the side effects of the corticosteroids by applying them topically. Dill and Bolstead[1] were among the first to use cortisone intranasally. Not surprisingly, since cortisone is not topically active, they found significant relief in less than half their patients with rhinitis. Better success was obtained by Pennypacker[2] who reported intranasal hydrocortisone was effective in 78% of his subjects treated. Others utilizing hydrocortisone or prednisolone applied intranasally as powders and snuffs also reported good to excellent results in the majority of patients treated. These methods never gained wide acceptance because of variable effectiveness, and the studies reported were not controlled.

Clinical Professor of Pediatrics, UCLA School of Medicine. Supported in part by a grant from Allergy Research Foundation, Inc., Los Angeles, CA.

The development of dexamethasone phosphate, a more potent topically active corticosteroid, and a method to deliver this hormone intranasally via an aerosol metered dose inhaler (Turbinaire®), ushered in a new era for the use of topical steroids in the treatment of rhinitis. Appropriately controlled studies with this aerosol preparation revealed significant improvement in the symptoms of allergic rhinitis[3] and improvement in nasal polyps.[4] Much of the improvement noted was attributed to the topical activity of the dexamethasone.[5] Despite its effectiveness as an aerosol in both allergic rhinitis and asthma, subsequent studies revealed significant systemic absorption of the dexamethasone with resultant suppression of the hypothalamic-pituitary-adrenal axis (PHA) even after short-term use, thus limiting its usefulness for the treatment of respiratory allergic disorders.[6–10]

In the 1970s a major advance in the management of rhinitis and asthma was made with the development and introduction of several new, highly active topical corticosteroids that had minimal to no systemic activity and could be administered via an aerosol or as a spray. Table I lists the topical corticosteroid preparations presently available or under investigation in the United States and elsewhere. Only beclomethasone dipropionate (BDP) and flunisolide (FI) presently are marketed for intranasal use in the United States. Budesonide (BUD) is available in most other countries. My associates and I have investigated BDP, FI, fluocortin butylester (FB), triamcinolone acetonide (TA), and fluticasone propionate (FP) for the treatment of allergic rhinitis. Based on our evaluation of these agents and review of the literature, we review their pharmacologic properties, chemical structure, possible mode of action, indications, dosage, delivery systems, side effects, and general

TABLE I

Newer Topical Corticosteroids

Beclomethasone dipropionate (Vanceril, Beclovent, Becotide, Beconase, Vancenase)

Flunisolide (Aerobid, Nasalide)

Fluocortin butylester

Triamcinolone acetonide (Azmacort)

Betamethasone valerate (Bextasol)

Budesonide (Pulmocort, Rhinocort)

Tixocortol

Dexamethasone isonicotinate

Fluticasone propionate (Flunase)

TABLE II

Comparative Topical Potencies

Corticosteroid	Topical Activity*
Hydrocortisone	1
Triamcinolone acetonide	1,000
Flunisolide	3,000
Beclomethasone dipropionate	5,000
Budesonide	10,000
Fluticasone propionate	20,000

* *Vasoconstrictor activity*

principles regarding their use for nasal respiratory disorders.

PATHOPHYSIOLOGY OF ALLERGIC RHINITIS

Recent progress in our understanding of the pathophysiologic mechanisms involved in both upper and lower respiratory allergic diseases has provided a more rational basis for the use of corticosteroids in the treatment of allergic rhinitis and asthma. It is now clear that an inflammatory response in the upper airway plays just as important a role in the pathogenesis of allergic rhinitis as it does in asthma.[11] Exposure to allergens causes release of mediators, which is accompanied by a surge of symptoms, the so-called early response. Three to 11 hours later many patients experience a second round of symptoms accompanied by mediator release and an influx of inflammatory cells (neutrophils, eosinophils, mononuclear, and basophils). Major basic protein from eosinophils also is released, contributing to the inflammatory response. Repeated exposure to an allergen often results in an augmented response to lesser amounts of allergen, a response termed "priming effect" and initially described by Connell in the late 1960s.[12] Pretreatment with corticosteroids has some effect on the early response but markedly diminishes the augmented response as well as the late-phase reaction.[13, 14]

PHARMACOLOGIC PROPERTIES

Several properties of the newer inhaled corticosteroids account for their ability to reduce the risk of untoward systemic glucocorticoid reactions: (1) They have potent topical activity that permits marked reduction in dosage requirements. (2) There is rapid first-pass hepatic degradation to metabolites with little or no glucocorticoid activity.[15-18] (3) There is greater inhibition of early phase reaction after antigen challenge after topical versus systemic corticosteroid therapy.[19]

After intranasal administration these drugs are absorbed via the respiratory tract, but a portion of the dose is swallowed. However, evidence has been presented this systemic absorption of the drug is unlikely to contribute to the beneficial effects on the nasal mucosa.[19-21] The approximate relative anti-inflammatory potencies of these corticosteroids compared with hydrocortisone, as determined by the vasoconstrictor assay, are shown in Table II. These topical corticosteroids have a vasoconstrictor activity several thousand times greater than that of hydrocortisone. Evidence showed that there is a good correlation between the ability of a corticosteroid to induce "vasoconstriction" in normal human skin and their anti-inflammmatory effects in skin disorders.[22, 23]

MECHANISM OF ACTION

Although our understanding of mechanisms by which corticosteroids provide their beneficial effect in asthma and nasal disorders has increased recently, our knowledge of the precise mechanisms involved remains incomplete. Several excellent reviews have been published about the mechanisms of action of corticosteroids in the treatment of asthma and allergic disorders.[24-29] Because topical corticosteroids exert their beneficial effects locally rather than through systemic absorption, the mechanisms involved in amelioration of symptoms after intranasal use are emphasized.

When administered topically or absorbed systemically, the free or unbound glucocorticoid molecules diffuse passively through the cell membrane, enter the cytoplasm, and bind to the steroid receptor. The steroid receptor complex moves into the cell nucleus, where it firmly attaches to nuclear binding sites on the DNA molecules. An increase in mRNA chain synthesis follows. The mRNA molecules then move into the cytoplasm, where they are translated by the ribosomes into formation of different proteins. One of these proteins induced in neutrophils is lipocortin (macrocortin). Lipocortin inhibits the release of arachidonic acid from phospholipids by its inhibitory activity on phospholipase A2. Arachidonic acid forms the substrate for the cyclooxygenase and lipoxygenase pathways, leading to the formation of the mediators prostaglandins and leukotrienes.

Other cellular activities of corticosteroids relevant to their efficacy in the treatment of rhinitis include the prevention of release of other inflammatory mediators. They inhibit release of IgE-mediated histamine from basophils and release of lysosomal enzymes and prostaglandins from neutrophils. Prostaglandin synthesis is thought to be partially responsible for the vasoconstrictor and antiedematous effects. The antiedematous effects of the corticosteroid also may be related to their influence on beta adrenergic receptors and inhibitory capacity on endothelial adherence of leukocytes.

It also has been observed that after intranasal administration of corticosteroids there is a reduction in the number of basophilic cells in the epithelial surface of nasal mucous membrane and the number of eosinophils in the nasal mucosa.[30] There is also a reduction in the sensitivity of irritant receptors and secretory response to the stimulation of cholinergic receptors.[31]

Previously it was thought the corticosteroids did not inhibit the allergen-induced early response.[32] Recent studies, however, have shown that prolonged treatment with topically applied corticosteroids have an inhibitory effect on the symptoms of early response.[33,14] Thus, in addition to their anti-inflammatory effects, topical corticosteroids potentially have prophylactic properties. The prevention or reduction in symptoms has been demonstrated by antigen challenge studies in asymptomatic hay fever patients to be due, at least in part, by decreasing the generation of inflammatory mediators.[19] Prevention of an increase in the influx and activation of eosinophils, neutrophils, and basophils also occur with both systemic and topical corticosteroids.[34] The precise mode of action by which these effects are produced is not well understood. The steroid-induced reduction in cellular influx has been postulated to be due to (1) reduced chemotactic activity, presumably due to decreased mediators; (2) a reduced responsiveness of the cells involved; and (3) a change in the endothelial-subendothelial environment that the cells traverse to reach the inflammatory focus.

Another beneficial effect of corticosteroids is to reduce hyperreactivity of the airways. In the lower airways, documentation of hyperreactivity by challenge with histamine, methacholine, or nonisotonic aerosols is standard procedure. Although nasal hyperreactivity has been demonstrated in selected patients, it cannot be used for diagnostic purposes because of overlapping results in normal subjects and rhinitis patients. Corticosteroids have been found to decrease nasal hyperreactivity, but the effect is weaker in the nose and not reported to occur in all subjects studies.[35] Thus, it is

unlikely this is an important mechanism by which topical corticosteroids exert their beneficial effects. On the other hand, reduction in specific allergen-induced reactivity can be blocked by even short-term oral and topical corticosteroids.[36]

PREPARATIONS

Beclomethasone Dipropionate

Beclomethasone dipropionate (Vancenase, Vancenase AQ, Beconase, Beconase AQ) was the first of the newer corticosteroids that clearly showed separation of topical activity from systemic effects. BDP differs from dexamethasone only by having a chlorine at the 9-a position, in place of a fluorine. It has potent glucocorticoid but weak mineralcorticoid activity. BDP is sparingly soluble. When administered intranasally, a portion of the drug is swallowed. Absorption occurs rapidly from all respiratory tissues, but is more slowly absorbed from the gastrointestinal tract. After absorption it is hydrolyzed by fecal esterases to beclomethasone 17-propionate. Further hydrolysis to beclomethasone and biotransformation by oxidative or reductive pathways results in inactive polar metabolites that are excreted via the bile. The elimination half-life is about 15 hours.

In the United States, both the Vancenase and Beconase inhalers are available as a freon-propelled metered dose aerosol unit that delivers about 42 μg drug with each actuation and as an aqueous formulation, .05%. The recommended dosage is one inhalation in each nostril two to four times a day (total dose 168 to 336 μg/day). The results of our studies of BDP showed that one inhalation into each nostril three times daily provided optimal symptomatic relief and that a higher dose or more frequent dosing was unnecessary[37] (see Figure 1). BDP is also available as a powder in other countries. Sidwell[38] has shown that there is no significant difference between the powder, aerosol, or aqueous forms in alleviating signs and symptoms of allergic rhinitis.

Flunisolide

Intranasal flunisolide, marketed under the trade name Nasalide in the United States and Syntaris in Europe, is a 0.25% aqueous solution administered by hand-activated pump delivering 25 μg per spray. The recommended starting dosage for adults in two sprays (50 μg) in each nostril two times a day (total dose 200 μg/day). If needed, the dosage may be increased to two sprays three times a day (total dose 300 μg/day). In children aged 6 to 14 years, the dosage is one spray in each nostril three times daily or two sprays in each nostril twice a day (total dose 150 to 200 μg/day). Absorption of FL occurs when given orally, but systemic bioavailability is only 21%, indicating an extensive first-pass liver metabolism. Fifty percent of the FL

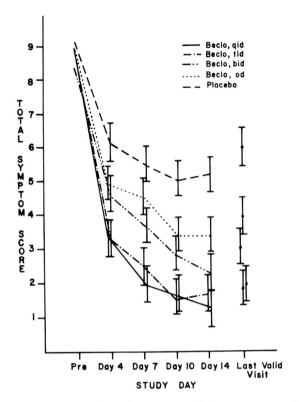

Figure 1. Mean total nasal symptom and sign scores over the 2-week study period. There was no statistical significant difference between t.i.d. and q.i.d. administration of BDP. Reprinted with permission by C.V. Mosby Company.

administered intranasally reaches the systemic circulation unmetabolized, but it is also rapidly metabolized to inactive metabolites. The half-life is also very short, about 1 to 2 hours.

In our double-blind placebo-controlled studies in 49 children aged 5 to 16 years, 80% of the patients receiving FL achieved either total or substantial control of their symptoms, in contrast to only 8% of the group receiving placebo. In addition, in those children receiving placebo about 71% did not benefit from the medication or their symptoms were aggravated. Similar results were found in 16% of the actively treated group. These results are shown graphically in Figure 2. Cortisol levels were measured and adrenocorticotropic hormone response tests were done before and after 12 weeks of active treatment with FL, and did not reveal any evidence of adrenal suppression.

Fluocortin Butylester

Fluocortin butylester is manufactured as a powder for insufflation through a specially designed Venturi tube that conforms to the shape of the nostrils. Clinical studies indicate FB is effective in treating rhinitis at a daily dosage of 2 to 4 mg given in two to four equally divided doses. After the ester undergoes hydrolysis, the resulting metabolite is inactive. Twenty-nine percent of the administered dose is bioavailable after bronchial inhalation; bioavailability after nasal inhalation has not been determined. The half-life of an intravenously administered dose of FB is three hours. Unlike BDP and FL, which are highly bound to serum proteins, FB is only 10% protein bound. Few systemic side effects have been reported; however, because FB is less potent than the other intranasal corticosteroids, a large dose is needed.

Our double-blind placebo-controlled studies in 30 children aged 6 to 16 years did not show any significant improvement as assessed by physician symptom-and-sign scores (including photographs of nasal mucous membranes taken via rhinoscopy before and after treatment), patient symptom-and-medication scores, blockage scores, and measurement of nasal airway resistance. However, others have reported a beneficial effect of FB in the treatment of allergic rhinitis.[39]

Budesonide

Budesonide (Rhinocort) is a nonhalogenated corticosteroid that has been shown to have a high ratio of topical to systemic activity over a wide dosage range. The reason for this favorable relation between therapeutic effect and side effects is that BUD is inactivated rapidly in the liver after absorption. Though BUD is available commercially in many countries as an aerosol for treatment of asthma and allergic rhinitis, investigation in the United States has been temporarily halted. BUD is administered by a freon-propelled metered-dose inhaler delivering about 50 μg per actuation. The recommended dosage is two puffs (100 μg) into each nostril twice daily (total dose 400 μg/day). This dosage can be halved once a good response is achieved. After oral ingestion, peak plasma concentrations of un-

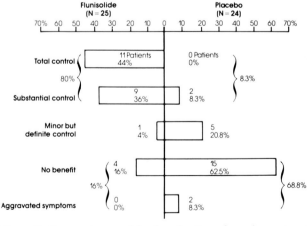

Figure 2. Comparison and final evaluation of nasal symptoms in 49 children. Reproduced by permission from a monograph, Siegel SC, ed. Current Concepts in Allergic Rhinitis, Part 1. 1986, 9–14.

changed BUD occur in about three hours, and within one hour after inhalation. BUD has a relatively short elimination half-life (about two hours) and high plasma clearance; this coupled with its rapid biotransformation in the liver to inactive metabolites and with its potent topical activity account for the good clinical results found by various investigators.[40]

Triamcinolone Acetonide

Triamcinolone acetonide (TA) is also a highly potent, nonpolar, water-insoluble halogenated topical corticosteroid developed in the United States. Although it is available as an aerosol (Azmacort) for the treatment of asthma, it is presently under investigation for the management of allergic rhinitis. The optimal dosage and frequency of administration has not been established for TA. In previous preliminary double-blind placebo-controlled studies in 205 patients with perennial allergic rhinitis, it was found that a daily dose of 200 μg (25 μg administered in each nostril four times a day) was effective and safe.[41] Additional studies using 100, 200, or 400 μg administered in each nostril once daily are under way. In a collaborative study reported by Grossman et al.[42] greater efficacy was found for the 200 μg per day treated group than in the subjects receiving 100 μg per day or placebo. Like the other topical corticosteroids, TA is rapidly metabolized in the liver, but it is less active topically than BDP, FL, or BUD.

Fluticasone Propionate

FP is the most recent glucocorticoid agent to have been developed for topical treatment. It has a spectrum of activity similar to BDP but is approximately twice as potent as BDP as indicated by the topical vasoconstrictor test. It is presently marketed under the trade name of (Flunase) in Europe and is under investigation in the United States. Clinical studies have shown it to be effective in the treatment of seasonal and perennial rhinitis.[43, 44] Pharmacokinetic studies have been performed by the intravenous and oral route. When administered intravenously its plasma half-life was 3.1 hours. It is rapidly cleared and has a low renal clearance, suggesting an extensive hepatic extraction or metabolism. FP has no effect on the hypothalamic-pituitary-adrenal axis when administered topically (200 μg q.d.) or orally (16 mg). This presumably is due to the extensive metabolism (first-pass metabolism) and due to its incomplete absorption from the gastrointestinal tract. Intranasal FP is well tolerated and was found to be equally effective when administered 200 μg once daily or 100 μg twice daily.[45] A higher dose of 400 μg administered twice a day was found by Meltzer et al.[43] to be slightly more effective in controlling nasal symptons than 200 μg or 100 μg used twice a day.

The structural formulas of the topical corticosteroid preparations used intranasally are shown in Figure 3a and 3b.

COMPARATIVE TREATMENTS

BDP, FL, and BUD have been compared with each other and with cromolyn sodium, antihistamines, and systemic corticosteroids in the symptomatic treatment of seasonal and perennial allergic rhinitis in a number of studies. The results of most of these studies showed that intranasal corticosteroid preparations were equally efficient; however, a few studies have suggested a marginally better effect with BUD versus BDP.[46–48] Such topical corticosteroid preparations as aqueous sprays, pressurized aerosols, or powders in comparative studies have shown equal efficacy. However, Orgel et al.[49] in comparing BDP aerosol with the aqueous for-

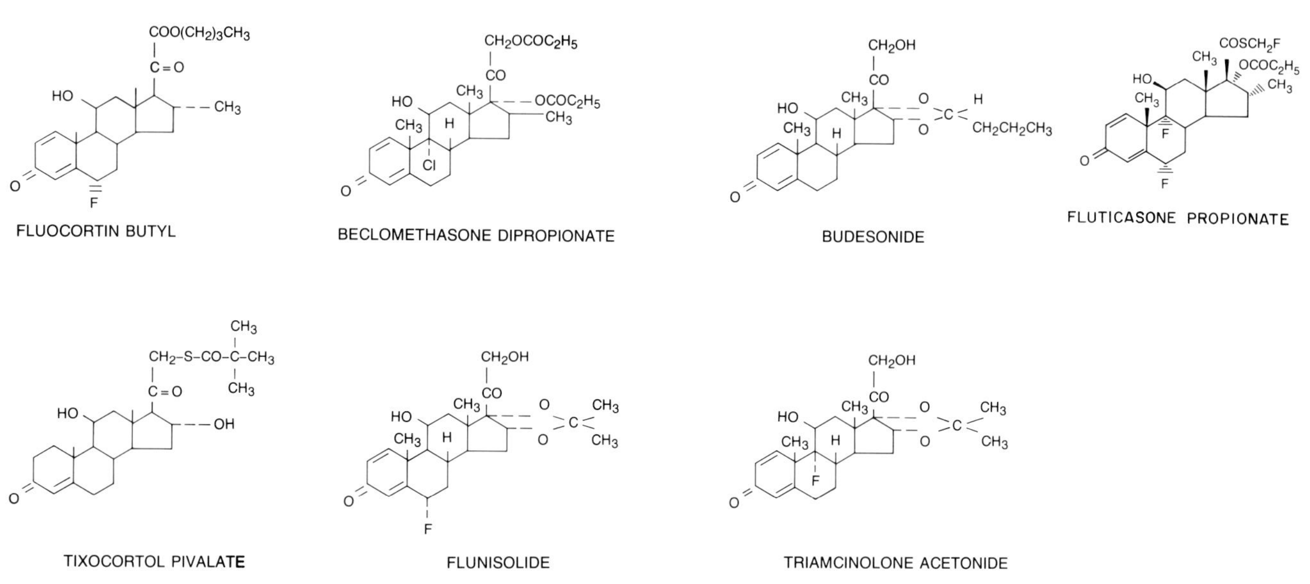

Figure 3a and 3b. Chemical structure of respiratory topical corticosteroids.

mulation found less nasal burning, pressure and sneezing with the aqueous preparation, which was preferred by 88% of the patients studied. Various modifications of nasal nozzles delivering aerosols also produce no difference in efficacy, but patients preferred a longer nozzle adapter.[50]

Comparison with Cromolyn Sodium

Most studies comparing intranasal cromolyn sodium with the topical corticosteroids have shown CS to be inferior in controlling nasal symptoms.[51-53] Based on nasal mucosal responses to allergen challenge, Pelikan[54] suggested that CS might be more helpful to patients with immediate responses to allergen challenge, whereas BDP would be more effective in preventing the delayed response. However, Pipkorn et al.[19] recently showed that topical FL inhibited the early-phase response to an antigen challenge as well as the late phase reaction.

Comparison with Antihistamines

Relatively few direct comparisons have been made between topical corticosteroids and antihistamines; often the two types of agents are administered together for additional relief of allergic symptoms, especially those involving the eyes. With the recent development of nonsedating and long-acting antihistamines, several investigators have reported their effectiveness in alleviating allergic symptoms, as compared with topical corticosteroids. Blackhouse et al.[55] found that FL nasal spray and terfenadine 60 mg twice daily were effective in reducing symptoms, but the combination treatment gave consistently better symptom relief. Sibbald et al.[56] in an open crossover trial comparing astemizole with intranasal aqueous BDP concluded the two drugs were equally effective in the symptomatic treatment of allergic rhinitis. Wood[57] also concluded that oral astemizole was as good as intranasal BDP and had the additional advantage of improved control of eye symptoms. On the other hand, Juniper et al.[58] and Salomonsson et al.[59] found corticosteroids provided better control of rhinitis than did astemizole. Beswick et al.[60] in a double-blind comparison of BDP and terfenadine also found that BDP was more likely to provide better overall control of nasal symptoms on days when pollen count was high. Dickson and Cruickshank[61] also found FL superior to terfenadine for the treatment of allergic rhinitis. Although we have not done drug studies comparing the effectiveness of the antihistamines with the topical corticosteroids, it is my clinical impression that the intranasal corticosteroids do provide greater relief of nasal symptoms in some patients. This opinion is based on the observation that patients failing to respond to the antihistamines experience additional improvement after the use of intranasal corticosteroids.

Comparison with Systemic Corticosteroids

There are few relevant clinical comparisons between systemic and intranasal topical glucocorticoid treatment. However, three recent studies making this comparison were published that provide some insight into the mechanisms of action of the topical corticosteroids. In the previously cited study by Pipkorn et al.,[19] the early-phase and the late-phase responses to antigen challenge were inhibited with topical FL, whereas two days of pretreatment with 20 mg prednisone administered three times a day for 48 hours had no effect on the early-phase reaction. This finding suggested to the authors that topical corticosteroids may provide an advantage over treatment with systemic glucocorticosteroids. Because systemic corticosteroid therapy has a limited role in the treatment of allergic rhinitis (except for short bursts), and topical corticosteroids have proved to be relatively devoid of systemic steroid side effects, a long-term study comparing systemic versus topical corticosteroid therapy probably will not be carried out. However, further nasal challenge studies with offending allergens should be done in allergic patients (e.g., asthma plus allergic rhinitis) needing long-term systemic glucocorticoid therapy, to determine whether the early phase reaction would be abated.

In another multicenter study the effectiveness of systemic FL was compared with topical FL.[20] Ninety-nine ragweed-sensitive patients were studied for four weeks during the ragweed season and randomly assigned to one of three treatment groups; intranasal placebo and oral FL 500 μg, both twice daily; oral placebo and intranasal FL 100 μg, both twice daily; and oral and intranasal placebo, both twice daily. Topical FL (200 μg/day) was statistically more effective in controlling allergic rhinitis manifestations than a systemic bioequivalent dose of 1000 μg orally administered FL. The oral dose effects were not significantly different from placebo, suggesting that the effects of topical FL are related to its local action rather than to systemic absorption.

Lindqvist et al.[21] have drawn similar conclusions from the effects of oral BD and topically applied BD in 96 patients with birch pollen allergic rhinitis. Topically applied BD significantly improved nasal symptoms, whereas the nasal symptoms of patients receiving orally administered BD were no different from those subjects receiving a placebo. These results also suggest that the effects of BD are dependent on its local action rather than to any systemic effect.

Pichler et al.[62] have compared the clinical efficacy of a single intramuscular dose of methylprednisolone acetate to topical BD in patients with seasonal allergic rhinitis. They concluded that acute symptoms of allergic rhinitis were ameliorated equally well by the two treatment regimens. Because of the greater potential for serious side effects with systemic methylprednisolone, I have preferred to use the topical corticosteroids in the management of my patients with allergic rhinitis.

PATIENT SELECTION

Indications for the use of intranasal corticosteroids in patients with rhinitis are listed in Table III. Topical corticosteroids have been shown to be highly effective in treating both seasonal and perennial allergic rhinitis. Complete control of nasal symptoms occurs in 60% to 90% of patients with comparable results in children and adults.[63] Topical corticosteroids improve the symptoms of itching, sneezing, rhinorrhea, and blockage, and in some instances relieve eye symptoms. In one recent study of intranasal BDP and FL the authors were surprised to find that symptoms of seasonal asthma were considerably reduced.[51]

Another form of rhinitis that responds extremely well to topical corticosteroids is eosinophilic rhinitis, also known as nonallergic rhinitis with eosinophilia (NARES).[64] These patients have no evidence of allergic disease by history, physical examination, skin tests, serum IgE levels, or in vitro tests for specific IgE antibodies (e.g., radioallergosorbent test [RAST], enzyme-linked immunosorbent assay [ELISA], and fluorescence allergosorbent test [FAST]).

Although the cause of nasal polyps remains obscure and their long-term treatment difficult, the use of topical corticosteroids has been shown to slow their growth, and in some patients to prevent recurrences after surgery, or even the necessity of surgery.[65-68]

Topical corticosteroids also can be used effectively for the treatment of rhinitis medicamentosa resulting from persistent use of topical vasoconstrictor agents. Although some patients with nonallergic rhinitis (vasomotor rhinitis) may respond well to treatment with these agents, in general the clinical response is poor. They are also ineffective for viral rhinitis.

ADVERSE EFFECTS

Although in the past the use of dexamethasone phosphate produced typical systemic side effects,[10] prolonged use of the newer topical corticosteroids has not been associated with systemic adverse effects, with the

TABLE III

Indications for Intranasal Topical Corticosteroids

Seasonal allergic rhinitis
Perennial allergic rhinitis
Nasal polyps
Eosinophilic nonallergic rhinitis (NARES)
Rhinitis medicamentosa
Nonallergic rhinitis (vasomotor rhinitis)

TABLE IV

Side Effects of Intranasal Corticosteroids

Transient symptoms
  Nasal irritation and stinging
  Sneezing
  Dryness
  Sore throat
Nasal bleeding
Candidiasis (unreported)
Adrenal suppression (? in 1 case)
Anatomic changes
  Atrophic (none reported)
  Septal perforation
  Nasal ulceration
Contact dermatitis

exception of one poorly documented recently reported case of adrenal suppression from intranasal BDP.[69] Local effects are quite common, but for the most part are inconsequential (Table IV) and include irritation in the form of stinging or burning, transient episodes of sneezing, dryness, and infrequent sore throat. Nasal burning and stinging is more prevalent with the use of FL. This effect has been attributed to the propylene glycol in the vehicle rather than the drug itself. A new formulation with less propylene glycol has been found to significantly decrease the severity and duration of nasal burning and stinging.[70]

Hemorrhagic crusting of the nasal septum may also occur, particularly when the spray is incorrectly directed toward the septum rather than in the sagittal plane. Although oropharyngeal candidiasis is a common compilation with the use of oral aerosolized topical corticosteroids, there have been no reports of nasal Candida albicans colonization. This finding may be related to the more rapid clearance of the topical corticosteroids by ciliated nasal epithelium. Evidence has also been presented that BUD and BDP have no adverse effects on mucociliary clearance.[71,72] Rhinoscopy and microscopic examination of biopsy specimens taken from the nasal mucous membranes of patients treated for as long as 5.5 years have not demonstrated any atrophic or metaplastic changes. Even more impressive is that no abnormal changes have been noted in bronchial biopsy tissue taken as long as 8 years after instituting oral BDP aerosol therapy.[73,74] Intranasal dexamethasone phosphate has been reported to cause nasal perforation.[10] Recently reports of nasal septal perforations with the newer topical corticosteroids have appeared in the literature. One such patient was a 9-year old girl who was being treated with FL, one spray twice daily for 7 months.[75] Schoetzel and Menzel[76] also observed eight patients with nasal perforation. It is of interest that one of these eight patients was using only a nasal decongestant spray, and two were not using any sprays at the time the defect was noted. Although cause and effect seems likely between the development of nasal perforation and the use of topical corticosteroids, this complication occurs rarely. Septum crusting or bleeding may be a predisposing factor to the development of septal perforation. Ulceration of the nasal mucosa has been reported related to BDP in only one patient,[77] and contact dermatitis in another patient, possibly related to intranasal BUD.[78]

PATIENT EDUCATION

For intranasal corticosteroid therapy to be successful, the patient should be educated in proper use of these medications. Thorough instruction in proper techniques of administration must be given, emphasizing that sprays or aerosols are to be administered onto the turbinates rather than against the septum. The nasal airway must be as open and clear as possible. Accordingly, the patient should be instructed to blow his or her nose gently before using the corticosteroid. Marked blockage of the nose, which frequently occurs with severe allergic rhinitis and with rhinitis medicamentosa, necessitates the use of a short burst of systemic prednisone, or prednisolone, for one to two weeks. In some patients with allergic rhinitis, temporary use of a topical decongestant also can be helpful to open the nasal passages.

The patient must understand that complete therapeutic effects are not likely to be achieved immediately. The physician should inform the patient that it takes three to ten days before full beneficial results of topical corticosteroids can be expected and that eye symptoms and postnasal drip are unlikely to respond to this form of treatment. The physician should also emphasize that the spray must be used regularly, and once the maximal benefit has been achieved, the dosage should be tapered gradually. Usually a twice daily regimen is equally effective and helps improve patient compliance.

When treating nasal polyps, the patient should be informed that polyps respond slowly and need constant treatment with the topical corticosteroid. Occasionally, a short burst of systemic corticosteroids may be necessary. In recalcitrant cases, surgical intervention may be needed.

When symptoms fail to respond to intranasal corticosteroid therapy after three weeks, the physician should be alerted to the possible cause; for example, the patient may be noncompliant or using the aerosol or spray improperly, the nasal passages may be too obstructed by the edematous turbinates and/or by a polyp or both to allow adequate penetration of the drug, or a nasal or sinus infection may be present. In the latter circumstance the use of a topical corticosteroid should be deferred until the infection is controlled.

REFERENCES

1. Dill JL, Bolstead DS. Observations on local use of cortisone in the nose in allergic rhinitis. Laryngoscope 61:415,1951.
2. Pennypacker GS. Hydrocortisone alcohol and the local treatment of hay fever: A preliminary study. J Allergy 25:513, 1954.
3. Norman PS, Winkenwerder WL. Suppression of hay fever symptoms with intranasal dexamethasone aerosol. J Allergy 36:284, 1965.
4. Report of Drug Committee of the American Academy of Allergy. A double-blind labeled study of dexamethasone nasal aerosol vs placebo in the treatment of nasal polyposis. J Allergy 41:10, 1968.
5. Norman PS, Winkenwerder WL, Murgatroyd GW, Parsons JW. Evidence for the local action of intranasal dexamethasone aerosols in the suppression of hay fever symptoms. J Allergy 38:93, 1966.
6. Michels MI, Smith RE, Heimlich EM. Adrenal suppression and intranasally applied steroids. Ann Allergy 25:569, 1974.
7. Norman PS, Winkenwerder WL, Agbayani BF, Migeon GJ. Adrenal function during the use of dexamethasone aerosols in the treatment of ragweed hay fever. J Allergy 40:57, 1967.
8. Crepea SB. Inhalation corticosteroid (dexamethasone PO4) management of chronically asthmatic children. J Allergy 34:119, 1963.
9. Siegel SC, Heimlich EM, Richards W, Kelley VC. Adrenal function in allergy. IV. Effect of dexamethasone aerosols in asthmatic children. Pediatrics 33:245, 1964.
10. Champion PK. Cushing syndrome secondary to abuse of dexamethasone nasal spray. Arch Intern Med 4:134, 1974.
11. Naclerio RM. Mechanisms of allergic rhinitis. J Respir Dis 10(Suppl):15, 1989.
12. Connell J. Quantitative intranasal pollen challenge. II. Effects of daily pollen challenge, environmental pollen exposure and placebo challenge on the nasal membrane. J Allergy 41:123, 1967.
13. Bascom R, Pipkorn U, Lichtenstein LM, Naclerio RM. The influx of inflammatory cells during the late response to antigen challenge: Effect of systemic steroid pretreatment. Am Rev Respir Dis 138:406, 1988.
14. Pipkorn U, Proud D, Schleimer RP, et al. Effects of short term systemic glucocorticoid treatment on human nasal mediator release after antigen challenge. J Clin Invest 80:957, 1987.
15. Martin E, Harrison C, Tanner RJN. Metabolism of beclomethasone dipropionate by animals and man. Postgrad Med 4(Suppl):11, 1975.
16. Anderson P, Ryrfeldt A. Biotransformation of the topical glucocorticoids, budesonide and beclomethasone dipropionate 17α 21-dipropionate in human liver and lung homogenate. J Pharmacol 36:763, 1984.
17. Chaplin MD, Rook W II, Swenson DW, Chu NI. Flunisolide metabolism and dynamics of a metabolite. Clin Pharmacol Ther 27:402, 1980.
18. Ryrfeldt A, Anderson P, Edspacher SS, Tannesson M, Davies D, Pauwels R. Pharmacokinetics and metabolism of budesonide, a selective glucocorticoid. Eur J Clin Pharmacol 22:86, 1982.
19. Pipkorn U, Proud D, Lichtenstein LM, Kagey-Sobotka A, Norman PS, Naclerio RM. Inhibition of mediator release in allergic rhinitis by pretreatment with topical glucocorticosteroids. N Engl J Med 316:1506, 1987.
20. Kwaselow A, McLean J, Busse W, et al. Comparison of

intranasal and oral flunisolide in the therapy of allergic rhinitis: Evidence for a topical effect. Allergy 40:363, 1985.

21. Lindqvist N, Andersson M, Bende M, Loth S, Pipkorn U. The clinical efficacy of budesonide in hayfever treatment is dependent on topical nasal application. Clin Exp Allergy 19:71, 1989.

22. Place VA, Velazquez JG, Burdick KH. Precise evaluation of topically applied corticosteroid potency. Modification of the Stoughton-McKenzie assay. Arch Dermatol 101:531, 1970.

23. McKenzie AW, Stoughton RB. Method for comparing percutaneous absorption of steroids. Arch Dermatol 86:608, 1962.

24. Townley RG, Suliaman F. The mechanism of corticosteroids in treating asthma. Ann Allergy 58:1, 1987.

25. Morris HG. Mechanisms of glucocorticoid action in pulmonary disease. Chest 88:1335, 1985.

26. Schleimer RP. The mechanisms of anti-inflammatory steroid action in allergic diseases. Am Rev Pharmacol Toxicol 25:381, 1985.

27. Kaliner M. Mechanisms of glucocorticosteroid action in bronchial asthma. J Allergy Clin Immunol 76:321, 1985.

28. Pauwels R. Mode of action of corticosteroids in asthma and rhinitis. Clin Allergy 16:281, 1986.

29. Schleimer RP, Claman HN, Oronsky A, eds. Anti-inflammatory Steroid Action: Basic and Clinical Aspects. San Diego: Academic Press, 1989.

30. Wihl JA. Topical corticosteroids and nasal reactivity. Eur J Respir Dis 63(Suppl 122)205, 1982.

31. Malm L, Wihl JA, Lamm CJ, Lindqvist N. Reduction of methacholine-induced nasal secretion by treatment with a new topical steroid in perennial non-allergic rhinitis. Allergy 36:209, 1981.

32. Pelikan Z. The effect of disodium cromoglycate and beclomethasone dipropionate on the late nasal mucosal response to allergen challenge. Ann Allergy 49:200, 1982.

33. Horak F, Matthew H. The protective action of fluocortin butylester (FCB) in the nasal antigen provocation test: A controlled double-blind crossover study. Ann Allergy 48:305, 1982.

34. Bascom R, Wachs M, Naclerio RM, Pipkorn U, Galli SJ, Lichtenstein LM. Basophil influx occurs after nasal antigen challenge: Effects of topical corticosteroid pretreatment. J Allergy Clin Immunol 81:580, 1988.

35. Okuda M, Senba O. Effect of beclomethasone dipropionate nasal spray on subjective and objective findings in perennial rhinitis. Clin Otolaryngol 53:12, 1980.

36. Andersson M, Andersson P, Pipkorn U. Topical glucocorticosteroids and allergen-induced increase in nasal reactivity: Relationship between treatment time and inhibitory effect. J Allergy Clin Immunol 82:1019, 1988.

37. Siegel SC, Katz RM, Rachelefsky GS, et al. Multicentric study of beclomethasone dipropionate nasal aerosol in adults with seasonal allergic rhinitis. J Allergy Clin Immunol 69:345, 1982.

38. Sidwell A. A comparison of the efficacy and tolerance of an aqueous beclomethasone dipropionate nasal spray with conventional pressurized spray. Curr Med Res Opin 8:659, 1983.

39. Hartley TF, Lieberman PL, Meltzer EO, Noyes JN, Pearlman DS, Tinkelman DG. Efficacy and tolerance of fluocortin butyl administered twice daily in adult patients with perennial rhinitis. J Allergy Clin Immunol 75:501, 1985.

40. Clissold SP, Heel RC. Budesonide: A preliminary review of its pharmacodynamic properties and therapeutic efficacy in asthma and rhinitis. Drugs 28:485, 1984.

41. Spector SL, Multicenter co-investigators. WHR-5029 (triamcinolone acetonide nasal aerosol) versus placebo in perennial allergic rhinitis (Abstract 71). Ann Allergy 58:296, 1987.

42. Grossman J, Bronsky E, Findley S, et al. WHR-5029 (triamcinolone acetonide nasal aerosol) versus placebo in perennial allergic rhinitis. New Engl Reg Allergy Proc 9:387, 1988.

43. Meltzer EO, Bronsky E, Grossman J, et al. A dose ranging study of fluticasone propionate aqueous intranasal spray in patients with seasonal allergic rhinitis. J Allergy Clin Immunol 83:279, 1989.

44. Van As A, Meltzer EO, Bronsky E, et al. A dose-tolerance study of intranasal fluticasone propionate aqueous nasal spray in the treatment of seasonal allergic rhinitis. J Allergy Clin Immunol 83:301, 1989.

45. Dolovitch J. Personal communication, 1989.

46. Pipkorn U, Rundkrantz H. Budesonide and beclomethasone dipropionate in hay fever: A single-blind comparison. Eur J Respir Dis 63(Suppl 122):211, 1982.

47. Samuelson A. A comparison between budesonide and beclomethasone dipropionate in patients with birch pollen induced hay fever. Folia Allergol Immunol Clin 30(Suppl 4):102, 1983.

48. Vanzieleghem MA, Juniper EF. A comparison of budesonide and beclomethasone dipropionate nasal aerosols in ragweed-induced rhinitis. J Allergy Clin Immunol 79:887, 1987.

49. Orgel HA, Meltzer EO, Kemp JP, Welch WJ. Clinical rhinomanometric and cytologic evaluation of seasonal allergic rhinitis treated with beclomethasone dipropionate as aqueous nasal spray or pressurized aerosol. J Allergy Clin Immunol 77:858, 1986.

50. Meltzer EO, Busse WW, Bush RK, Kemp JP, Orgel HA, Welch MJ. Beclomethasone dipropionate nasal aerosol spray in allergic rhinitis: A comparison of three daily doses. Ann Allergy 55:802, 1985.

51. Welsh PW, Stricker WE, Chu CP, et al. Efficacy of beclomethasone nasal solution, flunisolide, and cromolyn in relieving symptoms of ragweed allergy. Mayo Clin Proc 62:125, 1987.

52. Morrow-Brown H, Jackson FA, Porer GM. A comparison of beclomethasone dipropionate aqueous nasal spray and sodium cromoglycate nasal spray in the management of seasonal allergic rhinitis. Allergol Immunopathol 12:355, 1984.

53. Bjerrum P, Illum P. Treatment of seasonal allergic rhinitis with budesonide and disodium cromoglycate: A double-blind comparison between budesonide and disodium cromoglycate. Allergy 40:65, 1985.

54. Pelikan Z. The effects of disodium cromoglycate (DSCG) and beclomethasone dipropionate (BDA) on the delayed nasal mucosa response to allergen challenge. Ann Allergy 52:111, 1984.

55. Blackhouse CI, Finnamore VP, Gosden GW. Treatment of seasonal allergic rhinitis with flunisolide and terfenadine. J Int Med Res 14:35, 1986.

56. Sibbald B, Hilton S, D'Souza M. An open crossover trial comparing two doses of astemizole and beclomethasone dipropionate in the treatment of perennial rhinitis. Clin Allergy 16:203, 1986.

57. Wood SF. Oral antihistamine or nasal steroid in hay fever: A double-blind, double-dummy comparative study of once daily oral astemizole vs twice daily nasal beclomethasone dipropionate. Clin Allergy 16:195, 1986.

58. Juniper EF, Kline PA, Hargreave FE, Dolovitch J. Comparison of beclomethasone dipropionate aqueous spray, astemizole and the combination in the prophylactic treatment of ragweed-induced rhinoconjunctivitis. J Allergy Clin Immunol 83:627, 1989.

59. Salomonsson P, Gottberg L, Heliborn H, Norrlind K, Pegelow KO. Efficacy of oral antihistamine, astemizole, as compared to a nasal steroid spray. Allergy 43:214, 1988.

60. Beswick KBJ, Kenyon GS, Cherry JR. A comparative study of beclomethasone dipropionate aqueous nasal spray with terfenadine tablets in seasonal allergic rhinitis. Curr Med Res

Opin 9:560, 1985.

61. Dickson OJ, Cruickshank JM. Comparison of flunisolide nasal spray and terfenadine tablets in hay fever. Br J Clin Pract 38:416, 1984.

62. Pichler WJ, Klint T, Blaser M, et al. Clinical comparison of systemic methylprednisolone acetate versus topical budesonide in patients with seasonal allergic rhinitis. Allergy 43:87, 1988.

63. Pipkorn U, Norman PS, Middleton E. Topical steroids. In: Mygind N, Weeke B, eds. Allergic and Vasomotor Rhinitis: Clinical Aspects. Copenhagen: Munksgaard, 1986, p. 165.

64. Mullarkey MF, Hill JS, Webb DR. Allergic and non-allergic rhinitis: Their characteristics with attention to the meaning of nasal eosinophilia. J Allergy Clin Immunol 65:122, 1980.

65. Karlsson G, Runderantz H. A randomized trial of intranasal beclomethasone dipropionate after polypectomy. Rhinology 20:144, 1982.

66. Drettner B, Ebbesen A, Nilsson M. Prophylactic treatment with flunisolide after polypectomy. Rhinology 20:149, 1982.

67. Sorensen H, Mygind N, Pedersen CB, Prytz S. Long term treatment of nasal polyps with beclomethasone dipropionate aerosol. III. Morphological studies and conclusions. Acta Otolaryngol 82:260, 1976.

68. Chalton R, Mackay I, Wilson R, Cole P. Double-blind, placebo controlled trial of beclomethasone nasal drops for nasal polyposis. Br Med J 291:788, 1985.

69. Sorkins S, Warren D. Probable adrenal suppression from intranasal beclomethasone. J Fam Pract 22:449, 1986.

70. Greenbaum J, Leznoff A, Schulz J, Mazza J, Tobe A, Mitler D. Comparative tolerability of two formulations of Rhinalar (flunisolide) nasal spray in patients with seasonal allergic rhinitis. Ann Allergy 61:305, 1988.

71. Dechateau GSMJE, Zuidema J, Merkus HM. The in vitro and in vivo effect of a new non-halogenated corticosteroid-budesonide-aerosol on human ciliary epithelial function. Allergy 41:260, 1986.

72. Holmberg K, Pipkorn U. Influence of topical beclomethasone dipropionate suspension on human nasal mucociliary activity. Eur J Clin Pharmacol 30:625, 1986.

73. Broder I, Tarlo SM, Davies GM, et al. Safety and efficacy of long-term treatment with inhaled beclomethasone dipropionate in steroid-dependent asthma. Can Med Assoc J 136:129, 1987.

74. Pipkorn U, Pukander J, Suonpaa J, Makinen J, Lindqvist N. Long term safety of budesonide nasal aerosol: A 5-½ year follow up study. Clin Allergy 18:253, 1988.

75. Soderberg-Warner ML. Nasal septal perforation associated with topical corticosteroid therapy. J Pediatr 105:840, 1984.

76. Schoetzel EP, Menzel ML. Nasal sprays and perforation of the nasal septum. JAMA 253:2046, 1985.

77. Doble N. Reaction to beclomethasone Br Med J 290:518, 1985.

78. Medina B, Dahlberg E. Contact allergy to budesonide in a nasal spray. Contact Dermatitis 14:253, 1986.

Chapter XXVIII

Ocular, Nasal and Oral Cromolyn Sodium in the Management of Nonasthmatic Allergic Problems

Sheldon L. Spector, M.D.

ABSTRACT

The effectiveness of cromolyn sodium in various clinical situations continues to expand. Ocular cromolyn has been utilized in allergic eye conditions, as well as vernal conjunctivitis, atopic keratoconjunctivitis and giant papillary conjunctivitis. Nasal cromolyn has been successfully utilized in the treatment of allergic rhinitis of the seasonal and perennial types, and oral cromolyn has been employed in people with multiple food allergies and in unusual conditions such as systemic mastocytosis.

There has been a reawakening of the versatility of this agent in view of its effective blocking of both early and late phase allergic reactions, and its anti-inflammatory potential. Truly cromolyn is a useful agent, not only for its therapeutic efficacy but for its virtual lack of side effects.

INTRODUCTION

In the more than 20 years since Altounyan[1] recognized that cromolyn sodium effectively blocked allergic reactions in asthmatic subjects, several hundred clinical studies have examined the use of cromolyn as a prophylactic treatment of other allergic conditions.[2] *In vitro* and *in vivo* studies have shown that cromolyn sodium inhibits the degranulation of sensitized mast cells which occurs after various stimuli such as antigen challenge, and is thought to inhibit the release of his-

tamine and leukotrienes from mast cells as its main action.[3-5] Cromolyn is not thought to have intrinsic vasomotor or antihistaminic activity although recent studies have shown that it possesses indirect anti-inflammatory activity as well.[6]

OCULAR CROMOLYN

Ocular cromolyn (Opticrom®) is indicated in the treatment of certain allergic eye disorders such as superior limbic keratoconjunctivitis, vernal conjunctivitis, atopic keratoconjunctivitis, Type I allergic reactions such as hay fever, acute and chronic allergic conjunctivitis, and giant papillary conjunctivitis. Although the etiologic factor of many of these above-mentioned problems is often not known, airborne allergens or contact lenses have been implicated. Symptomatic response to therapy is usually evident within a few days, but longer treatment, for up to six weeks, is sometimes required. When symptomatic improvement has been established, therapy should be continued for as long as needed to sustain improvement. Perhaps the four commonest ocular allergies seen by allergists involving the conjunctivae are (a) the ocular manifestations of allergic rhinitis; (b) vernal keratoconjunctivitis; (c) atopic keratoconjunctivitis; and (d) giant papillary conjunctivitis. The common symptoms and signs of these four entities along with some specific studies substantiating the effectiveness of cromolyn in their treatment are given below.

Hay fever, i.e. allergic rhinitis is the most common problem seen by the practicing allergist. The major ocular symptoms are quite familiar and include mod-

Clinical Professor of Medicine, UCLA School of Medicine. Director Allergy Research, 11645 Wilshire Blvd, Suite 601, Los Angeles, CA 90425.

erate itching, tearing and burning. The symptoms are often greater than the signs since no clinically observable signs or only subtle conjunctival edema may be all that is present. There may be slight dilatation of the conjunctival vessels and minor swelling of the lids. Most of the reactions are thought to be due to Type I (Gell & Coombs) sensitivity to airborne allergens. Degranulation of mucosal mast cells in the conjunctivae can release pharmacologically active mediators that cause itching, edema and redness. Although late asthmatic and late rhinitic responses have now been described with exposure to allergen, late ocular reactions have only been postulated and their presence and possible importance are presently under consideration by various investigators. Differentiating features are "symptoms greater than signs," the lack of corneal involvement, and the presence of no more than a few eosinophils per high powered field in conjunctival scrapings.

Vernal keratoconjunctivitis is characterized by intense itching and tearing, a feeling of heat or tightness in the eyes, and the presence of photophobia. To go along with the above symptoms, ptosis and conjunctival injection may be prominent. Often there is a thick, ropy mucosal discharge, and on physical examination there are elevated giant papillae giving a cobblestone appearance to the upper tarsal plate. Corneal changes may also include shield-like vernal ulcers which may result in corneal scarring and/or plaque formation. There can be neovascularization and actual change in the curvature. Although pathogenetic mechanisms have not been fully defined, it is thought that Type I hypersensitivity reaction may be playing some role along with other undefined mechanisms that favor the recruitment of eosinophils and mast cells. Other differentiating factors include more frequent occurrence in young males, especially ages three to 25, a boy to girl ratio of three to one, and occurrence mainly in warmer climates. There are usually *more than* two to three eosinophils per high powered field in the conjunctival scrapings.

Atopic keratoconjunctivitis is often a perennial problem and may be looked upon as the ocular manifestation of chronic eczema. The patient has moderate to severe itching and the symptoms may be worse in the winter in areas of the country where pollens are dormant. There is burning and photophobia as has been described with vernal keratoconjunctivitis, with almost constant tearing. The major signs include a lichenification of the lid margins and a chronic macerated and indurated appearance of the lids. There may be hyperemia of the conjunctiva and frequent corneal involvement. Approximately 10% of these patients will have concomitant cataracts. Although the cause is not known, a combination of a Type I and Type IV immune reaction producing an exudative inflammation has been postulated. Unlike with vernal conjunctivitis, elderly patients are often afflicted. There are few eosin-

ophils on lid scrapings, and there is scarring and shrinkage of the fornix of the conjunctiva. Some of the changes may appear in areas of the skin other than the eyelids, manifesting as chronic eczema.

Giant papillary conjunctivitis is usually an iatrogenic disease[7] associated with foreign bodies in the eye.[8] I most often is associated with contact lens wear and has also been described after keratoplasty and cataract sutures. It may not be the material of the lens or prosthesis that causes the disease, but rather antigenic substances e.g. pollen particles adhering to the foreign body in the eye that are responsible.[9,10] In the patient with mild symptoms there may be minimal mucus, mild itching, and no change in vision. In the more severe situation there are abundant sheets of mucus so that the eyelids stick together, severe itching, pain on insertion of the lens, blurred vision even after lens removal, and the formation of giant papillae, along with erythema and edema of the upper tarsal conjunctiva. Generally if the contact lens is discontinued, symptoms abate. However, the majority of patients with giant papillary conjunctivitis secondary to contact lens wear do not want to give up their lenses.

Cromolyn sodium has been successfully used in all of the above-mentioned conditions. In the treatment of vernal conjunctivitis or atopic conjunctivitis, cromolyn sodium may be used concomitantly with corticosteroids, the latter for a short period of time, i.e. four to ten days. Although at one time 2% cromolyn sodium was utilized, the presently available cromolyn sodium 4% ophthalmic solution has proved to be more effective in many double-blind crossover studies. Two percent cromolyn sodium without preservative was found to be better than placebo in a study by Kray et al.[11] Interestingly in this study there was a trend for improvement in nasal allergy symptoms as well. Vakil et al[12] studied 2% vs. 4% Opticrom® in ragweed pollen-induced conjunctivitis in patients who previously had minimal relief with the 2% solution. Patients received one drop in each eye, four times a day for four weeks, and the comparisons showed that 4% solution was more effective than the 2% solution. There have been a few cases of adverse reactions to ocular cromolyn, two cases of acute chemotic reactions, with symptoms similar to the disease itself,[13] and one patient was described with a Type I reaction to cromolyn.[14] In the future we may see more use of an eye ointment containing cromolyn sodium since it is presently under active investigation. Ruggieri et al[15] described 31 patients with allergic eye disease who were given the ointment three times daily for four weeks, and the cromolyn ointment was significantly better than placebo and very well tolerated.

CROMOLYN SODIUM FOR NASAL DISEASE

Cromolyn is available for the treatment of allergic rhinitis in adults and children, six years of age and older. It has been successfully used in the treatment of seasonal and perennial allergic rhinitis. Cromolyn sodium has the ability to inhibit both the immediate phase and late phase asthmatic reactions. Now that both immediate and late phase reactions have been described in the nose, it has an expanded mechanism of action, especially in view of its anti-inflammatory properties. In fact, Pelikan et al[16,17] were able to block both early and late phase increases in nasal airway resistance by pretreating the nasal mucosa with cromolyn sodium.

Studies of the use of cromolyn in seasonal allergic rhinitis often employed a 2% solution rather than the 4% solution now employed in the United States.[18,19] Nevertheless, there was clinical improvement even with the lesser concentration of cromolyn. In certain studies patients who responded best to cromolyn were those with a high preseasonal anti-ragweed IgE and when therapy was initiated prior to the pollen season.[20,21] Typically there is a significant reduction in sneezing, rhinorrhea, nasal congestion and ocular irritation. Many investigators have also substantiated the usefulness of cromolyn in perennial allergic rhinitis; however, these patients are often more difficult to study since such patients often resemble those with nonallergic or vasomotor rhinitis. In one study[22] patients with strongly positive skin tests to perennial allergens such as epidermals and foods, and an elevated IgE level, had the best chance of having a good response to cromolyn. It is often difficult to differentiate the above mentioned patients from patients with nonallergic rhinitis with eosinophilia (NARES syndrome) since Nelson et al[23] found that cromolyn failed to relieve the sneezing, rhinorrhea and pruritus in patients with the NARES syndrome. In virtually all studies, intranasal cromolyn has proved to be remarkably free of side effects; virtually no patient has been taken off of cromolyn treatment because of an adverse reaction, despite the infrequent occurrence of mild nasal irritation, sore throat, headache or an unpleasant taste. I find it particularly useful in pregnant patients since the safety record of cromolyn would make it a logical choice in this group of patients as well. Cromolyn would not be expected to be useful in patients with nasal polyps and NARES syndrome, or patients with vasomotor rhinitis.

Cromolyn sodium often can be employed along with an antihistamine/decongestant. In fact, in a comparison study of cromolyn sodium and terfenadine in the treatment of seasonal allergic rhinitis, Lindsay-Miller et al[24] found that during the first week of treatment there was significantly greater relief of nasal symptoms with the combination, although cromolyn sodium alone tended to be more beneficial than terfenadine alone as time went on. Nasal cromolyn has been compared to topical steroids such as beclomethasone dipropionate and flunisolide.[16,17] Topical steroids might very well be the preferred agent for certain patients with nonallergic rhinitis or even nasal polyps. However,

nasal perforation has been described with the steroid preparations and not with cromolyn. In comparison studies of allergic and perennial rhinitis, both drugs are usually effective. In one study by Brown et al,[25] flunisolide proved more effective than cromolyn, yet Haguenauer[26] found no significant differences between a 2% intranasal solution of cromolyn sodium and beclomethasone dipropionate. Many of the comparison studies did not utilize the 4% cromolyn spray which is now the agent of choice in the United States. In any case, the risk to benefit ratio and patient population must always be assessed with the use of either agent and cromolyn sodium would appear to be the safer agent.

ORAL CROMOLYN FOR FOOD ALLERGY

No one would argue against the concept that the treatment of choice for food allergy is avoidance. On the other hand, some patients have multiple food allergies, making a recommendation of avoidance alone virtually impossible or even dangerous. Other patients find it difficult to assess the presence of certain foods in the diets they keep. Thus, pharmacologic treatment for patients with food allergies is sometimes indicated, especially when there is unavoidable or unintentional dietary exposure. Cromolyn sodium has been employed due to its presumed protective action against mast cell degranulation on the mucosal surface. Cromolyn, however, is thought to have additional modes of action as would be anticipated by its effectiveness in exercise-induced asthma and when mediators have not been conclusively shown to be released. Oral cromolyn in this respect has been shown in patients with food allergies to reduce the gut permeability to immune complexes.[27,28] There have been many European studies and some investigational work in North American on oral formulations of cromolyn sodium that have not yet been licensed. The lactose in such preparations has been removed in view of the potential worsening of symptoms in a patient with lactase deficiency who receives both lactose and cromolyn. Sogn has reviewed many of the studies of oral cromolyn.[29] There were 28 studies reported between 1973 and 1984 with almost 400 subjects in ages ranging from infancy to late adulthood. Twenty-one of those studies showed a role for the drug and seven showed no role. No trends are apparent from these studies as to what age group might show the best responder rate, or what dose would be optimal, since some have employed 100 mg of cromolyn sodium per day while others employed up to 1600 mg per day. Timing of the drug dosage seems important and should be given from 15 to 240 minutes prior to food challenge. In one double-blind placebo controlled study, Kocoshis and Gryboski[30] studied older children with gastrointestinal symptoms after milk, and found that five of seven subjects improved with the active therapy while only one of seven subjects improved with placebo. Unfortunately, there are still very few double-blind, placebo controlled challenge studies of cromolyn sodium use in food intolerance. However, in general, one might expect those patients with a documented response to food challenge by skin test, radioallergo-sorbent test, etc. to be in the responder groups. This was confirmed by Businco et al[31] and Molkhou and Waguet.[32]

Our group has studied oral cromolyn sodium employing two 100 mg capsules that were added to one-fourth of a glass of hot water and given one-half hour before meals, four times daily. This was an open study to gain some experience with oral cromolyn sodium prior to a subsequent double-blind controlled study. All patients had immediate positive skin tests to multiple foods before they were entered into the study. One of these patients was a 33-year old lady who had sought help from numerous physicians in the past, including a well-known clinical ecologist. In fact, she had become malnourished on the limited diet on which she had been placed. On oral cromolyn she gained back her weight by eating a reasonable diet, with improved well-being.

A 61-year old father of a physician experienced mainly sinus and nasal congestion, as well as migraines, yellow phlegm and inability to tolerate most foods. On oral cromolyn he had less chest tightness and nasal symptoms, along with his ability to eat small quantities of foods he could not eat before. Admittedly anecdotal reports such as these are of limited value. Many have been impressed enough to recommend a double-blind study of oral cromolyn sodium for future food-allergic patients. Such studies have been published.

Gerrard[33] studied 32 patients with adverse food reactions who were given cromolyn sodium vs placebo for two periods of seven days each. The cromolyn prevented adverse reactions in 24 patients (75%). The symptoms helped were gastrointestinal plus those involving the skeletal, vascular, and nervous systems. In an abstract given at a recent meeting, Pelikan et al[34] described 20 patients who had nasal symptoms after the ingestion of certain foods, who were given oral cromolyn. In his double-blind crossover study, oral cromolyn was found to be effective in both early and late responses due to the ingested food. He concluded that oral cromolyn was therefore a suitable drug for the prophylaxis of nasal complaints due to food allergy.

Oral cromolyn has been employed in certain patients with persistent diarrhea[35] and chronic proctitis with some limited success,[36] leading the authors to conclude that food allergy might be a possible responsible mechanism for these syndromes as well. However, there are many negative studies of patients with nonspecific gastrointestinal complaints, probably due to inappropriate patient selection.

Cromolyn has been employed in other situations that will only be briefly mentioned. A case report of a patient allergic to seminal fluid was presented in whom cromolyn sodium was employed as a vaginal cream and provided marked protection during intercourse.[37] Cromolyn also has been utilized in systemic mastocytoses with marked beneficial results.[38]

In summary, cromolyn sodium has shown itself to be a useful and versatile agent, with a remarkable safety profile, in patients with a variety of allergic conditions.

REFERENCES

1. Altounyan REC. Inhibition of experimental asthma by a new compound-disodium cromoglycate (Intal). Acta Allergol 22:487, 1967.
2. Berman BA, Ross RN. Cromolyn. Clin Rev Allergy 1:105, 1983.
3. Harries MG, Parkes PEG, Lessof MH et al. Role of bronchial irritant receptors in asthma. Lancet. 1:5–7, 1981.
4. Breslin FJ, McFadden ER, Ingram RH. The effects of cromolyn sodium on the airway response to hyperpnea and cold air in asthma. Am Rev Respir Dis 22:11–16, 1980.
5. Cox JSG, Beach JE, Blair AM et al. Disodium cromoglycate (Intal). Adv in Drug Res 5:115–196, 1970.
6. Kay AB, Walsh GM, Moqbel R et al. Disodium cromoglycate inhibits activation of human inflammatory cells in vitro. J Allergy Clin Immunol 80:1–8, 1987.
7. Mackie IA, Wright P. Giant papillary conjunctivitis—an iatrogenic disease resembling vernal conjunctivitis, in Pepys J. Edwards AM (eds): The mast cell: Its role in health and disease (Proc Int Symp Davos, Switzerland). London, Pitman Medical, 1979, pp 524–528.
8. Allansmith MR, Korb DR, Greiner JV et al. Giant papillary conjunctivitis in contact lens wearers. Am J Ophthalmol 83:697–708, 1977.
9. Fowler SA, Greiner JV, Allansmith MR. Soft contact lenses from patients with giant papillary conjunctivitis. Am J Ophthalmol 88:1056–1061, 1979.
10. Fowler SA, Greiner JV, Allansmith MR. Attachment of bacteria to soft contact lenses. Arch Ophthalmol 97:659–660, 1979.
11. Kray KT, Squire EN Jr, Tipton WR et al. Cromolyn sodium in seasonal allergic conjunctivitis. J Allergy Clin Immunol 76:623–627, 1985.
12. Vakil DV, Ayiomamitis A, Nizami RM. Treatment of seasonal conjunctivitis: comparison of 2% and 4% sodium cromoglycate ophthalmic solutions. Can J Ophthalmol 19:207–211, 1984.
13. Ostler HB. Acute chemotic reaction to cromolyn. Arch Ophthalmol 100:412–413, 1982.
14. Skarpaas IJ. An unexpected reaction towards disodium cromoglycate. Allergy 42:318–319, 1987.
15. Ruggieri ML, Scorcia G. Double-blind group comparative trial of sodium cromoglycate eye ointment and placebo in the treatment of allergic eye diseases. Ann Allergy 58:109–112, 1987.
16. Pelikan Z, Pelikan-Filipek J. The effects of disodium cromoglycate and beclomethasone dipropionate on the immediate response of the nasal mucosa to allergen challenge. Ann Allergy 49:283–292, 1982.
17. Pelikan Z. The effects of disodium cromoglycate and beclomethasone dipropionate on the late nasal mucosa response to allergen challenge. Ann Allergy 49:200–211, 1982.
18. Holopainen E. Effect of disodium cromoglycate on seasonal allergic rhinitis. Lancet 1:55–57, 1971.
19. Blair H, Herbert RL. Treatment of seasonal allergic rhinitis with 2% sodium cromoglycate solution. Clin Allergy 3:283–288, 1973.

20. Welsh PW, Yunginger JW, Kern EB. Treatment of ragweed hay fever with intranasal cromolyn solution. J Allergy Clin Immunol 57:241, 1976.

21. Welsh PW, Yunginger JW, Kern EB et al. Preseasonal IgE ragweed antibody level as predictor of response to therapy of ragweed hay fever with intranasal cromolyn sodium solution. J Allergy Clin Immunol 60:104–109, 1977.

22. Cohan RH, Bloom FL, Rhoades RB et al. Treatment of perennial allergic rhinitis with cromolyn sodium. J Allergy Clin Immunol 58:121–128, 1976.

23. Nelson BL, Jacob RI. Response of the nonallergic rhinitis with eosinophilia (NARES) syndrome to 4% cromolyn sodium nasal solution. J Allergy Clin Immunol 70:125–128, 1982.

24. Lindsay-Miller ACM, Chambers A. Group comparative trial of cromolyn sodium and terfenadine in the treatment of seasonal allergic rhinitis. Ann Allergy 58:28–32, 1987.

25. Brown HM, Engler C, English JR. A comparative trial of flunisolide and sodium cromoglycate nasal sprays in the treatment of seasonal allergic rhinitis. Clin Allergy 11:169–171, 1981.

26. Haguenauer JP. Controlled study of sodium cromoglycate and beclomethasone dipropionate in the local treatment of chronic aperiodic rhinitis. Revue Francaise d'Allergologie 21:167–169, 1981.

27. Brostoff J, Carini C, Wraith DG, Johns P. Production of IgE complexes by allergen challenge in atopic patients and the effect of sodium cromoglycate. Lancet 1:1268–1270, 1979.

28. Pagenelli R, Levinsky RJ, Brostoff J, Wraith DC. Immune complexes containing food proteins in normal and atopic subjects after oral challenge and effect of disodium cromoglycate on antigen absorption. Lancet 1:1270–1272, 1979.

29. Sogn D. Medications and their use in the treatment of adverse reactions to foods. J Allergy Clin Immunol 78:238–243, 1986.

30. Kocoshis S, Gryboski JD. Use of cromolyn in combined gastrointestinal allergy. JAMA 242:1169–1173, 1979.

31. Businco L, Cantani A, Benincori N et al. Effectiveness of oral sodium cromoglycate (SCG) in preventing food allergy in children. Ann Allergy 51:47–50, 1983.

32. Molkhou P, Waguet JC. Food allergy and atopic dermatitis in children: treatment with oral sodium cromoglycate. Ann Allergy 47:173–175, 1981.

33. Gerrard JW. Oral sodium cromoglycate its value in the treatment of adverse reactions to foods in gastrointestinal allergy. Ann Allergy 42:135–138, 1979.

34. Pelikan Z, Pelikan M. Protective effects of oral disodium cromoglycate (DSCG) on urticaria due to the food ingestion challenge. J Allergy Clin Immunol 81:251, 1988 (Abstract #334).

35. Bolin TD. Use of oral sodium cromoglycate in persistent diarrhea. Gut 21:848–850, 1980.

36. Sodium cromoglycate for use in the gut (Nasalcrom). Drug Ther Bull 17:10–12, 1979.

37. Goldenhersh MJ, Saxon A. Seminal fluid hypersensitivity: A new approach. J Allergy Clin Immunol (in press, 1988).

38. Soter NA, Austen KF, Wasserman SI. Oral disodium cromoglycate in the treatment of systemic mastocytosis. N Engl J Med 301:465–469, 1979.

Chapter XXIX

Anticholinergic Drugs for Rhinitis

Niels Mygind, M.D., and Peter Borum, M.D.

ABSTRACT

When the anticholinergic drug ipratropium bromide is given as a nasal spray, it can reach the glandular cholinoceptors and block the secretory response to methacholine. Nine placebo-controlled clinical trials have shown that the treatment significantly reduces watery rhinorrhea in patients with perennial rhinitis not responsive to other types of treatment. To avoid a sensation of nasal dryness as a side effect from spraying, it is important in the individual patient to match the dosage to the severity of hypersecretion. Ipratropium has no effect on sneezing or on nasal blockage.

Everyone has had watery rhinorrhea and has realized that it is a nuisance constantly to be aware of excess fluid in the nose, which irritates the nostrils and distracts one's attention from work and social activities. Other people find it unsavory and believe that it is potentially infectious.

When rhinorrhea is associated with sneezing, it is often caused by an allergic disease, and these patients can today be offered efficient treatment with nonsedating antihistamines and steroid sprays. This modern therapy, however, is usually not effective when rhinorrhea is the only symptom.[1] Until recently these patients could not be given any help, and, in the rare case, a patient with rhinorrhea can use hundreds of paper handkerchiefs daily.

For this reason we began more than 10 years ago to explore the potential efficacy of anticholinergic drugs for the treatment of watery rhinorrhea. Below is a summary of our findings, and an update on published

Otopathological Laboratory, Department of Otolaryngology, and Allergy Clinic, Department of Internal Medicine TTA, Rigshospitalet, DK-2200 Copenhagen, Denmark

work on intranasal administration of ipratropium bromide.

RATIONALE

It has been well established for a long time that the secretory activity of salivary glands can be inhibited by anticholinergic drugs, such as atropine. These agents can also reduce the secretory response to nervous stimulation of bronchial glands.[2] Thus, there was good reason to believe that blockage of nasal cholinoceptors could inhibit watery rhinorrhea. However, the degree of blockage could not be predicted, as we do not know to what extent nasal fluid is derived from nasal glands or from other sources (goblet cells in the nose, goblet cells and glands in the paranasal sinuses, lacrimal glands, exudation through blood vessels, and condensed water in the expiratory air). An anticholinergic nasal spray can only be expected to have effect on rhinorrhea, derived from nasal glands.

DRUG

Ipratropium bromide (ipratropium) is a quaternary derivative of isopropyl noratropine. It has a low lipid solubility and thus does not readily pass the blood-brain barrier and is poorly absorbed from the airway mucosa, as compared to atropine.[3] We have used ipratropium in the nose, because studies of asthma/bronchitis have shown a local bronchodilating effect in doses without systemic side effects.[4] The pressurized canister, used for inhalation, was equipped with a nozzle.

AIM OF THE STUDIES

These studies had a double purpose: first, to develop a drug for the treatment of watery rhinorrhea, and second, to analyze to what degree the nasal fluids are derived from nasal glands, and mediated by stimulation of cholinoceptors. Glands can be stimulated by other

TABLE I

Results of 9 Double-Blind, Placebo-Controlled Trials on Ipratropium Nasal Spray (80 μg q.i.d.)

	Preference: Ipr-No-Pl*	Symptom Reduction (%)	p Value
Borum et al.[6]	14-3-3	23	<0.01
Bok et al.[7]†	15-0-6	13	<0.035
Jokinen and Sipila[8]		33	<0.001
Malmberg et al.[9]‡	20-4-9	38	<0.01
von Haacke et al.[10]	15-2-3	28	<0.01
Sjogren and Juhasz[11]	8-3-1	11	<0.01
Knight et al.[12]	21-2-3	40	<0.0003
Dolovich et al.[13]	21-1-2	42	<0.00005
Kirkegaard et al.[14]		40	<0.001

* *Ipr, ipratropium; No, none; Pl, placebo.*
† *Half dose in some patients.*
‡ *Elderly patients.*

substances, which do not act by stimulation of this receptor type. Theoretically, it is a potential risk that the contribution of cholinoceptor-mediated fluid will be underestimated by this type of study, as there is no guarantee that local application of an anticholinergic drug will reach all of the 100,000 glands in the nose in a concentration that is sufficient for complete blockage of their receptors.

LABORATORY STUDIES

It was first shown that metacholine-induced rhinorrhea can be inhibited by pretreatment with intranasal ipratropium.[5] This demonstrates that the drug, given intranasally, does reach the glandular receptors. A similar result was obtained in patients with rhinitis, who react more vigorously to methacholine than normal subjects. The methacholine test was also used to show that the drug has a quick onset of action (maximum efficacy after 30 minutes), and a very long duration of action (8–12 hours). Based on these laboratory studies, in the clinical trials, two puffs of ipratropium, 20 μg into each nostril, four times daily, were given.

CLINICAL STUDIES IN PERENNIAL RHINITIS

In the first clinical trial, 20 patients with perennial rhinitis and watery rhinorrhea as a dominant symptom were studied; 15 preferred ipratropium and 2 the placebo spray.[6] Although the number of nose blowings was significantly reduced, there was no effect on sneezing and nasal blockage. Similar results have been obtained in eight further placebo-controlled trials.[7-14] However, the percent reduction of rhinorrhea, measured as the number of paper handkerchiefs used, has varied from 11 to 42% (Table I). This variation is probably due to differences in patient selection. The best therapeutic result was obtained in the study of Dolovich et al. in 1987,[13] and therefore their criteria for patient inclusion can be recommended (Table II).

In the study of Kirkegaard et al.[14] a very high ipratropium dose was used in order to define the maximum efficacy of this type of therapy. There was a mean reduction of symptoms of 55%, but at the expense of significant adverse effects (Table III). It was concluded that only a few patients with very severe rhinorrhea

TABLE II

Selection of Patients for Ipratropium Therapy According to Dolovich et al.[13]

1. Adults
2. Clear nasal discharge >1 hour each day
3. No major problem with nasal blockage
4. No known allergic basis for the rhinitis
5. No satisfactory response to antihistamine or steroid spray

TABLE III

Side Effects from Ipratropium in an Ordinary Dose and in a Very High Dose

Side Effect	Percentage of Patients			
	Run-in Period	Placebo	Ipratropium (80 μg q.i.d.)	Ipratropium (400 μg q.i.d.)
Dryness of nose	25	36	61†	72†
Dryness of mouth	39	28	42	78†
Dysuria	3	6	11	28†
Saccharine test (mean in min)	14.9	13.7	17.7	17.1

Adapted from Kirkegaard et al.[14]
† *p < 0.05.*

need a dosage higher than 320 μg/day (Table IV). Results of a few long-term trials have been published.[12,13,15] The efficacy of treatment did not decrease with time. On the contrary, most patients reduced the dosage considerably without loss of efficacy.

OTHER CLINICAL STUDIES

Exposure to cold air induces a runny nose in normal subjects. In order to find out to what extent it is caused by nasal hypersecretion, on the one hand, and by tearing and condensed expired water, on the other, 14 normal persons were pretreated with a single very high dosage of ipratropium, 400 μg, before exposure to cold air (walk around a frozen lake during winter).[16] A 73% reduction in the weight of nasal secretions clearly showed nasal hypersecretion to be the most important contributor to cold air-induced rhinorrhea. In this study it was also shown that the same was true for hot spicy soup-induced rhinorrhea (Table V).

In another placebo-controlled trial of volunteers with naturally occurring common colds,[17] ipratropium treatment reduced the number of nose blowings significantly during the first days of the disease (Table V). A very high ipratropium dosage was then given in order to define the maximum potential of this type of treatment in the common cold and to elucidate to what degree nasal glandular hypersecretion and stimulation of cholinoceptors contribute to the runny nose, caused by a virus infection.[18] A more than 50% reduction demonstrated that a glandular product is mainly responsible for rhinorrhea in this condition also (Table V). Again the maximum efficacy was obtained at the expense of significant local side effects (nasal dryness). A score for "aqueousness" of the nasal fluid discharge was significantly lower in the ipratropium group than in the placebo group. This indicates that while ipratropium can stop watery rhinorrhea almost completely, it ap-

pears to have little or no effect on the mucopurulent secretion. Consequently, this type of secretion seems not to be produced by stimulation of glandular cholinoceptors.

SIDE EFFECTS

There is no doubt that intranasal ipratropium can result in an unpleasant feeling of dryness in the nose, which has been described in most studies (Table III). This side effect usually disappeared when the patients in the long-term follow-up studies were allowed to adjust the dosage to their individual need.

Clinical experience since 1979 and three long-term studies have failed to show any serious local adverse effects (Table VI). It is of theoretical interest that the very high dose (400 μg q.i.d.) used by Kirkegaard *et*

TABLE IV

Examples of Patients Who Do Not Need Treatment (No. 13); Are Not Helped by It (No. 32); Require an Ordinary Dose (No. 1); and Require a High Dose (No. 4)*

Patient Number	Average Daily Number of Paper Handkerchiefs		
	Placebo	Ipratropium (80 μg q.i.d.)	Ipratropium (400 μg q.i.d.)
No. 13	4.3	2.4	1.9
No. 32	24.6	19.4	18.4
No. 1	14.9	4.9	4.0
No. 4	256	139	39.3

Adapted from Kirkegaard et al.[14]

TABLE V

Results of Other Ipratropium Studies

	Disease	Dosage	Symptom Reduction (%)	*p* Value
Ostberg et al.[16]	Cold air	400 μg	73	<0.001
	Spicy soup	400 μg	66	<0.001
Borum et al.[17]	Common cold	80 μg × 4	37	<0.001
Cerkez et al.[18]	Common cold	400 μg × 4	56	<0.001

TABLE VI

Parameters Studied during Long-Term Treatment with Ipratropium Nasal Spray

	Number of Patients	Mean Daily Dosage (μg)	Duration (mo)	Parameters
Borum et al.[15]	20	180	10–48	Rhinoscopy Metacholine test Olfactometry
Knight et al.[12]	19	≪400	12	Symptoms
Dolovich et al.[13]	24	90	12	Rhinoscopy

TABLE VII

Limitations for the Usefulness of Ipratropium Nasal Spray

1. No effect on itching, sneezing, blockage
2. Only effect on fluid formed in nasal glands (not tears, sinus secretion, goblet cell secretion, condensed water, or exudate)
3. Effect on watery rhinorrhea, not on viscous purulent secretions
4. Only partial effect (not all glands protected?)
5. Also reduction of physiological secretory activity
4. Local side effects (nasal dryness)

TABLE VIII

Optimal Use of Ipratropium Nasal Spray

1. Determine the severity of the disease (tissues/day during 1 week)
2. Match the dosage to symptom severity
3. Give one large dosage early in the morning (maximum 200 μg)
4. Administer smaller doses p.r.n. during the day especially before exposure to provoking factors

al.[14] resulted in a pronounced subjective feeling of nasal dryness but not in a reduction of mucociliary transport rate in the nose measured with the saccharine test. This dosage (400 μg q.i.d.) was associated with mild systemic side effects, which have not been observed with the ordinary dose (80 μg q.i.d.)(Table III).

CONCLUSIONS

It has been clearly shown that intranasal administration of ipratropium can reduce the amount of watery rhinorrhea in perennial nonallergic rhinitis. Studies have also demonstrated efficacy in cold air/hot spicy soup-induced rhinorrhea and in the common cold. Ipratropium seems to be a useful drug in selected patients (Table I), but it is a limitation that the treatment is monosymptomatic with no effect on sneezing or on nasal blockage (Table VII). As ipratropium can cause a sensation of nasal dryness, it is necessary to match the dosage to the severity of the symptom. Even a daily dosage of 320 μg can result in local side effects in a patient with slight, occasional rhinorrhea, but the same dose can be insufficient in a patient with profuse rhinorrhea. The clinical trials, using a standard dosage, have not been designed with due consideration given to this patient-to-patient variation. A further problem is that rhinorrhea varies considerably within the single patient, from time to time and during the day. As most patients have profuse rhinorrhea predominantly in the morning and a rather dry nose at night, it is probably preferable to give a high morning dose and only to supplement the treatment as required during the day

(Table VIII). This appears to give a better ratio between anti-rhinorrhea and adverse effects than a fixed q.i.d. dosage.

REFERENCES

1. Wihl J-A, Petersen BN, Petersen LN, Gundersen G, Bresson K, Mygind N. Effect of the nonsedative H1-receptor antagonist astemizole in perennial allergic and nonallergic rhinitis. J Allergy Clin Immunol 75:720–727, 1985.
2. Peatfield AC, Richardson PS. Evidence for non-cholinergic non-adrenergic nervous control of mucus secretion in the cat trachea. J Physiol 342:335–345, 1983.
3. Engelhardt A, Klupp H. The pharmacology and toxicology of a new tropane alkaloid derivative. Postgrad Med J 51(suppl 7):82–84, 1975.
4. Pakes GE, Brogden RN, Heel RC, Speight TM, Avery GS. Ipratropium bromide: a review of its pharmacological properties and therapeutic efficacy in asthma and chronic bronchitis. Drugs 20:237–266, 1980.
5. Borum P. Intranasal ipratropium. Inhibition of methacholine induced hypersecretion. Rhinology 16:225–233, 1978.
6. Borum P, Mygind N, Larsen FS. Ipratropium nasal spray: a new treatment for perennial rhinitis. Clin Otolaryngol 4:407–411, 1979.
7. Bok HE, van Wijngaarden HA, Cornelissen PJG. Intranasal ipratropium bromide for paroxysmal rhinorrhoea. Eur J Respir Dis 64(suppl 128):486–489, 1983.
8. Jokinen K, Sipila P. Intranasal ipratropium in the treatment of vasomotor rhinitis. Rhinology 21:341–345, 1983.
9. Malmberg H, Grahne B, Holopainen E, Binder E. Ipratropium (Atrovent) in the treatment of vasomotor rhinitis of elderly patients. Clin Otolaryngol 8:273–276, 1893.
10. von Haacke NP, Moore-Gillon V, Capel LH. Double blind cross over trial of ipratropium and placebo in chronic rhinorrhoea. Br Med J 287:1258–1259, 1983
11. Sjogren I, Juhasz J. Ipratropium in the treatment of patients with perennial rhinitis. Allergy 39:457–461, 1984.
12. Knight A, Kazim F, Salvatori VA. A trial of intranasal Atrovent versus placebo in the treatment of vasomotor rhinitis. Ann Allergy 57:348–354, 1986.
13. Dolovich J, Kennedy L, Vickerson F, Kazim F. Control of the hypersecretion of vasomotor rhinitis by topical ipratropium bromide. J Allergy Clin Immunol 80:274–278, 1987.
14. Kirkegaard J, Mygind N, Mølgaard F, Grahne B, Holopainen E, Malmberg H, Brondbo K, Rojne T. Ordinary and high-dose ipratropium in perennial nonallergic rhinitis. J Allergy Clin Immunol 79:585–590, 1987.
15. Borum P, Mygind N, Larsen FS. Ipratropium treatment for rhinorrhoea in patients with perennial rhinitis. An open follow-up study of efficacy and safety. Clin Otolaryngol 8:267–272, 1983.
16. Østberg B, Winther B, Mygind N. Cold air-induced rhinorrhea and high-dose ipratropium. Arch Otolaryngol 113:160–162, 1987.
17. Borum P, Olsen L, Winther B, Mygind N. Ipratropium nasal spray: a new treatment for rhinorrhoea in the common cold. Am Rev Respir Dis 123:418–420, 1981.
18. Cerkez V, Østberg B, Winther B, Borum P, Mygind N. Effect of high-dose ipratropium on watery rhinorrhea in the common cold. Use of a cholinoceptor antagonist as an indicator of reflex mediated hypersecretion. In preparation. □

Chapter XXX

Antibiotic Treatment of Rhinitis and Sinusitis

Donald N. MacKay, M.D.

ABSTRACT

With rare exception, the only microbial causes of rhinitis are viruses, and no effective treatment is available at present.

The most common organisms causing bacterial sinusitis are Pneumococci and Hemophilus influenzae. Accordingly, in a patient not allergic to penicillin, ampicillin or amoxicillin appear to be the antibiotics of choice in empirical treatment of bacterial sinusitis. In penicillin-allergic patients or in areas with a high incidence of β-lactamase producing H. influenzae, co-trimoxazole probably would be a better choice. Because organisms obtained by culture of nasal secretions do not correlate well with organisms obtained from sinuses by direct puncture aspiration, culture of nasal secretions is not recommended.

RHINITIS

The etiology of rhinitis is multifactorial, with viruses, allergies, and vasomotor rhinitis being the major contributors. Save for scleroma, a chronic granulomatous process found mainly in Eastern Europe involving the nose, sinuses, and upper airway (which is believed due to *Klebsiella rhinoscleromatis*) and the association of *Klebsiella ozaenae* with a rare form of chronic atrophic rhinitis, neither bacteria nor fungi have been implicated nor seriously suspected as agents causing the syndrome characterized by coryza.[1] Accordingly, until the recent past, antimicrobial agents have had no role in uncomplicated rhinitis.

However, in 1984 the use of zinc gluconate lozenges

Clinical Associate Professor of Medicine, Stanford University School of Medicine. Initially presented at the Spring 1982 meeting of the New England Society of Allergy.

was reported to significantly shorten the duration of symptoms of the common cold in a double-blind, placebo controlled study.[2] However, this study has been critized because the zinc gluconate lozenges left a distinct "aftertaste" in the patients and the study may therefore have been unblinded. Subsequently three more studies using either zinc gluconate[3,4] or zinc acetate[5] have been published, with all three showing no difference between zinc and placebo.

Rhinoviruses are the most frequent cause of the common cold, and long-term intranasal administration of alpha$_2$-interferon has been effective in the prophylaxis of these infections, even though this approach appears impractical due to the high rates of nasal intolerance to this compound during prolonged administration. Recently, alpha$_2$-interferon also has been shown to be effective in the postexposure prevention of rhinovirus colds in the family setting.[6,7] As "postexposure prophylaxis" may in fact be treatment, the question as to the efficacy of alpha$_2$-interfernon use after symptoms have developed should be answered. To date the author is unaware of published studies on this question.

Similarly a new synthetic antiviral drug, R61837, found effective in prophylaxis of rhinovirus colds, was not effective when used as treatment of an established infection.[8]

Numerous studies have failed to show effectiveness of Vitamin C in treatment of colds.[9]

SINUSITIS

Sinusitis, however, is a different matter. While most sinusitis appears to be a complication of a viral cold, several studies have implicated bacteria as the most common etiologic agents.[10-13] Therefore, antibiotics have an important role to play in the treatment of sinusitis. A note of caution must be inserted at this juncture, because most studies using antibiotics also have used a topical nasal vasoconstricting drug. Of greater significance is the paucity of studies comparing the use of antibiotics to a placebo, although when compared to patients who either stopped their antibiotic or were given a theoretically ineffective antibiotic, the effectiveness of correct therapy seemed convincing.[11]

What then, are the bacteria found in sinusitis, for successful treatment of a microbial disease requires knowledge of the causative organisms. Most of the information comes from studies done in acute sinusitis (and with two exceptions the maxillary sinus is the usual sinus studied) with the material obtained either at surgery or by direct aspiration by sinus puncture after careful sterilization of the nasal mucosa. Cultures of nasal secretions have been shown to correlate poorly with the results of direct sinus aspiration.[10,12,14] It has been suggested this may be due to normal flora multiplying faster than the true pathogens during the delay between collection of the specimen and streaking it on a culture plate, with subsequent overgrowth of normal flora obscuring the true pathogens.[15] If this latter point is valid, direct inoculation of culture media "at the bedside" might increase the usefulness of nasal cultures.

Gwaltney[1] has summarized the results of studies of acute maxillary sinusitis with the relative contribution of various microbes as shown in Table I. More recent studies have supported these findings.[16–18] Perhaps the

most surprising point about these studies is the fairly high percentage of H. influenzae infections in adults, with the isolation rate of this organism similar to that seen in children in most studies.[12] Except for gram-negative rods, the other bacteria isolated are commonly found as normal flora in healthy adults. Acute sinusitis due to anaerobic bacteria was often associated with dental disease.

Although apparently more common in the pre-antibiotic era, sphenoid sinusitis accounted for only 2.7% of cases of sinusitis seen at the Massachusetts Eye and Ear Infirmary and Massachusetts General Hospital between 1968 and 1980.[13] Unlike the studies with maxillary sinusitis summarized in Table I, Staphylococcus aureus was the most common cause of acute sphenoid sinusitis in this series, followed by S. pneumoniae, viridans and anaerobic streptococci, and gram-negative rods. H. influenzae was not seen in acute cases of sphenoid sinusitis but was found in one chronic case. A more recent study from Vancouver General Hospital also found Staphylococcus aureus and S. pneumoniae as the most common organisms, but H. influenzae was found as well.[19]

An earlier study by Frederich and Braude[20] (also not included in Table I) dealt with chronic sinusitis and showed a much higher recovery rate for anaerobes, with anaerobes being present in 43 of 62 cases in which a bacteria was isolated, 17 of the anaerobic isolates being accompanied by aerobic bacteria. In an additional 21 cases, no bacteria were found. Of the aerobic isolates, S. aureus was most frequent, with gram-negative rods and viridans streptococci also commonly found. Possibilities for the predominance of anaerobes in chronic sinusitis include chronic use of vasoconstricting drugs and the observation that the sinus-to-nose pressure gradient in chronic sinusitis is higher than in acute sinusitis — both factors that might impair blood supply and decrease oxygen tension in the involved sinus.[21]

Some special situations deserve comment. Diabetics with ketoacidosis and severely immunosuppressed patients may develop fungal sinusitis, particularly with Mucor or Rhizopus species. Pseudomonas aeruginosa is often found in patients with cystic fibrosis or Kartagener's syndrome.[22,23] Recently, nosocomial sinusitis due to gram-negative aerobic rods (as well as other bacteria) has been described, and is related to nasal intubation.[24] Treatment of these patients usually will be different from the patients described below.

Given the likely bacterial possibilities in a patient with acute sinusitis, ampicillin (or the closely related amoxicillin) has emerged as the favored drug for the treatment of sinusitis, as it should be effective against all the bacteria shown in Table I except for S. aureus, β-lactamase producing H. influenzae and Branhamella catarrhalis, some of the anaerobes, and many of the aerobic gram-negative rods (excluding H. influenzae).

TABLE I

Microbial Etiology of Acute Antral Sinusitis (after Gwaltney)[1]

Microbes	Mean Percent of Cases	
	Adults	Children
Bacteria		
S. pneumoniae	31	36
H. influenzae (unencapsulated)	21	23
S. pneumonia and H. influenzae	5	—
Anaerobic bacteria	6	—
S. aureus	4	—
S. pyogenes	2	2
B. catarrhalis	2	19
Gram-negative rods	9	2
Viruses		
Rhinovirus	15	—
Influenza virus	5	—
Parainfluenza virus	3	2
Adenovirus	—	2

Because reliable cultures cannot be obtained without direct sinus aspirate, it seems reasonable to initiate treatment on an empiric basis in most cases without resorting to culture, with ampicillin 500 mg q.i.d. or amoxicillin 500 mg t.i.d. orally for 10 days, plus a topical nasal decongestant. If the patient fails to respond, one of two possible options then should be considered. Either the antibiotic could be changed to a β-lactamase resistant drug (see below) or sinus puncture to obtain material for culture could be performed, and the material cultured both aerobically and anaerobically. Unless future investigation shows direct "bedside plating" of nasal cultures approaching the accuracy of sinus puncture and aspiration, this technique is not recommended.

In a small number of patients, the doses mentioned above may not be adequate. Using current standards for determining ampicillin/amoxicillin sensitivity, H. influenzae are considered sensitive by Baur-Kirby disc testing with minimum inhibitory concentrations that could exceed blood and sinus exudate concentrations when 2.0 grams of ampicillin orally per day are used.[25-27] Although studies suggest this dose is adequate,[11] one might consider doubling the dose of antibiotic in a patient who is not responding to treatment before resorting to sinus aspiration to obtain an adequate culture.

Because a small but significant number of sinus infections are caused by β-lactamase-producing organisms, there has been recent interest in using β-lactamase resistant antibiotics as initial treatment in sinusitis. Amoxicillin combined with the β-lactamase inhibitor clavulanic acid (Augmentin), should be superior to ampicillin or amoxicillin, as it would be effective against nearly all S. aureus as well as β-lactamase producing H. influenzae and Branhamella catarrhalis. However, the only study yet reported comparing Augmentin with amoxicillin failed to show any difference between the two drugs.[28] Cefaclor and cefuroxime axetil (an oral form of cefuroxime) have both been used in sinusitis but have only been compared with each other,[29] or in the case of cefuroxime axetil (in a study that included patients with otitis and pharyngitis), with Augmentin.[30] In the first of these studies, cefuroxime axetil 250 mg. B.I.D. was superior to cefaclor 500 mg T.I.D. In the second study, the drugs being compared were equally efficacious so at this point it is unknown if either would be superior to ampicillin or amoxicillin.

In patients with penicillin allergy, the use of co-trimoxazole (trimethoprim 80 mg plus sulfamethoxazole 400 mg) 2 tablets b.i.d. has been shown to be effective,[11] and might be the primary drug of choice in an area with a high incidence of β-lactamase producing H. influenzae that would be resistant to ampicillin or amoxicillin (unless combined with clavulanic acid). Tetracycline, 500 mg q.i.d., has been used in the past,

but Pneumococci and H. influenzae are no longer uniformly sensitive to it. If a β-lactamase positive H. influenzae is isolated, co-trimoxazole is probably the best choise for treatment, although cefaclor or cefuroxime axetil may prove equally effective.

Except for its lack of efficacy afgainst S. aureus, chloramphenicol should be unsurpassed in controlling sinusitis, but toxicity limits its usefulness to only the most unusual cases. In patients ill enough to be hospitalized, the second-generation cephalosporins, cefonocid or cefuroxime, could be used. Third generation cephalosporins, although effective, should not be needed save for the unusual case in which a gram-negative rod resistant to narrower spectrum drugs is suspected.

There is very little published experience with the newer quinolones. An Austrian study found ciprofloxacin slightly better than penicillin V in a study that included patients with otitis and peritonsillitis;[31] but did not compare it with ampicillin or amoxicillin, which should be more effective than penicillin V. Because pneumococci (and other streptococci) are less sensitive to quinolones than are most other organisms, at present the author would not use these drugs in acute sinusitis unless the infection were known to be due to a highly sensitive organism.

SUMMARY

Most cases of acute sinusitis are caused by bacteria, with S. pneumoniae and H. influenzae being the most common organisms isolated from direct sinus asperates. In view of the inaccuracy of nasal cultures, empiric treatment with ampicillin, amoxicillin, or co-trimoxazole is advocated.

REFERENCES

1. Gwaltney JM Jr. Sinusitis. In: Mandell, Douglas, Bennett, eds. Principles and Practice of Infectious Diseases. New York: John Wiley & Sons, pp. 369–372, 1231, 1985.
2. Eby GA, Davis DR, Halcomb WW. Reduction in duration of common colds by zinc gluconate lozenges in a double-blind study. Antimicrob Agents Chemother 25:20, 1984.
3. Farr BM, Conner EM, Betts RF, Oleske J, Minnefor A, Gwaltney JM. Two randomized controlled trials of zinc gluconate lozenge therapy of experimentally induced rhinovirus colds. Antimicrob Agents Chemother 31:1183–1187, 1987.
4. Smith DS, Helzner EC, Nuttall CE Jr, Collins M, Rofman BA, Ginsberg D, Goswick CB, Magner A. Failure of zinc gluconate in treatment of acute upper respiratory tract infections. Antimicrob Agents Chemother 33:646–648, 1989.
5. Douglas BM, Miles HB, Moore BW, Ryan P, Pinnock CB. Failure of effervescent zinc acetate lozenges to alter the course of upper respiratory tract infections in Australian adults. Antimicrob Agents Chemother 31:1263–1265, 1987.
6. Douglas RM, Moore BW, Miles HB, Davies LM, Grahm NMH, Ryan P, Worswick DA, Albrecht JK. Prophylactic efficacy of intranasal alpha$_2$-interferon against rhinovirus infections in the family setting. N Engl J Med 314:65–70, 1986.
7. Hayden FG, Albrecht JK, Kaiser DL, Gwaltney JM. Prevention of natural colds by contact prophylaxis with intranasal alpha$_2$-interferon. N Engl J Med 314:71–75, 1986.

8. Al-Nakib W, Higgins PG, Barrow GI, Tyrrell AJ, Andries K, Vanden Bussche G, Taylor N, Janssen PAJ. Suppression of colds in human volunteers challenged with rhinovirus by a new synthetic drug (R61837). Antimicrob Agents Chemother 33:522–525, 1989.

9. Sperber SJ, Hayden FG. Chemotherapy of rhinovirus colds. Antimicrob Agents Chemother 32:409–419, 1988.

10. Evans FO Jr, Sydnor BJ, Moore WEC et al. Sinusitis of the maxillary antrum. N Engl J Med 293:735–739, 1975.

11. Hamory BH, Sande MA, Sydnor A Jr, Seale DL, Gwaltney JM Jr. Etiology and antimicrobial therapy of acute maxillary sinusitis. J Infect Dis 139:197–202, 1979.

12. Wald ER, Milmoe GJ, Bowen A, Ledesma-Medina J, Salamon N, Bluestone CD. Acute maxillary sinusitis in children. N Engl J Med 304:749–754, 1981.

13. Lew D, Southwick FS, Montgomery WW, Weber AL, Baker AS. Sphenoid sinusitis. N Engl J Med 309:1149–1154, 1983.

14. Axelsson A, Brosson JE. The correlation between bacteriological findings in the nose and maxillary sinus in acute maxillary sinusitis. Laryngoscope 83:2003, 1973.

15. Scwartz RH, Rodriquez WJ. Letter to the editor. N Engl J Med 305:226, 1981.

16. Ylikoski J, Savolainen S, Jousimies-Somer H. The bacteriology of acute maxillary sinusitis. J Otorhinolaryngol Relat Spec (Switzerland) 51:175–181, 1989.

17. Berg O, Carenfelt C, Kronvall G. Bacteriology of maxillary sinusitis in relation to character of inflammation and prior treatment. Scand J Infect Dis 20(Suppl 5):511–516, 1988.

18. Nord CE. Efficacy of penicillin treatment in purulent maxillary sinusitis: A European multicenter trial. Infection 16 (Suppl 4):209–214, 1988.

19. Kibblewhite DJ, Cleland J, Mintz DR. Acute sphenoid sinusitis: Management strategies. J Otolaryngol 17(Suppl 4):159–163, 1988.

20. Frederick J, Braude AI. Anaerobic infection of the paranasal sinuses. N Engl J Med 290:135–137, 1974.

21. Drettner B, Lindholm CE. The borderline between acute rhinitis and sinusitis. Acta Otolaryngol 64:508, 1967.

22. Healy GB. Acute sinusitis in childhood. N Engl J Med 304:779, 1981.

23. Shapiro ED, Milmore GJ, Wald ER, Rodnan JB, Bowen A. Bacteriology of the maxillary sinuses in patients with cystic fibrosis. J Infect Dis 146:589–593, 1982.

24. Caplan ES, Hoyt NJ. Nosocomial sinusitis. JAMA 247:639–641, 1982.

25. Axelsson A, Brorson JE. The concentration of antibiotics in sinus secretions. Ann Otol Rhinol Laryngol 83:323, 1974.

26. Gilman AG, Goodman LS, Rall TW, Murad F. In: Goodman LS, Gilman AG, eds. The Pharmacological Basis of Therapeutics, 7th ed. New York: Macmillan, p. 1130, 1985.

27. The National Committee for Clinical Laboratory Standards. Performance standards for antimicrobial Disc Susceptibility Tests, 3rd Ed. 1984.

28. Wald ER, Chiponis D, Ledesma-Medina J. Comparative effectiveness of amoxicillin and amoxicillin-clavulanate potassium in acute paranasal sinus infections in children: A double-blind, placebo-controlled trial. Pediatrics 77:795–800, 1986.

29. Sydnor A Jr, Gwaltney JM Jr, Scheld WM. Cefuroxime axetil vs. cefaclor therapy of acute maxillary sinusitis (Abstract 327). Abstracts of the 1988 Interscience Conference on Antimicrobial Agents and Chemotherapy. 1988, p. 167.

30. Hebblethwaite EM, Brown GW, Cox DM. A comparison of the efficacy and safety of cefuroxime axetil and Augmentin in the treatment of upper respiratory tract infections. Drugs Exp Clin Res 13(Suppl 2):91–94, 1987.

31. Falser N, Mittermayer H, Weuta H. Antibacterial treatment of otitis and sinusitis with Ciprofloxacin and Penicillin V: A Comparison. Infection 16(Suppl 1):51–54, 1988.

Chapter XXXI

Functional Endoscopic Approach to Inflammatory Sinus Disease

David W. Kennedy, M.D.,* and S. James Zinreich, M.D.**

ABSTRACT

Endoscopic examination and pleuridirectional polytomography provided some important insights into the pathogenesis of inflammatory sinus disease. These insights have been further refined by the increasing utilization of endoscopy in medical therapy and surgical follow-up, and by the use of computed tomography for diagnosis. The aim of this paper is to review the current status of the diagnosis of chronic inflammatory sinus disease and of functional endoscopic surgical techniques. The impact of this approach on previously held theoretical and diagnostic concepts is evaluated. Technical modifications made since the surgery was first introduced in the United States and the lessons learned from close post-surgical endoscopic examination are presented.

The term "functional endoscopic sinus surgery" (FES) denotes an approach in which the major objective is the reestablishment of sinus ventilation and mucociliary clearance.[1] The surgery is tailored to the pathologic condition and varies in extent. A consistent

* *Philadelphia, Pennsylvania, Department of Otolaryngology Head and Neck Surgery, University of Pennsylvania Medical Center*
** *Assistant Professor, Neuroradiology Division of the Russell H. Morgan Department of Radiology and Radiological Sciences, The Johns Hopkins University, Baltimore, MD*

underlying principle is the removal of disease from the ostiomeatal complex, since these are the channels primarily involved in the majority of cases. The technique evolved primarily out of careful studies of mucociliary clearance and detailed nasal endoscopic evaluation by Messerklinger.[2-4] Although Proctor had long advocated the anterior ethmoid-middle meatal complex as the key to inflammatory sinus disease involving the other sinuses, the concept was contrary to much of the current teaching in the United States when introduced.[1,15] In order to differentiate the important theoretical and diagnostic concepts from other approaches, the term "functional endoscopic sinus surgery" was devised.[2]

Good supporting evidence existed for the concept that obstruction was both the critical event in the pathogenesis of inflammatory sinus disease and a major factor in the persistence of disease.[6-8] Anatomic evaluation demonstrated that this obstruction was most likely to occur within the narrow channels of the ostiomeatal complex and that anatomic variation within this area might be a significant predisposing factor. Additionally, the concept of the reversibility of secondary mucosal disease gained acceptance. Careful evaluation confirmed the presence of persistent inflammation in the ostiomeatal complex between episodes of acute infection. These findings further highlighted the necessity for meticulous diagnostic evaluation if early and underlying causes of disease were to be identified.[2]

FES, when introduced into the United States in 1984, brought the potential to significantly reduce morbidity when compared to traditional open approaches. While the incidence of complications has remained low in skilled hands, a high complication rate has been reported from those less familiar with endonasal surgery.[9-11] In general, early surgical results appear to be similar to those with other approaches. However, the relevance of any reported results must be questioned in the absence of an accepted staging system or the widespread adoption of routine endoscopic follow-up.[10]

METHODS
Diagnostic Evaluation

All patients complaining of chronic sinusitis undergo comprehensive nasal endoscopy. The examination is performed under topical anesthesia as part of the initial patient examination, using 30° or 70° rigid Hopkins telescopes (Karl Stortz Endoscopy America, Culver City, CA). The nasal recesses, including the middle meatus and its anatomic structures, are carefully examined. When significant disease is identified, medical therapy is typically initiated and the patient reevaluated.

Patients who show evidence of persistent disease following medical therapy, or in whom there is a well-documented history of recurrent infections, are selected for computed tomography (CT). Since the primary aim of CT is to visualize the underlying cause of disease rather than the secondary changes, the study is best performed after the patient has received appropriate medical therapy. The study is performed in the coronal plane without enhancement. The patient is placed in the prone position and scanned with 4-mm slices at 3-mm intervals. The images focus on only the paranasal sinus area, using a window width of approximately 2,000 and a center of approximately −200. Careful attention is given to the anatomy of the ostiomeatal complex, particularly with regard to the ventilatory and mucociliary clearance pathways of the major sinuses. Similarly, inflammatory disease is evaluated in the context of these relationships, rather than primarily on the basis of extent.

Therapeutic Intervention

Patients are selected for surgery based upon a combination of clinical history, endoscopic findings following medical therapy, and CT. Surgery is not performed based upon CT findings alone. Operative intervention is preferably performed under local anesthesia, typically on an outpatient basis. The surgeon sits alongside the supine patient, who is given intravenous sedation and monitored during the procedure. The extent of the surgery is varied according to the disease identified and is performed entirely under endoscopic visualization. Operative safety is maximized by using a 0°

telescope for the majority of the dissection and a deflected angle telescope only when necessary. Typically the surgery begins with an incision around the anterior and inferior attachment of the uncinate process. This structure is then removed to gain access to the ethmoidal infundibulum. Diseased ethmoid cells are then opened and removed using delicate forceps. The need for suction has been minimized by the use of suction forceps, which have also dramatically improved the ability to operate under direct visualization when bleeding is present (Fig. 1). The dissection is largely performed from anterior to posterior. The medial orbital wall and the roof of the ethmoid provide key landmarks and are skeletonized whenever more than very limited anterior ethmoid surgery is required. When severe disease precludes early identification of the ethmoid roof anteriorly, it is identified posteriorly after proceeding inferiorly into the posterior ethmoid or sphenoid sinus. Retrograde dissection is then performed along the skull base. In severe or recurrent nasal polyposis, a KTP-532 laser (Laserscope, San Jose, CA) or a Holmium-YAG laser may be helpful in allowing the removal of the bulk of intranasal polyps without bleeding. For the KTP-532 laser a sheath was created which holds the 400-μ quartz laser fiber alongside the telescope (Fig. 2). The fiber may be restricted to create a diffuse beam for coagulation or advanced to create a beam with a high power density ration for cutting. In general the polyps are removed with minimal bleeding by cutting them across the base, using the laser fiber in contact with the tissue. The beam is aimed by directing the telescope. Smoke is aspirated using either a separate suction or the suction forceps.

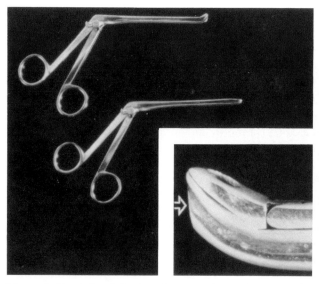

Figure 1. *Kennedy-Blakesly upbiting and straight suction forceps (Karl Stortz Endoscopy America, Culver City, CA). Inset shows the suction tube below the jaws. The opening of the suction tube is marked with an arrow.*

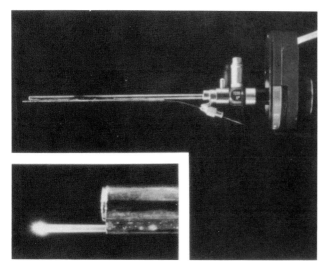

Figure 2. KTP-532 laser fiber attachment for the 0° telescope. Proximally the fiber is sheathed in black plastic in the area adjacent to the attachment. An eye safety filter protects the surgeon's eye used on the telescope and automatically brings a filter across the lens when the laser is fired. The surgeon's other eye is protected with a permanent filter. The tissue effect achieved is varied by advancing or retracting the fiber.

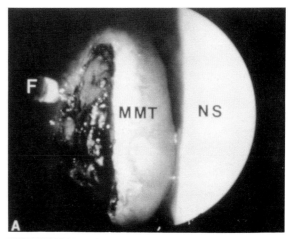

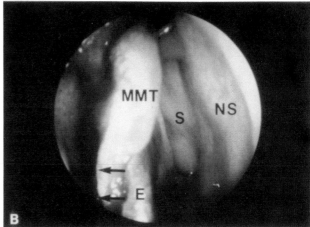

Figure 3. Excision of the lateral half of a massive concha bullosa (0° telescope, right nose). (A) The KTP-532 laser is used to incise the middle turbinate mucosa bloodlessly. The bone is then incised with sickle knife and scissors and the lateral half of the turbinate removed with forceps. NS, nasal septum; F, laser fiber; MMT, medial middle turbinate. (B) Following resection the remaining medial lamella of the middle turbinate (MMT) may be moved back into a more physiologic position (arrows) if the middle meatus is enormously widened. This provides a relatively normal middle turbinate. E, elevator; NS, nasal septum; S, sphenoid rostrum.

The operation is completed when all disease visualized on CT has been removed and the cells entered surgically are almost normal. Only in diffuse advanced disease is a complete sphenoethmoidectomy performed. In early disease the cells are merely opened so as to provide drainage and ventilation. In advanced or severe disease, however, all the cellular partitions are completely removed and every attempt is made to widely open both the frontal and maxillary sinuses. After middle meatal antrostomy is performed, disease may be removed from the maxillary sinus with right-angle forceps or with slim-angled biopsy forceps. Small-angled biopsy forceps may also be used to remove localized disease from the frontal sinus under direct endoscopic visualization.

The middle turbinate is generally preserved. If aerated, the lateral half of the middle turbinate may be removed and the medial lamella preserved (Fig. 3, A and B). Otherwise, the middle turbinate is sacrificed only when diffusely osteitic.

Usually no postoperative packing is placed. Occasionally, when heavy bleeding is encountered, or in an asthmatic patient when it is important to avoid the risk of postnasal discharge precipitating bronchospasm, a small cellulose sponge may be placed lateral to the middle turbinate. Unless there are complicating medical problems, the patient is typically discharged the same day.

Postoperatively the patient returns for regular cleaning of the operative field until the area has fully healed.

The cleaning is performed in the outpatient clinic under endoscopic visualization. If the maxillary sinus ostium was widened, it is suctioned free of blood and mucus until mucociliary clearance is reestablished. This is performed by introducing a curved suction tube through the middle meatal antrostomy under endoscopic visualization. The frontal sinus is similarly cleared of secretion. Any recurrent hypertrophic mucosa or, when possible, nonhealing areas of bone are removed under topical anesthesia as part of the routine follow-up visit. If a residual infected cell is identified, it is opened at this time under topical anesthesia. Post-operative antibiotic therapy is guided by culture. The duration of antibiotic therapy and, when indicated, oral steroid therapy, is determined by endoscopic examination.

RESULTS

Diagnostic

Nasal endoscopic and CT findings confirm that the ostiomeatal complex is the most frequent site of inflammatory sinus disease and that disease may persist in this area after the secondary sinus disease has resolved (Fig. 4). Nasal endoscopic examination consistently reveals significant but subtle evidence of disease which is not visible on anterior rhinoscopy, to the extent that the value of this diagnostic modality can no longer be seriously questioned (Fig. 5, A and B). Furthermore, the use of CT has allowed the incidence of concomitant

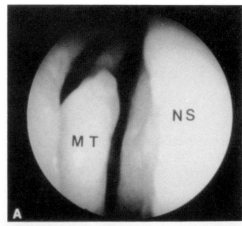

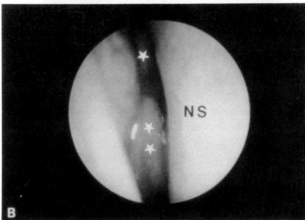

Figure 5. Patient with a complaint of chronic right nasal congestion and pain. (A) Examination from the front of the nose (30° telescope) demonstrates only a slight paradoxical curvature to the middle turbinate (MT). The middle meatus appears free of disease. NS, nasal septum. (B) More posterior endoscopic examination reveals polyps occluding the superior and supreme meatus and extending out into the nose (stars).

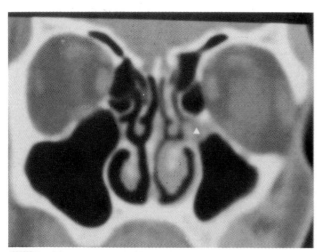

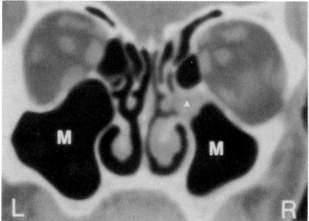

Figure 4. Sequential coronal CT slices of a patient with recurrent right maxillary sinusitis. The maxillary sinus disease has resolved, but disease persists in the ostiomeatal complex. A soft tissue density (triangle) obliterates the inferior middle meatus, hiatus semilunaris, ethmoidal infundibulum, and adjacent maxillary sinus (M).

anatomic variations and the extent of disease to be accurately recorded. In a study of 230 patients with chronic sinus complaints, we found that 78% had disease within the anterior ethmoid. The next most frequent site was in the maxillary sinus (66%). The posterior ethmoid cells were involved in only 31%, a strong argument against the necessity for a routine ethmoid dissection which begins posteriorly. Similarly the frontal sinus was only involved in 34% of patients and the sphenoid in 16%. At the time of the study, 16% of the patients had no evidence of inflammation. However, some of the patients had significant anatomic abnormalities which could possibly have been responsible for their prior recurrent disease. Therefore, 93% of the patients with radiologic evidence of inflammation at the time of the study had disease within the anterior ethmoid (Table I). Evaluation of the same CT studies also revealed a wide variety of anatomic variations. The most common variation was concha bullosa, which

TABLE I

CT of Chronic Sinusitis

Sites of Involvement with No Prior Surgery	Total (%) (*n* = 230)	Inflammatory Disease (%) (*n* = 193)
Anterior ethmoid	78	93
Maxillary	66	79
Frontal	34	41
Posterior ethmoid	31	38
Sphenoid	16	22

TABLE II

Incidence of Anatomic Variations (*n* = 230)

Variation	Incidence (%)
Concha bullosa (44% bilateral)	36
Septal deformity	21
Parodoxical middle turbinate	15
Haller cells	10
Large ethmoid bulla	8
Laterally deviated uncinate	3
Inferior turbinate bulla	1
Uncinate bulla	0.4

occurred in 36%. The second most frequent finding was a septal deformity. Other variations occurred with differing frequencies (Table II).

Therapeutic

Since this approach was introduced in the United States relatively recently, long-term statistical follow-up of patient outcome is not available. Additionally, the absence of any staging system for inflammatory sinus disease makes interstudy comparisons of limited value at best. However, preliminary information is encouraging. In a review of 95 ethmoid procedures in which endoscopic follow-up of 4 months duration or longer (mean 9 months) was present, we found that 92% of patients were either improved or asymptomatic. No patients were worse. In those patients in whom an antrostomy was performed, 98% were patent. Complications in this series were generally minor. There were no instances of cerebrospinal fluid rhinorrhea, diplopia, visual loss, or intraorbital hematoma. No patients required blood transfusion. The only significant complication was epiphora which developed in two patients some months following the procedure.[10]

Similar results have been reported from Europe, where the techniques have been practiced for considerably longer.[11,12] There again, in experienced hands, complication rates have been low and endoscopic techniques appear to be gaining increased acceptance. Stammberger[11] reported on 4,000 cases performed by Messerklinger and himself with only two cerebrospinal fluid leaks and one intraorbital hematoma. There were no cases of visual loss in the series.

Close endoscopic observation during the postoperative period demonstrates that those patients who later develop recurrent symptoms typically have endoscopic evidence of persistent disease continuing from the early postoperative period. In patients undergoing a complete sphenoethmoidectomy, persistent or recurrent disease appears to be most likely to occur in the area of the frontal recess. Even in the rare situation when polyps remain in the maxillary sinus after ethmoidectomy and middle meatal antrostomy, this persistent disease is rarely symptomatic or a cause of a secondary ethmoid recurrence.

DISCUSSION

By defining the techniques of CT evaluation of the paranasal sinuses, we have been able to improve recognition of ostiomeatal complex disease and confirm the endoscopic and radiographic observations of Messerklinger. In our experience both endoscopic and CT evaluation support the concept that the ostiomeatal complex is primarily responsible for inflammatory sinus disease and that anatomic abnormalities in this area predispose to obstruction (Fig. 6). The potential of this technique clearly lies in the ability to both identify early disease and to evaluate its clinical significance by meticulous diagnostic examination. On the other hand, the concept that the functional endoscopic approach is suitable only for limited disease is a myth. Indeed the most appropriate case for FES is one in which careful diagnostic evaluation demonstrates a limited underlying cause for widespread disease. In such a case, as in a frontal sinus mucocele arising from obstruction of the frontal recess, FES offers the greatest opportunity to reduce patient morbidity. Although the same surgical techniques are also applicable to a patient with diffuse polyposis, it is our experience that these patients still require a meticulous complete sphenoethmoidectomy. Thus, the operation performed endoscopically in these cases is similar to a standard intranasal sphenoethmoidectomy. There is therefore less potential to reduce morbidity, although the endoscopes still improve visualization. Whether or not the surgery is performed endoscopically, endoscopic postoperative examination demonstrates that these severe cases require more frequent and meticulous postoperative cleaning. Aggressive and sometimes prolonged antibiotic therapy and, in some situations, steroid therapy may be necessary if later recurrence is to be avoided.

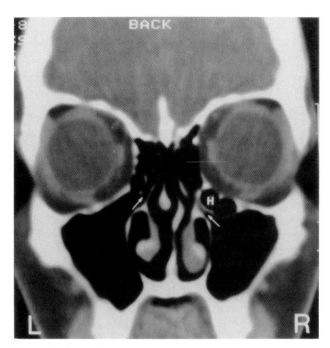

Figure 6. *Coronal CT scan through the infundibulae (arrows) of a patient with recurrent right maxillary sinusitis. The maxillary sinus disease has resolved but a Haller cell (H) is noted to be narrowing the right ethmoidal infundibulum. There is some persistent pacification within the infundibulum.*

Overall, the use of endoscopes during surgery has significantly aided us in reducing trauma and morbidity. Blood loss is reduced and the completeness of the surgery improved compared to the operating microscope. Although the use of suction irrigation devices has, to date, proved too traumatic, the development of suction forceps has dramatically improved our ability to obtain good visualization in the presence of bleeding. In our experience they have also helped to decrease operating time by reducing the necessity to alternate forceps with suction.

The ability of the KTP-532 laser to pass through small flexible quartz fibers has enabled the development of a variety of delivery devices for use in the nose and sinuses. The laser has, to date, been primarily of benefit in the treatment of patients with severe recurrent polyposis. It is important to initiate use of the laser at the start of the case. The aim is to prevent bleeding rather than to attempt hemostasis once bleeding is present. In the latter situation the laser has the tendency to char the extravasated blood on the surface rather than coagulating the bleeding sites. Care is required when introducing the endoscope with attached laser fiber, in order to avoid traumatizing the septal mucosa with the extended fiber. Typically, the polyp is grasped with suction forceps and cut along the base by bringing the fiber in contact with the tissue and advancing it slowly through the polyp mass. Power settings of 5–8 watts continuous have proven satisfactory. The KTP-532 laser has also proven beneficial in performing a bloodless resection of the lateral half of a concha bullosa and the division of extensive intranasal adhesions. Its usefulness in the maxillary sinus is still under evaluation, but should be enhanced by the development of new instrumentation. When a KTP-532 laser is not available, microcautery would appear to offer a possible alternative for use within the nose. Recent experience with the Holmium-YAG laser suggests this also has some utility on endoscopic sinus surgery. This laser has a particular affinity for vaporization of bone and thus is especially appropriate in this area.

Wide experience with anatomical dissection has demonstrated a wide variety of anatomic and pathologic variations and confirmed the concept that the surgery must be performed under direct vision. Although the incidence of bony optic nerve dehiscence appears to be very low in anatomic specimens, the incidence of bony dehiscence of the carotid artery appears to be higher than previously reported. A detailed study to evaluate the incidence of this variation is underway, but initial results suggest that some degree of bony dehiscence of the carotid occurs in 20–30% of adult anatomic specimens. In the presence of disease, the frequency of bony dehiscence of the medial orbital wall is high. Since orbital fat can, on occasion, appear similar to mucosal disease, this observation argues for routine early skeletonization of the medial orbital wall and, in view of the markedly increased pain sensitivity of the orbital contents, for the use of local anesthesia.

Should diffuse bleeding occur to the extent that good visualization is impossible, even with the use of suction forceps, a temporary pack may be utilized. Although the use of a pack or neurosurgical sponge soaked in a vasoconstrictive solution was originally advocated, soaking the pack in a slurry of microfibrillar collagen [Avitene, Alcon (Puerto Rico) Inc., Humacao, Puerto Rico] also has been found to be efficacious.[13] Loose microfibrillar collagen is mixed with saline solution to form a pasty suspension in which the packing material is immersed. While this provides excellent hemostasis, the problem of removing excess collagen, after hemostasis has been obtained, is avoided. Similarly, if hemorrhage occurs from violation of the anterior or posterior ethmoid artery, microfibrillar collagen has proven effective. In this instance a ball of microfibrillar collagen is applied directly to the bleeding site, followed immediately by a wet cotton ball. After the bleeding has been controlled, the cotton ball and excess collagen are removed.

Careful endoscopic postsurgical follow-up has, in several cases, demonstrated the importance of ensuring that the iatrogenic middle meatal antrostomy connects with the natural ostium of the maxillary sinus. Persistence of maxillary sinus disease has been noted in several cases in which the middle meatal antrostomy was not brought far enough anteriorly. In this situation disease may persist in the area of the natural ostium of the maxillary sinus and the resultant mucoid discharge recirculates into the maxillary sinus through the antrostomy (Fig. 7, A and B).

The observation that patients who develop late recurrent disease typically have early endoscopic evidence of persistent disease has led us to greatly intensify postoperative care. Endoscopic examination of these patients may reveal small osteitic bony spicules surrounded by regenerated hypertrophic mucosa, or, in some cases, large areas of persistent low-grade mucosal inflammation. Occasionally, areas of the medial orbital wall are soft, osteitic and nonhealing. The most common area for disease persistence and recurrence appears to be the frontal recess, even when this area is cleaned meticulously under endoscopic control. It is possible to remove disease from this area more completely using endoscopes with deflected angles of view than by any other method (with the exception of transfrontal eth-

moidectomy). The observation that disease tends to persist or recur in this area therefore argues strongly in favor of the use of telescopes for at least this portion of the procedure if recurrence is to be minimized.

Any residual disease or hypertrophic regenerating mucosa identified during the postoperative period is cleaned under topical anesthesia as part of the outpatient follow-up visit. Frequently a small area of bony osteitis will be identified underneath the mucosa and this is then also resected. The frequency of follow-up during the healing period is dependent on the severity of disease and the postoperative endoscopic findings. Patients with limited disease may require minimal cleaning and heal rapidly, but patients with severe longstanding diffuse disease and extensive osteitis may require long-term follow-up and frequent cleaning if late recurrence is to be avoided. Postoperative medical therapy is similarly based on the endoscopic appearance following surgery. The use of normal saline sprays is usually initiated in the postoperative period. However, if severe crusting is present, saline irrigations may be required. The patients are typically given broad spectrum antibiotic coverage in the early postoperative

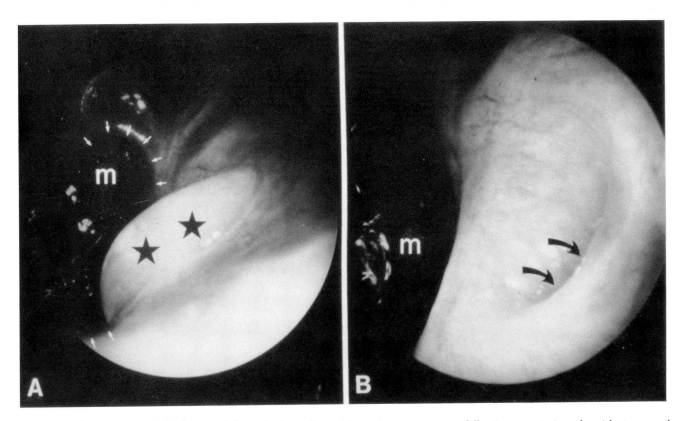

Figure 7. *Endoscopic view (70° telescope, left nose) of a patient with persistent symptoms following an anterior ethmoidectomy and middle meatal antrostomy. (A) Examination reveals thick mucus (stars) arising from the natural ostium of the maxillary and reentering the sinus through the iatrogenic middle meatal antrostomy (arrows). M, maxillary sinus. (B) After the mucus has been suctioned away, the natural ostium of the maxillary sinus can be identified (curved arrows). It becomes clear that the middle meatal antrostomy does not connect with the natural ostium.*

period. In the presence of severe infection, or endoscopic evidence of persistent inflammation, antibiotic therapy is aggressive and may be prolonged. Aerobic and anaerobic mucosal cultures are used as a guide to therapy. Anaerobic coverage is usually considered important even in the absence of definitive culture.[14-16] Again, however, the endoscopic appearance of the mucosa provides the most important therapeutic guide. Similarly, the appearance of the mucosa aids in the titration of oral steroid therapy when this is indicated, providing a significantly more sensitive method of evaluation for persistent disease than reliance on patient symptoms.

For the future, the problem of training others in FES must be overcome if unacceptably high complication rates are to be avoided. We are currently equipping a permanent endoscopic laboratory for resident anatomic dissection. However, in the operating room even the addition of a small CCD camera and beam splitter adds significant weight to the telescope. This makes the endoscope more traumatic to the mucosa, particularly in the hands of an inexperienced surgeon. Lighter and more light-sensitive cameras and beam splitters are essential if a good level of intraoperative visualization is to be achieved.

CONCLUSION

The use of routine comprehensive nasal endoscopy and advanced CT techniques had dramatically improved our ability to identify disease within the critical area of the ostiomeatal complex, and this is the greatest advantage of the functional endoscopic approach. During the postoperative period endoscopic examination dramatically improves our ability to identify residual disease. Careful evaluation during this period supports the necessity for aggressive postoperative medical and surgical treatment.

The use of endoscopes at surgery is subordinate to their use for diagnosis and postoperative care. Functional endoscopic surgery is of greatest benefit when careful diagnosis demonstrates a limited medically irreversible cause for extensive disease, and this cause can be removed endoscopically. Widely differing complication rates have occurred, demonstrating that endoscopic surgical techniques are not for every otolar-

yngologist. This will probably remain true even as the surgical approach continues to replace traditional techniques in our residency training programs, and therefore it will be important to provide experience with standard surgical techniques. In well-trained hands, however, FES offers major advantages in reducing operative morbidity and improving intraoperative visualization. The surgery is facilitated by the use of suction forceps and the KTP-532 laser.

REFERENCES

1. Kennedy DW, Zinreich SJ, Rosenbaum A, Johns ME. Functional endoscopic sinus surgery: theory and diagnostic evaluation. Arch Otolaryngol 111:576–582, 1985.
2. Messerklinger W. Endoscopy of the Nose. Munich: Urban and Schwartzenberg, 1978.
3. Messerklinger W. On the drainage of the normal frontal sinuses of man. Acta Otolaryngol 63:176–181, 1967.
4. Messerklinger W. Uber die Drainage der Menschlichen Nasennebenholen unter Normalen und Pathologischen Bendingungen: II. Mitteilung: Die Stirnhohle und ihr Ausfuhrungssystem. Monatsschr Ohrenheilkd 101:313–326, 1967.
5. Proctor DF. The nose, paranasal sinuses and pharynx. In: Walters W, ed. Lewis-Walters Practice of Surgery, Vol. 4. Hagerstown: WF Prior Co., 1966 pp 1–37.
6. Carenfelt C. Pathogensis of sinus empyema. Ann Otol Rhinol Laryngol 88:16–20, 1979.
7. Aust R, Drettner B. Oxygen tension in the human maxillary sinus under normal and pathological conditions. Acta Otolaryngol (Stockh) 78:264–269, 1974.
8. Drettner B. The obstructed maxillary ostoium. Rhinology 5:100, 1967.
9. Stankiewicz JA. Complications of endoscopic intranasal ethmoidectomy. Laryngoscope 97:1270–1273, 1987.
10. Kennedy DW et al. Endoscopic middle meatal antrostomy: theory, technique and patency. Laryngoscope 97(suppl 43):No 8, Part 3, August 1987.
11. Stammberger H. Endoscopic sinus surgery: complications and results. Paper presented before the American Rhinologic Society, September 18, 1987.
12. Wigand ME. Transnasal ethmoidectomy under endoscopical control. Rhinology 19:7, 1981.
13. Kennedy DW. Surgery of the sinuses. In: Johns ME, ed. Complications in Head and Neck Surgery, Vol II. New York: BC Decker Inc, 1986.
14. Brook I. Bacteriologic features of chronic sinusitis in children. JAMA 246:967–969, 1981.
15. Karma P, Jokipii L, Sipilä P, Luotonen J, Jokipii AMM. Bacteria in chronic maxillary sinusitis. Arch Otolaryngol 105:386–290, 1979.
16. Su W-Y, Liu C, Hung S-Y, Tsai W-F. Bacteriological study in chronic maxillary sinusitis. Laryngoscope 93:931–934, 1981. □

Chapter XXXII

Controlled Studies of Immunotherapy in Allergic Rhinitis — A Critical Review

William Franklin, M.D.

ABSTRACT

Evidence from twelve controlled studies of good experimental design, using the principles of random assignment of patients, placebo control and blind evaluation, supports the conclusion that immunotherapy can be effective in allergic rhinitis, and that this effect is specific and dose related. Ragweed pollen, grass pollen, tree pollen, cat dander, and mites have been studied, but the effect is probably more general. Whether to use immunotherapy and which extracts to use, cannot be answered entirely by such studies and requires clinical judgment.

Injections of grass pollen extract were first reported to be effective in hayfever over seventy years ago.[1] The premise that specific substances in the environment, generally harmless, caused symptoms in susceptible individuals and that injections of extracts of these substances over a long period of time would alleviate symptoms became widely held before specific IgE and IgG were recognized as factors in the process. At first, this approach was called desensitization, but when it became clear that skin reactivity was not depleted by the process, the term hyposensitization was substituted. We now recognize the possible role of specific IgG blocking antibodies, and regulatory T cells, and the failure of clinical response to correlate well with any immunologic parameter. The term immunotherapy does not commit itself to which immunologic mechanism may be responsible for clinical response and is therefore more appropriate. This

One Hawthorne Place, Boston, MA 02114.

subject has been well reviewed by experienced allergists who draw somewhat differing conclusions.[2,3]

During the first half of this century no adequately controlled studies of this form of treatment were carried out. Based on uncontrolled observations of patients, however, using the patients' recollections of the past as a comparison, a consensus was formed which may be termed "standard immunotherapy." This may be briefly stated as follows: treatment to tolerance with extracts of pollens, dust and molds over a period of months was effective in both allergic rhinitis and asthma, but not in atopic dermatitis.

At the same time, other 'unconventional techniques' of immunotherapy were gaining adherents — low doses given coseasonally or perennially with the expectation that a prompt relief of symptoms would occur.[4] This scheme had variations, based on the use of skin titrations to determine the correct dose to achieve the desired result. Others were using immunotherapy in conditions other than asthma and rhinitis, sometimes administering small doses of foods to patients who had no evidence of an abnormal immunologic response to the food, in the hope of provoking symptoms and then relieving those same symptoms.

Even physicians who were otherwise in the main stream of allergy treated patients with bacterial vaccines in the belief that allergy to bacterial flora in the respiratory tract played a role in causing asthma or rhinitis and that injections of vaccines made from these organisms would help relieve these conditions in the long run. No well-controlled studies supporting their efficacy have appeared. The lack of credibility of these techniques has been transferred to immunotherapy in general by the rest of the medical profession and the public.

Allergists failed to fully appreciate the importance of factors other than the treatment itself that could lead to an apparently successful therapeutic result. It would be well to review some of these factors listed in Table 1. They are especially important in the case of a treatment that is only partially effective over a prolonged period of time in a chronic fluctuating disease that can be influenced by many varying factors in the environment.

Patients expect treatment to be effective and will assume that they would be worse without it. Physicians also assume that treatment is effective and will explain away their failures and take credit for their successes. It is not known whether there is a real "placebo" effect in such a chronic form of treatment similar to that which may be related to endorphins in acute treatment.

The decision to begin immunotherapy is often made after a relatively bad season. The next season may be less severe. Regular visits to the physician for injections may permit better regulation of symptoms with medication and better environmental control than would occur without such frequent contacts. Many patients with the common allergic syndromes improve spontaneously over a period of years, and this might occur coincidentally with treatment.

Although most of these factors tend to favor the conclusion that treatment is effective, bias can work both ways. Patients and physicians may conclude that anything less than full relief of symptoms represents treatment failure or attribute too much to the use of drugs.

The need for controlled studies was finally recognized, and reports of studies began to appear. The experimental design varied and some of these studies had serious flaws. The major requirements of a properly done study are listed in Table II.

I. SELECTION OF SENSITIVE CASES.

If immunotherapy is specific, then only those patients whose symptoms are primarily due to the allergen being studied could be expected to show a significant response. It may be difficult to accurately define such patients. Most patients are selected on the basis of a consistent history and positive skin tests. However, other allergens may be causing symptoms at the same time. For example, during the ragweed season symptoms may also be due to dust, mites and molds, as well as other weeds. Furthermore, many patients with the common allergic syndromes also have symptoms on a non-allergic basis. These factors may mask any effect of specific immunotherapy. To get around this problem, patients with pollen sensitivity have been selected for study who have little or no trouble at other seasons. Such an approach does not work with dust, mites or other ubiquitous allergens. The use of provocative tests may increase the odds that the patient's symptoms can be produced by the allergen in question, but does not guarantee that the allergen is the major cause of symptoms. Most studies will therefore include some patients whose symptoms are at least in part due to other factors, which may obscure the effect of treatment.

II. RANDOM ASSIGNMENT.

It is essential that all patients be selected from the same pool and, then, randomly assigned to treatment or control groups. This is true of all controlled studies, whether of immunotherapy or any other form of treatment. Pairing prior to assignment helps to assure equal sized groups and may permit matching of cardinal characteristics, which is important if the total number of patients is small. It is the hope that factors which cannot be paired will balance out if the groups are large enough. Comparison of patients who come in for treatment in one season with those who present themselves in another season is not valid. Nor is it valid to compare patients who opt for

Table I.

Factors Other Than Effect of Treatment Which May Lead to Favorable Results.

1. Patient bias
2. Physician bias
3. Placebo effect
4. Seasonal variation
5. Concomitant use of other measures
6. Natural history of disease

Table II.

Essential Features of Well Controlled Study of Immunotherapy.

1. Selection of sensitive cases
2. Random assignment
3. Placebo control
4. Adequate dose
5. Blind evaluation
6. Sensitive index of response
7. Adequate analysis of data

treatment with those who reject treatment for any of a variety of reasons.

III. PLACEBO CONTROL.

The placebo effect has been shown to have a chemical basis in certain therapeutic situations. Whether or not endorphins play a role in allergic syndromes, it is possible that other mechanisms may operate. It is, therefore, important that patients do not know which form of treatment is given. All groups should feel that there is a chance that they are receiving either active or inactive treatment. Furthermore, unless the placebo is indistinguishable from the real treatment to both patient and staff, it is too easy for the "blindfold to slip."

When a new form of immunotherapy is compared with standard immunotherapy, it is important to design the study so that it will not be apparent who gets the new form of treatment. Otherwise the dictum "Use the new drugs while they still have the power to cure" may operate.

IV. BLIND EVALUATION.

Bias can have a major influence on the patient's and physician's evaluation not only of symptoms, but even physical findings and laboratory studies. Procedures as seemingly objective as the counting of white cells[5,6] can be misinterpreted by a biased observer. The "cytotoxic test" for allergy is a case in point.[7] It is doubtful that a quantitive system for scoring symptoms and medication can eliminate the need for blind evaluation on the part of both the patient and observer (double blind).

V. ADEQUATE DOSAGE.

Intuition leads one to believe that there must be a dose response curve for immunotherapy and that even if some forms of immuntherapy prove to be effective, some of the low dose regimens would not be. There is evidence that the dose response curve is not flat even at what is considered high dose immunotherapy, and negative studies which use much lower doses should not be considered evidence that immunotherapy per se is ineffective.

VI. SENSITIVE INDEX OF RESPONSE.

Immunotherapy may be only partially effective in a large proportion of patients. Too blunt an index of response may fail to detect any difference between effective treatment and control. Various quantitative symptom and medication scores have been devised to permit more ready discrimination between patients and to permit better statistical analysis.

VII. ADEQUATE STATISTICAL ANALYSIS.

It is important to show the significance of any differences that may be observed. In most studies of immunotherapy, there is difficulty in assembling large enough samples of sensitive cases. Because of the great variability in response and the inability to exclude non-sensitive cases, even an effective form of immunotherapy might produce a response which differs from the controls of a "p" value greater than 0.05. It is better to report the actual "p" value than merely to state that the results are not significant. This helps the design of future studies. Furthermore, if the two studies of the same allergen show a "p" value of less than 0.2, then the combined probability becomes significant.

No matter how carefully designed, it is possible for studies to be biased. Two modifications of "Murphy's Law" apply to controlled studies.
1. If the "Blindfold" can drop, it will.
2. If bias can creep in, it will.
It is important to make sure that if the treatment that one patient is receiving becomes apparent, it will not identify the entire group. If patients are paired, and each member of the pair assigned to treatment or controlled groups, then identification of one member of the pair identifies only the other member and not any other subject in the study. Patients should have individual treatment extracts. If possible, whoever assigns the patients to treatment groups and keeps the "code" until it is broken should have nothing to do with the evaluation of patients. Preferably evaluators should be different from those giving treatment. These precautions ought to be stated in the paper.

There are not many studies which fulfill all of the above criteria. However, I believe that there are conclusions that can be drawn from those studies which seem adequately controlled. These are listed in Table III.[8-19]

There is overwhelming evidence that immunotherapy with ragweed pollen extract is effective. The first study by Lowell and Franklin[9], in 1963, compared patients treated with multiple allergens with those treated with a placebo. The treated patients did better than the controls during the ragweed season, but the difference was not statistically significant until the third season of treatment. This study included patients with symptoms due to a wide variety of allergens. In a second study[10], previously treated patients were selected who were observed to have both a clear-cut rise in symptoms during the ragweed season and a symptom-free period at some other time of the year. Thus, all patients demonstrated a major contribution from ragweed and a minimal contribution from any perennial allergen or from coincident non-allergic rhinitis. The treated group was given a mixture of all allergens which were deemed clinically significant, including ragweed. The control group was treated with other allergens, but not ragweed. This study showed that treatment was not only effective, but specific. A third study[12] compared the effect of high doses of ragweed with

Table III. — Controlled Studies of Immunotherapy in Rhinitis*

Year	Authors	Allergen	Placebo or Control	Case Selection	Max Dose	Evaluation Index	Patients	Control	"p"
1954	Frankland Augustin	(2) Grass	(3)	HST (4) O Sy off season	20,000 Noon units	Sy Score	100	100	0.001
1963	Lowell Franklin	Multiple	CGH	HST	0.2-0.5cc 1/30 w/v	Sy & drug score	53	59	0.01-0.05
1965	Lowell Franklin	Ragweed	CGH & other allergens	HST Sy while treated	0.1-0.5cc 1:100 to 1:20	Sy & drug score	12	12	0.01
1966	Fontana Holt Mainland	Ragweed	Tannic acid & glycerine	HST	?? 1-2cmm swelling	Sy free days drug need	35	35	<0.05
1967	Franklin Lowell	Ragweed	Ragweed low dose + CGH	HST Sy while treated	0.3 1/50 vs 0.3 1/1000	Sy & drug score	12	13	0.025
1967	Lichtenstein Norman Winkenwerder	Ragweed AgE	Buffered saline & histamine	HST Histamine release	2815 μg total	Sy score Histamine release	22	18	0.01
1969	Reisman Wicher Arbesman	Ragweed AgE	Ragweed	HST	24,000 vs 7000 AgE	Sy & drug score	18	18	0.3 (NS)
1969	Sadan (1) et al	Ragweed	Minimal dose of Ragweed	HST Histamine release	3500 PNU	Sy Score	17	18	<0.001
1976	Pence et al	Mountain cedar	CGH	HST	0.3 1/50 w/v	Sy score	17	15	<0.01
1978	Warner et al	Tyrosine absorbed mites	Tyrosine Suspension	HST + bronchial challenge	400 Noon Units	Sy & drug score + Subjective	23	22	<0.05
1980	Van Metre	Ragweed	CGH + low dose ragweed	HST 0 ST molds 0 Sy JulOctNov	0.3 cc 1/100 (11.1 μg AgE)	Sy score	15	14 15	<0.01
1981	Grammer et al	Polymer Ragweed	CGH	HST	6250 PNU (125 μg AgE)	Sy score	21	21	0.02

Legend.

* *Employing random assignment, placebo control and blind evaluation.*

1. *Not explicitly stated that assignment was random or evaluation blind.*

2. *AgE = antigen E*

3. *CGH = caramelized glucose and histamine*

4. *HST — history and skin tests*

5. *Sy-Symptom*

doses $\frac{1}{20}$th as large. All patients selected were treated with high doses of ragweed up until June. In June, the patients were randomly assigned to a low dose or a high dose group. The low dose group was given a comprehensive mixture with only $\frac{1}{20}$th the ragweed concentration. The high dose group received the treatment mixture at full doses of ragweed. There was a significant difference in symptom scores during the subsequent ragweed season. This indicated not only that dosage was important, but that the effect of dose wore off within a three month period. It also confirmed that treatment was specific.

The efficacy of immunotherapy with ragweed pollen extract and the importance of dosage was confirmed by the investigators at Johns Hopkins.[13] They failed to detect the difference between treated and controlled groups at low dosage, but when they switched to high doses of ragweed antigen E, they noted a clear-cut difference. Although not statistically significant, there is evidence that antigen E is somewhat less effective than whole ragweed extract, based on one well controlled study.[15] Another study from Johns Hopkins showed that high dose treatment with ragweed pollen extract was effective in children.[14] However, it was not explicitly stated that assignment was random or that evaluation was blind. In a double blind, randomly assigned, placebo controlled study designed primarily to study the Rinkel technique of low dosage immunotherapy, Van Metre[19] and his associates showed that patients treated by this technique did no better than a placebo-treated group, whereas the control group treated with high doses of ragweed extract, did much better.

The one controlled study which draws different conclusions[11] used symptom-free days to evaluate response without regard to whether symptoms might have been reduced in frequency or severity without disappearing entirely. This is too blunt an index for the evaluation of treatment which is only partially effective. Furthermore, their method of analysis ignored "p" values of less than 0.05 in their largest group. Finally, the doses given were not explicitly stated. They stopped advancing the dose if there was one or two centimeter local swelling. This may result in a maintenance dose too low to give a full effect.

Recently an excellent controlled study[18] showed that polymerized ragweed is effective. This study, however, does not tell us whether it is more or less effective than treatment with unpolymerized extract. The potential advantage of this approach makes it most important to compare the two methods directly, preferably using, in addition, a placebo control with all three groups randomly assigned from the same pool of patients.

The first well-controlled study of immunotherapy in rhinitis[8] showed that grass pollen is effective 43 years after Noon's initial study. There is also excellent evidence[16] that treatment with mountain cedar pollen is effective.

The only evidence that immunotherapy with dust has an effect in rhinitis comes from a study of asthmatics[17], selected by inhalational challenge with extracts of dermatophagoides pteronyssinus, the house dust mite. Forty-five of the fifty-one patients also had rhinitis, and this was significantly improved following treatment.

There is evidence that animal dander immunotherapy is effective in asthma.[20–22] but no studies have been done in rhinitis.

Since there is good evidence that immunotherapy is effective with dust antigens and cat dander as well as ragweed, grass and tree pollens, it is probably reasonable to assume that it would be effective against other clinically important allergens that produce positive immediate wheal and flare reactions or specific IgE. It will be difficult to prove the efficacy of all the allergens currently in use. Because treatment is specific, it is important to include all significant allergens. However, since the effect is dose related, putting too many allergens in a treatment mixture may dilute each one too much.

Perhaps more important than which allergens to use is which patients to treat. Unfortunately, controlled studies are easier to do on the patients who may need immunotherapy the least. Patients with symptoms limited to a single pollen season may not need to be burdened with a prolonged program of injections if they can be kept comfortable with a drug regimen, even if that regimen includes steroids for a short period. Patients with perennial symptoms are more in need of help. Many of these patients react by skin test to pollens, dust, molds and danders. We generally include all of these in a comprehensive treatment mixture, if exposure cannot be avoided. But it is impossible to define the role of each.

I believe that it is time for allergists to leave the question of whether immunotherapy is effective in rhinitis, and study how to make it better. How much? How often? For what duration? We need to answer these questions. We also do not know when treatment becomes effective.

Finally, we must consider the adverse effects of immunotherapy. Immediate local and systemic reactions are a constant problem. In a retrospective survey completed at times by unrelated third parties, rare deaths have been reported especially in unskilled hands.[23] It is hoped that modified allergens may reduce this risk which often prevents achieving adequate dosage levels. In most controlled studies, apparent systemic reactions have occurred in the placebo-treated group. In the study using polymerized ragweed[18], systemic reactions seem to be reduced.

Modifications of allergenic extracts may prove to be safer and even more effective than plain aqueous extracts, but each modification will require controlled studies employing the principles discussed before it can

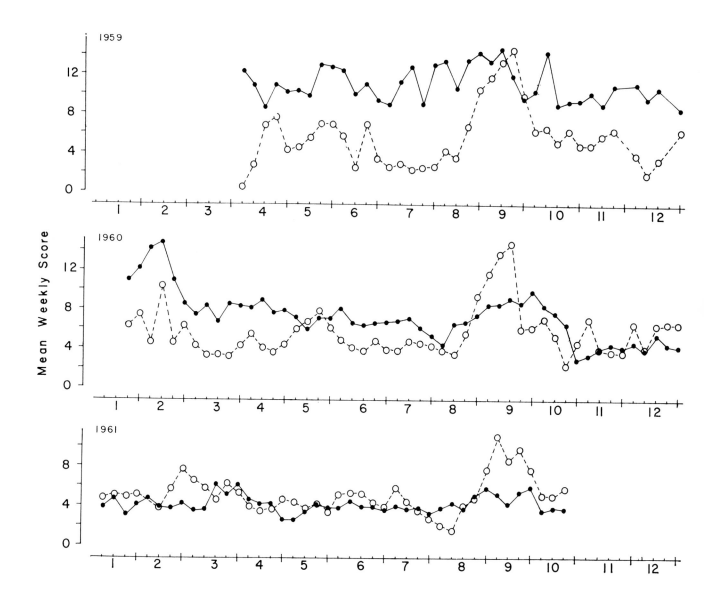

Figure 1. *Solid dots and lines represent the treated group, and the circles and the broken lines represent the untreated group. Numbers on the horizontal axis are months of the year. (Printed with permission from J Allergy Clin Immunol 34:165, 1963.)*

be accepted for clinical use.

There has been great concern that prolonged high dose immunotherapy might lead to adverse effects from circulating immune complexes. So far there is no evidence that this occurs, nor have any other long term effects been noted.

Some patients seem to be made symptomatically worse, at least early in the course of immunotherapy. That this may not be a rare phenomenon is suggested by the data shown in Figure 1, taken from our first study of immunotherapy. The treated group had a much higher symptom score than the control group during the first year of treatment. Some patients claim that they develop year-round symptoms while being treated, whereas they had only seasonal symptoms before.

Whether immunotherapy should be used or not' depends largely on how well patients can be controlled by other measures. More effective and safer forms of immunotherapy will increase the indications for its use; whereas, if new drugs become available that are better tolerated and more effective, the need for immunotherapy will be less. At the present state of the art, however, the motto "Allergists can do it better" applies for many patients.

REFERENCES

1. Noon L. Prophylactic innoculation against hayfever. Lancet 1:1572, 1911.
2. Patterson R, Lieberman P, Irons JS, Pruzansky JJ, Melam HL, Metzger WJ, Zeiss CR. Immunotherapy. In: Allergy Principles and Practice. Middleton EJ, Reed CE, Ellis EF (Eds.) St. Louis, MO, CV Mosby Co., 1978, pp 2:877.
3. Norman PS. Using immunotherapy to treat respiratory allergy. J Respir Dis 3:25, 1982.
4. Rinkel HJ. The management of clinical allergy. Part III. Inhalant allergy therapy. Arch Otolaryngol 77:205, 1963.
5. Squier TL, Lee HJ. Lysis in vitro of sensitized leukocytes by ragweed antigen. J Allergy Clin Immunol 18:156, 1947.
6. Franklin W, Lowell FC. Failure of ragweed pollen extract to destroy white cells from ragweed-sensitive patients. J Allergy Clin Immunol 20:375, 1949.
7. American Academy of Allergy. Position statements — Controversial techniques. Cytotoxic testing. J Allergy Clin Immunol 67:333, 1981.
8. Frankland EW, Augustin R. Prophylaxis of summer hayfever and asthma. A controlled trial comparing crude grass pollen extracts with isolated main protein components. Lancet 1:1055, 1954.
9. Lowell FC, Franklin W. "Double blind" study of treatment with aqueous allergenic extracts in cases of allergic rhinitis. J Allergy Clin Immunol 34:165, 1963.
10. Lowell FC, Franklin W. A double-blind study of the effectiveness and specificity of injection therapy in ragweed hayfever. N Engl J Med 273:675, 1965.
11. Fontana VJ, Holt LE, Mainland D. Effectiveness of hyposensitization therapy in ragweed hayfever in children. JAMA 201:915, 1967.
12. Franklin W, Lowell FC. Comparison of two dosages of ragweed extract in the treatment of pollenosis. JAMA 201:915, 1967.
13. Lichtenstein LM, Norman PS, Winkenwerder W. Clinical and in vitro studies on the role of immunotherapy in ragweed hayfever. Am J Med 44:514, 1968.
14. Sadan N, Rhyne MB, Melits ED, Goldstein EO, Levy DA, Lichtenstein L. Immunotherapy of pollenosis in children: investigation of the immunologic basis of clinical improvement. N Engl J Med 280:623, 1969.
15. Reisman RE, Wicher K, Arbesman CE. Immunotherapy with antigen E. J Allergy 44:82, 1969.
16. Pence HL, Mitchell DQ, Greeley RL, Updegraff BR, Selfridge HD. Immunotherapy for mountain cedar pollenosis. J Allergy Clin Immunol 58:39, 1976.
17. Warner JO, Soothill JF, Price JF, Hey EN. Controlled trial of hyposensitization to dermatophagoides pteronyssinus in children with asthma. Lancet 2:912, 1978.
18. Grammer LC, Zeiss CR, Suszko IM, Shaughnessy MA, Patterson R. A double-blind, placebo-controlled trial of polymerized whole ragweed for immunotherapy of ragweed allergy. J Allergy Clin Immunol 69:494, 1982.
19. Van Metre TE, Adkinson NF, Amodio KJ, Lichtenstein LM, Mardiney MR, Norman PS, Rosenberg GL, Sobotka AK, Valentine MD. Comparative study of the effectiveness of the Rinkel method and the current standard method of immunotherapy for ragweed pollen hayfever. J Allergy Clin Immunol 66:500, 1980.
20. Taylor WW, Ohman JL, Lowell FC. Immunotherapy in cat induced asthma. J Allergy Clin Immunol 61:283, 1978.
21. Ohman JL, Findlay SR, Leitermann --. Immunotherapy in cat-induced asthma. J Allergy Clin Immunol 74:230–239, 1984.
22. Creticos PS, Norman PS. Immunotherapy with allergens. JAMA 258:2874–2880, 1987.
23. Luckey RF, Benedict LM, Turkeltraub PC et al. Fatalities from immunotherapy (It) and skin testing (St). J Allergy Clin Immunol 79:660–677, 1987.

Chapter XXXIII
Modified Antigens and the Immune Response

T. P. King, Ph.D.

ABSTRACT

A brief review is given of the types of chemically modified antigens that have been studied as possible reagents for immunotherapy in allergic diseases. The modified antigens retain the property of native antigens to induce suppression of specific IgE levels in sensitized mice, and this suppression is dependent on the dose and on the immune state of the mice.

Patients usually can be treated with larger doses of the modified antigens than the native antigens because of their reduced allergenicity. Patients treated with modified or native antigens show similar changes of their specific IgE and IgG levels.

The use of modified antigens, such as bacterial toxoids and attenuated viruses, is a common practice for the control of infectious diseases. However, the use of modified antigens for the treatment of allergic diseases is not yet a common procedure. Among the early reports on the use of modified pollen extracts for the treatment of hay fever were those by Carter in 1935,[1] Cooke and colleagues in 1936,[2,3] and Naterman in 1938.[4] Since that time, there has been continued interest in this area of research in different laboratories.[5-19] Recent studies received new impetus from findings in mice[20] and rats,[21] to the effect that the specific IgE antibody responses are more readily suppressed on increasing antigen dose than are the specific IgG antibody responses. Better understanding of the cellular mechanism for regulation of IgE antibody synthesis[22-24] also stimulated such studies.

The types of modifications that have been tried to reduce the allergic activity of the antigens while retaining the immunogenic activity can be divided into three broad categories: (1) physical adsorption to a carrier to permit slow but continuous release of antigens, (2) chemical change of the structures of antigens to alter the number and/or the nature of antigenic determinants, and (3) a combination of physical adsorption and chemical changes of the antigens. In the first category of physical adsorption, we have alum adsorbed pollen extracts[3,6] and vegetable[4] and mineral oil[5] emulsions of pollen extracts. Two representative examples in the third category of modified antigens are the alum precipitated pyridine pollen extracts[7] and the tyrosine absorbed glutaraldehyde polymerized pollen extracts.[8]

The second category of chemically modified antigens can be divided further into four types: (1) denatured antigens on heat,[3] alkali,[7] or urea treatments;[9,10] (2) antigen fragments obtained by chemical degradation;[11,12] (3) antigens polymerized by treatment with formaldehyde[1,3,13] or glutaraldehyde,[8,14] and (4) conjugates of antigens with nonimmunogenic polymers such as alkoxypolyethylene glycols (PEG),[15-17] and copolymer of D-glutamic acid and D-lysine (DGL),[15,18] or antigen conjugates with lectins[19] or immunoglobulins.[19]

Depending on the extent and the type of their modification, the modified antigens show varying degrees of reduction of allergenic activity in humans. The denatured antigens show several thousandfold or greater decrease in allergenic activity. They apparently lack the antigenic determinants of the native antigen recognized by the host's antigen-specific B-cells, since they do not combine with animal or human antibodies that are specific for the native antigens. The denatured antigens are thought to retain the antigenic determinants of the native antigens that are recognized by the host's antigen-specific T-cells, since the denatured antigens induce suppression of antigen-specific IgE antibody responses

Professor, Rockefeller University, New York, New York

in mice.[10] Similarly, antigen fragments obtained on proteolysis were indicated to retain the T-cell specific determinants of the native antigen;[11] such fragments were reported to induce suppression of IgE responses specific for the intact antigen although they were only capable of inducing antibody responses specific for the fragments.[12] The polymerized antigens and conjugates of antigens with different polymers show varying decreases of allergenic activity ranging from severalfold to a hundredfold. These decreases probably are associated with changes in antigenic valency of modified antigens, and/or their affinities for antibodies, on introduction of bulky groups into the antigen molecules. It is generally accepted that the allergenic activity depends on the interaction of a multivalent antigen with cell-bound IgE antibodies.[25]

Laboratory studies suggest that some modified antigens, such as alkoxyPEG or DGL-coupled ragweed antigen E[15,16] are less immunogenic on a molar basis for specific antibody responses in mice than are the native antigens, but they are slightly more effective in inducing IgE antibody suppression than are the native antigens. The duration and the degree of suppression of IgE antibody response were found to depend on the dose and the immune state of the mice. The strongest suppression was observed with unprimed or weakly primed mice that had very low antibody levels at the time of treatment, while the weakest suppression was observed with primed mice that had high antibody levels at the time of treatment.[15]

Antibody response of IgE isotype, like those of other IgG isotypes, is under the control of helper and suppressor T-cells. The different degrees of suppression of IgE responses observed on treatment of primed or weakly primed mice probably reflect their relative levels of helper and suppressor T-cells. Primed mice have elevated levels of antigen-specific helper T-cells, while the weakly primed mice do not. Therefore it is difficult to induce the antigen-specific suppressor T-cells in primed mice without concomitantly expanding the antigen-specific helper T-cells.[22]

In the past ten years or so, there have been several reports on the treatment of hay fever patients with modified ragweed antigens, namely alum-adsorbed,[6] formaldehyde-treated,[26] glutaraldehyde-treated,[14] urea-denatured,[27] DGL-coupled,[28] and alkoxyPEG-coupled ragweed antigens.[28] The following generalizations may be stated: Hay fever patients usually can be treated with greater cumulative doses of these modified pollen antigens in fewer injections than those of the native pollen antigens, and they show symptom relief comparable to those of patients treated with the native antigens. Patients treated with modified antigens show changes in their antigen-specific IgE and IgE antibody responses similar to those treated with the native antigens. Following one year of treatment, the patients' specific IgE antibody level usually rises by fivefold or less while their specific IgG antibody level increases twentyfold or more. However, patients treated with modified antigens and, in particular, conjugates of antigen E with alkoxyPEG appear to show a smaller increase in IgE level than do those treated with native antigens.[28] On further treatment, the specific IgE antibody level slowly decreases while the patients' specific IgG levels reach a plateau value. With the cumulative yearly dosage of hundred-μg amounts of ragweed antigen E used, there is no obvious relationship between the dosage level and the antibody responses. Results from patients treated with urea-denatured ragweed antigen[27] are an exception. In contrast to the above generalization drawn from results with other modified antigens, patients treated with denatured antigen did not show significant changes in their specific IgE or IgG antibody levels or their symptom relief.

The minimum dose of modified or native ragweed antigen E required to give observable suppression of specific IgE antibody level in a mouse was about 25 μg,[15] which is equivalent to a dose of about 25 mg for a human of 150 lb body weight. This difference in dose between human and mouse may be a factor as to why only a limited degree of suppression of IgE antibody level was observed in humans after treatment with less than mg amounts of native or modified antigen. Another possible explanation for the difference in findings between the laboratory and the clinic may be that it is difficult to induce selectively antigen-specific suppressor T-cells in patients without expanding further their helper T-cells just as is the case with antigen-primed mice.

Although the known types of modified antigens are safer to use in humans than are the native antigens, their efficacy in reducing allergic symptoms or in altering the specific IgE and IgG antibody levels has not yet been significantly better than that of the native antigens. Nor has the treatment with modified antigens at the present stage provided us with a clearer understanding of the association of symptom relief with changes in specific IgE and IgG antibody levels. It is doubtful that treatment doses of modified or native antigens in their present form can be sufficiently increased in humans to approach those used in mice to obtain near complete suppression of IgE antibody response.

Antibody synthesis is regulated by the interaction of B cells with different subsets of helper and suppressor T-cells.[24] These T-cells may be antigen-specific, or antigen-nonspecific but Ig-specific, and they each have different cell-surface markers.[29] If antigens can be chemically modified to bind selectively the appropriate suppressor T-cells, this can be a way to improve immunosuppressive activities of antigens without increasing their effective dose. The cellular uptake of a protein can be greatly enhanced when it can bind with specific cell surface receptors; indeed, such receptor-mediated uptakes are operative at extremely low protein concentration, i.e., picomolar, 10^{-12}M. This scheme of receptor-mediated protein uptake has been exploited to synthesize pharmacological reagents exhibiting cell type-specific activities.[30] Whether such modified antigen for targeted delivery will be effective for suppression of IgE response remains to be tested.

REFERENCES

1. Carter EB. Detoxified pollen extract. U.S. Patent 2010808. Nov. 5, 1935. Chem Abstr 30:575, 1936.
2. Cooke RA, Stull A, Hebald S, Loveless M, Sherman WB. A preliminary report on the preparation and use of modified (denatured) extracts in the treatment of allergic conditions. J Allergy 8:278, 1937.
3. Stull A, Cooke RA, Sherman WB, Hebald S, Hampton SF. Experimental and clinical study of fresh and modified pollen extracts. J Allergy 11:439–465, 1940.
4. Naterman HL. The treatment of hay fever by injections of pollen extract emulsified in lanolin and olive oil. N Engl J Med 218:797–802, 1938.
5. Arbesman CE, Reisman RE. Repository therapy. J Allergy 34:39–47, 1963.
6. Norman PS, Lichtenstein LM. Comparisons of alum-precipitated and unprecipitated aqueous ragweed pollen extracts in the treatment of hay fever. J Allergy Clin Immunol 61:384–389, 1978.
7. Fuchs AM, Strauss MB. The clinical evaluation and the preparation and standardization of suspensions of a new water insoluble whole ragweed pollen complex. J Allergy 30:66–82, 1959.
8. Johansson SG, Miller AC, Mullen N et al. Glutaraldehyde-pollen tyrosine: Clinical and immunological studies. Clin Allergy 4:255–263, 1974.
9. Naterman HL. Formalinized pollen protein precipitates with tannic acid or urea in desensitization treatment. J Allergy 36:226–233, 1965.
10. Takatsu K, Ishizaka K, King TP. Immunogenic properties of modified antigen E. III. Effect of repeated injections of modified antigen on immunocompetent cells specific for native antigen. J Immunol 115:1469–1476, 1975.
11. Mackerheide A, Pesce A, Michael JG. Modulation of the IgE immune response to BSA by fragments of the antigen. I. Suppression by free fragments and by fragments conjugated to homologous gamma-globulin. Cell Immunol 59:392–398, 1981.
12. Ferguson TA, Peters T Jr, Reed R, Pesce AJ, Michael JG. Immunoregulatory properties of antigenic fragments from bovine serum albumin. Cell Immunol 78:1–12, 1983.
13. Marsh DG. Allergens and the genetics of allergy. In: Sela M, ed. The Antigens, Vol. III. New York: Academic Press, pp 271–359, 1972.
14. Hendrix SG, Patterson R, Zeiss CR, et al. A multi-institutional trial of polymerized whole ragweed for immunotherapy of ragweed allergy. J Allergy Clin Immunol 66:486–494, 1980.
15. King TP, Kochoumian L, Chiorazzi N. Immunological properties of conjugates of ragweed pollen antigen E with methoxypolyethylene glycol or a copolymer of D-glutamic acid and D-lysine. J Exp Med 149:424–435, 1979.
16. King TP, Weiner C. Immunologic properties of conjugates of ragweed antigen E with various alkoxypolyethylene glycols. Int Arch Allergy Appl Immunol 66:439–446, 1981.
17. Lee WY, Sehon AH, Åkerblom E. Suppression of reaginic antibodies with modified allergens. IV. Induction of suppressor T-cells by conjugates of polyethylene glycol (PEG) and monomethoxy PEG with ovalbumin. Int Arch Allergy Appl Immunol 64:100–117, 1981.
18. Liu FT, Bogowitz CA, Bargatze RF, Zinnecker M, Katz LR, Katz DH. Immunologic tolerance to allergenic determinants: Properties of tolerance induced in mice treated with conjugates of protein and a synthetic copolymer of D-glutamic acid and D-lysine (D-GL). J Immunol 123:2456–2465, 1979.
19. King TP, Giallongo A. Some immunochemical studies of native and modified allergens. In: Bostrom H, Ljungstedt N, eds. Theoretical and Clinical Aspects of Allergic Diseases. Stockholm: Almqvist & Wiksell International, pp 215–232, 1983.
20. Levine BB, Vaz NM. Effect of combinations of inbred strain, antigen, and antigen dose on immune responsiveness and reagin production in the mouse. A potential mouse model for immune aspects of human atopic allergy. Int Arch Allergy Appl Immunol 39:156–171, 1970.
21. Jarrett EE. Stimuli for the production and control of IgE in rats. Immunol Rev 41:52–76, 1978.
22. Ishizaka K. Twenty years with IgE: From the identification of IgE to regulatory factors for the IgE response. J Immunol 135:i–x, 1985.
23. Katz DH. Regulation of the IgE system: Experimental and clinical aspects. Allergy 39:81–106, 1984.
24. Tada T. Help, suppression and specific factors. In: Paul WE, ed. Fundamental Immunology. New York: Raven Press, pp 481–517, 1984.
25. Ishizaka K. Experimental anaphylaxis and reaginic hypersensitivity. In: Samter M, ed. Immunological Diseases, Part I. Boston: Little Brown & Co., pp 164–182, 1978.
26. Norman PS, Lichtenstein LM, Kagey-Sobotka A, Marsh DG. Controlled evaluation of allergoid in the immunotherapy of ragweed hay fever. J Allergy Clin Immunol 70:248–260, 1982.
27. Norman PS, Ishizaka K, Lichtenstein LM, Adkinson NF. Treatment of ragweed hay fever with urea-denatured antigen E. J Allergy Clin Immunol 66:336–341, 1980.
28. Norman PS, King TP, Alexander JF, Kagey-Sobotka A, Lichtenstein LM. Immunologic responses to conjugates of antigen E in patients with ragweed hay fever. J Allergy Clin Immunol 73:782–789, 1984.
29. Cantor H. T Lymphocytes. In: Paul WE, ed. Fundamental Immunology. New York: Raven Press, pp 57–70, 1984.
30. Neville DM Jr, Chang TM. Receptor-mediated protein transport into cells. Curr Top Membr Transp 10:66–150, 1978.

Chapter XXXIV
The Pediatric Aspects of Allergic Rhinitis

Irving W. Bailit, M. D.

ABSTRACT

Allergic rhinitis is the most common atopic disorder in the child and one which usually follows the child into adulthood. Rhinitis may predispose the child to increased incidence of otitis media, serous otitis and chronic sinusitis. Rhinitis in childhood is more likely to be of allergic origin and, therefore, more responsive to both medical management and immunotherapy. Early recognition and treatment is of paramount importance in reducing morbidity and complications.

The allergic child is destined by virtue of his genetic inheritance to produce allergic (IgE) antibodies to various foods and/or inhalants. The most common target of this antigen-antibody interaction is the nose. This atopic susceptibility causes increased mucosal permeability of the antigen and the production of specific reaginic antibodies

Although allergic rhinitis (AR) does not affect longevity, it may have a profound effect on speech, hearing and learning ability of the child. The allergic nose also provides a suitable milieu for secondary infections of the ears, sinuses and the lower respiratory tract.

Associate in Allergy at Children's Hospital, Boston, Mass.
Clinical Instructor in Pediatrics at Harvard Medical School.

INCIDENCE

Approximately 10-20% of children have AR, and 22% have significant secondary disease.[1] Symptoms may appear as early as the first year but more commonly occur between ages 5-10 with the peak years between 10-20.

Viner and Jackman[2] studied over 1200 cases of chronic rhinitis and found 31.5% began before the age of 10 with established allergic causes in 64%. Studies among toddlers with acute and recurrent respiratory symptoms have uncovered underlying AR in over 50%.[3] In one large pediatric clinic,[4] 10% of AR diagnoses were in children below the age of 2 years, and 75% were in those less than 10 years. This data supports the fact that allergic disease of the nose is a common childhood affliction and one that may often be misdiagnosed and mismanaged.

NATURAL HISTORY

In a study of the natural appearance of allergic symptoms in infants and preschool children, Orgel[5] found rhinorrhea rather than eczema to be the earliest symptom, often associated with a positive family history of allergy, nasal eosinophilia, positive skin tests and elevation of serum IgE.

During the first two years, food may play a causative role. With increasing age, inhalants, both seasonal and perennial, become the foremost provocateurs of allergic sensitization. The earliest allergens are the household (dust mites, animals and molds). The incidence of seasonal AR increases after five years of age.

CLINICAL MANIFESTATIONS

Children exhibit classic symptoms of clear nasal secretions, congestion of the nasal turbinates, paroxysmal

277

bouts of sneezing and itching of the nose, eyes, ears and palate. Reluctance to blow the nose produces forceful backward sniffling. Conjunctival itching, redness, tearing and periorbital edema are noted during seasonal exacerbations and on exposure to animal pets.

Perennial symptoms tend to be less acute and may include frequent sore throats, increased postnasal secretions and throat clearing, recurrent nosebleeds, decreased hearing and night cough.

PHYSICAL FINDINGS

In seasonal rhinitis, typical findings consist of pale distended nasal turbinates, profuse watery rhinorrhea and frequent swiping and twitching of the nose (allergic salute). The conjunctivae become injected with increased tearing and swelling of the lids.

Chronic perennial allergy may cause obligatory mouth breathing, a gaping facies and clear to mucoid nasal secretions. Frequent swiping of the nose with upward thrusts from the heel of the hand will eventually produce a transverse nasal crease. Other features sometimes present are Dennie's line, a line fold of the lower lid extending from the medial epicanthus, and lymphoid hypertrophy of Waldeyer's ring (tonsils, adenoids, posterior pharynx). Engorgement of the nasal turbinates causes increased venous stasis and darkened circles under the eyes (allergic shiners).

Nasal polyps occur infrequently (<0.1%) with nasal allergy, especially in children. Serous otitis is a common finding and may require pneumatic otoscopy for diagnosis.

DIAGNOSIS

A comprehensive history and physical examination, followed by confirmatory laboratory studies and skin testing, will identify the allergic child and the specific offending allergens.

A positive family history is present in 50% of allergic children. There is frequently an associated history of atopic dermatitis, food allergy, wheezing or recurrent respiratory infections. Salient information should include a detailed description of symptoms, the time, place and season of occurrence, known causes, response to medication, and complications. The environmental history should disclose the potential allergens within the home, school and neighborhood. The role of non-allergic stimuli such as weather changes, chilling, activity, smoke, aerosols, and fumes should be clearly defined.

In the very young, a dietary history may uncover an etiologic relationship to nasal symptoms. The toddler crawling on carpeted floors has an intimate relationship with dust mites and animal danders. The child's bedroom is usually cluttered with a myriad of books, stuffed animals, banners, etc. The use of vaporizers enhances the mold population of the bedroom.

LABORATORY STUDIES

The demonstration of nasal eosinophils is a simple office procedure and serves to distinguish allergic rhinitis and eosinophilic non-allergic rhinitis from infectious or vasomotor rhinitis. The finding of at least 10-15% eosinophils is diagnostic. However, careful search and multiple samples may be necessary. Eosinophils will be reduced or absent during inactive clinical periods, in the presence of superimposed infection, or with food allergy. Malmberg[6] described an excellent relationship between active AR and eosinophils, especially in children (40/44). Infants up to 3 months may have nasal eosinophils unrelated to atopy.

Serum IgE levels are frequently elevated in AR, but this test is not sufficiently accurate to distinguish allergic from non-allergic rhinitis. Serum IgE levels over 20 I.U./ ml at one year of age and 100 I.U./ml at 3 years have proven to be accurate for prediction and diagnosis of allergic disease in children. However, serum IgE levels are seldom necessary for diagnosis.

Children presenting with recurrent upper respiratory infections should have quantitative immunoglobulins to rule out immunodeficiency.

SKIN TESTING

No child is too young to skin test if the history and physical findings suggest atopy. However, testing should be restricted to those allergens to which the child is exposed and compatible with the clinical history. Prick testing is the preferred method of testing followed by intracutaneous testing when indicated. RAST testing is less accurate and five times more expensive and should be used only under special circumstances when skin testing is not possible.

DIFFERENTIAL DIAGNOSES

Upper respiratory infection, either primary or secondary to underlying allergy, is the most important condition to be differentiated from nasal allergy. The nature of the secretions (clear or purulent), the duration of illness, study of nasal secretions (smear and culture), associated systemic manifestations, and localized foci of infection in the ears, sinuses, or pharynx all serve as guidelines for making this distinction.

Obstruction of nasal airways may result from congenital choanal atresia, foreign bodies, nasopharyngeal tumors, and most commonly from hypertrophied adenoids. A lateral x-ray of the nasopharynx may be required for diagnosis.

Eosinophilic non-allergic rhinitis is characterized by the absence of allergic history, absence of specific IgE antibodies on skin testing, and the presence of nasal eosinophilia. Although adult onset is more probable, it may begin in childhood.

Vasomotor rhinitis is rarely seen in the pediatric age

group. Profuse rhinorrhea and nasal obstruction in the absence of allergic history or positive skin tests or nasal eosinophils would suggest this diagnosis.

Nasal polyps are rarely seen in children. Approximately 10-20% of children with cystic fibrosis have nasal polyps associated with chronic nasal infection and sinusitis. A sweat test should be performed on all children and young adults with nasal polyps. In older children, one may see nasal polyps associated with aspirin hypersensitivity and asthma (ASA triad).

Rhinitis medicamentosa may be related to the overuse of topical vasoconstrictor medication with resultant rebound swelling of the nasal turbinates. Children are rarely exposed to systemic medication that would cause similar findings.

COMPLICATIONS

Sinusitis is a common sequela to nasal allergy. Rachelefsky[7] studied a group of 70 allergic children with chronic nasal symptoms and found 53% with abnormal sinus films including 21% with complete opacity. Persistent purulent nasal discharge and cough are the most common presenting symptoms. A Water's view of the sinuses is usually sufficient for diagnosis. Cultures of sinus aspiration are most often positive for Streptococcus pneumoniae or Haemophilus influenza.

Otitis media and middle ear effusions occur more frequently in allergic children (20-30% incidence). Earlier reports of higher incidence were not on random populations. Studies to implicate the middle ear as a direct allergic shock organ have been either inconclusive or negative. The physical changes of AR may cause eustachian tube obstruction and dysfunction, and middle ear effusion. Serous otitis is not an allergic disease but is a complication of nasal allergy.[8]

Increased lymphoid tissue of the nasopharynx is frequently associated with perennial nasal allergy. A history of multiple adenoidectomy should suggest this relationship.

In contrast to previous higher estimates, the epidemiologic studies of Smith[9] noted the transition of AR to bronchial asthma in only 5-10% of patients with AR. However, the transition from asthma to AR was found with greater frequency. Kawabori[10] found abnormal exercise tolerance on pulmonary function testing in up to 40% of nonasthmatic atopic children on free running. Decreased pulmonary function has been found on methacholine challenge in nasal allergy.

Perennial allergic rhinitis may cause facial abnormalities such as malocclusion, high arched palate, and underdevelopment of the midface. These physical changes are not reversible with allergic therapy.

TREATMENT

Realistic therapeutic goals should be directed toward achieving maximum symptomatic control where complete cure is not usually possible. The greater likelihood of allergy as the primary cause of rhinitis in childhood increases the response to the various modalities of allergic management.

Environmental control: The avoidance and elimination of proven or suspected environmental allergens is a basic concept of care (animals, feathers, molds and dust mites). The child's bedroom is a repository for many of these allergens. Detailed instructions for preparing the environment may be found elsewhere. The indoor environment should be adequately humidified (40%) during the winter heating season. HEPA air cleaners are the most effective to reduce airborne particulates, but they are not usually necessary. Air conditioning of the bedroom will decrease the pollen and the dust mite population. The avoidance of cigarette smoke, aerosols and other irritants are protective measures. The school also holds various perils (pets, plants, chalk dust) which may be aggravants. If foods are suspected, eliminate the food for 10 days and follow with food challenge.

Pharmacologic management: The antihistamines continue to be the primary agents directed toward symptom control. In competition with histamine for the H_1 receptors, they show variable effect on pruritis, sneezing and rhinorrhea, and less effect on congestion and conjunctival symptoms. Whether given singly or combined with oral decongestants, the results are unpredictable. Rotation among the different classes of antihistamines may be necessary to offset lack of response, tachyphylaxis or soporific side effects. They are less effective for perennial rhinitis. Children often tolerate this group of drugs better than adults. The newer second-generation antihistamines (H_1) offer benefits without sedative and anticholinergic side effects. Terfenidine (seldane) and astemizole (hismanal) are available and loratadine and ceterizine await arrival. These preparations are well tolerated by older children but may require supplementary oral decongestants. Bothersome eye symptoms may require liquid tears or topical vasoconstrictor-antihistamine preparations. Oral decongestants (pseudoephedrine and phenylpropanolamine) may be used alone where congestion is the primary problem. Topical vasoconstrictors should be discouraged.

Cromolyn sodium is administered as a 4% nasal solution (Nasalcrom) or as an ophthalmic (Opticrom) preparation has proven effective in controlling AR especially in the presence of increased eosinophils and elevated IgE. Nasalcrom is most effective when administered prophylactically one to two weeks before the onset of pollen season. Comparison trials with cromolyn and nasal beclomethasone have shown cromolyn to be the less effective preparation.[11]

The next sequence of pharmacologic management is the topical corticosteroids, beclomethasone (Beconase, Vancenase) and flunisolide (Nasalide). These agents are very effective, especially in children in offering effective control of both seasonal and perennial allergy. There have been many studies in children describing a 70–90% response rate.[12,13] Children can be controlled on 100–150 mg/day of flunisolide or 200–400 mg/day of beclomethasone. It is important that initial trial be extended to two weeks before evaluation of effectiveness. Studies with these two preparations have shown comparable results. These drugs are well tolerated by children and may cause only minor irritation or bleeding. The beclomethasone preparations are now available as aqueous preparations (Beconase Aq, Vancenase Aq) delivered by a pump spray rather than by chemical propellants. These preparations are often less irritating to the child. They do not cause overt systemic corticoid effects, candidiasis or atrophic changes in the nose. Aerosolized dexamethasone is an effective agent; however, systemic absorption and suppression of the hypothalmus-pituitary axis should limit use to 2–3 week periods.

Oral corticosteroids are only rarely necessary. Short bursts of prednisone may be needed for severe uncontrolled symptoms during the peak of a pollen season or for initial control of rhinitis medicamentosa or nasal polyps, substituting with topical beclomethasone or flunisolide after a 2-week course of prednisone.

Associated ear and sinus infections are best treated with ampicillin or amoxicillin. In cases of organism resistance or penicillin sensitivity, consider cefaclor, erythromycin with sulfisoxazole, or trimethoprim and sulfamethoxazole. Treatment should be continued for three weeks.

Immunotherapy: For children with proven allergic hypersensitivity unresponsive or intolerant to medical management, immunotherapy remains an effective means of control. This is especially true for seasonal rhinitis due to pollens and less true for dust mites and molds. Several controlled studies on pollen immunotherapy in children have demonstrated success rates of over 80%. Improvement has been associated with elevation of IgG blocking antibody and decrease of basophil histamine release. Aqueous extracts at highest tolerated dose on a perennial program offer the optimum clinical response. Newer aldehyde modified and polymerized extracts may someday increase the ease and response to treatment.

Indications for immunotherapy are based on 1. identification of allergic antibody and correlation with clinical history; 2. severe protracted symptoms unresponsive to environmental control measures or to antihistamines/decongestants; and 3. associated wheezing.

Children with allergic rhinitis seldom outgrow their nasal allergy (<10%) and most will spend a major part of their lifetime coping with this condition. Therefore, it becomes incumbent on the physician to recognize and treat the child early so as to offer maximum comfort and reduce complications.

REFERENCES

1. Zeiger R, Schatz M. Chronic rhinitis: a practical approach to diagnosis and treatment. Part I: Diagnosis. Imm and Allergy Practice 4:17-32, 1982.
2. Viner A, Jackman N. Retrospective survey of 1271 patients diagnosed as perennial rhinitis. Clin Allergy 6:251-259, 1976.
3. Holzel A. The allergic toddler. Practitioner 200:369, 1968.
4. Church J. Allergic rhinitis. Clin Pediatrics 19:655-659, 1976.
5. Orgel H, Kemp J, Meltzer E, et al. Atopy and IgE in a pediatric allergy practice. Ann Allergy 39:161-168, 1977.
6. Malmberg H, Holopainen E. Nasal smear as a screening test for immediate type of nasal allergy. Allergy 34:331, 1979.
7. Rachelefsky G, Goldberg M, Katz R, Boris G, Gyepes M, Shapiro M, Michey M, Finegold S, Siegel S. Sinus disease in children with respiratory allergy. J All Clin Imm 61:310-314, 1978.
8. Reisman R, Bernstein J. Allergy and secretory otitis media. Ped Clin N Am 22:251-257, 1975.
9. Smith JM. A five-year prospective survey of rural children with asthma and hayfever. J Allergy 47:23-30, 1971.
10. Kawabori I, Pierson W, Conquest L, et al. Incidence of exercise induced asthma in childhood. J All Clin Imm 58:447, 1976.
11. Brown H, Engler C, English J. Comparative trial of flunisolide and sodium cromoglycate nasal sprays in the treatment of allergic rhinitis. Clin All 11:169-173, 1981.
12. Sarsfield J, Thomson G. Flunisolide nasal spray for perennial rhinitis in children. Brit Med J 2:95-97, 1979.
13. Strem E, Austrian S, Geller G, Johnson J, Crepea S. Flunisolide nasal spray for the treatment of children with seasonal allergic rhinitis. Ann All 41:145-149, 1978.
14. Hill D, Connally D, Vorath J. Beclomethasone dipropionate aerosol in the treatment of children with severe perennial rhinitis. Med J Aust 2:603-4, 1978. □

PROCEDURES

Chapter XXXV

Allergy Skin Tests: Methodology and Comparisons

S. David Miller, M.D.,* Donald E. Klein, M.D.**

ABSTRACT

Allergy skin testing to detect specific IgE antibody remains an essential part of the work-up in patients suspected of suffering from an allergic-based disease. Proper attention to performance skills, understanding the limitations of skin testing, and the correct interpretation of results increase the yield of this important diagnostic tool. Finally, correlating skin testing results with a comprehensive history and physical exam enhances the ability to diagnose diseases with an allergic etiology.

HISTORICAL PERSPECTIVE

Since their introduction in the 1960s by Charles Harrison Blackely,[1] skin tests have been used as a diagnostic tool in allergic diseases. He noted that after applying sprinkled rye grass pollen to a scarified portion of his forearm, there developed a pruritic swelling surrounded by erythema that was eventually followed by a late cutaneous reaction. Von Pirquet's use of the scratch test with tuberculin (1907) and Schick's intracutaneous test with diphtheria were influential in promoting the broad use of skin testing in detecting immunologic-related diseases. Sir Thomas Lewis theorized that the puncture technique might be used as a method for diagnosing allergic diseases.[2] In 1911 Robert A. Cooke first employed intracutaneous testing as a

diagnostic tool in general atopic diseases. Schloss (1912) extended skin testing for the identification of suspected reactions to food allergens. For many years after their introduction, there was marked variability in allergy testing due to the use of various instruments, applications, and interpretations. In recent years, investigators have made attempts at standardization with application devices, methods (prick, intracutaneous), and testing materials (extracts, diluents), and proposed refinements of these procedures. Although introduced over 100 years ago, these diagnostic procedures (with recent modifications) remain important diagnostic tools in the evaluation of allergic diseases.

Skin testing is useful for the diagnosis of specific allergic diseases and atopic conditions. For example, skin testing facilitates detection of inhalant allergic states (allergic rhinitis, allergen-induced bronchospasm/asthma) secondary to pollens, danders, dust, and mold. Skin testing also can be applied in the diagnosis of food, antibiotic,[3] and *Hymenoptera* sensitivity.[4] Because skin testing offers the advantage of simplicity of technique, rapidity of performance, low cost, and high sensitivity,[5] it has become a major tool in the diagnosis of allergic-based diseases.

To the inexperienced practitioner, skin testing may appear to be a simple procedure that anyone can do with minimal instruction. Improper performance and/or interpretation can lead to false-positive and false-negative results. Skin testing is done to confirm a clinical suspicion of an allergic disease. As in any other diagnostic test, it is an important adjunct used in conjunction with and subordinate to a complete clinical history and physical exam. The latter two done by experienced and trained allergists are most important in making a clinical diagnosis of specific allergy

*Fellow, Division of Allergy and Immunology, Brown University Program in Medicine, and Pediatrics, Rhode Island Hospital, Providence Rhode Island.
**Clinical Associate Professor of Pediatrics; Director, Division of Allergy and Immunology, Department of Pediatrics, Rhode Island Hospital, Providence, Rhode Island.

with skin testing acting as a confirmatory aid in the diagnosis.

PATHOPHYSIOLOGIC BASIS OF SKIN TESTING

Immediate Hypersensitivity

Skin testing is employed to detect a Type 1 immunological reaction or immediate hypersensitivity. The skin sensitizing antibody (in the past called reagin) eventually determined to be immunoglobulin E (IgE), was only identified in the past 25 years.[6] IgE-mediated dermatologic responses to antigens clinically present as the classic wheal-and-flare response. This is often seen within 15–30 minutes of the application of the suspected antigen on a prepared skin site. On the cellular level, IgE antibody molecules are attached to the surface of tissue mast cells. When two IgE molecules are cross-linked by a specific antigen on the surface of the mast cell, a series of enzymatic events is initiated causing an influx of calcium, with degranulation and subsequent activation of phospholipase A2. With degranulation, the release of a variety of active mediators including histamine, ECF-A, prostaglandins and leukotrienes (formally known as SRS-A) occurs. Histamine, a potent vasoactive amine, is thought to be primarily responsible for the vasodilatation (flare), and the subsequent increase in capillary permeability (leading to the wheal) observed in positive skin reactions.

The intensity of the immediate response in sensitized individuals is related to several factors. These include (1) the amount of allergen injected or applied, (2) the degree of sensitization of the cutaneous mast cells, which is related to the amount of circulating specific IgE, (3) the reactivity to the mediators released during the degranulation of the mast cells,[7] and (4) the concomitant use of antihistamines and vasoconstrictors.

LATE ALLERGIC RESPONSE (LAR)

The immediate dermatologic response may be followed by a late-phase reaction consisting of a non-specific inflammatory, edematous reaction occurring within 6–8 hours and persisting for up to 24–48 hours.[8] The histologic picture consists of mast cell degranulation with the progressive cellular infiltration of neutrophils, eosinophils, and basophils, with or without fibrin deposition.

SKIN TESTING TECHNIQUES

The ability to diagnose hypersensitivity to specific antigens is first evaluated by a comprehensive history, taking into account the patients' symptoms in relation to their environmental and seasonal history. Familiarizing oneself with the home, environmental, occupational, and regional exposures helps identify the appropriate antigens to be selected for confirmatory skin testing.

Prior to testing, certain precautions should be taken (Table I).

Testing Extracts

Historically, physicians prepared their own extracts for testing in their office from raw materials (dried pollens, dust samples, food stuffs, and animal pelts). Methods to standardize extracts have ranged from labeling extracts in protein nitrogen units (PNU) to weight per volume (W/V). None of these units relate to the biologic potency of the materials. Attempts to quantitate this potency (in correlation with the *in vitro* RAST test), have produced the Allergy Unit (AU) as the current standardized unit for specific extracts (dust mite, cat). Recent data show that variability even exist among extracts from different manufacturers,[9] indicating the need for universal standardization.

At present commercially available extracts contain either 50% glycerol or human serum albumin as a stabilizing agent. Studies have shown there are nonspecific irritative effects induced by the glycerol that can occur in 16–50% of the population, depending on the concentration used.[10,11] A safe concentration of glycerol

---

TABLE I

Skin Testing Precautions

1. Skin tests should never be performed unless a physician is immediately available to treat systemic manifestations.
2. Have emergency equipment and medications readily available.
3. Do not test the patients if marked allergic symptoms are present.
4. Determine the diagnostic value of the allergic extracts used and assess their stability.
5. Be certain that test concentrations are appropriate.
6. Include a positive and negative control solution.
7. Perform tests on normal skin.
8. Evaluate the patient for dermatographism.
9. Determine and record medications taken by the patient and the time of the last dose.
10. Be aware of other medical conditions and medications the patient may be taking for them (i.e., beta-blockers, MAO inhibitors).
11. Record the reactions at the proper time.

Modified from Mansmann HC. Allergic tests in clinical diagnosis. In, Bierman CW, Pearlman DS (eds). Allergic Diseases of Infancy, Childhood and Adolescence. 1st Ed. Philadelphia, PA: W.B. Saunders Co., 1980, p. 293.

in the extract used for intradermal testing should be less than 2%.[10,11]

With the extensive number of extracts available for testing, physicians must avoid the ineffective, unsafe extracts once used (i.e., cigarette smoke, chalk, newsprint, etc.).[12] On the basis of the patient's history, the physician should select the extracts most appropriate for testing to confirm the clinical suspicion of an allergic-based disease.

SKIN TESTING METHODS

There are two basic approaches to allergy skin testing. These include the (1) epicutaneous (scratch, puncture, and prick methods) and (2) intracutaneous (intradermal) method. The testing site usually is cleaned with alcohol and should be totally dry before skin tests are applied.

EPICUTANEOUS TESTING

The epicutaneous tests can be performed in a variety of ways with several instruments:

Scratch Testing. With the scratch test, an abrasion is made on the superficial epidermis, and the testing extract is applied directly to the site. The tester must be careful to avoid drawing blood due to the increased possibility of obtaining false positive results, and contaminating the testing stock solutions with blood borne viruses (hepatitis, HIV). A disposable scarifier should be used.

Puncture Testing. The puncture test is performed by first placing the allergy extract on the skin surface. A disposable sterile needle or other sharp instrument is passed through the drop of testing extract into the superficial epidermis, allowing a few microliters of fluid to penetrate the puncture site. Care again must be taken to avoid drawing blood. A separate needle or repeatedly cleaned needle should be used for each puncture.

Prick Testing. This method of testing is similar to the puncture test with only minor variations. A drop of testing extract is applied to the skin surface and a sharp disposable instrument is passed through the extract and into the skin at a 45 degree angle. The skin is then lifted by the point of the instrument, thus creating a small break in the epidermis allowing entry of the allergen. Some of the many instruments used in prick testing include the standard gauge hypodermic needle, lancets (i.e., Morrow Brown, Allergy Pricker), bifurcated scarifiers, and Multitest devices. It is difficult to quantify the amount of testing extract actually introduced by the prick method. This variability of the skin response is dependent on the reliability of the device, the depth of puncture, the proper application of the device, and the force and duration of the puncture as performed by the tester.[13]

Many studies have assessed the differences between testing devices. Bosamba[14] analyzed the differences be-

tween several devices and found that the Allergy Pricker had the highest degree of reproducibility while the Morrow Brown and the standard gauge hypodermic needle displayed discrepancies within the same patient and from tester to tester. Preliminary results with the newer Phazets (lancets dipped in standardized extracts and subsequently applied to the skin) are equally effective as the modified prick testing method. Despite its limitations, the prick test is considered the most reliable of the available epicutaneous tests.[7] Some of the common errors in epicutaneous testing are described in Table II.

INTRACUTANEOUS TESTING

The intradermal test is performed by introducing testing extract into the intracutaneous area of the skin. This usually is accomplished by injection volumes of approximately 0.01 to 0.05 ml, raising a superficial bleb of 3 mm in diameter. The tester should take care not to penetrate the superficial layers of the dermis. Some of the common errors in intradermal testing are noted in Table III.

Intradermal testing is considered more sensitive than epicutaneous testing because the skin reaction is dependent on the actual dose of the extract injected. On this account, it is imperative to use more dilute extracts when performing intradermal testing. This is especially important as there is an increased incidence of symptemic anaphylaxis associated with intracutaneous testing.[15] To reduce the incidence of serious side effects (in patients with initial negative epicutaneous tests), the American Academy of Allergy and Immunology recently recommended the use of intracutaneous testing

---

TABLE II

Common Errors in Epicutaneous Testing

1. Tests are too close together, so that overlapping reactions cannot be separated visually.
2. Technique is not identical for each site, i.e., different lengths of scratches or varying intensity of scratch or puncture.
3. Too much allergen solution, which causes spreading from the site.
4. Too many tests done at a time.
5. Patient not checked for a reaction frequently enough after testing. It is particularly important to check highly sensitized individuals early, and wipe away allergen if reaction develops rapidly.

Modified from Mansmann HC. Allergic tests in clinical diagnosis. In, Bierman CW, Pearlman DS (eds). Allergic Diseases of Infancy, Childhood and Adolescence. 1st Ed. Philadelphia, PA: W.B. Saunders Co., 1980, p. 294.

TABLE III

Common Errors in Intradermal Testing

1. Tests sites are too close together.
2. Too large a volume is injected.
3. Concentration is higher than necessary.
4. Person performing test neglects to prevent or observe "splash" resulting from air injection.
5. Antigen is injected subcutaneously instead of intradermally.
6. Intracutaneous bleeding site read as an adequate test.
7. Too many tests done at a time.

Mansmann HC. Allergy tests in clinical diagnosis. In, Bierman CW, Pearlman DS (eds). Allergic Diseases of Infancy, Childhood and Adolescence. 1st Ed. Philadelphia, PA: W.B. Saunders Co., 1980, p. 295.

extracts ranging from a hundred thousand-fold dilutions of the concentrated extract solution used in the epicutaneous testing.[13]

COMPARISONS OF TESTING METHODS

Some of the advantages of each method of testing is shown in Table IV. In general, prick testing is less sensitive than intradermal tests. Intracutaneous testing provides increased sensitivity and reproducibility due to the constant amount of extract introduced into the skin. However, the degree of false positives are higher with intradermal testing due to an irritant effect from the testing solution. Therefore, positive results must be correlated with the patient's history. Prick testing is considered convenient, better tolerated by the patient,

and less expensive than intradermal testing. Most clinicians use the epicutaneous tests as one component of the initial screening work-up and proceed to intradermal testing to confirm a negative prick test, if the patient's clinical history warrants.

Whatever method of skin testing is chosen, a positive and negative control should be applied. This positive control usually consists of histamine or other releasers of mast cell mediators such as opioids and the substance 48/80. The negative control preferably should be the diluent of the initial extract.

GRADING OF SKIN TEST RESULTS

The immediate response to skin testing usually induces a response to histamine within 10 minutes, and 15–20 minutes for the allergen response.[16] Most studies recommend recording the results of testing approximately 20 minutes from the time of application. The presence of wheal and flare is the criteria for a positive skin test. Various indices using the wheal or both the wheal and flare provide a grading system for interpretation. For prick testing, these include measurements of diameters, comparisons with histamine controls (the histamine equivalent prick [HEP]), and recently the measurement of geographic areas (as defined by the perpendicular diameters of the area of a wheal reaction).[17] At this time, no universal agreement exists as to a specific standard for interpretation and recording of results. The proposed use of standardized extracts in testing may facilitate a consensus for interpretation of epicutaneous testing in the future.

As for intracutaneous testing, the same controversy over the grading of the skin response persists as noted with prick testing. A grading system widely in use in present clinical settings is shown in Table V.

TABLE IV

Advantages of Each Method of Skin Testing

Prick Testing	Intradermal Testing
1. Positive and negative more clearly distinguishable	1. Increased sensitivity
2. Safety	2. Better reproducibility
3. Speed	
4. Simplicity	
5. Little discomfort	
6. Many tests in one session	
7. Stability of extracts	
8. Positives correlate better with clinical disease	

Nelson HA. Diagnostic procedures in allergy skin testing. Ann Allergy 51:412, 1983.

TABLE V

Grading System to Measure Skin Reactions with Intradermal Tests

Grade	Erythema	Wheal
0	<5 mm	<5 mm
±	5–10 mm	5–10 mm
1+	11–20 mm	5–10 mm
2+	21–30 mm	5–10 mm
3+	31–40 mm	5–10 mm or with pseudopods
or	>40 mm	
4+		>15 mm or with many pseudopods

Reproduced by permission from Norman PS. In vivo methods of study of allergy. In Middleton E Jr, Reed CE, Ellis EF (eds). Allergy: Principles and Practice, 2 ed. St. Louis: The C.V. Mosby Co. 1983, p. 297.

FACTORS AFFECTING THE SKIN TEST

Several factors interfere with the performance of skin testing, including:

Medications. Antihistamines are the most often cited medications that interfere with skin testing. For the more common antihistamine preparations, their withdrawal for 24 to 48 hours prior to testing usually eliminates any suppression of results. However, with the introduction of the newer antihistamines with their longer half lives, the period of withdrawal of the medication may extend as long as two to three weeks. Table VI summarizes the different medications and the duration of suppression. If one is in doubt about the possible interference of a medication, a control histamine response can be used to gauge skin reactivity.

Area of the Body. Where the skin test is placed on the body has been shown to affect the results of skin testing due to the different reactivity of body areas.[18] The back is more reactive than the forearm.[19] A reason for the difference in sensitivity may be related to the number of mast cells in the area of testing.[20]

Age. Infants usually manifest less reactivity than do adult patients.[21] Recent evidence shows that there is a progressive increase in reactivity from infancy through adulthood. Reactivity then declines at age 50 and levels off by the age of 60.[22]

Circadian Rhythms. Reactivity to histamine and allergen has been shown to be influenced by the time of testing. The peak time of sensitivity appears to be in the late evening hours and the lowest in the early morning hours.[23] Recently, Vichyanond and Nelson[24] studied the reactivity of ragweed sensitive patients during morning and afternoon hours. They demonstrated that reactivity for ragweed and histamine was slightly higher in the morning hours (8 a.m.), than those results obtained during the late afternoon hours (4 p.m.). However, the difference in results was not statistically significant. They concluded that any changes that may occur during the clinical hours of most physicians should not interfere with the interpretation of skin testing results.

INTERPRETATION OF SKIN TEST RESULTS

The presence of a positive skin test by itself does not mean that the patient is clinically allergic. In fact, Lindsblad and Farr[10] demonstrated various rates of positivity (by ID testing) to house dust and pollens in patients with no history of allergic symptoms. Curran and Goldman[25] reported that one third of asymptomatic patients tested with a positive family history of allergy displayed positive skin tests. However, the presence of positive skin tests may have predictive value in the asymptomatic patient. Hagy and Settipane[26] showed that in a population of skin test positive, non-allergic patients the incidence of allergic rhinitis reached 18.2% after three years, and after seven years this rose to 32%.

To assess the value of skin testing adequately, the practitioner must be attentive to the etiologies of false positive and negative results. These may occur as a result of improper testing materials and techniques, and patient-related factors.

False Positive Results. This type of error may occur as a result of (1) tests placed too close together with the development of a nonspecific enhancement through an axonal reflex from a neighboring positive reaction. For this reason it is recommended that skin tests be placed at least 5 cm apart,[16] (2) an irritant effect secondary to a stabilizing agent added to the extract (i.e., glycerol), and (3) dermatographism.

False Negative Results. A false negative reaction can occur because of (1) procedural error where the allergen is not delivered in sufficient quantity to the appropriate skin area, (2) the skin reaction is suppressed by medications, and (3) extracts are of poor initial quality or lose their potency (either due to time or improper storage and or preservation).

IN VIVO VERSUS *IN VITRO* TESTING

In vitro diagnostic studies (see Chapter IV) provide good correlation with skin testing results to common allergens.[27-29] A recent study demonstrated that skin testing more closely correlated to clinical symptoms than to *in vitro* tests.[30] The most common discrepancy

TABLE VI

Suppression of Skin Test Results by Various Medications

Drug	Duration of Suppression (days)
Antihistamines	
Chlorpheniramine	3
Diphenhydramine	3
Promethazine	3
Tripelennamine	3
Astemizole	5–40
Clemasine	1–10
Hydroxyzine	1–10
Corticosteroids	
Methylprednisolone	0
Prednisone	0
Beclomethasone	0
Theophylline	
Aminophylline	0
Cromolyn	
Cromolyn Sodium	0
Beta Agonist	
Inhaled	0
Oral	0

TABLE VII

In vivo and *in vitro* Testing

	Advantages	Disadvantages
Skin Testing	Sensitivity Rapid Results Inexpensive Technically easy Wide variety of allergens Long established	Time consuming Uncomfortable Dependent on skin condition Affected by drugs Risk of reaction Difficult quality control
In vitro Testing	Safe Independent of skin condition Not affected by drugs Less time consuming Less discomfort	Not as sensitive Delayed results More expensive Technically more complex Difficult to control quality Variability of lab performance

Ownby D. Allergy testing: In vivo *versus* in vitro *testing. Pediatr Clin North Am. 35(5):1007, 1988.*

noted in these studies is a positive skin test with a negative RAST study. Van der Zee and colleagues[31] theorized that this is most likely due to circulating IgE that is either in low quantity or specificity, which cannot be detected by present methods. In addition, mast cells with their high content of IgE are found in tissues rather than blood.

Some of the advantages and disadvantages of *in vivo* and *in vitro* testing are outlined in Table VII. *In vitro* testing is most useful in specific instances, including (1) patients who have skin conditions (i.e., atopic dermatitis, eczema) where the performance of skin testing would be difficult, (2) those patients who are unable to stop medications (i.e., beta blockers, antihistamines, MAO inhibitors) that would interfere with skin reactivity or put the patient at risk if they were to suffer an untoward reaction, (3) those suspected individuals who are considered at risk for systemic reactions if skin testing were to be performed, (4) patients who are at a considerable distance from a skin testing center, or (5) patients who emotionally cannot tolerate *in vivo* testing.

REFERENCES

1. Taylor G, Walker J. Charles Harrison Blackley (1820–1900). Clin Allergy 3:103, 1973.
2. Lewis T. Vascular reactions of skin to injury; reaction to stroking; urticaria and factitia. Heart 11:119–39, 1924.
3. Levine DB, Zolov DM. Prediction of penicillin allergy by immunological tests. J Allergy 43:231, 1969.
4. Hunt JK, Valentine MD, Sobotka AK, Lichtenstein LM. Diagnosis of allergy to stinging insects by skin testing with *Hymenoptera* venoms. Ann Intern Med 85:56, 1976.
5. From the Practice Standards Committee, the American Academy of Allergy and Immunology; reviewed and revised March 1983. Position statement. Skin testing and radioallergosorbent testing (RAST) for diagnosis of specific allergens responsible for IgE-mediated disease. J Allergy Clin Immunol 72:515, 1983.
6. Ishizaka K, Ishizaka T, Hornbrook MM. Physiochemical properties of reaginic antibody. IV. Presence of a unique immunoglobulin as a carrier of reaginic activity. J Immunol 97:75–85, 1966.
7. Nelson HS. Diagnostic procedures in allergy. I. Allergy skin testing. Ann Allergy 51:411, 1983.
8. Dolovitch J, Hargreave FE, Chalmers R, et al. Late cutaneous allergic responses in isolated IgE-dependent reactions. J Allergy Clin Immunol 52:38, 1973.
9. Eichler I, Gotz M, Jarisch R, Eichler HG, Moss R. Reproducibility of skin prick testing with allergen extracts from different manufacturers. Allergy 43:458–463, 1988.
10. Lindblad JH, Farr, RS. The incidence of positive intradermal reactions and the demonstration of skin sensitizing antibody to extracts of ragweed and dust in humans without history of rhinitis or asthma. J Allergy 32:392, 1961.
11. Menardo JL, Bosquet J, Bataille A et al. Effects of diluents on skin tests. Ann Allergy 51:535, 1983.
12. Schaffer M, Sisk LC. Allergen extracts: A review of their safety and efficacy. Ann Allergy 52:2–14, 1984.
13. Bernstein, IL. Relevant in vivo and in vitro diagnostic tests of IgE-dependent reactions (immediate hypersensitivity): Proceedings of the Task Force on Guidelines for Standardizing Old and New Technologies Used for the Diagnosis and Treatment of Allergic Diseases. J Allergy Clin Immunol 82:487–507, 1988.
14. Basomba A, Saster A, Pelaez A et al. Standardization of the prick test. Allergy 40:395–399, 1982.
15. Lockey RF, Benedict LM, Turkeltaub PC, Bukantz SC. Fatalities from immunotherapy (IT) and skin testing (ST). J Allergy Clin Immunol 79:660–677, 1987.
16. Voorhorst R. Perfection of skin test technique. Allergy 35:247, 1980.
17. Vohlonen I, Terho EO, Koivikko A et al. Reproducibility of the skin prick test. Allergy 44:525–531, 1989.
18. Bowman KL. Pertinent factors influencing comparative skin tests on the arm. J Allergy 7:39, 1935.
19. Alexander HL, McConnel FS. The variability of skin reactions in allergy. J Allergy 2:23, 1930.
20. Eady RAJ. The mast cell in diseases of the skin. In: Pepys J, Edwards AM, ed. The Mast Cell: Its Role in Health and Disease. Bath, England: Pittman Medical, p. 544, 1979.
21. Carey TN, Gay LN. Skin reactions in infants: Susceptibility of the skin of the newborn to passive atopic sensitization: Comparison with reaction to histamine. J Allergy 5:488, 1934.
22. Skassa-Brociek W, Manderscheid JC, Michel FB, Bousquet J. Skin test reactivity to histamine from infancy to old age. J Allergy Clin Immunol 80:711–716, 1987.
23. Lee RE, Smolensky MH, Leach CS, McGovern JP. Circadian rhythms in cutaneous reactivity to histamine and selected antigens, including phase relationship to urinary cortisol excretion. Ann Allergy 38:231, 1969.
24. Vichyanond P, Nelson HS. Circadian variation of skin reactivity

and allergy skin test. J Allergy Clin Immunol 83:1101–1106, 1989.

25. Curran WS, Goldman G. The incidence of immediate reacting allergy skin test in a "normal" adult population. Ann Intern Med 55:777, 1961.

26. Hagy GW, Settipane GA. Risk factors for developing asthma and allergic rhinitis. A seven year follow-up study of college students. J Allergy Clin Immunol 58:330, 1976.

27. Brown WG, Halonen MJ, Kaltenborn WT, Barbee RA. The relationship of respiratory allergy, skin test reactivity and serum IgE in a community population sample. J Allergy Clin Immunol 63:328, 1979.

28. Berg TLO, Johansson SGO. Allergy diagnosis with the radioallergosorbent test: A comparison with the results of skin and provocative tests in an unselected group of children. J Allergy Clin Immunol 54:209, 1974.

29. Bryant PH, Burns MW, Lazarus L. The correlation between skin tests, bronchial provocation tests and serum level of IgE specific for common allergens in patients with asthma. Clin Allergy 5:145, 1975.

30. Kalliel JN, Goldstein BM, Braman SS, Settipane GA. High frequency of atopic asthma in a pulmonary clinic population. Chest 96:1336–1340, 1989.

31. VanderZee JS, de Groot H, van Swieten P et al. Discrepancies between skin test and IgE antibody assays: Study of histamine release, complement activation in vitro and occurrence of allergen-specific IgG. J Allergy Clin Immunol 82:270–281, 1988.

Chapter XXXVI

Nasal Cytology in Clinical Practice

Eli O. Meltzer, M.D.,* and Alfredo A. Jalowayski, Ph.D.**

ABSTRACT

Analysis of the nasal cytology provides information regarding the pathophysiology and response to therapy of the airway. This paper reviews the techniques for obtaining and interpreting specimens. The discussion focuses on the epithelial and inflammatory cells and the patterns seen in allergic, infectious and structural nasal disorders.

The management of patients with nasal diseases requires an effective and complete history and physical examination. Analysis of the nasal cytology can provide additional useful information in the differential diagnosis and progress assessments. This includes assisting in:

1. distinguishing between inflammatory and noninflammatory rhinopathies (Table I);
2. distinguishing between allergic, nonallergic, and infectious rhinitis;
3. distinguishing between bacterial and viral infections;
4. classifying the cellular response to an infection;
5. obtaining rapid detection of the causative pathogen;
6. evaluating cilia function and ultrastructure;
7. following the course of a disease; and
8. evaluating the response to treatment.

The purpose of this paper is to describe the techniques for obtaining, processing, and interpreting the nasal cytology.

---

* *Clinical Professor of Pediatrics, Division of Allergy and Immunology, University of California, San Diego and Allergy and Asthma Medical Group and Research Center, San Diego, CA*
** *Director of Pediatric Respiratory Unit and Rapid Diagnostic Laboratory, Department of Pediatrics, University of California, San Diego, San Diego, CA*

MATERIALS AND METHODS

Equipment and Supplies for Obtaining the Specimens

The various materials utilized in the process of collecting the appropriate specimen are the following: a headlamp or a Welch Allen illuminator ring and clean specula of different sizes; sterile nasal scrapers (Rhinoprobe, Synbiotics Corporation, San Diego, CA) and nasopharyngeal swabs (Calgi-swab); microslides, frosted end one side or preferably two-ring (12mm) Cel-Line microscopic slides; a fixative: 95% ethyl alcohol; Hank's balanced salt solution (HBSS) with antibiotics; and forms to be stamped with patient's name, labels, etc.

Sampling Methods

Various techniques have been used for obtaining uniform and adequate nasal cytologic specimens (Table II).[1] A technique which permits examination of both the superficial mucosa and secretions would be preferred.[2] Such a nasal specimen can, with minimal trauma, be rather easily obtained by scraping the mucosal surface in the middle third of the inferior turbinate.[3–5] Additional sampling of the superficial mucosa from the middle turbinate or nasapharynx may occasionally be necessary to document the presence or absence of eosinophilic or basophilic disease.

Collection Procedures

1. The purpose of the test and the procedure for its collection should be explained to the patient and/or parent. This will enhance cooperation. The patient will experience a feather-like whisk sensation, tearing, and sometimes sneezing. Reassure the patient that the sampling should not cause any bleeding and minimal pain.
2. Instruct the patient to clear the nose of excess secretions. In infants, a rubber bulb syringe may be used to aspirate excess mucus. Rarely, aspiration with an 8-French suction catheter attached to a manual or wall suction device may be necessary. Eliminating

the extra mucus is important as the focus of the sample is the superficial epithelial cells, not the secretions.

3. Position the patient so that the internal nose can be seen. Have the patient's occiput rest back against a firm surface. If necessary, obtain assistance with positioning a young child. If the septum is deviated or one side is more obstructed, choose the most patent side for sampling.

4. Select the proper size speculum, insert it into the nasal vestibule, and gently dilate the soft nostril. Take care not to press medially against the septum or to insert the speculum into the nasal valve area as these will be uncomfortable for the patient. With infants and young children, it is usually not necessary to use a speculum and, because their nares are so small, there is no room for both the speculum and the Rhino-probe. Adequate visualization of the anterior aspect of the nasal airway in these children can usually be obtained by resting the fingers against the forehead and lifting the nostril tip with the thumb.

TABLE I

Classification of Chronic Rhinopathies

Inflammatory Rhinitis
Eosinophilic allergic rhinitis
    Seasonal
    Perennial
Eosinophilic nonallergic rhinitis
Infectious rhinitis
    Viral
    Bacterial
    Fungal
Nasal polyposis
Nasal mastocytosis
Atrophic rhinitis

Noninflammatory Rhinitis
Vasomotor rhinitis
    Autonomic dysfunction
    Associated with systemic conditions, e.g., pregnancy or thyroid disease
Rhinitis medicamentosus
    Local sympathomimetic overuse
    Systemic medications, e.g., antihypertensives or contraceptives

Structure-Related Rhinitis
Anatomic deformities, e.g., septal deviations, ciliary disorders
Obstruction, e.g., adenoidal hypertrophy, foreign body or tumors

---

5. Under direct visual inspection, identify the anterior bulb of the inferior turbinate. Flex and bend the Rhino-probe so that it will curve between the septum and the anterior bulb.

6. Maneuver the disposable Rhino-probe 2–3 cm posteriorly and gently press the cupped tip of the probe on the mucosal surface of the medial aspect of the inferior turbinate.

7. Two or three times make a short scraping of the epithelial membrane before withdrawing the probe.

Processing Procedures for Nasal Cytogram

1. Transfer the specimen to a labeled slide. Lightly, without squashing, spread the contents of the cupped tip over a small area of a plain slide or within the ring area of circled slides. Some tilting of the cupped tip and tapping may be necessary to make the wet specimen attach to the glass. The collected specimen should be visible to the naked eye on the microscope slide.

2. Before it dries, quickly flood the slide or place it in a jar containing 95% ethyl alcohol. At any time after 1 minute in the fixative, the slide is ready for staining.

3. Staining may be achieved with the Wright-Giemsa Dip Method as follows:
   a. Remove the slide(s) from the jar and drain the excess alcohol, but do not allow the cells to air dry.
   b. Dip the slide(s) in Wright-Giemsa (Volu-Sol) stain for 10–15 seconds.
   c. Drain the excess stain, then dip the slide(s) in Volu-Sol buffer for 15–30 seconds.
   d. Drain the excess buffer, then dip the slide(s) in Volu-Sol hematology rinse for 4–5 seconds, using quick dips, or flood slides with Rinse contained in a squeeze plastic bottle with nozzle and delivery tube.
   e. Drain the excess rinse and air-dry the specimens. An alternative to steps b, c, and d above is to obtain the ampules of stain available through Synbiotics. They recommend staining for 1 minute or longer, then washing the stain from the slide using a gentle stream of distilled water. Specimens that have been fixed in alcohol and then allowed to air-dry for transport purposes will also require 1 minute or longer staining time.

4. To examine the nasal cytogram, add a drop of immersion oil to the specimen. Scan the whole specimen at low power (×100) to determine if the specimen has an adequate number of nonsquamous epithelial cells and a good stain quality.

Processing Procedure for Viral Detection

1. Place the cupped tip of the Rhino-probe turbinate specimen into the HBSS. Twirl the probe's handle to dislodge the material. When cells are collected,

TABLE II

Nasal Cytologic Sampling Methods

A. Type of Specimen
1. Nose blowing: secretion
2. Scraping: superficial epithelium ± secretions
3. Biopsy: mucosa + submucosa

B. Collection Techniques and Comments

1. Nose blowing	Expelled secretions only
	Frequency contamination with dead cells, bacteria
	Less optimal staining due to mucus
2. Scraping	All cellular constituents
Cotton-tipped	Cell adherence, degranulation
	Discomfort
Calcium alginate (Calgi-swab)	Cell distortion, disruption
	Discomfort
Flexible plastic scoop (Rhino-probe)	Excellent specimens
	Minimal discomfort without anesthesia
3. Biopsy	Anesthesia required
	Discomfort, occasional bleeding

C. Sites of Nasal Mucosal Sampling
Inferior turbinate

Anterior bulb	Frequent bacteria/neutrophil artifacts, rare eosinophil
Middle third	Respiratory epithelium with esoinophils + basophilic cells
Middle turbinate	> yield of eosinophils (2-fold)
Superior turbinate	Visualizations hard, stimulate nasal cardiac reflex
Septum	Bleeding, rare eosinophil

D. Limitations
1. Only semiquantitative
   Sampling errors
   Grading systems
   Percent of Cells
   Number per high power field
   Scale (Pluses)
2. Temporal effects (allergen exposure, infections, etc.)

Nasal Cytologic Sampling Methods

3. False negative eosinophilia or basophilia
   Inadequate sample: watery secretion, anterior bulb
   Infection
   Systemic steroid
   Local steroid

E. Cellular Constituents of Collection Specimens

Cell or Tissue	Collection Technique		
	Secretion	Scraping	Biopsy
Ciliated epithelium	No	Yes	Yes
Goblet	No	Yes	Yes
Eosinophils	Yes	Yes	Yes
Basophils	Yes	Yes	Yes
Mast Cells	Rare	Yes	Yes
Neutrophil	Yes	Yes	Yes
Submucosa	No	No	Yes
Bacterial artifact	Frequent	Infrequent	Infrequent

they usually go into solution rather readily as white flakes of material, in contrast to mucus which usually floats to the top.
2. Cap, label, and place the vial in a container of ice.
3. A nasopharyngeal specimen can be obtained inserting a Calgi-swab into one of the nares past the turbinates. After a gentle rotation along the mucosal lining, the swab is withdrawn.
4. The tip of the swab is then placed into a second tube of HBSS or viral transport medium and the remainder of the metal shaft is cut with a nail clipper. Cap, label, and place the vial in ice.

Processing Procedures for Cilia Function and Ultrastructure
1. After scraping the medial portion of the inferior turbinate with the Rhino-probe, place the contents in HBSS warmed to room temperature. Twirl the handle a few times to remove the mucosal specimen from the probe's tip.
2. Use a Pasteur pipette to aspirate the pieces of mucosa and transfer them to a welled microscope slide with a drop or two of the HBSS. Place a coverslip

over the well and under light microscopy observe the beating ciliated epithelial cells.

3. The same sample, or preferably a different one, can be studied by electron microscopy. Place the specimen in a small conical plastic test tube containing 2.5% glutaraldehyde in phosphate buffer (0.1 M) at pH 7.3 for 1–2 hours or longer.

4. Refrigerate sample and arrange with electron microscopy laboratory for processing.

DISCUSSION

The nasal cytogram should be read by a properly trained individual. The diagnostic interpretation must be done by a physician familiar with nasal diseases: A). The various cell types seen in the stained specimen are described in Table III. B). The nasal cytogram should be graded at high power (oil immersion, ×1000) as a mean of cells per 10 high power fields, or qualitatively on a scale of 0–4+ as suggested in Table IV. C). The analysis of the nasal cytogram has both diagnostic and therapeutic clinical significance. A review of this follows.

Normal

The normal nasal mucosal cytology of infants, children, and adults consists of numerous epithelial cells including ciliated columnar, nonciliated columnar, goblet, and basal cells. There are usually no eosinophils or basophilic cells within the superficial layer above the basement membrane; however, a few neutrophils and bacteria can be seen.[3,6,7] Patients with chronic nasal disease due to noninflammatory or structural rhinitis typically have a normal cytogram unless several mechanisms coexist. For example, patients with rhinitis medicamentosus may have normal findings suggesting a physiologic process, whereas others may have a variety of histologic abnormalities.

Eosinophilic Cells

Increased numbers of eosinophils are found in the nasal mucosa in active allergic nasal disease.[6–8] In university students, school children, and infants, a highly significant correlation has been shown with nasal secretion eosinophilia and evidence of allergy such as nose rubbing, sneezing, sniffing, runny nose, and wet and swollen turbinates.[9,10] Significant increases in nasal secretion eosinophilia occurs within 30 minutes after a positive nasal allergen challenge.[11] The degree of nasal eosinophilia appears to relate to the extent of allergic exposure and symptoms in allergic rhinitis.[12] Significant decreases have been documented following symptom improvement due to topical nasal steroid therapy.[13–15] Because with nasal allergy the change from normal to active manifestations of disease is often gradual, the

---

TABLE III

Cell Morphology

1. **Epithelial Cells:** Five cell types can be seen: squamous (anterior aspects of turbinates), ciliated columnar, nonciliated columnar, goblet and basal cells; the latter give rise to columnar and goblet cells. The normal columnar to goblet ratio is 5:1.

2. **Eosinophils:** Slightly larger than neutrophils. Usually have bilobed blue-staining nucleus. Cytoplasm filled with distinct large granules, which are eosinophilic and stain reddish-orange in this procedure. Not common in epithelium and nasal secretions under normal conditions.

3. **Basophils:** Contain conspicuous, large or coarse, densely purple-staining basophilic granules. These cells have bilobed nucleus and are on average smaller than the mast cells described below.

4. **Neutrophils:** Similar in appearance as in blood smear. They have multilobed blue-purplish nuclei with clear or lightly pink-stained and finely granulated cytoplasm. Polymorphonuclear leukocytes are classified as neutrophils. A small number can be found in normal nasal mucosa.

5. **Bacteria:** Stain dark blue; often cocci and rods are present. A small number of bacterial cells are normally present. When bacteria are seen, along with many squamous epithelial cells, most likely the sample was taken too far anteriorly, resulting in a contaminated specimen which provides no clinical relevance. During bacterial infection many bacteria can be seen within neutrophils.

6. **Goblet Cells:** Have foamy, vacuous appearance with the nucleus displaced toward the basal part of the cell.

7. **Ciliocytophthoria:** Epithelial cells infected by virus may demonstrate clumping of chromatin material, an appearance of clear area (halo) surrounding nuclear material, or splitting of cells into ciliated portion (tufts) and nuclear portion.

8. **Mononuclear Cells:** Lymphocytes and monocytes appear morphologically similar to these cell types in blood smears.

9. **Plasma Cells:** Large and egg-shaped with abundant basophilic cytoplasm and small spherical nucleus. Infrequent in nasal mucosa or mucus.

10. **Mast Cells:** May take many shapes. Nucleus is oval in shape and may be obscured by secretory granules which are large and stain purplish.

occurrence of eosinophils in secretion samples of subjects with no history of allergic rhinitis and in those with a history of chronic, nonallergic rhinitis may represent mild, unnoticed nasal allergy. In eosinophilic nonallergic rhinitis conditions, the nasal secretions contain large numbers of eosinophils and the nasal mucosa has a marked infiltration of eosinophils. Many of these eosinophils appear ruptured with the consequent scattering of numerous eosinophilic granules within the nasal mucosa.

Regional differences of eosinophils in the nose of patients with perennial rhinitis have been observed.[16,17] In a study of 30 adult patients with allergic rhinitis and/or polyps, nasal eosinophils were found in 90% of the specimens obtained from the ethmoid region, maxillary sinus mucosa, and polyps; 80 and 40% of specimens from the middle and inferior turbinates, respectively; and 50% of nasal secretions. Eosinophils were identified in at least one sampling site from all of the patients.[16] In 14 adults with perennial allergic rhinitis, Gristwood[17] noted eosinophils in 100% of nasal specimens obtained from both the middle and inferior turbinates with the former evidencing significantly more cells (24 versus 9 eosinophils per high power field).

Miller et al.[18] confirmed the diagnostic usefulness of the nasal smear for eosinophils in 167 children. Significant nasal smear eosinophilia ($\geq 4\%$) was observed by either nose blowing or scraping techniques in 69, 11, and 7% of children, respectively, with either seasonal allergic rhinitis ($n = 42$), or nonallergic controls ($n = 70$). The nose blowing and scraping techniques evidenced an equal sensitivity of 70% and specificity of 94%; however, almost 40% of children could not provide blown specimens. The reliability of the method, as measured by intraspecimen variation, intra- and interobserver reliability, was 85, 90, and 93%, respectively. Wright or Hansel staining methods were equally effective.[18]

Surveying for possible variability of eosinophil detection from both nostrils, Kaufman et al.[19] found a concordance between nostrils for the absence or presence ($>8\%$) of nasal secretion eosinophils in 90 and 80%, respectively, but with an overall detection rate for eosinophils $>90\%$. Nevertheless, most studies urge strongly that multiple nasal specimens be obtained before ruling out the presence of nasal eosinophils.[4,11,16,17,20,21]

Basophilic Cells

The normal basophilic cell content of the nose is about 200–400 cells/cu mm of mucosa[22]; however, the great majority of these cells are located within the lamina propria. Some patients with chronic rhinitis have more than 2,000 basophilic cells/cu mm as the only histologic abnormality. They are classified as having "nasal mastocytosis." [23] Basophilic cells have been identified as being biologically active in allergy with the basophil leukocytes constituting the majority of the basophilic cells in mucosal scrapings[24] and in the nasal secretions.[25] As the number of basophilic cells increases, the nasal symptoms become more severe and provocative challenge responses usually become stronger. However, nasal reactivity to allergen challenge can also increase without a concomitant increase in the number of surface basophilic cells.[26] Their number frequently increases during the pollen season and decreases in the nasal secretions during the off season in patients with pollinosis and after successful immunotherapy or following topical nasal steroid therapy. These results suggest that the appearance of the basophilic cell in nasal secretions is related to their significance in nasal allergy. The number of basophils also correlates with nasal eosinophilia in allergic rhinitis.[27] Salas et al.[28] have further shown that both these cells and their total highly correlate to the natural log of the serum IgE level. A quantification of basophilic cells must be included in any complete nasal cytology workup. The finding of these cells and/or eosinophils increases the sensitivity of the test for confirming an allergic diagnosis to nearly 80%.[29]

Neutrophils and Bacteria

Neutrophils and bacteria, many of them intracellular, are usually increased with acute, subacute, and chronic bacterial infection, whether it is nasopharyngitis or sinusitis.[30,31] Gill and Neiburger[32] reported that a statistically greater number of patients had abnormal sinus x-rays (opacification, air fluid level, mucosal thickening >6 mm in adults or >4 mm in children, cystic or polypoid changes or asymmetric clouding) when >5 polymorphonuclear leukocytes/high power field was found on their nasal cytology. As a predictor of sinus pathology, >5 polymorphonuclear leukocytes/high power field on nasal cytology was 84% sensitive and 40% specific. Infection, and the consequent increase in neutrophils affect both the relative and the absolute number of eosinophils in the secretion sample.[8] Infections make the turbinates hyperemic and swollen, which may partially explain why only half of the patients with nasal allergy have a pale nasal mucosa. Irritants or chemicals also can induce a nasal neutrophilia without bacteria.

Goblet Cells

Patients with chronic rhinitis have significantly more goblet cells in mucosal scrapings than normal individuals. They are found in the largest number in patients with pronounced nasal obstruction and may ex-

TABLE IV

A Guide for Grading Nasal Cytograms

Quantitative Analysis	Semi-quantitative Analysis	Grade
A. Epithelial cells		
N/A	Normal morphology	N
N/A	Abnormal morphology	A
N/A	Ciliocytophthoria	CCP
B. Eosinophils, neutrophils		
0*	None	0
0.1–1.0*	Occasional cells	½+
1.1–5.0*	A few scattered cells or small clumps	1+
6.0–15.0*	A moderate number of cells and larger clumps	2+
16.0–20.0*	Larger clumps of cells which, however, do not cover the entire field	3+
>20.0*	Large clumps of cells covering the entire field	4+
C. Basophilic cells		
0	None	0
0.1–0.3*	Occasional	½+
0.4–1.0*	A few scattered	1+
1.1–3.0*	Moderate number	2+
3.1–6.0*	Many easily seen	3+
>6.0*	Larger number, as many as 25 per high power field	4+
D. Bacteria		
N/A†	None seen	0
N/A†	Occasional clump	1+
N/A†	Moderate amount	2+
N/A†	Many easily seen	3+
N/A†	Large amounts covering the entire field	4+
E. Goblet cells‡		
0–24%	None, occasional to few cells	1+
25–49%	A moderate number	2+
50–74%	Many easily seen	3+
75–100%	Large number, may cover entire field	4+

* Mean of cells per 10 high power fields (×1000).
† Note presence of intracellular bacteria.
‡ Ratio of goblet cells to epithelial cells, expressed as percent.

plain the common clinical observation of a viscid nasal secretion in these cases.[33] Both in perennial and seasonal rhinitis, an increase in goblet cells has been significantly correlated with secretion eosinophilia.[34] Increased numbers of goblet cells are also reportedly seen in patients with selective IgA deficiency[35] and in the vasomotor rhinitis due to the cold, dry, somewhat polluted air found in winter in Denver, Colorado.[36]

Viral Detection

Ciliated epithelial cells undergo distinctive destructive changes termed "ciliocytophthoria" in the presence of viruses. The features of the cytopathic effects of the viruses include clumping of the nuclear chromatin material, margination of the pyknotic chromatin mass attached to inclusion material within the nucleus, increased granulation of the cytoplasm, halo formation around the nucleus, constriction of the ciliated cell, and finally separation of the nucleus-containing basal portion from the ciliated apical portion.[37] Examination of the nasal cytogram for ciliocytophthoria can be helpful in identifying a response to a viral infection by comparison with allergic or bacterial inflammation.

A guide for interpreting the nasal cytogram is presented in Table V.

The epithelial cells can also be evaluated for specific viral infections by viral cultures, immunofluorescent tests, and most recently by a peroxidase-antiperoxidase assay. This latter test has been used successfully for the rapid diagnosis of respiratory syncytial virus, parainfluenza, influenza, and adenoviral infections of the respiratory tract. It is more convenient to perform than immunofluorescence because the color reaction and cell morphology are easily observable by light microscopy.[38] Obtaining epithelial samples with the Rhino-probe allows for a large enough specimen to analyze for multiple viruses.

Cilia Function and Ultrastructure

Surgical biopsy of nasal or bronchial mucosa and cytologic brushing techniques have been used to obtain ciliated respiratory cells for functional and ultrastructural analysis. These methods are traumatic, requiring anesthesia and are unsuitable for repeated use in children.

The Rhino-probe scraping method is a safe and nontraumatic procedure that can be used to screen young children suspected of having ciliary abnormalities.[39] The method provides sufficient nasal respiratory ciliated epithelial cells for both functional and ultrastructural analysis. On light microscopic examination, cilia which beat with a sweeping and rapid whip-like motion[40] most likely have normal ultrastructure. Cilia

TABLE V

The Interpretation of Nasal Cytograms

Cellular Type	Diagnostic Classification
Increased eosinophils (1–4+)	Allergy Nonallergic rhinitis with eosinophilia Aspirin sensitivity
Increased basophils (1–4+)	Allergy Nonallergic rhinitis with eosinophilia Aspirin sensitivity Nonallergic rhinitis with basophilia/ primary nasal mastocytosis
Increased neutrophils (2–4+) With intracellular bacteria With ciliocytophthoria With fungi With no bacteria	 Nasopharyngitis or sinusitis Viral upper respiratory infection Fungal upper respiratory infection Irritant reaction or rhinitis medicamentosus (?)
Increased goblet cells (3–4+)	Allergy Infection Vasomotor (?) IgA deficiency

with missing dynein arms or other ultrastructural defects either do not move at all or appear to quiver and move stiffly. These types of specimens require ultrastructural analyses to determine the exact defect. This procedure greatly reduces the cost of screening patients for the immotile cilia syndrome.

The diagnosis of the immotile cilia syndrome is based on ultrastructural analysis of cilia by transmission electron microscopy. Several ultrastructural defects have been reported in patients with recurrent upper and lower respiratory tract infections. Missing dynein arms,[41] spoke defects,[42] and transposition of microtubules[43] can contribute to abnormal function of the mucociliary transport system, predisposing these patients to recurrent infections.

REFERENCES

1. Meltzer EO, Schatz M, Zeiger RS. Allergic and nonallergic rhinitis, In: Middleton E Jr, Reed CE, Ellis EF, eds. Allergy: Principles and Practice, 3rd ed. St. Louis: The C.V. Mosby Company, 1988, p. 1253.
2. Angel-Solano G, Shturman R. Comparative cytology of nasal secretions and nasal mucosa in allergic rhinitis. Ann Allergy 56:521, 1986.
3. Cohen GA, MacPherson GA, Golembesky HE, Jalowayski AA, O'Connor RD. Normal nasal cytology in infancy. Ann Allergy 54:112, 1985.
4. Zeiger RS, Jalowayski AA, Schatz M. Chronic rhinitis: only half a diagnosis. Diagnosis 5:91, 1983.
5. Jalowayski AA, Zeiger RS. Examination of nasal or conjunctival epithelial specimens. In: Lawlor GJ Jr, Fischer TJ, eds. Manual of Allergy and Immunology, 2nd ed. Boston: Little, Brown and Company, 1988, p. 432.
6. Bryan MP, Bryan WTK. Cytologic diagnosis in allergic disorders. Otolaryngol Clin North Am 7:637, 1974.
7. Bickmore JT. Nasal cytology in allergy and infection. ORL Allergy 40:39, 1978.
8. Hansel FK. Observations on the cytology of the secretions in allergy of the nose and paranasal sinuses. J Allergy 5:357, 1934.
9. Malmberg H. Symptoms of chronic and allergic rhinitis and occurrence of nasal secretion granulocytes in university students, school children and infants. Allergy 34:389, 1979.
10. Murray AB, Anderson DO. The Epidemiologic relationship of clinical nasal allergy to eosinophils and to goblet cells in the nasal smear. J Allergy 43:1, 1969.
11. Pelikan Z. The changes in the nasal secretions of eosinophils during the immediate nasal response to allergen challenge. J Allergy Clin Immunol 72:657, 1983.
12. Hansel FK. Cytologic diagnosis in respiratory allergy and infection. Ann Allergy 24:564, 1966.
13. Elkhalil M, Fiore L, Bellioni P, Cantani A, Corgiolu M, Businco L. Evaluation of nasal and blood eosinophilia in children suffering from perennial allergic rhinitis treated with beclomethasone dipropionate. Allergol Immunopathol (Madr) 11:225, 1983.
14. Mygind N. Topical steroid treatment for allergic rhinitis and allied conditions. Clin Otolaryngol 7:343, 1982.
15. Orgel HA, Meltzer EO, Kemp JP, Welch MJ. Clinical rhino-

manometric and cytologic evaluation of seasonal allergic rhinitis treated with beclomethasone dipropionate as aqueous nasal spray or pressurized aerosol. J Allergy Clin Immunol 77:858, 1986.

16. Vaheri E. Nasal allergy with special reference to eosinophilia and histopathology. Acta Allergol 10:203, 1956.

17. Gristwood RE. Observations on the hisopathology of allergic rhinitis: regional differences in mucosal eosinophilia. J Laryngosc Otol 49:270, 1982.

18. Miller RE, Paradise JL, Friday GA, Fireman P, Voith D. The nasal smear for eosinophils. Its value in children with seasonal allergic rhinitis. Am J Dis Child 136:1009, 1982.

19. Kaufman HS, Rosen I, Shaposhnikov N, Wei M. Nasal eosinophilia. Ann Allergy 49:270, 1982.

20. Malmberg H, Holopainen E. Nasal smear as a screening test for immediate-type nasal allergy. Allergy 34:331, 1979.

21. Mullarkey MF, Hill JS, Webb DR. Allergic and nonallergic rhinitis: their characterization with attention to the meaning of nasal eosinophilia. J Allergy Clin Immunol 65:122, 1980.

22. Connell JT. Nasal disease: mechanisms and classification. Ann Allergy 50:227, 1983.

23. Connell JT. Nasal mastocytosis. J Allergy 43:182, 1969.

24. Jalowayski AA, Maes TE, Wasserman SI, Zeiger RS. Histochemical differentiation of the human nasal mucosa mast cells from basophil leukocytes. J Allergy Clin Immunol 71:89, 1983.

25. Okuda M, Kawabori S, Otsuka H. Electron microscope study of basophilic cells in allergic nasal secretions. Arch Otorhinolaryngol 221:215, 1978.

26. Wihl J-Å, Brofeldt S, Grønborg H, Borum P, Mygind N. Blind study of basophilic cells in nasal smears from patients with grass pollen hay fever. Eur J Respir Dis 64(suppl128):383, 1983.

27. Okuda M, Otsuka H. Basophilic cells in allergic nasal secretions. Arch Otorhinolaryngol 214:283, 1977.

28. Salas A, Wilson N, Hamburger RN. Relation of serum IgE level to the cells observed in nasal cytogram. Ann Allergy 60:175, 1988.

29. Lang DM, Howland WC, Stevenson DD. Sensitivity and features of nasal cytology in diagnosis of allergic (IgE-mediated) rhinitis. Ann Allergy 60:176, 1988.

30. Bryan WTK, Bryan MP. Cytological diagnosis in otolaryngology. Am Acad Ophthalmol Otolaryngol Trans 63:597, 1959.

31. Anderson H. Practical nasal cytology: key to the problem nose. ORL Allergy 41:51, 1979.

32. Gill F, Neiburger J. Nasal smear cytology in chronic sinusitis. Ann Allergy 60:175, 1988.

33. Mygind N, Viner AS, Jackman N. Histology of nasal mucosa in normals and in patients with perennial rhinitis. Rhinology 12:131, 1974.

34. Binder E, Holopainen H, Malmberg H, Salo OP. Clinical findings in patients with allergic rhinitis. Rhinology 22:255, 1984.

35. Karlsson G, Hansson H-Å, Petruon B, Björkander J, Hanson LÅ. Goblet cell number in the nasal mucosa relates to cell-mediated immunity in patients with antibody deficiency syndromes. Int Arch Allergy Appl Immunol 78:86, 1985.

36. Silvers WS. Personal communication.

37. Bryan WTK, Bryan MP, Smith CA. Human ciliated epithelial cells in nasal secretions. Morphologic and histochemical aspects. Ann Otol Rhinol Laryngol 73:474, 1964.

38. Jalowayski AA, England BL, Temm CJ, Nunemacher TJ, Bastian JF, MacPherson GA, Danner WM, Straube RC, Connor JD. Peroxidase-antiperoxidase assay for rapid detection of respiratory syncytial virus in nasal epithelial specimens from infants and children. J Clin Microbiol 25:722, 1987.

39. Jalowayski AA. Work in progress.

40. Rossman CM, Forrest JB, Newhouse MT. Motile cilia in "immotile cilia" syndrome. Lancet 1:1360, 1980.

41. Afzelius BA. A human syndrome caused by immotile cilia. Science 193:317, 1976.

42. Sturgess JM, Chao J, Wong J, Aspin N, Turner JAP. Cilia with defective radial spokes: a cause of human respiratory disease. N Engl J Med 300:53, 1979.

43. Sturgess JM, Chao J, Turner JAP. Transposition of ciliary microtubules. Another cause of impaired ciliary motility. N Engl J Med 303:318, 1980.

Chapter XXXVII

CT Scan of the Paranasal Sinuses

Jan Malat, M.D.

ABSTRACT

Direct coronal CT (computed tomography) is the most accurate examination for evaluation of the paranasal sinuses. Its capability to demonstrate detailed paranasal sinus anatomy and the relationship between fine structures of the ostiomeatal unit makes CT examination an important part of the preoperative planning. Minimal soft tissue swelling, anatomic variants such as concha bullosa, deviated nasal septum, paradoxical turbinates, etc. may obstruct infundibulum of the maxillary sinus and cause sinusitis. Coronal CT scan not only may help diagnose such conditions but also may represent a road map for endoscopic surgery. Several common pathologic conditions and techniques are presented.

R ecent advances in functional endoscopic sinus surgery brought new understanding of the anatomy of the paranasal sinuses. Direct visualization of detailed anatomy of the paranasal sinuses is possible by high-resolution direct coronal CT scan images. Meticulous radiographic delineation of the small structures of the ostiomeatal unit, coupled with endoscopic evaluation, provides detailed preoperative information regarding morphology and pathology of the paranasal sinuses.[1] This information is important for decrease of intra- and postoperative complications. It is mandatory to obtain direct coronal CT images prior to an operation to guarantee the operative success.

Proctor (1966) stressed the importance of ethmoid sinuses as a key problem in infectious sinusitis. He pointed out that persistent infection in the ethmoid sinuses is usually the reason for failure of therapy directed at any of the other paranasal sinuses.[2]

Messerklinger (1967) studying mucociliary drainage of the paranasal sinuses, showed that apposition of mucosal surfaces causes ventilatory disturbance of the ostiomeatal unit.[3] He showed that apposition of abutting mucociliary surfaces within the paranasal sinuses

Clinical Assistant Professor, Yale University School of Medicine, MRI and Neuroradiology Consultant, Southern Massachusetts Hospitals Consortium, Fall River, Massachusetts

forms an anatomic substrate for disrupting sinonasal drainage.[1,3] The resulting retention of secretion leads to inflammation and infection. It was shown that the infundibulum in the middle meatus is most frequently affected by anatomic variations such as: concha bullosa, deviated septum, paradoxical turbinate, etc. The final results are obstruction of this natural mucociliary clearance, retention of the mucous inside the sinuses, and, therefore, formation of substrates for chronic sinusitis.

These findings led to development of a new surgical technique aimed toward this area. Advances in development of the endoscopic equipment and direct visualization by high-resolution CT scan led to successful management of chronic sinusitis.[1,4,5]

AVAILABLE DIAGNOSTIC PROCEDURES

C urrent technology offers several diagnostic modalities for demonstration of paranasal sinus pathology.
1. Routine x-rays
2. Pluridirectional tomography
3. MRI (Magnetic Resonance Imaging)
4. CT (Computed Tomography)

Routine x-rays are the least expensive and most readily available examination. They consist of four views in the upright and supine positions. Paranasal sinuses usually are well visualized. Increased density in sinus cavities indicates advanced sinusitis. Air-fluid levels are demonstrated in the case of acute sinusitis. This examination is technique dependent and lacks demonstration of fine bone and mucosal details.

Pluridirectional tomography may demonstrate bone structures in better detail. It usually is reserved for patients with facial trauma and congenital abnormality. CT scan replaced wider use of tomography in the majority of cases.

MRI is very sensitive in demonstrating paranasal sinus pathology. Multiple orthogonal views may be obtained without changing the patient's position. It is suitable for cases where complications are suspected. Invasion of brain or orbits is better demonstrated by MRI than by CT scan. MRI is not optimal for bony structures and, therefore, cannot be used for preoperative planning.

CT scan is the optimal diagnostic method for demonstration of sinus anatomy and pathology.[1,2,3] High resolution coronal or axial images routinely demonstrate anatomical details desired for endoscopic surgery. The latest developments of 3-D technologies promise further improvement in preoperative evaluation of paranasal sinuses. The rest of this chapter deals with computed tomography.

COMPUTER TOMOGRAPHY TECHNIQUE

Thin section (4–5 mm) contiguous scans are used from the middle of the nasal bone to the most posterior portion of the sphenoid sinus (Figure 1). If more detailed anatomy or 3-D reconstructions is desired, thinner sections may be obtained.

Inherited problems of bone or metallic artifact from dental fillings are usually overcome by coronal technique. Off-coronal images also may be attained by different gantry or patient position. This technique may be used for patients who are unable to assume prone position for direct coronal scans.

Magnified images should be obtained using 2,000 window widths and centered to −200 level. Saved data may be used later for high-resolution images (Figure 2).

COMPUTER TOMOGRAPHY ANATOMY

The anatomy of the paranasal sinuses and particularly the ostiomeatal unit are well-visualized by coronal CT.[1,2,3] The most anterior sections include frontal sinus and anterior nasal fossae. More posterior sections show middle and inferior turbinate. Nasolacrimal duct and canal are usually demonstrated at this level. It is located laterally and slightly superior to the inferior turbinate. It is at this level, or at slightly more posterior sections, where the infundibulum and maxillary sinus ostium are seen. The infundibulum is a channellike structure connecting the maxillary sinus and hiatus semilunaris. It is bounded laterally by the inferomedial orbit, superiorly by the hiatus semilunaris and ethmoidal bulla, medially by the uncinate process, and inferiorly by the maxillary sinus as the sinus funnels into it[1] (Figure 3).

Hiatus semilunaris is the half-moon shaped area of the maxillary sinus drainage. It is bounded by ethmoidal bulla, medial bony orbit, uncinate process, and middle meatus.

The middle turbinate lies inferomedial to the anterior ethmoid air cells. It is attached vertically to the cribriform plate and connected to the lamina papyaracea through the bony strut, the basal lamella. The basal lamella is oriented from anteromedially to posterolat-

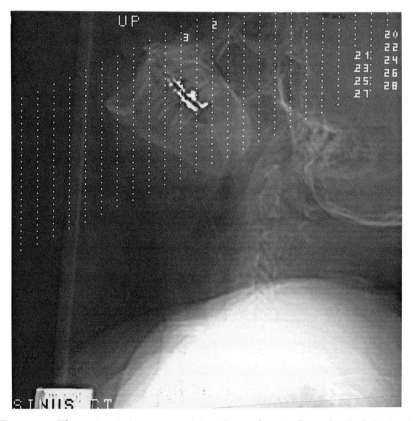

Figure 1. Topogram. The patient is in prone position. Cursor lines indicate level of obtained images.

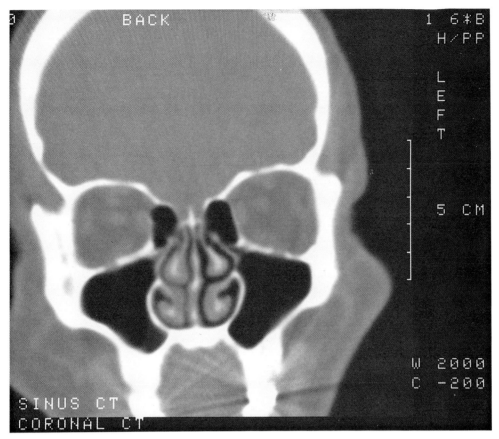

Figure 2. Sinus technique (2000/−200) adequately shows bone structures and soft tissues.

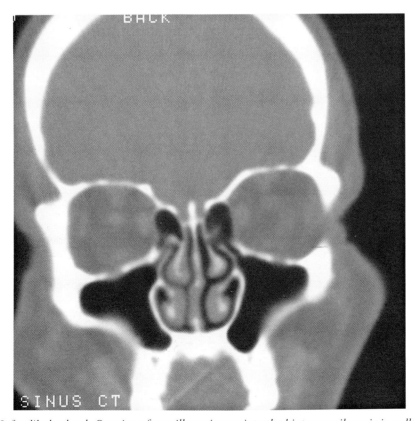

Figure 3. Infundibular level. Opening of maxillary sinuses into the hiatus semilunaris is well visualized.

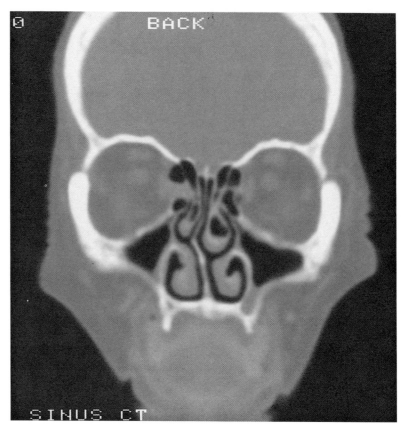

Figure 4a. *Bilateral concha bullosa. Asymmetric aeration of both middle turbinates. There is deviation of uncinate process laterally. Both infundibula are narrowed.*

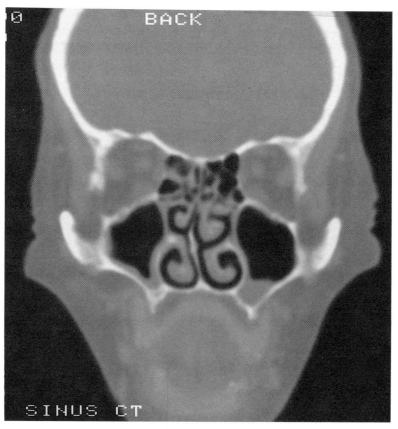

Figure 4b. *More posterior level shows bilateral maxillary sinusitis.*

erally to become situated behind the ethmoidal bulla. The space between the ethmoidal bulla and basal lamella is called the sinus lateralis.[1]

Ethmoidal bulla consists of clusters of air cells of variable size and shape. It is bordered inferomedially by the infundibulum and hiatus semilunaris, laterally by the lamina papyracea, and superoposteriorly by the sinus lateralis.

The frontal recess drains the frontal sinus. The ostium of the frontal sinus usually opens into the middle meatus medial to the uncinate process.

Maxillary sinus ostium and infundibulum, hiatus semilunaris, middle turbinate, ethmoidal bulla, and frontal recess form the ostiomeatal unit (or complex). Anatomical changes, trauma, or even subtle mucosal thickening in the unit may be responsible for secondary inflammatory changes in the maxillary sinus.

Further posterior sections demonstrate posterior ethmoidal compartments separated from the maxillary sinus by the ethmoidal maxillary plate. They are separated from the orbit by the lamina papyracea.

Sphenoid sinus is demonstrated on the most posterior sections. Asymmetrical septations in relationship to the posterior ethmoids as well as nasopharynx and sella turcica are well visualized by direct coronal CT scans.

ANATOMICAL VARIANTS

Variability of paranasal sinus anatomy is well known. There is virtually no identical appearance of anatomy among different cases: its unique appearance for each individual reminds one of thumbprints. The most common variant is asymmetric aeration of middle turbinate (concha bullosa). Excessive expansion of aerated turbinate may obstruct the infundibulum or form mucocele. Deviated septum due to trauma or congenital predisposition is the second most common anatomic reason for obstructed infundibulum. Paradoxical rotation of middle turbinate, lateral deviation of the uncinate process, and excessive ethmoidal bulla formation may be responsible for abnormal drainage of the ostiomeatal complex (Figures 4a, 5, 6). It is important to recognize such variation to prevent surgical complications (Figures 6a and b).

PATHOLOGY

Subtle inflammatory changes or allergic reaction may be responsible for mucosal thickening in the ostiomeatal complex area. As noted previously, such changes may be followed by obstruction of natural maxillary sinus drainage and subsequent chronic infections. Soft

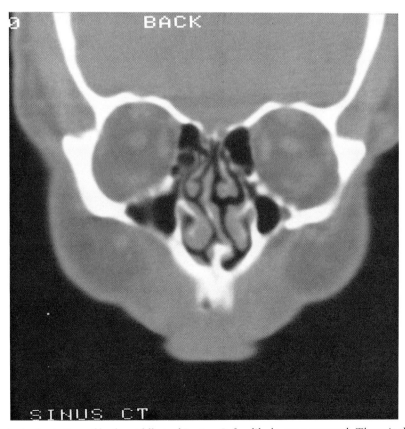

Figure 5. *Paradoxical rotation of both middle turbinates. Infundibula are narrowed. There is deviated septum.*

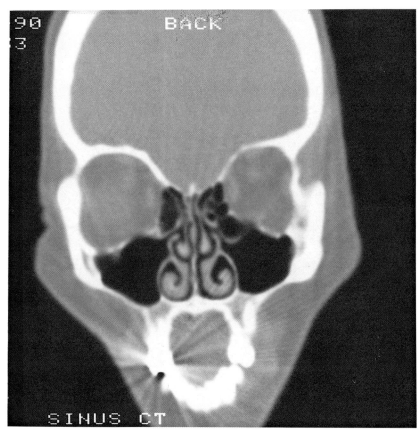

Figure 6a. Abnormal enlargement of the left anterior ethmoidal bulla with narrowing of the left infundibulum.

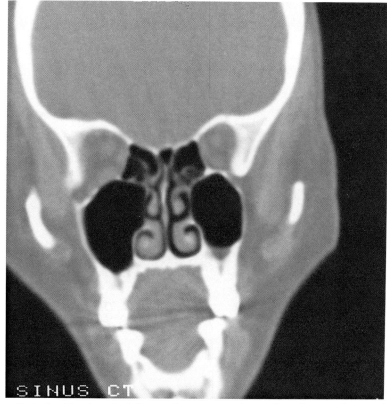

Figure 6b. Small air fluid level in the left maxillary sinus indicate disturbance of mucociliary drainage.

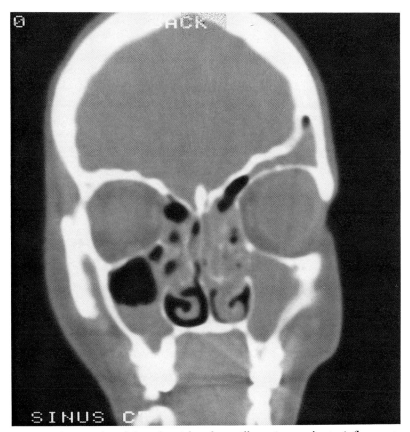

Figure 7. *Extensive opacity of the ethmoid and maxillary sinuses due to inflammatory polyps.*

tissue thickening in the middle meatus is most frequent. It may be unilateral or, in the majority of cases, asymmetrically bilateral (Figure 7). This is a crucial point in preoperative CT diagnosis. Early recognition of infundibular compromise may prevent subsequent maxillary sinusitis. In some cases, extensive obliteration of the whole ostiomeatal unit is demonstrated. In that event, anatomy may be completely obscured by inflammatory masses.

CT scan is also helpful in follow-up studies after surgery or for screening of patients who are not surgical candidates.

REFERENCES

1. Zinreich SJ, Kennedy DW, Rosenbaum AE et al. Paranasal sinuses: CT imaging requirements for endoscopic surgery. Radiology 163:769–775, 1987.
2. Rice DH, Achaffer SD. Endoscopic Paranasal Sinus Surgery. New York: Raven Press, 1988.
3. Messerklinger, W. On the drainage of the normal frontal sinus of man. Acta Otolaryngol 63:176–181, 1967.
4. Kennedy DW, Zinreich SJ, Rosenbaum AE, Johns ME. Functional endoscopic sinus surgery, theory, and diagnostic evaluation. Arch Otolaryngol 111:576–582, 1985.
5. Stammberger H. Endoscopic endonasal surgery—Concepts in treatment of recurring rhinosinusitis. Part 1. Anatomic and pathophysiologic considerations. Otolaryngol Head Neck Surg 94:143–155, 1986.

Chapter XXXVIII

Magnetic Resonance Imaging (MRI) of the Nasal Airway

Philip Cole, M.D.,* James S. J. Haight, M.D.,* Kensai Naito, M.D.,* and Walter Kucharczyk, M.D.**

ABSTRACT

Magnetic resonance imaging was used to demonstrate both erectile tissues and airway lumen of the nasal cavities together with their responses to lateral recumbent postures and to topical decongestant. The inferior turbinate and the anterior septal body responded to lateral recumbency by swelling in the inferior nasal cavity and reciprocal shrinking in the superior side and both responded to topical decongestant by shrinking. Converse changes in airway lumen took place in each case. In the untreated nose erectile tissues of the lateral nasal wall appeared to adapt to septal irregularities and to maintain a uniform width of the airway lumen in the more patent side. Erectile tissues on the lateral nasal wall anterior to the inferior turbinate and medially on the anterior septum were seen to intrude on the constricted region of the nasal valve where their potential to exert a critical influence on airflow resistance was evident.

This report is concerned with configuration and dimensions of erectile tissues and the nasal airways of a healthy human adult and their responses to posture and to decongestant as depicted by magnetic resonance imaging. A previous computed tomographic x-ray study of the effects of vasoactive substances demonstrated the distribution of erectile tissues in the nasal cavities and indicated their role in regulating the dimensions of the airway and its resistance to airflow.[1] The present study enabled more lengthy and repeated imaging to be undertaken without exposure of the subject to ionizing radiation.

---

* Department of Otolaryngology Airflow Laboratory, St. Michael's Hospital, Toronto, Ontario
** Department of Radiology, The Toronto Hospital, Toronto, Ontario

METHODS

Subject

One of the authors (JSJH), a healthy male aged 43 years with no nasal symptoms and unremarkable clinical findings on rhinoscopic examination, was the subject of this study.

Magnetic Resonance Imaging

All imaging was performed on a 1.5 Tesla superconducting magnetic resonance imager (Signa, General Electric Medical Systems, Milwaukee, WI).

Coronal and axial images were obtained with the subject in each of three recumbent positions: dorsal, left lateral, and right lateral. The dorsal recumbent position was repeated after application of topical decongestant. The imaging parameters were spin echo 600/20 (TR/TE), 256×256 matrix, 16 cm field of view (equaling in-plane resolution of approximately 0.6 $\times$ 0.6 mm) and 5 mm thick sections.

Assessment of Erectile Tissues and the Airway

The cross-sectional areas of the mucosa and airway of the nose were obtained from coronal images at each of four reference planes: posterior, middle, anterior, and septal body. All measurements were obtained by outlining the area of interest of the image on the video display terminal and then using manufacturer-supplied software to determine the surface area of the enclosed region automatically as outlined on the image.

Experiments

The subject assumed a dorsal recumbent posture on the imaging table. Following a minimum period of 30 minutes for equilibration with ambient conditions and posture, sagittal magnetic resonance imaging views were obtained to determine and adjust precise head position. The head was then fixed by foam packing and axial and coronal tomograms were obtained. The sequence was repeated with the subject in left lateral and right lateral recumbency and finally in the dorsal posture following topical application of the decongestant, 0.1% xylometazoline.[2] In each posture the matching head position was confirmed by sagittal views before tomography.

RESULTS

Figures 1 and 2 show the lumen of the nasal airways outlined by fixed and erectile tissues as the subject lies in dorsal recumbency. Much of the asymmetry between right and left sides probably results from the phase of the spontaneous nasal cycle.[3] On each side the lumen of the airway (Figs. 1 and 4) extends laterally into the middle and inferior meatus with a transverse dimension 3 mm throughout both vertical and horizontal sections.[4] Its width is remarkably uniform on the more patent side. Figure 4 shows that assumption of a lateral recumbent posture results in narrowing of the airway lumen of the inferior cavity and widening that of the superior cavity.[5] Cross-sectional areas of both mucosa and airway lumen and their postural and decongestant responses are shown in Figures 3 and 4 and in Table I. Although mucosal cross-section is less clearly delineated by the imaging process than airway lumen, measurements confirm the visual impression that mucosal volume changes take place throughout the length of the inferior turbinate and also in the septal erectile body (Table I). The inferior turbinate and the anterior septal body responded to lateral recumbency by swelling in the inferior nasal cavity and reciprocal shrinking in the superior side. Both responded to topical decongestant by shrinking.

DISCUSSION

The postural responses of erectile mucosa and their effects on nasal airway lumen demonstrated in Figure 4 are consistent with airflow studies which have shown reciprocal adjustments in patency of the nasal cavities in response to lateral recumbent postures.[5] In addition, the extent of the erectile component of the mucosa may be gauged from comparison between untreated and decongested noses (Figs. 3 and 4).

Axial and coronal views are, respectively, parallel with and perpendicular to the main caval airstream,[4] which is approximately horizontal in the upright subject. In cadaver studies Swift and Proctor[6] have shown the main inspirator airstream to be concentrated in the mid-portion between roof and floor of the narrow, sinuous cleft of the caval lumen depicted in Figures 1 to 4.[4] By contrast, expiration is widely dispersed. In the

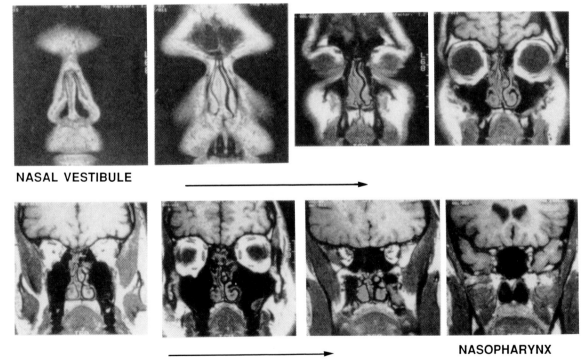

NASAL VESTIBULE

NASOPHARYNX

Figure 1. Coronal sections of nasal cavities from vestibule to nasopharynx. Note regular width of patent airway, adaptation of lateral to medial walls, septal and lateral erectile mucosa in anterior nose.

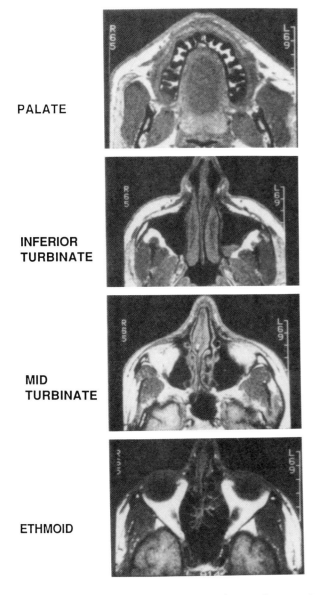

Figure 2. Axial sections of nasal cavities from palate to ethmoids. Note prominent septal erectile tissue above the level of the inferior turbinate and anterior to middle turbinate.

PALATE

INFERIOR TURBINATE

MID TURBINATE

ETHMOID

recognized clinical finding of turbinate expansion corresponding with a septal concavity is clearly demonstrated by the adaptation of the lateral wall mucosa to septal irregularities which may be seen in these magnetic resonance imaging studies. The mucosa maintains a uniform width of the more patent airway lumen despite the irregularities.

The importance of erectile tissues to airway patency is most apparent in the anterior nose where the septal body and the anterior end of the inferior turbinate intrude on the narrowed lumen of the nasal valve[7] Here is a critical segment of the nasal airway where respiratory airflow resistances[7] and linear velocities[6] exceed by far those generated at any other location in the respiratory passages. At this constricted site a pathological intrusion on the lumen is less readily accommodated than in the nasal cavum[8,9] and transmural pressures of inspiratory airflow, which are augmented by pathological narrowing,[10,11] are exerted on compliant walls of the anterior nose and may increase narrowing further and limit flow.

The size and site of the erectile body of the anterior septum,[1,12] so prominently demonstrated by tomography, is usually unremarkable on rhinoscopic or conventional x-ray examination and although it may well contribute to nasal obstruction, it is seldom included in surgical procedures directed toward reduction of obstructive erectile tissues. Comparably, erectile tissue anterior to the bony inferior turbinate (Fig. 3) does not attract much therapeutic attention. The adenovascular body of the posterior septum which has been described[13] is not evident in this subject.

Mucosal dysfunction is a common cause of nasal obstruction and its effects may be exacerbated by structural abnormality. In the course of a lifetime few people escape obstructive nasal symptoms from infective, allergic, or less specific rhinitis in acute, recurrent, or chronic forms.[14] Analysis of results from 1000 patients referred to our pediatric nasal clinic demonstrated mucosal swelling which was substantially reduced by topical decongestant in two-thirds of the cases of chronic nasal obstruction.[15]

Nasal obstruction impairs the quality of life and may have pathological consequences. It is aggravated by recumbency[16] and leads to micro-arousals[17] and breathing disorders in sleep.[18] Furthermore, it promotes mouth breathing and in chronic form it is commonly associated with oral and dental pathology and abnormalities of facial growth.[19] It is reported also to exert a measurably adverse effect on pulmonary function which can be reversed by relief of the obstruction.[20]

The narrow confines of the nasal airways exhibit their vulnerability to mucosal dysfunction and consequent obstruction more strikingly by tomographic studies than by anterior rhinoscopy or plain x-rays.

anterior nose both coronal and axial views are oblique to the direction of much of the airway, which turns through almost 90° in this region, the views are oblique also to the caudal edge of the upper lateral cartilage which defines the entrance to the nasal valve. Interpretation of tissue and airway relationships from coronal and axial views are more speculative here than in the cavum. Nevertheless, it can be seen that accumulations of erectile tissue of the septum and lateral nasal wall are prominent in this region.

Physiologically active erectile mucosa of the anterior septum and the lateral nasal walls together with more stable tissues delineate the airway boundaries. The well

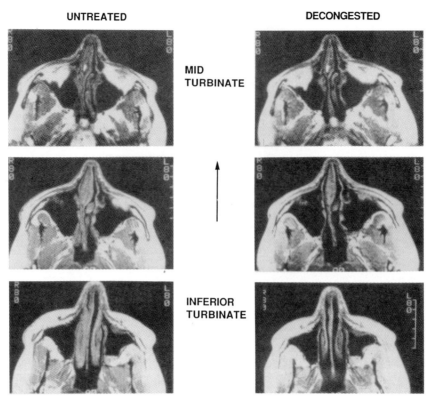

UNTREATED **DECONGESTED**

MID TURBINATE

INFERIOR TURBINATE

Figure 3. *Axial sections of inferior and middle tubinates. Comparison between untreated and decongested states emphasizes erectile tissue of anterior lateral wall in close proximity with that of the septum.*

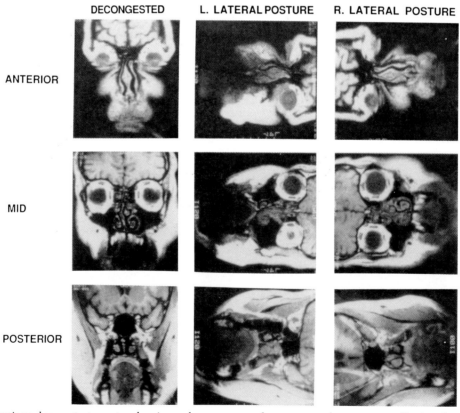

DECONGESTED **L. LATERAL POSTURE** **R. LATERAL POSTURE**

ANTERIOR

MID

POSTERIOR

Figure 4. *Coronal sections demonstrate postural reciprocal responses and response to decongestant affecting the anterior septal body the anterior lateral wall and both the inferior middle turbinates.*

TABLE I

Cross-Sectional Areas of Nasal Lumen in mm² (Coronal Views)

Intervention	Site	Mucosa Right	Mucosa Left	Airway Right	Airway Left
Left lateral posture	Posterior	52	110	170	47
	Mid	158	194	102	3
	Anterior	32	57	115	54
	Septal body	28	98		
Right lateral posture	Posterior	102	57	81	139
	Mid	96	92	9	136
	Anterior	51	49	16	78
	Septal body	168	91		
Decongestant	Posterior	40	48	135	172
	Mid	38	91	99	158
	Anterior	20	27	93	151
	Septal body	34	28		

REFERENCES

1. Cole P, Haight JSJ, Cooper PW, Kassel EE. A computed tomographic study of nasal mucosa: effects of vasoactive substances. J Otolaryngol 12:58–60, 1983.
2. Bende M. Vascular effects of topical oxymetazoline on human nasal mucosa. J Laryngol Otol Rhinol 100:285–288, 1986.
3. Cole P, Haight JSJ. Posture and the nasal cycle. Ann Otol Rhinol Laryngol 95:233–237, 1986.
4. Proctor DF. The upper airway. In: Proctor DF, Andersen IB, eds. The Nose. Upper Airway Physiology and the Atmospheric Environment. Amsterdam: Elsevier Biomedical Press, 1982, Chap 2.
5. Haight JSJ, Cole P. Reciprocating nasal airflow resistances. Acta Otolaryngol (Stockh) 97:93–98, 1984.
6. Swift DL, Proctor DF. Access of air to the respiratory tract. In: Respiratory Defense Mechanisms, New York, Marcel Dekker, 1977.
7. Haight JSJ, Cole P. Site and function of the nasal valve. Laryngoscope 93:49–55, 1983.
8. Chaban R, Cole P, Naito K. Simulated septal deviations. Arch Otolaryngol Head Neck Surg 114:413–415, 1988.
9. Cole P, Chaban R, Naito K, Oprysk D. The obstructive nasal septum. Arch Otolaryngol Head Neck Surg 114:410–412, 1988.
10. Bridger GP. Physiology of the nasal valve. Arch Otolaryngol 92:543–553, 1970.
11. Bridger GP, Proctor DF. Maximum inspiratory flow and nasal resistance. Ann Otol 79:481–488, 1970.
12. Wustrow F. Schwellkorper am Septum nasi. Z Anat Entwicklges 116:139–142, 1951.
13. Haight JSJ, Cole P, Cooper PW, Kassel EE. The choana and nasal obstruction. J Otolaryngol 14:99–102, 1985.
14. Mygind N, Weeke B. Allergic and Vasomotor Rhinitis: Clinical Aspects. Copenhagen: Munksgaard, 1985.
15. Parker L. Thesis, Faculty of Dentistry, University of Toronto, 1986.
16. Rundcrantz H. Posture and congestion of nasal mucosa in allergic rhinitis. Acta Otolaryngol (Stockh) 58:283–287, 1985.
17. Lavie P, Gertner R, Zomer J, Podoshin L. Breathing disorders in sleep associated with microarousals in patients with allergic rhinitis. Acta Otolaryngol (Stockh) 92:529–533, 1981.
18. McNicholas WT, Tarlo S, Cole P, Zamel N, Rutherford R, Griffin D, Phillipson A. Obstructive apneas during sleep in patients with allergic rhinitis. Am Rev Respir Dis 126:625–628, 1982.
19. McNamara JA Jr, Ribbens KA. Nasorespiratory Function and Craniofacial Growth. Ann Arbor, MI: Center for Human Growth and Development, The University of Michigan.
20. Ogura JH, Harvey JE. Naso-pulmonary mechanisms: experimental evidence of influence of the upper airways on the lower. Acta Otolaryngol (Stockh) 71:123–132, 1971. ☐

Chapter XXXIX
Nasal Patency and Its Assessment

Philip Cole, M.D.

ABSTRACT

The propagation of nasal airflow resistance and its indispensable role in the modification of inspiratory air is described. Aerodynamic features and principles of rhinomanometric techniques which are commonly involved in the assessment of nasal patency are outlined. The clinical value of rhinomanometry is discussed in the light of the Toronto experience with several thousand patients.

The nasal cavities provide the principal portal for the passage of respiratory air, yet they present at least as great a resistance to breathing as the combined airflow resistances of the remaining segments of the respiratory tract.[1] Resistance of the nasal passages results from airflow characteristics which are essential for adequate modification of respiratory air.

In health almost all nasal resistance is confined to a narrowed segment of only a few millimeters in length which is situated in the anterior nose.[2] Orifice flow through this narrowed region introduces inertial disturbances which disrupt the laminar pattern with which inspiratory air enters the nasal vestibule.[3] The disturbances are entrained to the bronchi,[4] and they enable rapid and substantial exchanges to take place by contact between air and mucosa. The exchanges would be much less effective in the nose and large diameter upper airways under laminar flow conditions. By contrast, in small diameter airways, where airflow is slow and laminar and distances between midstream and mucosa are short, exchanges by slower processes of diffusion and convection play a greater part.

In order to maintain alveolar function, adequate modification of inspiratory air is essential. It involves thermal and aqueous exchanges between air and mucosa, entrapment of particulates, and solution of soluble gases.[5] Energy is required to promote and maintain the inertial disturbances of respiratory air necessary for these exchanges in the nose and larger airways, and it is manifested as resistance.

RHINOMANOMETRY

Nasal patency is measured by rhinomanometry, a system of measurement in which transnasal airflow and pressure are determined to provide an objective index, and rhinomanometric methods of proved value in physiological studies are extended increasingly to clinical assessment of the nasal airways.

Objective assessment provides useful documentation, it aids diagnosis and clinical management decisions, and it is available for the monitoring of therapy and as medico-legal evidence. This paper is concerned with clinical rhinomanometry and particular reference will be made to techniques employed and experience gained in the Airflow Laboratories of the Department of Otolaryngology, University of Toronto.

Passive rhinomanometric methods in which air is forced or drawn through the nasal passages by apparatus situated outside the subject have been applied to humans and are especially useful in animal studies, but this presentation will be confined to active methods employing the subject's respiratory airflow which are more usual in the clinical setting.

Early workers in the field of active rhinomanometry recorded separate tracings of concurrent transnasal airflow and differential pressures against time as subjects breathed through the nose. They assessed nasal respiratory function from inspection and from measurements of the recordings.[6] Today it is more common, and indeed, it is a recommendation of the International Committee on Standardization of Rhinomanometry[7] that recordings are made as an *x-y* plot of concurrent transnasal flow and pressure signals. Flow and pressure values are determined at a designated point or points on the resulting sigmoid tracing and patency is expressed in reciprocal form as resistance, a ratio between the coordinates ($\Delta P/\dot{V} = R_n$).

Department of Otolaryngology, Airflow Laboratories, University of Toronto, Toronto, Ontario, Canada

Several feasible alternatives to resistance, also derived from pressure and flow measurements, have been used for assessment of nasal patency. Derived units include conductance ($\dot{V}/\Delta P$, the reciprocal of resistance), power ($\Delta P \times \dot{V}$ in watts), work ($\Delta P \times V$ in joules) and effective cross-sectional area

$$\dot{V}/k\left[\frac{2(\Delta P)}{d}\right]\cdot {}^{1/2}$$

where d = density of air.[8,9]

Maximum expiratory flow assessment has been used also: it offers the advantages of simple and inexpensive instrumental requirements but it entails the disadvantages of effort dependence. In addition, there have been many attempts to apply or improve on Röhrer's equation,[10] $P = k_1 \dot{V} + k_2 \dot{V}^2$, by different mathematical transformations for description of the pressure/flow curve[11] and for calculation of patency, but general mathematical agreement has not been achieved. In the absence of such agreement, empirical methods prevail and resistance measurements similar to those recommended by the International Committee on Standardization of Rhinomanometry (ISCR) are widely used.

The Pressure/Flow Curve

Three main methods are utilized for transnasal pressure detection: pressures are conducted via a small tube inserted a) through closed lips to the oropharynx, b) along the floor of a nasal cavity to the nasopharynx, or c) sealed in one nasal vestibule as the subject breathes through the other. A transducer converts the pressure signal to an electrical analog for recording. Similar pressure values are produced by all three methods, but care must be taken to avoid interference with the compliant valvular portion of the anterior nose which contributes almost a half to resistance of the nose in health.[2]

Transnasal airflow is detected by a pneumotach incorporated in a facemask or in a head-out body plethysmograph; the signals are transduced for recording and similar results can be obtained by the two methods.[12] Again, care must be taken to avoid interference with the compliant anterior nose by pressure of the mask on facial tissues, a risk obviated by the plethysmographic method.

An x-y plot of concurrent pressure and flow is displayed, usually by an oscilloscope, and it takes the sigmoid form shown diagrammatically in Figure 1. As the subject breathes the course of the sigmoid curve exhibits remarkable consistency. This course is altered by change in nasal patency; a decrease rotates it toward the pressure axis or an increase rotates it toward the flow axis. Therefore, the ratio of the coordinates of any given point on the curve increases or decreases together with changes in patency. The ratio provides an index of patency.

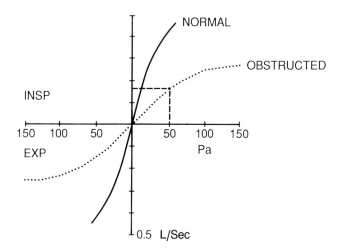

Figure 1. *Pressure and flow values are recorded and processed manually or electronically. Microprocessor computation from digitized values provides rapid and convenient data display, hard copy, and capability of storage and retrieval.*

A study of a large number of subjects with differing nasal patencies has shown that their pressure/flow curves can be arranged about an origin in radial order. Since these curves rarely cross,[13] numerical comparisons of patency similar to those obtained from a single subject by $P/\dot{V}$ measurements can be made between subjects also.

The preceding comments outline general principles of rhinomanometry as it is performed in many centers throughout the world. There are differences in technique and choice of equipment, but they are probably less important than the differences which prevail in methods of obtaining a $P/\dot{V}$ ratio from the sigmoid pressure/flow curve. Members of the ICSR are making efforts to resolve this problem by recommending internationally acceptable rhinomanometric standards so that investigators can more readily assess and compare results from different centers. A $P/\dot{V}$ ratio calculated at a point on the curve corresponding with a transnasal pressure of 100 Pa is widely accepted in Japan, and this standard is included in the provisional recommendations of the ISCR. Greater transnasal pressures are less frequently achieved by resting breaths in healthy Occidental or Oriental noses when subjects breathe through both nasal cavities.[14]

Use of a Microcomputer

A microcomputer can simplify the acquisition and processing of rhinomanometric data. Digitization of transnasal pressure and flow signals enables computation of several nasal and respiratory variables to be performed with a programmed microcomputer, and results can be displayed and printed. In addition to hard copy, disk storage of data is convenient for future reference and further processing.

Nasal patency in terms of work, power, effective cross-sectional area, conductance, and resistance is readily obtained by digital computation. Resistances can be averaged or acquired at separate predetermined points on the pressure/flow curve and comparisons made between different simultaneous measurements. In addition, other respiratory parameters, e.g., frequency, tidal volume, inspiratory and expiratory duration, peak pressures, and flow, etc. are easily computed.

A standard desktop microcomputer is adequate for clinic and laboratory rhinomanometry, but a small dedicated microcomputer with miniaturized equipment has proved more convenient for fieldwork.

The Toronto Experience

Fieldwork rhinomanometry has been performed with almost 5,000 subjects.[15] Nasal airflow is measured by means of a pneumotach incorporated in a facemask and transnasal pressures via a per-oral tube to the oropharynx. Pressure and flow signals are tranduced (Validyne MP45 transducers and CD101 carrier demodulators) and digitized at 50 Hz by an a/d converter of our own construction. Averaged resistance is computed from the digitized values by an inexpensive programmed microcomputer (Rockwell AIM65) from 5 consecutive nasal breaths which are monitored for synchrony of pressure and flow signals by paired LED arrays. Averaged ΔP and $\dot{V}$ values from 50 Hz sampling avoid the limitations imposed by calculations dependent upon predetermined points on the pressure/flow curve. This method accommodates all conditions of transnasal pressure and flow of respiratory air. The equipment is assembled as a rugged and portable miniaturized package. Three identical units have been in use for about 3 years; regular calibration has confirmed their stability and satisfactory results have been acquired from 85% of subjects tested.

Laboratory rhinomanometry is conducted in two adult clinics, a pediatric clinic, and a research laboratory. About 6,000 patients including 2,000 children and many volunteer subjects have been tested. Analysis of 1,000 consecutive referred pediatric patients shows a test failure rate of only 1.4%.

Laboratory techniques differ from those used in the field, but the principles are unchanged. In place of a facemask the subject is seated in a head-out body plethysmograph[16] which incorporates a large laminar flow element[17] for measurement of respiratory airflow (Fig. 2). This has proved to be more convenient, comfortable, and foolproof than a facemask; moreover, construction specifications are not particularly demanding and maintainance requirements are negligible. Calibration procedure is simple and it has shown the system to retain stability without readjustment during periods of several months of almost daily use. In addition, the subject's face is entirely unobscured which

is useful for the observer (e.g., for alar retraction or video studies, etc.) and kind to the patient. Children find the experience to be fun.

In pediatric patients, who may have obstruction from adenoid tissue, transnasal pressures are detected via a per-oral tube through closed lips to the oropharynx. This requires cooperation from the patient and persistance from the technician, but acceptable results can be obtained in almost all cases. In the adult, whose nasopharynx is not obstructed, the procedure is simpler. A fine catheter (Infant Feeding Tube 7F) lubricated with lidocaine gel is passed along the floor of the wider nasal cavity to the nasopharynx and secured to the upper lip with adhesive tape. Measurements have shown that the presence of a catheter of these dimensions along the floor of the nose produces no obstructive artefact and the catheter conducts the pressure signal adequately.

Pressure and flow signals are conditioned and processed in a manner similar to that described above for rhinomanometry in the field and an IBM-PC or compatible microcomputer is used in each of our laboratories. These microcomputers are not dedicated only to

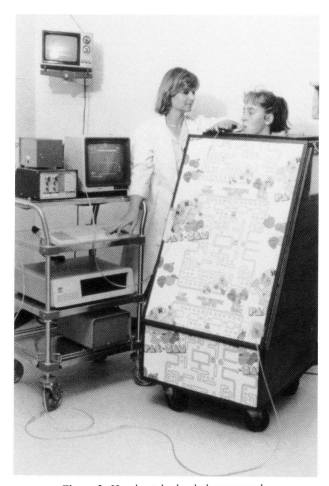

Figure 2. Head out body plethysmograph.

airflow studies, they are used also for the usual purposes of word processing, data base analysis, spreadsheets, etc. They will accept several data acquisition programs which have been developed for assessment of nasal patency and other variables of the extrapulmonary airways.

Our rhinomanometric results show substantial agreement with those of other workers[18] and correspond with resistance values which have been obtained at a transnasal pressure of 100 Pa.[19]

Procedural Details

Following the period required for documentation, history taking and clinical examination, the patient, acclimatized to a comfortable environment and at rest, is seated in the body plethysmograph with the head protruding through a fine dental dam diaphragm which provides a neck seal. The per-oral or per-nasal pressure detecting catheter is placed in position, transducer connections are completed and the x-y pressure/flow tracing is monitored as the subject breathes through the nose. When this tracing shows a regularly repeating and stable sigmoid course, a data acquisition program is activated to compute resistance. Five measurements of averaged resistance are acquired and displayed and if the coefficient of variation exceeds their mean by >8% aberrant results are rejected and repeated. If greater precision is required a smaller coefficient of variation is chosen.

Resistances are obtained from the combined nasal cavities of the untreated nose and, by occluding alternate sides, from each nasal cavity separately. The mucosa is then decongested by topical application of 0.1% xylometazoline and the measurements are repeated. Decongestion abolishes the nasal cycle, and it enables the magnitude of the mucovascular component of resistance to be assessed and the residual fixed components of resistance of the two nasal cavities to be measured separately and compared. Finally, resistances are measured, on each side separately, with wide alar retraction to minimize valvular resistance and to determine the residual resistance of each bony nasal cavity.

Resistive contributions of the compliant anterior nose, the bony cavum, and the vascular component of the mucosa are compared with the ranges of resistances established from healthy noses.

RESULTS AND COMMENTS

A few observations which result from our experience and might interest the reader are cited below; however, they are limited in number and content by the scope of the paper.

The healthy nose of an adult at rest in a comfortable environment has a resistance to respiratory airflow of the combined nasal cavities in the range of 2.0 ± 0.5 cm H_2O/L/sec (Pa/cm^3/sec × 10). This shows little change from day to day,[20] but there is a gradual trend from the higher toward the lower limits of the range throughout adult life. These resistance values are approximately halved by topical decongestant and they are increased in most cases by structural abnormality and by mucosal disease.

Children exhibit much greater intersubject variation of nasal resistance than adults and although generally resistances are higher, we have found many young children with resistances within the adult range. Of 1,000 consecutive referred pediatric patients aged 4 to 16 years, 15% demonstrated fixed adenoidal obstruction and 40% obstructive mucosal swelling which responded to decongestant.

Almost one-fifth of adult patients complaining of nasal obstruction at the time of examination had an unremarkable appearance of the nasal cavities and a resistance <2.5 cm H_2O/L/sec. In several cases complaints of nasal stuffiness accompanied exceptionally low resistance. In general, patients' assessment of the severity of obstruction at the time of examination was poorly correlated with resistance, even the acute effects of a decongestant were not invariably recognized and the presence of common aromatic substances produced misleading perceptions of nasal patency.

Septal deviations in the nasal cavum, which appeared large to rhinoscopy, were usually not obstructive and, by contrast, much smaller deviations in the anterior nose caused severe obstruction in many cases.

CONCLUSION

The present writer concludes, in common with many rhinologists, that wide international acceptance of appropriate rhinomanometric standards will improve the utility and credibility of this form of investigation of nasal function. Furthermore, in addition to the well established role of rhinomanometry in research, it has a practical application in clinical practice.

REFERENCES

1. Ferris BJ, Mead J, Opie LH. Partitioning of respiratory flow resistance in man. J Appl Physiol 19:653–658, 1964.
2. Haight JSJ, Cole P. The site and function of the nasal valve. Laryngoscope 93:49–55, 1983.
3. Swift DL, Proctor DF. Access of air to the respiratory tract. In: Respiratory Defense Mechanisms. New York: Marcel Decker, 1977, chap. 3.
4. Beekmans JM, Shephard RJ. Computer calculations of exercise dead space. Respiration 28:236–256, 1971.
5. Proctor DF, Andersen IB, eds. The Nose: Upper Airway Physiology and the Atmospheric Environment. Eds: Amsterdam: Elsevier Biomedical Press, 1982.
6. Cottle MH. Rhino-sphygmo-manometry: an aid in physical diagnosis. Int Rhinol 6:7–26, 1968.
7. Clement PAR. Committee Report on Standardization of Rhinomanometry, 1983.
8. Connell JT. An instrument for measuring the effective cross-

sectional nasal airway. J Allergy 37:127–134, 1966.

9. Warren DW. A quantitative technique for assessing nasal airway impairment. Am J Orthod Dentofacial Orthop 86:306–314, 1984.

10. Rohrer F. Der Stromungs weiderstand in den menlichen Atmenwegen und der Einfluss der unregelmassigen Verzweigung des bronchial Systems auf dem Atmungsverlauf in verschiedenen Lungenbezirken. Pflügers Arch 162:225–299, 1915.

11. Pallanch JF. Nasal Resistance. Thesis, University of Minnesota, 1984.

12. Cole P, Havas T. Nasal resistance to respiratory airflow: a plethysmographic alternative to the face mask. Rhinology 25:159–166, 1987.

13. Broms P. Rhinomanometry. Thesis, University of Lund, 1980.

14. Ohki M, Hasegawa M. Studies of transnasal pressure and airflow values in a Japanese population. Rhinology 24:277–282, 1986.

15. Broder I, Corey P, Cole P, Mintz S, Lipa M, Nethercott J. Health status of residents in homes insulated with urea formaldehyde. In: Walkinshaw DS, ed. Indoor Air Quality in Cold Climates: Hazards and Abatement Measures Air Pollution Control Association, Pittsburgh, PA, 1986, pp. 155–166.

16. Niinimaa V, Cole P, Mintz S, Shephard RJ. A head-out body plethysmograph. J Appl Physiol 47:1336–1339, 1979.

17. Griffin PM, Zamel N. Volume-displacement body plethysmograph using a large flowmeter without pressure compensation. J Appl Physiol 47:1127–1130, 1979.

18. McCaffrey TV, Kern EB. Clinical evaluation of nasal obstruction. Arch Otolaryngol 105:542–545, 1979.

19. Cole P, Havas TE. Resistance to respiratory airflow of the nasal passages: comparisons between different common methods of calculation. Rhinology 24:163–173, 1986.

20. Cole P, Fastag O, Forsyth R. Variability in nasal resistance measurements. J Otolaryngol 9:309–315, 1980. □

Chapter XL

Flexible Fiberoptic Endoscopy of the Upper Airway

William K. Dolen, M.D.*, John C. Selner, M.D.**

ABSTRACT

Fiberoptic rhinolaryngoscopy is a safe, convenient, and affordable means by which any physician may examine the upper airway. Although rhinoscopic findings in uncomplicated allergic rhinitis are uninformative, therapeutic decisions (including institution of allergen immunotherapy) are sometimes made in patients with allergic rhinitis significantly complicated by anatomic nasal obstruction or other conditions primarily managed by surgery. Comprehensive examination is indicated when allergy is not a satisfactory explanation for patient symptoms or when response to management is not satisfactory.

We believe the procedure, used as an adjunct to routine upper airway examination, should not add substantial cost to a medical evaluation. We suggest that rhinolaryngoscopy should be taught early in the course of training in allergy or otolaryngology, where it can be used as a means of teaching upper airway anatomy and pathology as well as a way of facilitating collaboration, rather than competition, with other specialists. Thoughtful use of rhinolaryngoscopy will result in early and appropriate requests for consultation.

Routine physical examination of the upper airway usually consists of inspection of the anterior structures of the nares with an otoscope and pharyngeal examination with a tongue depressor. These traditional methods limit the extent to which physicians can evaluate symptoms referable to structures of the upper airway. Thus, therapeutic decisions often are made on the basis of presenting symptoms. Use of a nasal speculum and a bright, focused light source permits examination of most of the inferior structures of the nasal passage and part of the nasopharynx; nasopharyngeal and laryngeal mirrors facilitate inspection of the phar-

* *Clinical Assistant Professor of Medicine*
** *Clinical Professor of Pediatrics*
University of Colorado Center for the Health Sciences, Denver, CO

ynx and larynx. Although a skilled examiner can examine most adults and many children without local anesthesia, sedation, or restraint, most physicians have not developed these skills. Those who have often are rewarded with only a fleeting glimpse of important structures. These conventional methods, even under the best of conditions, do not permit careful examination of the recessed structures of the upper airway, such as the ostia of the paranasal sinuses, the sphenoethmoidal recess, and the Eustachian tube orifice.

The medical and industrial development of flexible fiberoptic technology has provided a safe, convenient, and affordable alternative to traditional methods for any physician interested in comprehensive examination of the upper airway. The flexible fiberoptic rhinolaryngoscope places the physician who evaluates and manages patients with upper airway complaints at the same advantage as his pulmonary and gastroenterology colleagues who routinely perform endoscopy.[1-4]

HISTORY OF UPPER AIRWAY ENDOSCOPY

Instrumentation for upper airway endoscopy is derived from that ordinally designed for examination of the gastrointestinal tract, the urinary bladder, and the lower airway.[5] Kussmaul first performed gastrointestinal endoscopy on sword swallowers in 1868, employing a rigid metal tube and a light source fueled by a mixture of alcohol and turpentine. By the turn of the century, a more practical instrument illuminated by an incandescent light had been developed.

These rigid instruments required considerable skill and experience for use, were uncomfortable for patients, and could not be employed to examine recessed areas. It was thus necessary to construct a flexible endoscope. Conveying an image requires that light be transmitted through a bundle of small glass fibers, but light leakage from fiber to fiber in the course of travel results in considerable loss of image quality. Curtiss, Peters, and Hirschowitz developed a method whereby optical glass can be clad with glass of a lower refractive index and pulled into a thin fiber. In 1956, they successfully transmitted "a bright spot of light" from one room to another in the physics department of the University of Michigan. Two months later, a primitive flexible fiberscope was employed to inspect a duodenal ulcer in the wife of a dental student.[6] Industrial applications requiring great flexibility for inspection of automobile engine parts without dismantling resulted in further improvements in maneuverability and image quality. For use in examination of the upper airway, the flexible fiberscope required miniaturization. Modern instruments contain as many as 1200 bundles in an endoscope of 3.5 mm diameter.

The optically excellent Hopkins nasal endoscopes permit extensive examination of the nasal cavities and portions of the nasopharynx, as well as high quality photography of the structures examined. The cost of a set of these rigid instruments and the relative difficulty in learning to use them has limited their use for routine office examination; they are primarily used for endoscopic sinus surgery.

INDICATIONS FOR ENDOSCOPIC UPPER AIRWAY EXAMINATION

Modern fiberoptic instruments can be used in patients of any age; a limited examination can be performed even in premature infants. Nearly any symptom referable to the upper airway and not explained by routine examination is a relative indication for endoscopy (Table I).

TABLE I

Indications for Upper Airway Endoscopy[4]

General
    Any symptom or complaint referable to the upper airway
Nose and nasopharynx
    Nasal obstruction (particularly if unilateral)
    Snoring, mouthbreathing
    Anosmia
    Headaches, facial pain
    Epistaxis
    Rhinorrhea
    Sinusitis
    Earache, recurrent, or chronic otitis media
    Regional adenopathy
    Assessment of results of surgical intervention
Hypopharynx and larynx
    Dysphagia or globus
    Hoarseness or other changes in voice quality
    Chronic cough
    Atypical asthma (laryngeal dysfunction)

METHOD

The endoscope (Figure 1) was designed to be held in one hand, leaving the other hand free to manipulate the patient's head and control depth of insertion of the endoscope. At the Allergy Respiratory Institute of Colorado (ARI), we routinely videotape examinations to review examination findings with the patient, parents, and other physicians. The patient is seated in an examination chair with an adjustable headrest, and the height of the chair is adjusted to bring the floor of the nasal passage to the level of the rhinolaryngoscope, which is attached to a video camera suspended from the ceiling on a movable track (Figure 2). Output from the video camera is fed into a videocassette recorder and a color video monitor (Figure 3). While viewing the video image, the examiner adjusts the patient's head position and guides the endoscope with the left hand, using the right hand to manipulate the endoscope-camera unit, and using the thumb of the right hand to direct the course of the endoscope tip.

Following a routine nasal speculum examination, the nasal mucosa are decongested with topical oxymetazoline. Pharyngeal and laryngeal anesthesia are not necessary; the nasal passage is anesthetized with 4% xylocaine solution. The endoscope is lubricated for small children or patients with dry mucosa.

A comprehensive endoscopic evaluation includes examination of the nasal septum, the turbinates, the meati of the turbinates, the roof and floor of the nasal cavity, and the anterior and posterior choanae. Structures of the nasopharynx, such as the torus tubarius, the eustachian tube orifice, Rosenmüller's fossa, and the adenoidal pad may easily be inspected. Without need for laryngeal anesthesia, it is possible to examine the pharyngeal walls, soft palate, posterior tongue, lingual tonsils, epiglottis and associated structures, arytenoid cartilages, and the true and false vocal cords in phonation and quiet respiration.

FINDINGS

Fiberoptic examination may produce pertinent positive as well as negative findings. A summary of findings encountered in the examination of thousands of patients is presented in Table II. The information obtained from fiberoptic examination almost always directly influences interpretation of patient complaints, permitting the development of an informed differential diagnosis, cost-effective ordering of further diagnostic studies, and selection of appropriate treatment strategies.

Figure 4 is a photograph of the left nasal cavity of a child undergoing psychiatric evaluation for sleep disturbance and severe behavior problems. There was an "adenoidal facies" and disturbed maxillary growth. The patient was undergoing orthodontic corrective measures, including use of a palate expander. The septum is

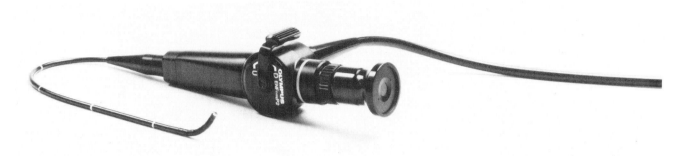

Figure 1. The Olympus ENF-P2 flexible fiberoptic rhinolaryngoscope. Photograph courtesy of Olympus Corporation, Lake Success, NY.

located at 9 o'clock; at 11 o'clock is the posterior margin of the middle turbinate. There is extreme adenoidal hyperplasia, with herniation of adenoidal tissue anteriorly through the choana, resulting in complete obstruction. This child had obstructive sleep apnea without cardiopulmonary compromise,[7] and symptoms were relieved by adenoidectomy.

QUANTITATIVE ENDOSCOPIC EVALUATION OF NASAL PATENCY

A number of subjective and objective methods for evaluation of nasal patency have been used to assess the result of nasal challenge or therapeutic intervention. No single method appears satisfactory for all circumstances; a combination of symptom scoring and rhinomanometry is often used. The effect of medication and provocation challenge on the nasal mucosa can be observed directly by endoscopy and videotaped.

A simple modification of the basic rhinoscopic technique permits estimation of cross-sectional nasal airway area at the level of the anterior portion of the inferior turbinate.[8] The study subject is positioned as usual, and the endoscope tip is placed on the nasal floor at the anterior portion of the inferior turbinate. The endoscope tip is flexed as necessary to bring the nasal sep-

Figure 2. Positioning of patient, examiner, and equipment for fiberoptic rhinolaryngoscopy as performed at ARI. The endoscope is attached to a video camera suspended from the ceiling. The examiner stands to the patient's right.[2]

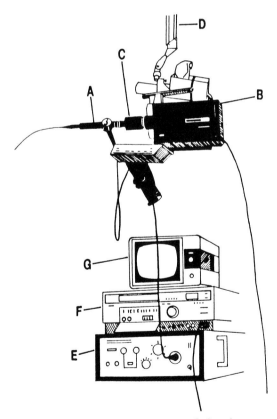

Figure 3. Equipment for videotaping of rhinolaryngoscopic examinations: (A) fiberoptic endoscope (B) video camera (C) camera mount for endoscope (D) overhead suspension apparatus connected to a sliding ceiling mount (E) endoscopic light source (F) videocassette recorder (G) color video monitor.[2]

TABLE II

Findings and pathology Evident on Fiberoptic Rhinolaryngoscopy in Clinical Practice.[4]

Region	Findings
Mucosa	Mucus (clear vs. purulent)
	Color, vascular changes
	Inflammation, cobblestoning
	Mucosal atrophy or ulceration
Nasal cavity	
Turbinates	Bony or mucosal hypertrophy
	Compression from septal deviation
	Surgical resection
	Clefting (horizontal and sagittal)
	Polypoidal degeneration
	Concha bullosa
Septum	Deviation, dislocation
	Perforation, spurs, ulcers
	Maxillary ridge
Polyps	Paranasal sinus origination
	Squamous metaplasia
	Papillomas, tumors
Paranasal sinuses	Purulent mucus draining from a sinus ostium
	Direct inspection of maxillary sinus
	Postoperative evaluation of sinus surgery
Nasopharynx and superior oropharynx	
Choana	Atresia or stenosis (unilateral or bilateral)
Eustachian tube orifice	Cysts
	Prominent tubal tonsil
	Edematous obstruction
	Postsurgical scarring and retraction
Adenoids	Adenoiditis, Rathke's pouch cyst
	Hyperplasia, anterior herniation through choana
Pharyngeal wall	Osteophytes, carotid aneurysm
	Constrictor muscle spasm
Malignancies	Carcinomas originating in Rosenmüller's fossa
Oropharynx, hypopharynx, larynx	
Posterior tongue	Cystic circumvallate papillae, mucoceles
	Papillomata, Candida infection
Lingual tonsils	Hypertrophy, infection
Epiglottis	Edema, positional deformity
	Inflammation of petiole
Glottis	Erythema, edema, laryngocele
Arytenoids	Contact ulcers, edema
Vocal cords	Polyps, nodules, papillomata, granulomas
	Reinke's edema
	Contact ulcers, webs, paralysis
	Vocal cord adduction syndrome[11]

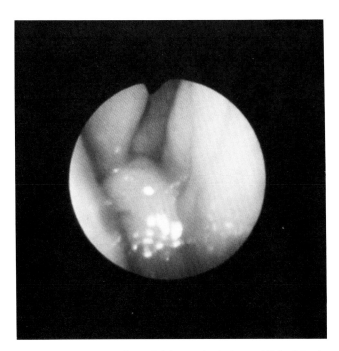

Figure 4. Massive adenoidal hyperplasia in a child with obstructive sleep apnea. (Photograph reproduced from Selner et al.[4]; used with permission.)

tum, inferior turbinate, and nasal floor into view simultaneously. These structures in this view, called a "fixed point," are used as the basis for cross-sectional airway measurements. The distance from the tip of the endoscope to the opening of the nostril is measured and recorded, and a rubber O ring is inserted on the endoscope at this point to ensure that the endoscope will remain in place and at a constant depth during the examination.

A video recording is made with the endoscope in correct position. At a later time, the recordings are replayed. An image is frozen on the video monitor using the stop frame mode of the videocassette recorder, and the image is traced onto a transparency placed on the monitor screen. The area of the tracing is measured with a computer digitizer. For subsequent examinations, consistency of endoscope placement is achieved by use of a constant depth of insertion of the endoscope tip as well as use of the nasal floor and septum for orientation. This method produces results comparable to those from anterior rhinomanometry[8] and that correlate well with subjective symptoms of airway obstruction.[9]

COMPLICATIONS

In nearly 3,000 examinations, there has been one episode of epistaxis, requiring temporary pressure and ice application. On two occasions, contact of the endoscope with the nasal mucosa has triggered marked coughing spasms. Syncopal episodes, probably vasovagal in nature, have occurred about ten times, primarily in young adult males. Consequently, we do not believe that a signed informed consent document should be required for this procedure. It is the only endoscopic procedure exempt from the informed consent requirement by our statewide, physician-run liability corporation.

CONCLUSION

The clinical usefulness of fiberoptic upper airway examination has been questioned.[10] Indeed, rhinoscopic findings in uncomplicated allergic rhinitis are quite uninformative. All too often, however, therapeutic decisions, including institution of allergen immunotherapy, are made for patients with allergic rhinitis significantly complicated by anatomic nasal obstruction or other conditions primarily managed by surgery. Comprehensive examination is indicated when allergy is not a satisfactory explanation for patient symptoms or when response to management is not satisfactory.

We believe that nearly any motivated physician can learn to integrate fiberoptic rhinolaryngoscopy into an office practice. We think the procedure, when used as an adjunct to routine upper airway examination, should not add substantial cost to a medical evaluation.

We suggest that rhinolaryngoscopy should be taught early in the course of training in allergy or otolaryngology, where the procedure can be used as a means of teaching upper airway anatomy and pathology as well as a means of facilitating collaboration, rather than competition, with other specialists. Thoughtful use of rhinolaryngoscopy will result in early and appropriate requests for consultation.

REFERENCES

1. Rohr A, Hassner A, Saxon A. Rhinopharyngoscopy for the evaluation of allergic-immunologic disorders. Ann Allergy 50:380, 1983.
2. Selner JC, Koepke JW. Rhinolaryngoscopy in the allergy office. Ann Allergy 54:479, 1985.
3. Lancer JM, Jones AS. Flexible fibreoptic rhinolaryngoscopy: Results of 338 consecutive examinations. J Laryngol Otol 99:771, 1985.
4. Selner JC, Dolen WK, Spofford B, Koepke JW. Rhinolaryngoscopy, 2nd Ed. Denver: Allergy Respiratory Institute of Colorado, 1989.
5. Hirschowitz BI. A personal history of the fiberscope. Gastroenterology 76:864, 1979.
6. Curtiss LE, Hirschowitz BI, Peters CW. A long fiberscope for internal medical examinations. J Am Optical Soc 46:1030, 1956.
7. Brouillette RT, Fernbach SK, Hunt CE. Obstructive sleep apnea in infants and children. J Pediatr 100:31, 1982.
8. Zedalis D, Dolen WK, Selner JC, et al. Evaluation of nasal patency by fiberoptic rhinoscopy. J Allergy Clin Immunol 83:973, 1989.
9. Selner JC, Wiener MB, Koepke JW et al. Rhinoscopy: Cross sectional area measurements of nasal patency comparison with nasal symptoms (Abstract). J Allergy Clin Immunol 79:233, 1987.
10. Schumacher MJ. Flexible nasopharyngoscopy: A procedure for allergists? J Allergy Clin Immunol 82:909, 1988.
11. Christopher KL, Wood RP, Eckert RC et al. Vocal cord dysfunction presenting as asthma. N Engl J Med 308:1566, 1983.

Chapter XLI

Nasal Provocation Testing

Minoru Okuda, M.D.

ABSTRACT

Nasal provocation testing is employed to evaluate the sensitivity of nasal mucous membrane to allergen, mediators of the type I allergy, autonomotropic drug and so on. From our experimental results, nasal provocation should be performed by application of a fixed size of surface area of the bilateral inferior turbinate visually using a rhinoscope and then nasal response produced should be assessed by rhinoscopy together with counting the number of sneezes or with a rhinomanometer. For this purpose, the paper disc method was practically useful due to easiness of application, reliability of test result, and minimum side effect.

Nasal provocation testing is normally employed to evaluate the sensitivity of the nasal mucous membrane to allergen, mediators of the type I allergy, autonomotropic drug, and so on. Its diagnostic value for allergies, however, is still controversial. Some investigators have found this test to be an important diagnostic tool for confirmation of the accuracy of a skin test and nonspecific hyperreactivity of the nose; others state that it gives little additional information. Such confusion may result from a lack of standardization of this test. Therefore, I would like to contribute to establishing the international standardization of a nasal provocation test by summarizing briefly the result of our study of this problem.[1-3]

PRINCIPLE OF METHODOLOGY OF NASAL PROVOCATION

Nasal responses to allergen, histamine, and another provoking agents varied depending on the site in the nasal cavity, the nasal side, and the size of the nasal mucosal surface to be provoked.[1]

Both the inferior turbinate and agger nasi were more sensitive than the septum or middle turbinate because of different densities of the nerves, vessels, and secretory glands in the mucosa (Table I).

The side differences in the sensitivity to allergen or histamine were observed in 60% of patients examined with allergic rhinitis and were not well correlated with the side of stimulation, the side of septal deviation, degree of swelling, and color of the inferior turbinate stimulated (Table II). In addition, positive responses were frequent with simultaneous provocation of both sides more than with provocation to one side selected at random (Table III).

Two different sized areas of the inferior turbinate were provoked with the same concentration of histamine and the nasal response produced was revealed to be stronger with provocation to the wider surface (Table IV).

The intensity of stimulants (concentration of provoking agents) was also an important factor in changing the degree of nasal response. In the application of allergen to the inferior turbinate in a series of increasing concentrations, the accumulation curve of positive responses was obtained. The number of positive responses increased as the concentrations were increased and

TABLE I

Four-Site Differences in Sensitivity to Histamine*

Site According to Greatest Sensitivity	No. of Cases
Inferior turbinate and agger nasi	9
Agger nasi	6
Inferior turbinate	3
Inferior turbinate, agger nasi, middle turbinate	2
Nasal septum	1

Both inferior turbinate and agger nasi were the most sensitive in 21 patients with house dust allergy ($p < 0.001$, t test).

Department of Otolaryngology, Nippon Medical School, Tokyo, Japan

325

TABLE II

Side Differences in Sensitivity to Histamine and Allergen*

	Histamine	Allergen
Right > left	6 (19.4%)	18 (30.0%)
Right = left	11 (35.5%)	25 (41.7%)
Right < left	14 (45.1%)	17 (28.3%)

* There were side differences in the sensitivity to histamine and allergen in each patients although sometimes a side and sometimes one side is more sensitive than the other.

TABLE IV

Size Difference of the Surface Area in Sensitivity to Histamine*

Size	Number of Discs
>3	0
=3	5
<3	15

* The size of the surface area of the nasal mucous membrane stimulated were expressed by the number of paper discs. The larger the size, the stronger the nasal response (p < 0.025, t test).

finally reached a plateau (Fig. 1). Based on the above results, it could be concluded that nasal provocation should be performed at a fixed size of the nasal mucosa on both sides of the nose by the iteration method. This principle is referred to as the three S system.

FORM OF THE PROVOKING AGENT

The provoking agents are usually solid or liquid. Either form could be used for the 3-S system of provocation if the delivery system was adequate.

We developed a paper disc method for nasal provocation. The provoking allergen extract in different doses is contained in a round paper disc (Toyo-Roshi No 5), 3 mm in diameter, and is dried and stored for later use, or 10 μl of liquid agents of different concentrations are absorbed by the same paper disc immediately before use. This method is useful for the 3-S system of provocation, because it is easy to stimulate a fixed site and the fixed size of the nasal mucosa. Since the agent contained in the disc is dried and stored, the stability of the agent increases (Table V). Powder form is also recommended if quantitative provocation is to be performed. We took 3 mg of allergen powder on a small spoon and placed it on the surface of the inferior turbinate so as not to irritate the nasal mucosa or risk having the powder blown out by heavy breathing. A

positive response was more frequent with this method than with the paper disc method (Table VI), and nonspecific response was minimum. The freeze-dried powder, however, has disadvantages as a result of being hygroscopic. It sometimes becomes wet by absorption of water, or causes a severe response since the allergen extract is quickly and totally dissolved in the nasal fluid in contrast to the slow elution of allergen from the disc in the paper disc method.

DELIVERY OF THE PROVOKING AGENT

Provoking agents are delivered to the nasal cavity by visual or nonvisual means (Table VII).

Blind spraying, or dropping of the test solution into the nose, or sniffing a powder, which are generally used by doctors other than otolaryngologists, is not recommended, since the distribution of agents would not be consistent in the site and size of the nasal mucosa.

We sprayed a liquid radio-opaque agent (iodamide

TABLE III

Differences in Incidence of Positive Reaction between Both Side and Right Fixed Side Challenge with Allergen in 114 Patients with House Dust Allergy*

Side	Incidence (%)
Both	64.0
Right	33.3

* Positive reactions occurred in both side challenge more frequently than in right side only (p < 0.001, χ^2 test).

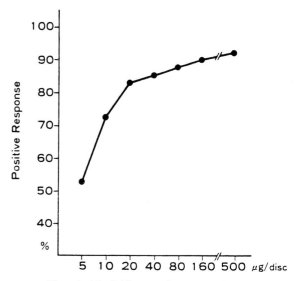

Figure 1. Accumulation curve of positive response. The curve reached peak allergen concentration of 20 μg/disc (N = 40).

326

TABLE V

Stability of Allergen in Paper Disc*

	Total N (μg)				Protein N (μg)			
	0	3 Mo	6 Mo	12 Mo	0	3 Mo	6 Mo	12 Mo
2–8°C	8.98	9.00	9.20	8.76	3.31	3.22	3.20	3.05
Room temperature	8.98	9.02	8.91	9.12	3.31	3.25	3.20	3.04
37°C	8.98	9.00	8.91	8.65	3.31	3.27	3.35	3.20

Allergen paper disc stored at 2–8°C, room temperature or 37°C. Total N and protein N were not decreased for 3, 6 or 12 months.

meglumine) into the nasal cavities of normal individuals and patients with allergic rhinitis and then examined the distribution by computer x-ray tomography. The results were quite unsatisfactory since the distributions were not uniform and random (Table VIII).

Even if a quantitative provocation was performed visually with an atomizer the distribution of the test solution would be inconsistent since the form of the nasal cavities of patients with allergic or hypertrophic rhinitis is different from person to person due to the different degrees of swelling of the nasal mucosa. Therefore, to perform the 3 S system of provocation, test agents, contained in a paper disc or similar material, or powdered agents should be delivered to a fixed site of a consistent size on the bilateral inferior turbinate. Otherwise, a constant volume of test solution could be dropped through a fine needle onto the mucosal surface. In this case, however, the solution dropped would easily flow down to the nasal floor from the inferior turbinate. Each method, however, has adavantages and disadavantages in application, onset of response, side effects, positive response, titration test, nonspecific reaction, and preservation of material (Table IX).

TABLE VI

Differences in Positive Provocation Reaction between the Paper Disc Method and Challenge with Freeze-Dried Allergen Powder*

Disc	Powder†	No. of Cases
Negative	Negative	14
Positive	Positive	31
Positive	Negative	2
Negative	Positive	6

The results of both method agree in 84.9%.
† House dust powder: about 3 mg (protein N 12 μg/mg).

DOSE OF THE PROVOKING AGENT

For the 3 S system of provocation, titration is preferred, since the nasal sensitivity differs greatly from patient to patient, and a higher concentration of test agents induces a stronger reaction. Other advantages of the titration method are minimum consumption of allergen, expression of nasal sensitivity by the value of thresholds, and ease in judging positive response.

On the other hand, a method of provocation using a fixed single amount of test agents and involving evaluation of the degree of response produced is also useful because it saves time. For this purpose our allergen paper disc method is preferable since a fixed single dose of allergen in a disc elutes slowly and diffuses into nasal

TABLE VII

Nasal Provocation with Allergens and Pharmacological Agents

Physical Conditions	Delivery into the Nose
1. Particles	
Powders	Natural inhalation
Particles in carriers (paper, cotton, etc.)	Injection with a compressor, rubber bulb, etc.
	Sniff
	Insertion with a pincette, spoon, etc.
2. Solution	
Aerosol	Spray with an atomizer, nebulizer, etc.
Liquid	Dropping with a pipette, syringe, etc.
Liquid in carriers (paper, cotton, etc.)	Insertion with a pincette
3. Gas	Active inhalation
	Passive inhalation with a rubber bulb, etc.

TABLE VIII

Distribution of Radio-opaque Agent in Computed Tomography of the Nose After Quantitative Nonvisual Spray with Iodamide Meglumine Solution into the Nose*

Nose	N	Inferior turbinate	Middle turbinate	Septum	Epipharynx
		Anterior Parts			
Normal	6	6	1	6	0
Allergic or hypertrophic rhinitis	5	5	1	3	1

There was no deposition of the agent on the posterior parts of the inferior and middle turbinate and of the septum.

secretion until the amount of allergen eluted becomes necessary to produce nasal symptoms.

To confirm this experimentally, we placed paper discs with allergen on the surface of CNBr activated paper discs which were filled with phosphate-buffered saline solution. We then collected the latter discs at 1-, 2-, 3-, 5-, 10-, and 30-minute intervals. After the paper discs were collected, the amount of allergen eluted and transferred from the allergen paper discs was measured by means of enzyme-linked immunosorbent test to see how much allergen was eluted (Fig. 2). We found that allergen eluted from the paper disc slowly in time-dependent manner (Fig. 3). We examined the correlation of the degree of response to a fixed single dose of allergen with the end-point value of allergen and found a good correlation ($r = 0.744$) between these two methods (Fig. 4).

ASSESSMENT OF THE RESPONSE

The main nasal symptoms to be provoked are sneezing, hypersecretion, and nasal blockage, each of which is objectively assessed. The number of sneezes

can be counted; hypersecretion can be assessed by measuring volume or weight of nasal secretion collected by suction into tubes, blowing the nose with paper or by other methods; nasal blockage can be assessed by measuring the nasal airway resistance (NAR) with a rhinomanometer.

Practically however, we need to express the result of provocation in one figure. For this purpose, a judging method has been proposed and used by us, which is referred to as the rhinoscopic method.[2] The responses were graded by sneezing or itchiness increase in nasal secretion, and swelling of the nasal mucosa Appearance of more than two of these symptoms is regarded as positive; appearance of two is classed as 1+; appearance of three with less than five sneezes as 2+ and with more than six sneezes as 3+.

This method is simple and time-saving and requires neither special equipment nor the patient's cooperation, but it has the disadvantages of being subjective and requiring an experienced examiner. Rhinomanometry is widely used for total assessment of nasal response in spite of the fact that it only evaluates nasal blockage,

TABLE IX

Characteristics of Different Provocation Methods

Methods	Application (the 3 S System)	Onset of Response	Side Effects	Incidence of Positive Response	Titration Test	Nonspecific Reaction	Preservation
Paper disc with a pincette	Easy	Slow	Minimum	Moderate	Easy (unnecessary)	Slight	Good
Powder with a spoon	Not easy	Quick	Sometimes severe	High	Difficult	Minimum	Good
Solution with a syringe	Difficult	Quick	Sometimes severe	Low	Easy	Minimum	No good

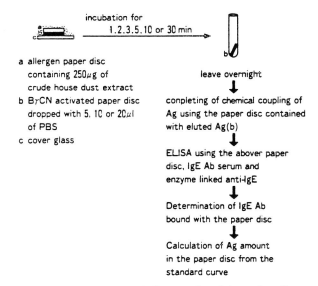

a allergen paper disc
  containing 250μg of
  crude house dust extract
b BγCN activated paper disc
  dropped with 5, 10 or 20μl
  of PBS
c cover glass

incubation for
1.2.3.5.10 or 30 min

leave overnight

↓

conpleting of chemical coupling of
Ag using the paper disc contained
with eluted Ag(b)

↓

ELISA using the abover paper
disc, IgE Ab serum and
enzyme linked anti-IgE

↓

Determination of IgE Ab
bound with the paper disc

↓

Calculation of Ag amount
in the paper disc from the
standard curve

Figure 2. *Determination of allergen eluted from the allergen paper disc.*

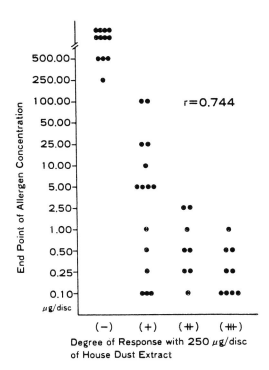

Figure 4. *Relationships between end-point test and fixed single dose test (250 μg/disc) in provocation. The end-points correlated well with the degree of reaction by single dose allergen (r = 0.744, p < 0.01).*

which is only one of the nasal symptoms in provocation. To elucidate the value of rhinomanometry in the general assessment of nasal response, we examined the response of provocation by the allergen paper disc method in the same patients with allergic rhinitis simultaneously by both rhinoscopy and rhinomanometry, and the results were compared. Rhinomanometry was performed by the active anterior method, using a rhinomanometer (MPR-1100, Nihon-Koden). Changes in NAR measured were expressed as the ratio of allergen/control provocation and changes of 20% or more

were judged as positive, since spontaneous changes in NAR were mostly below 20%. As a result, positive response rates were the same (56.0%) for both methods and the agreement rate of each method was 72%. Contradictory results were obtained in 14 of 50 patients (Table X).

Rhinomanometry is completely objective and can be used by doctors or nurses who are not familiar with rhinoscopy, but the disadvantages are that it needs special expensive equipment, the patient's cooperation,

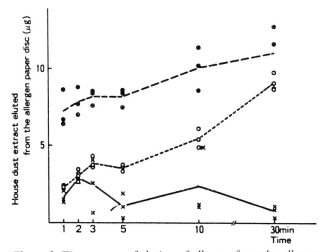

Figure 3. *Time course of elution of allergen from the allergen paper disc in 5 μl (×), 10 μl; (●), or 20 μl (○) of phosphate-buffered saline solution. The amounts of allergen eluted were determined by enzyme-linked immunosorbent assay. Time-dependent elutions were observed.*

TABLE X

Assessment of Nasal Response in the Comparison of Rhinoscopy with Rhinomanometry*

Rhinoscopy Degree	Rhinomanometry	
	Positive	Negative
3+	6	2
2+	8	2
1+	7	3
0	7	15

* *Positive response rate by rhinoscopy was the same as that by rhinomanometry (56.0%), and the agreement rate was 72.0%. Contradictory results were obtained in 14 patients (28.0%).*

329

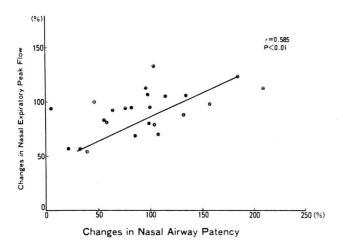

Figure 5. *Changes in nasal patency after provocation.*

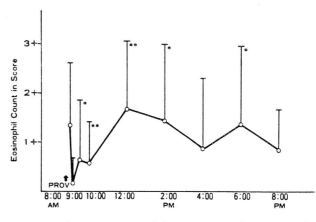

Figure 6. *Change in eosinophil count in nasal secretion after allergen provocation to patients with Japanese cedar pollinosis. The eosinophil count decreased immediately after provocation and then increased (N = 14, *p < 0.05, **p < 0.01).*

and a longer testing time. The results were invalid for many children, and even for adults who have highly congested noses that they are unable to breath through. The value of NAR differs depending on the instrument used.

Instead of a rhinomanometer, a handy peak flow meter with a nose mask (mini-wright peak flow meter) is sometimes used for measuring a change in the patency of the nasal cavity. Correlation of the results by rhinomanometry with those by the peak flow meter were good in simultaneously measuring the change after nasal provocation (Fig. 5).

There are additional methods to assess the nasal provocation response.

To evaluate nasal response the measurement of nasal blood flow was examined. However, it is not a recommended method because it requires expensive equipment, is time consuming, and involves complicated procedures (Table XI).

To confirm whether or not the response produced is allergic we sometimes examine the number of eosinophil leukocytes in the nasal secretion. In this case, we have to collect the nasal secretion 2–3 hours after provocation, since the number reaches its peak at this time (Fig. 6).

FACTORS INFLUENCING NASAL RESPONSE

Nasal provocation reaction was affected by many different factors.

Decreases in the response were induced by administration of anti-allergic drugs (histamine antagonist, cromolyn sodium, ketotifen, tranilast, and topical steroid, etc.), long-term immunotherapy (Table XII), topical adrenergic stimulant (for nasal blockage only) and cholinergic blockade (for secretion only) (Table XIII), warm stimulation on the leg (Fig. 7), and during the off-season of pollinosis (Fig. 8). On the other hand, increases in the response were induced by administration of adrenergic blockade (for nasal blockage only) and cholinergic stimulant (for secretion only) (Table XIII), block of the stellatum ganglion of the neck, cold stimulation on the leg (Fig. 7), and, during the in-season of pollinosis (Fig. 8).

RELIABILITY OF THE TEST

The reliability of the disc method and rhinoscopic assessment was studied by a comparison of test results with a patient's history as to causative allergen, serum IgE antibody level and the effect of treatment.

TABLE XI

Changes in Nasal Blood Flow (ml/min/g) after Provocation to the Allergic Nasal Mucosa*

	N	0	1 Min	5 Min	10 Min	15 Min
Histamine	18	1.39 ± 0.34	1.30 ± 0.26	1.22 ± 0.35**	1.30 ± 0.31	1.36 ± 0.20
Allergen	27	1.42 ± 0.27		1.26 ± 0.23***	1.33 ± 0.27	

* *Blood flow in the nasal mucosa decreased by provocation with histamine and allergen.*
** *P < 0.05.*
*** *P < 0.01.*

TABLE XII

Decreases in the Degree of Provocation Reaction after Treatment with DSCG or Beclomethasone or Immunotherapy with Allergen*

	No. of Cases	Decrease (%)	Increase (%)	Significance
DSCG	48	60.4	0.02	$p < 0.01$
Placebo	54	18.5	0.02	
Beclomethasone	47	72.9	0.04	$p < 0.001$
Placebo	42	21.0	0	
Immunotherapy	89	75.3	3.4	$p < 0.01$†

* *Decreases in the degree of provocation were obtained after the treatments in association with significant improvement of subjective symptoms.*
† *Comparison of provocation responses before and after treatment. r = 0.4337.*

Of the 87 patients with both a positive history and skin test including Japanese cedar, timothy, orchard grass and ragweed, a positive provocation reaction was obtained in 79.3% of them, while of the 24 patients with a positive history but a negative skin test this reaction was obtained in only 4.1%. On the other hand, of the 29 patients with a negative history and a positive skin test, positive provocation was obtained in 48.3%, while of 30 patients with both a negative history and skin test 0% showed positive provocation (Table XIV). The presence of patients with a positive history and skin test but a negative provocation suggested the clinical diagnostic value of the provocation test rather than its false reaction. Negative provocation but positive skin test in the patients with a positive history was caused by a

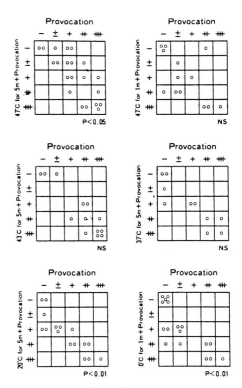

Figure 7. *Comparison of nasal provocation reactions without pretreatment with those with warm or cold stimulation on leg before provocation. Cold treatment (0°C for 1 minute and 20°C for 5 minutes) increased nasal response, while warm (47°C for 5 minutes) decreased it.*

lower sensitivity of the nose to allergen and chemical mediators released. The relationship between the serum IgE antibody level determined by radioallergosorbent test (RAST) and the degree of provocation reaction was examined in house dust allergy patients and a statisti-

TABLE XIII

Effects of Autonomotropic Drugs on Nasal Provocation Reaction to Allergen*

	Dose	N	Sneezes	Nasal Secretion	Nasal Airway Resistance
Phenylephrine	3.2 mg	16	NE	NE	Decreased
Phentolamine	1.0 mg	13	NE	NE	Increased
Isoproterenol	400 µg	23	NE	NE	Increased
Propranolol	100 ng	25	NE	NE	NE
Methacholine	2 or 6 mg	26	NE	Increased	NE
Ipratropium	140 µg	13	NE	Decreased	NE

* *Nasal secretion decreased by pretreatment with topical cholinergic blockade and increased by pretreatment with topical cholinergic stimulant. Nasal airway resistance decreased by pretreatment with topical α_1-stimulant and increased by pretreatment with topical α_1-blockade and α_2-stimulant.*
† *NE, not significantly effective.*

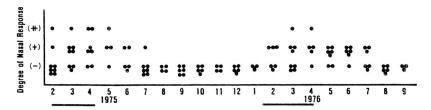

Figure 8. Seasonal changes in the degree of nasal response to offending antigen in patients with Sugi pollinosis. Black bars indicate the pollen season. Nasal responses increased during the period of the season and a few months after the season.

cally significant correlation was found between them ($r = 0.2755$, $p < 0.05$) (Table XV and Fig. 9).

Changes in provocation responses were examined after administration of either cromolyn sodium (DSCG) or placebo 4 times a day for 4 weeks. A significant difference in the decrease of the degree of response ($p < 0.01$) was found between DSCG and placebo. The changes were also examined after beclomethasone treatment (4 times a day for 2 weeks) and results similar to those of DSCG were obtained. Immunotherapy for 1 year also decreased the provocation reaction in house dust allergy patients. These results of the study gave actual evidence that the present provocation test is reliable and available clinically (Tables XII, XIV, and XV). Furthermore, reproducibility of this provocation method was studied. In terms of difference in examiners the patients with a positive skin reaction to house dust were examined in 5 different ENT clinics in Japan by the rhinoscopic method, and there was no difference in the rate of positive response among them (Table XVI).

Reproducibility of this method was also studied by consecutively repeating provocation with an allergen paper disc 4 times every 5 minutes, 4 times every 30 minutes, 2 times every hour, 4 times every 6 hours, 2 times every day and 4 times every week. The degree of nasal responses evaluated by the rhinoscopy method

were classed as follows negative is zero, 1+ is one, 2+ is two, and 3+ is three, and the total scores were averaged in each provocation of each group. As a result there was no significant difference in the provocation of any group, showing a tendency of increase in response after repeated testing (Table XVII). This indicated a good reproducibility of the paper disc method, but provided a question as to why the sensitivity of nasal mucosa to allergen did not change spontaneously or after repeated provocation in which the first provocation affects the results of the second test by increasing nonspecific reactivity or specific reactivity.

SIDE EFFECTS

The paper disc method was widely used in Japan for 25 years in numerous patients with allergic rhinitis. No systemic reaction has been seen since the amount of allergen necessary for a response is eluted from the disc, and, if the symptoms occurred, allergen is removed from the nose quickly. A reason for minimal side effects may also be that the surface area to be stimulated is limited (7 mm^2). Unlike the paper disc method, the spray of allergen solution sometimes induced edematous swelling of the soft palate and epipharynx or asthma, since allergen entered deeply into the pharynx and trachea and was absorbed quickly without any inhibition by the onset of nasal symptoms as seen in

TABLE XIV

Relationships between History, Skin Test, and Provocation to Allergen Paper Disc in Pollinosis*

History	Skin Test	Japanese Cedar	Timothy or/ and Orchard Grass	Ragweed	Total
Positive	Positive	73.2% (41)	84.8% (34)	83.3% (12)	79.3% (87)
Positive	Negative	9.0% (11)	0 (9)	0 (4)	4.1% (24)
Negative	Positive	60.0% (10)	62.0% (8)	27.2% (11)	48.3% (29)
Negative	Negative	0 (10)	0 (10)	0 (10)	0 (30)

* The results of provocations were well correlated to those of patient history or skin test.
† Numbers in parentheses are number of cases.

TABLE XV

Relationships between Allergen Provocation and Other Tests*

Tests	No. of Cases	Correlation Coefficient	Significance
Histamine provocation	166	0.3385	$p < 0.01$
Basophil count	117	0.3284	$p < 0.01$
RAST	65	0.2755	$p < 0.05$
End-point of skin test	74	0.1522	NS
End-point of provocation	44	0.7438	$p < 0.01$

* Provocation by paper disc method correlated well with histamine provocation, basophil counts in nasal secretion, RAST, and end-point of allergen provocation, but not with end-point of skin reaction.

allergen paper disc provocation. However, the test agent solution contained in the paper disc rarely induced a systemic effect. When the nose was provoked with a histamine paper disc, asthma-like symptoms occurred in one asthmatic patient, possibly due to quick absorption of histamine into the circulation.

In spite of the many advantages of the paper disc

method, there was a nonspecific irritation of the nose by the paper disc. Of 288 allergy patients examined, 28 showed a slight nasal irritation (itching, sneezing, and secretion) upon application of the control disc without allergen (Table XVIII). This irritation was rather frequent in patients below the age of 20. It appeared within a short time (within 30 seconds) after the start of testing, and the amount of watery secretions and swelling of the mucosa were less for the degree of sneezing when compared with specific response to allergen. Therefore, differentiation of nonspecific reaction from specific reaction is not difficult. If the differentiation is difficult, we have to repeat the test again on another day.

CLINICAL SIGNIFICANCE OF NASAL PROVOCATION

The provocation test is useful practically, because it is the only test which can give information on local sensitivity to allergen. In spite of this advantage, there are many objections to this test: it is time-consuming, involves the risk of systemic anaphylactic reaction, and often gives both false positive and false negative reactions. In addition, the test is only semiquantitative, the

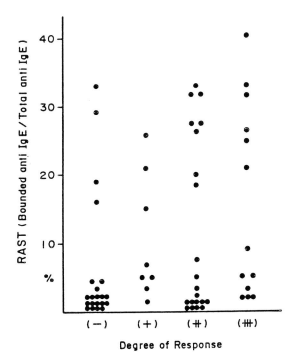

Relationships between RAST and Provocation

They correlated well.
(r = 0.2755 , P < 0.05)

Figure 9. Relationships between RAST and provocation. They correlated (r = 0.2755, p < 0.05).

TABLE XVI

Difference in Positive Provocation Among Five Different Clinics in House Dust Allergy*

	No. of Patients	Positive Response (%)
A	34	73.5
B	54	74.1
C	159	62.9
D	34	55.9
E	25	84.0

* There was no difference in positive response rate among five different clinics (NS, χ^2 test).

TABLE XVII

Changes in Provocation Reaction by Repeated Challenges at Different Time Intervals*

Interval	No. of Challenges	N	1	2	3	4	Significance
5 min	4	20	1.60 ± 0.88	1.50 ± 0.94	1.60 ± 0.88	1.45 ± 0.82	NS
30 min	4	19	2.10 ± 0.73	2.05 ± 0.84	2.15 ± 0.83	2.15 ± 0.76	NS
1 hr	2	14	1.00 ± 0.96	1.07 ± 1.14			NS
6 hr	4	14	0.92 ± 1.07	1.14 ± 0.77	1.07 ± 1.07	1.21 ± 0.81	NS
1 day	2	16	1.18 ± 1.32	1.06 ± 1.28			NS
1 wk	4	13	1.69 ± 0.85	1.53 ± 0.87	1.23 ± 0.83	1.53 ± 0.66	NS

* There was no difference in nasal provocation reaction by repeated challenges in different time intervals.

result varies from time to time, and measurements are seldom strictly objective. The present test method proposed by us can overcome these problems. The test time is less than 10 minutes, and no systemic reaction occurs. The test results correlate well with the history of the patients, IgE antibody level in serum, and effects of drug showing that the test results are reliable. Occasionally contradictory results to skin test and history of patient is obtained, but it may indicate that the nasal sensitivity to allergen differs from the skin sensitivity. Reproducibility is satisfactory and side effects are minimal. For complete removal of nonspecific irritation, however, the improvement of material to contain allergen is necessary. For this purpose use of allergen powder is recommended as previously described.

It is true that evaluation of provocation is semiquantitative and not strictly objective if our rhinoscopic criteria are used for positive standardization. The same applied, however, to the skin test and RAST. The rhinomanometric assessment is suitable as an objective test.

We routinely use the nasal provocation tests in confirmation of results of the skin test, in selection of allergens for immunotherapy when many allergens showed positive in the skin test, in follow-up of treatment, in the examination of drug effects, and as a test for nonspecific hyperreactivity.

In conclusion, nasal provocation should be performed: 1) by application of a fixed amount of provoking agent, 2) to the fixed size of surface area of the bilateral inferior turbinate, 3) visually using a rhinoscope, and then nasal response produced should be assessed by 4) rhinoscopical change together with the number of sneezes or by rhinomanometer. For this purpose the paper disc or powder method is useful.

TABLE XVIII

Nonspecific Reaction to Control Disc*

	Ages						
	~10	~20	~30	~40	~50	~60	Total
No. of cases	77	63	52	55	28	10	288
Positive response (%)	16.8	14.2	3.8	5.1	0	10	9.7 (mean)
Positive response to histamine	68	57	65	60	47	55	

* Nonspecific irritation to control disc without allergen was seen in 9.7% of patients with age differences which were not marked in histamine provocation.

REFERENCES

1. Okuda M. Basic study of nasal provocation test. Arch Oto-Rhino-Laryngol 214:241–246, 1977.
2. Okuda M. Basic study of nasal provocation test. Arch Oto-Rhino-Laryngol 218:203–207, 1978.
3. Okuda M. Nasal provocation. In: Oehling A, et al., eds. Advances in Allergology and Immunology. New York: Pergamon Press, 1980, pp 125–131. □

Chapter XLII

Experience in Counting Ciliary Beat Frequency from Vital Cytologic Sampling

T. Deitmer, M.D. and S. Phadhana-anek, M.D.

ABSTRACT

From a viable cytologic brush biopsy of the respiratory epithelium you can get an insight into the functional state of the epithelial cell layer, especially of the ciliated cells. We report on our experience of several hundred sampling procedures from the nasal and bronchial mucosa. The technique of the method is described, including the microphotometric apparatus to determine the ciliary beat frequency. We stress the importance of checking the ciliary beat frequency of the 10 most active cells of one preparation to get representative results. Futhermore it is decisive to watch them over a period of 10 seconds, considering the time shift of the ciliary beat frequency. Putting the cell solution into a counting chamber gives the possibility of differentiating viable and dead ciliated cells as well as squamous cells in the sample. These results proved to yield a good picture of the functional state of the sampled respiratory mucosal site.

During endoscopy of the nose or the tracheobronchial system we are not aware of the existence nor the necessity of the ciliated epithelium as the main motor of the mucociliary system. This mucociliary system provides a permanent cleansing of the surfaces of the respiratory tract, which is exposed to ubiquitous airborne pollution. As many of the diseases of the nose and the lungs result from exposure to the air, this cleansing is of great clinical importance. Our knowledge is rather scanty regarding the functional reactions of the ciliated epithelium during viral or bacterial infec-

Universität Münster, Klinik und Poliklinik für Hals-Nasen- und Ohrenheilkunde, Münster, Federal Republic of Germany

tions, physical stress, and tumors or carcinogenesis; furthermore, the functional effects of our therapeutical efforts are of importance.

The assessment of functional changes is best achieved by *in vivo* studies. Hybbinette and Mercke[1], Lindberg et al.[2,3], Mercke et al.,[4] and Reimer et al.[5,6] used an animal model for *in vivo* studies in measuring the ciliary activity from the opened maxillary antrum of a rabbit. Similar studies were done by Reimer et al.[5,6] in humans during a Caldwell-Luc procedure with highly sophisticated equipment not suitable for routine clinical testing.

Despite the central function of the ciliated cell in the defense of the respiratory tract, we have few and not well-established methods to assess its functional state. Measuring the ciliary function by a vital cytologic sampling from respiratory mucosa seemed to be a practicable and promising method.[7,8] We want to report on our experience with it from several studies and clinical routine.

METHODS

To harvest the cells we prefer a nylon brush of about 2 mm diameter as it is used in flexible bronchoscopy.[9–11] The use of curettes and sharp forceps or other rigid instruments involves the possibility of lesions and inconvenience for the patient.[12]

The brush is introduced into the nose under visual control. The mid portions of the nose, i.e., about 1 cm behind the head of the inferior turbinate should be reached, as squamous metaplasia is usual in the anterior parts of nasal cavities. In our experience the sampling procedure with rotating and brushing can be well tolerated without local anesthesia. Although it is known from *in vitro* studies that local anesthetics can be harmful to the ciliary function[13] Rutland et al.[14] demonstrated that there was no difference of ciliary beat rate if a nose was anesthetised or not. We see no problem in avoiding local anesthetics, although it is of greater importance for sampling in the bronchial tree during flexible endoscopy.

After withdrawal from the nose the brush is agitated in 100 μl of Dulbecco's modified medium, which is suitable for short duration cultures. From a study with varying examination times we know that when using this culture medium without antibiotics the examination should be done within ½ hour because of bacterial growth. The effects of bacterial products on the ciliary function are well known[15,16] and must be avoided. The choice of culture medium should take into account that viscosity is able to slow down ciliary action.[17]

In the literature there are varying recommendations concerning temperature for culture and examination. It is well known that ciliary action is temperature dependent rising from 10°C to a maximum activity at 37°C and reaching a reversible arrest at about 40°C. From 45 to 50°C and higher the arrest is irreversible.[10,18–23] We prefer a temperature of 37°C as physiologic, assuming the same temperature in the ciliary layer of the nose and the bronchi. The temperature is provided by a water bath during culture and should be maintained by a heated stage during microscopy. The cell solution is pleased in a counting chamber (Fuchs-Rosenthal) with a depth of 200 μm. This depth is acceptable for a good microscopic survey despite the lack of depth of focus giving enough room for free ciliary movement. The counting chamber enables us to count cells in a known volume to assess the efficacy of the sampling procedure. For examination we use a Zeiss phase-contrast microscope with magnifications up to 1000 times. The path of the light is divided by a beam splitter and a narrow beam is directed onto a phototransistor. Other authors use a photomultiplier,[10,11,20] but we have had good results with a phototransistor and a custom made automatic gain control. The power

supply with 9 V DC from a battery is much simpler than high voltage for a photomultiplier (Fig. 1). It seems to us of great importance to use a diaphragm which allows a spot size of only a few micrometers for the photosensitive area in the focus plane. A larger spot yields a better photocurrent but shows undulations resulting not only from the varying activity of the movement of one cell but from a whole cell group. The amplified photocurrent is fed into a low pass filter, which eliminates frequencies of more than 40 Hz and thus cuts off as well the 50 Hz from the main frequency introduced by the illumination of the microscope. The amplified signal is displayed on a scope together with the trigger level of a counter connected in parallel. The gain must be controlled in a manner that the undulations produced by a moving cell in focus can trigger the counter which has a counter gate time of 1 second, giving the ciliary beat frequency directly in Hertz. It cannot be denied that the highly sensitive equipment can produce minor artificial waves. These can be held at a gain below trigger level. For counting the ciliary beat frequency we must look for cells that are adherent to each other or to a basement membrane.[24] With a fixed cell body one is able to count the ciliary action of the ciliary border. Focusing on a cell floating free in the medium is difficult and can result in measuring a resonance frequency not only dependent on the ciliary action but also on the mass of the cell body which moves together with the cilia.

RESULTS

Counting ciliary beat frequency during several studies in about 200 tests showed us that a cytologic sample cannot be characterized by a single measurement. We learned that in a sample the cells are working at different levels of activity. Even measuring only the most active cells brings about no uniform frequency between the different cells. Another problem arises in the time shift of ciliary frequency. This should be taken into account and the measurement should be performed on an individual cell for at least 10 consecutive seconds in the same position. We prefer to list the data of 10 individual, most active cells of a preparation for 10 seconds each. The data are entered in a form (Fig. 2) and then into a computer to calculate mean values and standard deviations. In Figure 2 the mean values and standard deviations of the 10 cells during a time of 10 seconds are given. From these 100 values a mean value and standard deviation can be calculated, which characterises the ciliary activity of the whole preparation. Comparisons between samples can be made using these data and convenient statistical tests. Using the counting chamber we had the further advantage of being able to count the cells in our preparation. Under phase microscopy it is easy to recognize active and dead

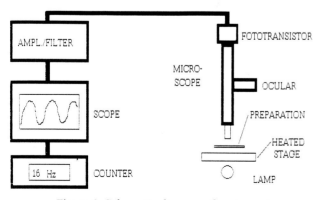

Figure 1. Schematic diagram of equipment.

Beat Frequency (Hz) of Cells

sec										
13	9	12	15	13	14	14	12	13	11
13	9	12	15	11	12	14	13	11	12
13	9	12	15	14	12	13	13	13	14
11	13	12	15	12	13	12	13	13	13
11	13	12	14	14	13	16	13	12	11
11	13	12	14	12	13	16	12	13	14
11	13	12	14	13	14	14	13	13	14
11	13	12	15	10	12	14	13	13	12
11	13	12	13	10	13	14	14	13	11
11	13	13	14	11	13	15	13	12	14
11.6	11.8	12.1	14.4	12.0	12.9	14.0	12.9	12.6	12.6	Mean
0.96	1.93	0.31	0.69	1.49	0.73	1.24	0.56	0.69	1.34	SD

Mean of all cells: 12.69 Hz
SD of all cells: 0.915 Hz

Figure 2. Data sheet of a preparation.

ciliated cells as well as squamous cells representing the important epithelial cells of the mucosa. We counted the different cells in a known volume and thus were able to calculate the total number of harvested epithelial cells and give the percentage of active and dead ciliated cells and of squamous cells. An example of such a cell differentiation is given in Figure 3. During a study of vital cytologic sampling from the trachea of tracheotomized patients we found an overwhelming majority of squamous cells in our samples as a sign of the well-known squamous metaplasia of the trachea in such conditions.

DISCUSSION

Vital cytologic sampling does not provide the standardized circumstances of *in vitro* testing. We cannot watch a single cell changing its activity under altered conditions. Therefore, it is of more importance to find a good, valid characterization of the whole sample.

Cell Differentiation		Counted Volume	Absolute Number	Relative Number (%)
Viable ciliated cells	47		188	38
Dead ciliated cells	69	0.25 ml	276	56
Squamous cells	7		28	6

Total cell count: 492

Figure 3. Example of cell differentiation.

From our experience we have to emphasize that the ciliary activity of a vital cytologic sample cannot be represented by a single measurement of a single cell. The time shift of ciliary frequency was demonstrated by Kennedy and Duckett,[20] who performed a fast Fourier transformation on the signal of several seconds. They found a shift of several Hertz.

Whereas ciliary beat frequency seems to be a good parameter for pharmacologic and certain physical tests upon the ciliated epithelium *in vitro*, it is unsuitable in *in vivo* tests. Often no significant differences can be calculated using our proposed evaluation, which we think is representative of the reality of ciliary beating. We saw a more sensitive tool in counting the percentage of active and dead ciliated cells as proposed by other authors.[24-26] We believe that noxious influences on the ciliated cells by chemical or physical stress or disease do not lead to a proportional decay in ciliary activity, but it is probable that a cell will work at the inborn beat rate as long as possible and then rapidly fall to death. Thus, there will be a greater chance to measure by counting the dead cells than by counting the ciliary beat frequency of the last 10 most active cells of the preparation. On the other hand, measuring 10 randomly chosen cells of the preparation will bring about more arbitrary faulty results.

For vital cytologic sampling we therefore propose that not only the ciliary beat frequency of the 10 most active cells of a preparation be counted for 10 seconds but also the percentage of dead and live ciliated and squamous cells be determined.

REFERENCES

1. Hybbinette JC, Mercke U. A method for evaluating the effect of pharmacological substances on mucociliary activity *in vivo*. Acta Otolaryngol 93:151–159, 1982.
2. Lindberg S, Hybbinette JC, Mercke U. Effects of neuropeptides on mucociliary activity. Ann Otol Rhinol Laryngol 95:94–100, 1986.
3. Lindberg S, Dolata J, Mercke U. Nasal exposure to airway irritants triggers a mucociliary defence reflex in the rabbit maxillary sinus. Acta Otolaryngol 104:552–560, 1987.
4. Mercke U, Lindberg S, Dolata J. The role of neuorokinine A and calcitonine gene related peptide in the mucociliary defence of the rabbit maxillary sinus. Rhinology 25:89–93, 1987.
5. Reimer A, Toremalm NG. The mucociliary activity of the upper respiratory tract. Acta Otolaryngol 86:283–288, 1978.
6. Reimer A, Mecklenburg C von, Toremalm NG. The mucociliary activity of the upper respiratory tract. III. A functional and morphological study on human and animal material with special reference to maxillary sinus disease. Acta Otolaryngol Suppl 355, 1978.
7. Dalham T, Rylander R. Frequency of ciliary beat measured by a phtotosensitive cell. Nature 196:592–599, 1962.
8. Hilding AC. The common cold. Arch Otolaryngol 12:133–137, 1930.
9. Carson JL, Collier AM, Shih-Chin SH. Acquired ciliary defects in nasal epithelium of children with acute viral upper respiratory infections. N Engl J Med 312:463–468, 1985.
10. Konietzko N, Nakhosteen JA, Mizera W, Kasparek R, Hesse H. Ciliary beat frequency of biopsy samples taken from normal persons and patients with various lung diseases. Chest 80: Suppl Dec, 1981.
11. Yager J, Tzeng-Ming C, Dulfano MJ. Measurement of frequency of ciliary beats of human respiratory epithelium. Chest 73:627–633, 1978.
12. Duchateau GSMJE, Graamans K, Zuidema J, Merkus FWHM. Correlation between nasal ciliary beat frequency and mucus transport rate in volunteers. Laryngoscope 95:854–859, 1985.
13. Mostow SR, Dreisin RB, Manawadu BR, Marc La Force F. Adverse effects of lidocaine and methylparabene on tracheal ciliary activity. Laryngoscope 89:1697–1700, 1979
14. Rutland J, Griffin W, Cole P. Nasal brushing and measurement of ciliary beat frequency. Chest 80(Suppl):865–867, 1981.
15. Hingley ST, Hastie AT, Higgins ML, Kueppers F. Effect of pseudomonade proteases on mammalian ciliary activity. Am Rev Respir Dis 132(Suppl 4A):73, 1986.
16. Wilson R, Roberts D, Cole P. Effects of bacterial products on human ciliary function. Thorax 40:125–131, 1985.
17. Ohashi Y, Nakai Y, Zushi K, Muraoka M, Minowa Y, Harada H, Masutani H. Enhancement of ciliary action by a β-adrenergic stimulant. Acta Otolaryngol 97:49–59, 1983.
18. Dixon WE, Inchley O. The cilioscribe, an instrument for recording the activity of cilia. J Physiol (Lond) 32:395–400, 1905.
19. Engelmann TW. Flimmeruhr und Flimmermühle. Zwei Apparate zum Registrieren der Flimmerbewegung. Pflügers Arch Gesamte Physiol 15:493–510, 1877.
20. Kennedy JR, Duckett KE. The study of ciliary frequencies with an optical spectrum analysis system. Exp Cell Res 135:147–156, 1981.
21. Mercke U. The influence of temperature on mucociliary activity. Acta Otolaryngol 78:253–258, 1974.
22. Proetz AW. Applied Physiology of the Nose. St. Louis, Annals Publishing Company, 1953.
23. Toremalm NG, Mercke U, Reimer A. The mucociliary activity of the upper respiratory tract. Rhinology 13:113–120, 1975.
24. Lopez-Vidriero MT. Objective criteria for measuring ciliary beat frequency *in vitro*. Am Rev Respir. Dis 125(Suppl 4):244, 1982.
25. Baum GL, Roth Y, Teichtahl H, Ahronson E, Priel Z. Ciliary beat frequency of respiratory mucosal cells: comparison of nasal and tracheal sampling sites. Am Rev Respir Dis 125(Suppl 4):244, 1982.
26. Pedersen M, Sakakura Y, Winther B, Brofeldt S, Mygind N. Nasal mucociliary transport, number of ciliated cells and beating patterns in naturally acquired common colds. Eur J Respir Dis 64(Suppl 128):355–364, 1983. □

Index

Note: Page numbers in ***italics*** refer to figures. Page numbers followed by t refer to tables.

Brachyfacial skeleton, 89
Bradykinin, 35, 107, 137
Branhamella catarrhalis, 254
Bronchial mucosa, sampling procedures, 335
Bronchoconstriction
　exercise-induced, 121
　nasal stimulation and, 139
Bronchonasal reflex, 140
Bronchoprovocation, testing for asthma, 121
Bronchospasm, aspirin intolerance in asthma and, 180t
Budesonide, 234

Calcitonin gene-related peptide, 137
Calcium ionophores, 21
Candida sp., yeastlike vegetative cell, *64*f
Candidiasis, 212
Capsaicin, 137
Carbachol, 121
Carotid artery, external branches, 79
Cartilagenous deformities, 165
Cell morphology, 294t
Cerebrospinal fluid, leakage into nose, 203
Cetirizine, 226
Children, allergic rhinitis in, 277–280
Chlorpheniramine, 105, 107
Churg-Strauss syndrome, 173
Chymotryptic protease, 20
Cigarette smoke, 137
Ciliary beats, counting, 10, 335–338
Cladosporium, 66, 68, 69
Cladosporium cladosporioides, *70*f
Cladosporium herbarum, *70*f
Clemastine, 107
Clonidine, 137
Cocaine, 108
Coccidiodomycosis, 200
Codeine, 21
Computed tomography, paranasal sinuses, 9, 299–305
Concanavalin A, 21
Contraceptives, 162
Contrast media, 21
Coprinus comatus, *70*f
Corticosteroids
　eosinophilic nonallergic rhinitis, 169
　topical, 8, 231–240
　　chemical structure, *235*f
　　comparison with systemic, 236
Cromolyn sodium, 8, 107–108, 235, 241–245
　allergic rhinitis and, 242
　food allergy and, 243
　ocular, 241
Crutch reflex, 140
Cryptococcus neuformans, 211
Curvularia, 70, *71*f
Cyclooxygenase, pathway metabolites, 29

Cystic fibrosis, 173
Cytogram, nasal, 292
　interpretation, 296t, 297t
Cytologic sampling, ciliary beat frequency from, 335–338
Cytology, nasal, 9
Cytomegalovirus rhinitis, 210

Daldinia concentrica, *71*f
Decongestants, 8
　chronic rhinitis treatment, 219–223
　topical and oral, 220t
Dentofacial development, 6, 85–93
Dermatophagoides fairnae, 5
Dermatophagoides pteronyssinus, 5
Dextran, 21
Drugs, olfaction and, 99
Dyskinetic cilia syndrome, 202–203
Dysosmia, 98

Endocrine disorders, nasal manifestations of, 199
Endoscopy
　flexible fiberoptic, upper airway, 319–323
　inflammatory sinus disease, 257–262
Environment, nose and, 115
Eosinophil chemotactic factors
　anaphylaxis, 17, 176
　oligopeptides, 20
Eosinophil-derived substances, 21
Eosinophilic disease, 163
　nonallergic rhinitis, 169–171
Ephedrine, 108
Epithelial abnormalities, 162
Exercise, 22
Exercise reflex, 140

Fenoterol, 108
Fiberoptic rhinolaryngoscopy, 319, 322t
Flunisolide, 234
Fluocortin butylester, 234
α-Fluoromethylhistidine, 33
Fluticasone propionate, 235
Food challenges
　gustatory rhinitis, 191–195
　　specific foods, 192t
　　symptoms after, 193t
Formaldehyde, 137
Formylmethionyl peptides, 21
Functional endoscopic sinus surgery, 257–262
Fungal spores, 54
　allergenicity, 55
Fungi
　common skin tests, 55t
　diseases caused by, 54
　identification and biology, 63–75
　nasal challenges, 107